Useful Units in Radiology

SI Prefixes

Factor	Prefix	Symbol
10^{18}	Exa	E
10^{15}	Peta	P
10^{12}	Tera	T
10^{9}	Giga	G
10^{6}	Mega	M
10^{3}	Kilo	k
10^{2}	Hecto	h
10^{1}	Deca	da
10^{-1}	Deci	d
10^{-2}	Centi	c
10^{-3}	Milli	m
10^{-6}	Micro	μ
10^{-9}	Nano	n
10^{-12}	Pico	p
10^{-15}	Femto	f
10^{-18}	Atto	a

SI Base Units

Quantity	Name	Symbol
Length	Meter	m
Mass	Kilogram	kg
Time	Second	s
Electric current	Ampere	A

SI Derived Units Expressed in Terms of Base Units

Quantity	SI UNIT Name	Symbol
Area	Square meter	m^2
Volume	Cubic meter	m^3
Speed, velocity	Meter per second	m/s
Acceleration	Meter per second squared	m/s^2
Density, mass density	Kilogram per cubic meter	kg/m^3
Current density	Ampere per square meter	A/m^2
Concentration (of amount of substance)	Mole per cubic meter	$mole/m^3$
Specific volume	Cubic meter per kilogram	m^3/kg

Special Quantities of Radiologic Science and Their Associated Special Units

Quantity	CUSTOMARY UNIT Name	Symbol	SI UNIT Name	Symbol
Exposure	roentgen	R	air kerma	Gy_a
Absorbed dose	rad	rad	gray	Gy_1
Effective dose	rem	rem	seivert	Sv
Radioactivity	curie	Ci	becquerel	Bq

Multiply	R	by	0.01	to obtain	Gy_a
Multiply	rad	by	0.01	to obtain	Gy_t
Multiply	rem	by	0.01	to obtain	Sv
Multiply	Ci	by	3.7×10^{10}	to obtain	Bq
Multiply	R	by	2.58×10^{-4}	to obtain	C/kg

RADIOLOGIC SCIENCE for TECHNOLOGISTS

Physics, Biology, and Protection

Eighth Edition

RADIOLOGIC SCIENCE for TECHNOLOGISTS

Physics, Biology, and Protection

Stewart C. Bushong, Sc.D., FACR, FACMP

Professor of Radiologic Science
Baylor College of Medicine
Houston, Texas

With more than 750 illustrations

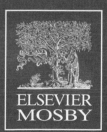

ELSEVIER
MOSBY

ELSEVIER
MOSBY

11830 Westline Industrial Drive
St. Louis, Missouri 63146

NOTICE

Radiology is an ever-changing field. Standard safety precautions must be followed, but as new research and clinical experience broaden our knowledge, changes in treatment and drug therapy may become necessary or appropriate. Readers are advised to check the most current product information provided by the manufacturer of each drug to be administered to verify the recommended dose, the method and duration of administration, and contraindications. It is the responsibility of the licensed prescriber, relying on experience and knowledge of the patient, to determine dosages and the best treatment for each individual patient. Neither the publisher nor the author assumes any liability for any injury and/or damage to persons or property arising from this publication.

Previous editions copyrighted 2001, 1997, 1993, 1988, 1984, 1980, 1975

International Standard Book Number 0-323-02555-2

Acquisitions Editor: Jeanne Wilke
Developmental Editor: Rebecca Swisher
Publishing Services Manager: Linda McKinley
Project Manager: Rich Barber
Designer: Teresa McBryan
Editorial Assistant: Katherine Tomber

Printed in the United States

Last digit is the print number: 9   8   7   6   5   4   3   2   1

Reviewers

Alberto Bello, MEd, RT (R) (CV)
Assistant Provost/Associate Professor
Oregon Institute of Technology
Klamath Falls, Oregon

Jacqueline Gallet, PhD
Diagnostic Imaging Physicist
Cancer Care Manitoba
Winnipeg, Manitoba
Canada

Edward J. Goldschmidt, Jr., MS, DABMP
Medical Physicist
Cooper Health System
Camden, New Jersey

Gerald L. Graddy, MS, RT (R)
Associate Professor of Radiography
Jackson State Community College
Jackson, Tennessee

John H. Harper, PhD
Physics Instructor
Angelina College
Lufkin, Texas

Deborah Hughes-Schroth, MBA, BSRT (R) (M)
Director, School of Radiologic Science
St. Anthony Hospitals
Denver, Colorado

R. Paul King, MS, DABR
Radiological Physicist
Jeff Anderson Regional Medical Center
Meridian, Mississippi

Robert A. Luke, PhD
Professor and Physics Department Chair
Boise State University
Boise, Idaho

Thomas Piccoli, DABMP, DABR
Medical Physicist
Monmouth Medical Center
Long Branch, New Jersey

John G. Wolodzko, MSc, PhD
Certified Medical Physicist
Yardley, Pennsylvania

This book is dedicated to the 827 Houston Community College radiography student TOOLS who endured my medical physics classes, my easy exams, my lousy jokes, and my stupid hats since I began doing this in 1972. They gave me much grief but much more pleasure, and many have become lasting close friends.

Aboozar Farahnaz 1991 - Abraham Koshy 1995 - Abraham Christina 2000 - Abraham Aleyamma 2003 - Acklin Mark 1990 - Agee Jacqueline 1984 - Aguila Fred 1976 - Aguillar Corina 2001 - Aimadeddine Sabah 1998 - Akhter Shameem 1997 - Akshar Nadia 2000 - Alam Saira 1993 - Alexander Blessy 1999 - Alford Michael 1986 - Allahar Yasmin 1984 - Allen Vincent 1986 - Allen Angela 1995 - Alummoottil Jimmi 1985 - Alvarado Ricardo 1984 - Alvarado Rosalinda 1990 - Amos Lamont 1995 - Amos Gwendolyn 1998 - Anderson Sandra 1976 - Andrassy Stephanie 2001 - Aquerre Anita 1987 - Ashburn Laura 1976 - Atkinson Elaine 1998 - Awad Aghaby 1985 - Bagget Joseph 1997 - Bailey Jennifer 2002 - Baker Christi 1998 - Balderas Juan 2000 - Balderas Noelia 2001 - Ball Russell 1989 - Ballard Barbara 1997 - Banahan Lynne 1992 - Barbee Norma 1987 - Barbre David 2003 - Barker Gerald 1985 - Barnes Willie 1983 - Barstow Christine 2000 - Bass Gerald 1995 - Bauer Todd 1991 - Beago Tara 1989 - Beal Sandra 1990 - Beeson James 1997 - Beheler Rhonda 1991 - Behler Gregory 1999 - Beissel Shea 1999 - Benamar Aziz 1993 - Benedict Carole 1990 - Benefiel Paula 1979 - Benfer Sherry 1994 - Berry Donna 1978 - Bertram Mary Ann 1996 - Best Lori 1994 - Bierstedt Willie 1979 - Billeck Joanne 1999 - Birmingham Cindy 1997 - Blackburn Christie 1993 - Blansett Barbara 1986 - Bolton Jamie 1984 - Bouldin Richard 1983 - Boyd Charles 1986 - Bradford Andrea 1999 - Braggs Karen 1994 - Brannon Pamela 1997 - Brantley Ray 1992 - Braun Rhonda 1999 - Bravo David 2001 - Brewer Mary 1994 - Brick Joanne 1990 - Brimble Brian 1992 - Brito Pablo 1998 - Broadnax Edward 1977 - Broadnax Sherri 1989 - Brokaw Jared 2003 - Brooks Constance 1977 - Brooks Alice 1980 - Brooks Madelon 1982 - Brooks Patrick 1989 - Brooks Mara 1991 - Brooks Udunna 1992 - Brown Beverly 1976 - Brown David 1982 - Brown Patricia 1983 - Brown Regina 1988 - Brown Jim 1988 - Brown Richard 1999 - Bryan Cloteal 1994 - Bryer Ronda 1992 - Buentello Alma 1994 - Burrell Rae Angela 2001 - Byrne Tess 1991 - Cabrera Alfred 1991 - Cade Anthony 1988 - Caldwell Diana 1973 - Camp Judy 1975 - Cantrell Melissa 1999 - Cantu Yvonne 1984 - Capizzo Michael 1998 - Carey LaWana 1995 - Carlson Julie 1997 - Carmona Sarah 1991 - Carpenter Jana 1979 - Carpenter Brandi 1997 - Carpenter Matthew 1999 - Carr James 1980 - Carr Betty 1990 - Carter Pamela 1976 - Castillo Rogelio 1978 - Castro Carlos 2002 - Cavazos Larry 1982 - Cervando Pena 1991 - Cespedes Raul 1996 - Chagolla Andrea 2000 - Chapa Olivia 1974 - Chapel Mary 2000 - Chase Carolyn 1991 - Chavez Rudy 1980 - Chavez Mariah 2003 - Cheeks Gregory 1980 - Chester Corelle 1995 - Cheung Sophia 2002 - Churchwell Alan 1999 - Cieslewicz Sandra 1978 - Cisneros Denise 2000 - Clark Cathy 1975 - Clark Charlotte 1992 - Clark Marilyn 1994 - Clement Lennox 1987 - Cline Nancy 1991 - Cline Patricia 1997 - Codina Richard 1991 - Cohn James 1998 - Coleman Kathy 1993 - Collins Cynthia 1978 - Collins Patricia 1999 - Conly Marinnia 1981 - Conran Mark 1988 - Cook Charles 1976 - Cooper James 1989 - Cooper Joyce 1989 - Corvin Lynne 2001 - Cotton Anthony 1994 - Cotton Ronna 1999 - Covey Sandra 1992 - Coward Kimberly 1986 - Crawford Janet 1986 - Crawford Joella 1994 - Crawley Betsy 1995 - Creech Edward 1991 - Cronkright Philip 1994 - Cruiz Margarita 1974 - Cruz Norma 1978 - Cruz Irene 1994 - Cullum Jaclyn 1998 - Cummings Helen 1974 - Cunningham Cathy 1985 - Dabo Braima 1998 - Daly Marilyn 1976 - Daniels Barbara 1985 - Daniels Janet 1990 - Dao Joy 2001 - Darden Nina 1992 - Darrah Marcia 1974 - Davis Andrea 1976 - Davis Erica 1984 - Davis Reginald 1984 - Davis Lee 1985 - Davis Keidra 1999 - De Ocampo Levi 2001 - Deary Marc 1993 - Dees Kimberely 1984 - Desai Galvan 1990 - Desai Vimalkumar 1995 - Desso Rosheena 1995 - Dezalia Lori 1994 - Dezalia Lori 1994 - Diaz Ronald 1995 - Dickey Tracy 1990 - Dickson Sarah 1996 - Diosdado Sylvia 1997 - Dixon Ethel 1976 - Do Hoan 1994 - Do Khai 1988 - Do Hung 1989 - Dobbins Tina 1982 - Dockery Belinda 1976 - Docz Nancy 1995 - Doherty Linda 1998 - Dohme Bethany 1987 - Doyle Cranford 1991 - Doyle Hoan 1994 - Doyle Leigh 1996 - Drabek Marie 1999 - Druckhammer Linda 1979 - Dubois Danielle 1997 - Duhon Lyle 1987 - Duong Lan 2000 - Dutton Lucy 1997 - Ebey Dale 1986 - Eddington Lucille 1983 - Edinger Heidi 2001 - Edison Denise 1986 - Eirven Shelia 1985 - Ekanem Joshua 1995 - Ekechi Chiekezi 1994 - El Rafaie Razan 2002 - Elassi Farid 2002 - Ellis Charles 1990 - Ellis Allisson 2001 - Elsayegh Shireen 2003 - Emami Debra 1982 - Equia Edward 1979 - Escamillo Yolanda 1975 - Escobar Patricia 1977 - Esparza Sherie 2002 - Espinosa Concepcion 1983 - Esquivel Juanita 1992 - Eubanks Shannon 2001 - Evans Marilyn 1987 - Evans Leslie 1993 - Evans Anita 1994 - Falconer Karen 1979 - Falconer Gary 2001 - Falconer Gareth 2002 - Faldyn Darrell 1983 - Farrar Cynthia 1970 - Farrar John 1976 - Farris Janice 1979 - Faz Alma 2003 - Fedee George 2001 - Fernandez Bertha 1981 - Fernandez Alain 1996 - Ferrell Elizabeth 1985 - Figgs Tabatha 1992 - Filler Martina 1993 - Fitzpatrick Kristi 2000 - Flannelly Mary 1982 - Flores Rene 1991 - Florio Walter 1974 - Folds Karen 1984 - Ford Debra 1981 - Fortune' Michelle 1983 - Foster Velvet 1998 - Fowler Marilyn 1996 - Fox Robin 1996 - Francois Anthony 2003 - Franklin Gwendolyn 1977 - Free Phillip 1987 - Freeman Angie 2000 - Funderburk John 1991 - Galatian Janet 1974 - Galindo Lina 1999 - Gamboa Hector 1992 - Garcia Joel 1987 - Garcia Rosa 1990 - Garcia Adam 1999 - Garcia Genevieve 1999 - Garcia Claudia 2001 - Garcia Lisbeth 2001 - Garcia Lori 2001 - Gardner Jeff 2003 - Garmon Julia 1992 - Garrett Marsha 1978 - Garza Rolando 1980 - Garza Cynthia 1991 - Garza Joel 1997 - Gebremichael Yohannes 1999 - Gebremichael Rediet 2003 - Geevarghese Matthew 1986 - George Teresa 1987 - Gerino Norman 1988 - Gervais Joseph 1995 - Ghadiminejad Shahnaz 2002 - Ghorbani Majgan 2001 - Glaser Angela 1994 - Glenn Delma 1977 - Godarzi Mahnaz 1996 - Godet Johannes 1996 - Godines Claudio 2000 - Goldberg Harold 2002 - Goldsby Kathleen 1980 - Golyer Duanne 1993 - Gomez Jose Angel 1984 - Gonzales Nelly 1975 - Gonzales Josie 1981 - Gonzales Patsy 1979 - Gonzalez Frances 1979 - Gonzalez Nickie 1999 - Gonzalez Estella 2003 - Goodman Frances 1977 - Graham Gayle 1987 - Green IV Quincy 2001 - Greenleaf Regina 1991 - Gregg Carol 1979 - Guajardo Donato 1998 - Guerra Janie 1995 - Guerra Lisbeth 2001 - Gunter Terry 1985 - Gurn Candis 1996 - Gurrola Joseph 1991 - Gustofson Andrea 1990 - Gutierrez Marissa 2001 - Guy Kimberely 1999 - Hablitz Garrett 1988 - Haeber Robin 1997 - Hahn Kathleen 1977 - Hahn Mike 1997 - Hall Karen 1991 - Hall Barbara 1998 - Hamilton Damon 1997 - Hamilton Roberto 2003 - Harget Martin 1991 - Hargrave Laura 1987 - Harper Gregory 1989 - Harrell Vanita 1982 - Harris Debra 1977 - Harris Sandra Jo 1978 - Harris Greta 1979 - Harris Diedria 1992 - Harrison Mathea 1981 - Hartnett Rosemarie 1999 - Haspel Stephanie 1997 - Hawkins Jennie 1975 - Hawthorne Cynthia 1981 - Hayes Myra 1986 - Hebert Joan 1997 - Hedgepeth James 1995 - Henry Gloria 1980 - Herbert Joanne 1996 - Heren Daniel 1997 - Hern Melissa 2003 - Hernandez Marco 1990 - Hernandez Jorge 2001 - Herrera Sandra 2002 - Herrington Rebecca 2002 - Hershkowitz Rachel 1994 - Higgins Niki 1996 - Hightower Andrea 1984 - Hill Melanie 1996 - Hinz Elizabeth 1992 - Hitt Hugh 1991 - Hivale Ronald 1982 - Ho Elizabeth-Minh 2000 - Hobkirk David 1989 - Holbrook Cynthia 1987 - Holley Edora 1985 - Holmes April 1984 - Holmes Christopher 1996 - Holt Yesenia 2001 - Holub Kay 1975 - Honea Rosemary 1983 - Horsley George 1990 - Houston Jeanetta 1992 - Hrncir Leon 1976 - Huebner Angie 1989 - Hughes Rex 1991 - Huntley Kelly 2002 - Hurtado Vicki 1996 - Hutcherson Paul 1978 - Huynh Nancy 1993 - Imhoff Phillip 1985 - Jack Montrell 1998 - Jackson Eva 1977 - Jackson Tashie 1983 - Jackson Gale 1988 - Jackson Shavonn 2001 - Jeanpierre Tanya 1999 - Jeffries Janice 1977 - John Maureen 1974 - Johnson Sandra 1975 - Johnson Andrew 1977 - Johnson Marilyn 1979 - Johnson Raymond 1979 - Johnson Charlotte 1985 - Johnson Roderic 1988 - Johnson Niki 1997 - Jones Mary Alice 1977 - Jones Stephanie 1982 - Jones John 1989 - Jones Eddie 2000 - Jordan Sharon Lee 1982 - Jordan Cindy 1998 - Karl Riana 1993 - Karl Donald 1996 - Kasmiersky Anna 1979 - Kees Floyd 1976 - Keeter Amanda 2000 - Keistler John 1985 - Kennedy Donna 1982 - Kessee Nancy 1979 - Killian Rosalie 1983 - Kneer Daniel 1991 - Knepp Jeanette 2003 - Knipes Linda 1995 - Knox Colleen 1991 -

Kocian Laura 1993 - Koenst Ann 2003 - Kosters Brian 1989 - Kulcak Karen 1991 - La Son T. 1997 - LaCour Tammy 1991 - Lacy Wanda 1995 - LaFell Kathalyn 1979 - Laffert Dale 1981 - Lagway Denise 1982 - Lagway John 1983 - LaJune Reanette 1994 - Lake Jeffrey 1990 - Lalmansingh Andrew 1999 - Landa Isabel 2002 - Lane Bruce 1994 - Lanka Indira 1995 - Larson Lisa 1991 - Lathrop Alisha 1999 - Lauve Christi 1996 - Lavigne Camille 1996 - Lawrence Kristopher 2003 - Lazo Melissa 1989 - Le Andrew 1996 - LeBlanc Sharon 1991 - Lee Rosalyn 1979 - Lee Rickie 1983 - Lemons Yvette 1983 - Leonard Lawrence 1987 - Lesniak Lidia 1997 - Lester Donnie 1987 - Leverne Douglas 1992 - Lewis Larry 1977 - Lewis Lisa 1988 - Lewis William 1997 - Libert Kari-Lynn 1993 - Libreros Monica 1994 - Lightfoot Roderick 1996 - Lillie Doren 1984 - Lindsey Jennifer 1983 - Lindsey Keith 1985 - Linne Jennifer 2001 - Lipton Stephen 1992 - Llanas Hector 1987 - Locke Richard 1995 - Lonergan Ryan 1990 - Longoria Mona 2003 - Lopez Mona 1976 - Lopez Lourdes 1989 - Lopez Concepcion 1995 - Lopez Christina 1999 - Lorrance Lisa 1997 - Love Michael 1985 - Lui Hung-Wen 2000 - Luke Elizabeth 1986 - Luna Judy 1979 - Lupu Valeria 1992 - Lussier Joseph 2001 - Lynch Sharon 1992 - Machado Wanda 1992 - Mack Arnetta 1993 - Magers Janice 1994 - Mahtabfar Kurosh 2000 - Maldonado Isidra 1979 - Malone Charlotte 1990 - Malveaux Virgia 1986 - Marotta Tracy 1994 - Martin Phillip 1984 - Martin Amanda 2003 - Mason Larry 1986 - Mason Regina 1987 - Mason Richard 1992 - Matuszak Barbara 1996 - Mayorga Walter 1987 - McCool Kevin 1987 - McDaniel John 1993 - McDonald Rick 2001 - McIntyre Tammy 1997 - McKeel Lee 1995 - McKentiel Gwendolyn 1973 - Meacham Mary 2001 - Medina Oscar 1999 - Medina Adrian 2003 - Mehta Bina 1990 - Melendez Ricardo 1978 - Melendez Larry 1982 - Mendieta Vicente 1998 - Mendieta Marilu 1999 - Mendiola Carlos 1979 - Mendoza Gloria 1979 - Mendoza Norman 1991 - Mendoza Gary 1993 - Menefee Misty 2000 - Mercer Robin 1976 - Merritt Kenneth 1989 - Merritt Andrea 1997 - Mesa Kimberely 1998 - Mijares Neil 1992 - Milburn E.S. III 1993 - Miles Carlessia 1999 - Miller Susan 1977 - Miller Steve 1986 - Miller Toni 1990 - Miller Bruce 1992 - Mills Karman 1991 - Mills LaShawn 2001 - Milton Judy 1988 - Minter Theresa 1979 - Mitcham Alyson 2001 - Mitchell Charles 2001 - Modest Penny 1983 - Mohammed Shaieeza 1983 - Mohammed Adrane 1995 - Mohammed Adam 2001 - Monge Doris 2001 - Monroe Shannan 1999 - Montgomery Cardene 1990 - Montgomery Kristi 1994 - Montoya Roman 1976 - Moore William 1982 - Moorer Millicent 1976 - Moreland Ann 1977 - Moreno Alma 2001 - Morris Katherine 1981 - Mosley Mary 2003 - Moss Cheryl 1980 - Moura Mario 1995 - Moyer Mark 1994 - Muehr Mary 1975 - Muniz Leo 1996 - Munoz Carlos 1979 - Munoz Yvette 1992 - Munoz Edward 1994 - Mushtaq Lisa 2001 - Narcisse Dana 1990 - Nasir Sadia 2001 - Nedhif Mohamed 1996 - Neicheril Dolly 2003 - Neumann Rochelle 1999 - NgSaye Camille 1992 - Nguyen Teresa 1992 - Nguyen Son T. 1996 - Nguyen Dung 1997 - Nguyen Phuc 1997 - Nguyen Liz 1998 - Nguyen My 1998 - Nguyen Thuy 1998 - Nguyen Jaclynn 1999 - Nguyen Anne 2000 - Nguyen Mark 2001 - Nichols Lisa 1990 - Noble Cheryl 1985 - Nobles Catherine 1990 - Nolan Carl 1996 - Norman Demetra 1992 - Norton Sherri 1991 - Nost Margaret 1984 - Novitski Karin 1991 - Okoronkwo Victoria 2000 - Olivier Velda 1995 - Onda Kelli 2000 - Ontiveros Angelina 1996 - Ortega Francelia 1992 - Oveal Alexander 1989 - Ovieda Cristi 1998 - Owens Algretta 1999 - Pack Jeff 1992 - Padilla Carolyn 1982 - Pappan Daniel 1985 - Patel Taru 1990 - Patel Minesh 1996 - Patterson Tawnee 1997 - Peckham Karen 1978 - Pennie William 2003 - Pepin Brenda 1977 - Perez Feli 1974 - Perez Jose 1999 - Perez Robert 2001 - Perkins Monique 1991 - Perrone Lauri 1993 - Perry Robert 1978 - Pesson Cydney 1981 - Peters Douglas 1982 - Petterson Macye 1990 - Pham Thanh 1987 - Pham Thu 2002 - Phan Hoang-Ha 1994 - Phan Ngoc Hong 1998 - Phillips Roy 1984 - Pierce Samantha 2003 - Pina Kathy 1986 - Pittman LaTanya 1980 - Pohler Deborah 1976 - Pollack William 1976 - Pollard Jessie 1998 - Pool Tara 1997 - Porras Sylvia 1981 - Porter Mildred 1975 - Posten David 1997 - Potter Mary 1985 - Powell Linda 1977 - Powell Hollyann 1994 - Power Lupita 1990 - Preston Genevieve 1988 - Profita Julie 1991 - Puckett Robin 1998 - Puebla Lorelei 1998 - Pugh James 1987 - Pulido Margaret 1978 - Putnam Brenda 1976 - Pye Frances 1980 - Quinn Dion 2001 - Raja Sahar 2000 - Rajan Soju 2003 - Ramos Randolph 1996 - Ramos Frank 1999 - Randolph Melvina 1983 - Rangel Maria 2002 - Ratliff Mary 1992 - Rawlins A.K. 1992 - Rayburn Cathy 1978 - Redor Jason 1996 - Reed Barbara 1987 - Reid Deborah 1994 - Rendon Denise 1977 - Renken Allison 1995 - Resendez Juana 1985 - Rezaie Nora 2003 - Rhodes Susan 1997 - Rhodes Tracy 2000 - Ribera Ann Marie 1975 - Richardson Nathaniel 1987 - Riddle Deborah 2001 - Rincones Estella 1993 - Riojas Toribio 1996 - Rivera Juan 1973 - Rivera Antonio 1999 - Roberts Tyronne 1986 - Roberts Joshua 1999 - Robinson Gwendolyn 1979 - Rodgers Regina 1987 - Rodriquez Miguel 1987 - Rodriquez Jose 1989 - Rodriquez Roberto 1991 - Rodriquez Naghieli 1996 - Roe Jill 1988 - Rogue Ricardo 2001 - Rojas Alicia 1983 - Rollins Floyd 1991 - Romo Seferino 1982 - Ronsonette Michael 1997 - Ross Cheryl 1981 - Ross Melissa 1997 - Rozell Tanya 1997 - Ruiz David 1979 - Russ Grace 1994 - Ryan Ellen 1976 - Rychlik Marie 2000 - Saenz Erin 1993 - Sanchez Mary 1976 - Sanders Rhonda 1992 - Sargent Sharon 1991 - Sargent Nicole 1996 - Savoy Miles 1994 - Scalise Joseph 1995 - Schlaich Arlene 1994 - Schlear Yon 1993 - Schmitt Allen 1988 - Schnyder Tim 1991 - Schultz Rebecca 1981 - Scott Wendy 1991 - Scurlock Earl 1980 - Semien Cynthia 1986 - Sepulveda Monica 1991 - Sergent Melvina 1982 - Shah Shraddha 2001 - Shalilesh Manibhai 1981 - Shields Rickey 1985 - Shows Courtney 1998 - Shrum Brenda 1993 - Sias Marilyn 1990 - Simon Brenda 1983 - Simons Mitchell 1993 - Sims Jeff 1993 - Sirman Kenneth 1988 - Skelley Renee 1997 - Smith Flora 1976 - Smith Ann 1983 - Smith Zendia 1983 - Smither Roy 1983 - Snoddy Cheryl 1993 - Sorensen Kay 1976 - Sosa Robert 1978 - Sousa Joanne 1978 - Speck Eric 1992 - Spero Jill 1997 - St. Vigne James 1985 - Stanton Inka 2001 - Starr John 1993 - Staude Kathleen 1982 - Steinbeck Sylvia 1992 - Steinway Debra 1989 - Stephens Jane 1975 - Sterans Kelsir 1983 - Sterling Ronnie 1980 - Stewart Ernest 1981 - Stiff Timothy 1993 - Stills Sharon 1980 - Stock Maria 1993 - Stokes Ben 1991 - Strickland Sandra 1974 - Strum Nicole 1992 - Styron Judith 1993 - Sullivan Deborah 1976 - Surman Dianna 1976 - Sutherland Lisa 1996 - Tanner Yolanda 1991 - Tanner Otis 1994 - Tansiongco Nancy 1996 - Tapley Darla 1992 - Taylor Carolyn 1979 - Taylor Joanne 1979 - Taylor Yvette 1991 - Taylor Samantha 2003 - Terrell Dane 1985 - Terry Monie 1980 - Thomas Theresa 1981 - Thomas James 1982 - Thomas Andrew 1994 - Thompson Marie 1977 - Thompson Kathleen 1981 - Thompson Ginger 1982 - Thompson Patricia 2000 - Thorn Lavell 1996 - Thrasher Anika 1990 - Tibodeaux Paul 1978 - Titus Matthew 1985 - Tolman Sandra 1995 - Towson Rachel 1995 - Towson Rachel 1995 - Toy Sally 2002 - Tran hanh 1988 - Tran Thuy 1994 - Tran Kathy 1998 - Trapp Dee 1978 - Troy Jeffrey 1995 - Tucker Theresa 1988 - Tully Linda 1985 - Tunstall Terrie 1980 - Tupper Margaret 1983 - Turner Rita 1983 - Turner Bernadette 1989 - Turner John 1991 - Tyznik John 1992 - Ubah Dorathy 2002 - Umeh Judith 2001 - Valdez Sandra 1991 - Valentin Jeffrey 1996 - Valladares Jose 2001 - Vallarta Angel 1993 - Valle Jorge 1993 - Vallery Christine 1983 - Van Antwerp Patrice 1979 - Varghese Chacko 1986 - Vargos Enrique 1987 - Vasquez San Juanita 1979 - Venissat Jonathan 1989 - Vickers Catherine 1996 - Vigil Claudia 1992 - Villaganos Anita 1979 - Villarreal Juan 1979 - Villarreal Victor 2000 - Vinagre Norbet 1996 - Vinuzea Ivan 1995 - Vitelli Trinidad 1979 - Vitonne Christine 1977 - Vo Cam 1993 - Wade Chivato 1989 - Wageick John 1985 - Walker Anita 1984 - Walkingstick Melanni 1991 - Wallace Annias 1983 - Wallace Antoinette 1983 - Wallace Tracy 1987 - Waller Debra 1976 - Warhol Tammy 2001 - Warren Alice 1977 - Warren Kimberlie 1985 - Warshaw Risa 1997 - Washburn Robin 1997 - Watson Velma 1997 - Watts Jeffery 1979 - Watts Glyna 1992 - Wedelich Virginia 1978 - Wesley Joe 1981 - West Phyllis 1985 - Wheeler Rhea 1991 - Wheeler Kirk 1997 - White Deborah 1977 - White Gerald 1988 - White Tim 1990 - White Doris 1997 - Whitfield Shelley 2002 - Whitsett Judith 1996 - Wiggins Sandra 1990 - Wilke Christie 1991 - Wilke David 1995 - Williams Velma 1976 - Williams Gregory 1976 - Williams Janet 1976 - Williams Teresa 1985 - Williams Tracy 1987 - Williams Shirrele 1989 - Willis Kim 1990 - Wilson Louis 1976 - Wilson Christopher 1987 - Wilson Shanta 1999 - Windrum Lancer 1993 - Withrow Joni 1997 - Womack Linda 1989 - Woodson Steve 1992 - Workman David 1973 - Wren Anthony 1994 - Wright Teresa 1984 - Wunderlick Catherine 1981 - Zarosky Elizabeth 1973 - Zeisig Fred 1994

HOUSTON COMMUNITY COLLEGE

viii

Preface

PURPOSE AND CONTENT

The purpose of *Radiologic Science for Technologists: Physics, Biology, and Protection* is threefold: to convey a working knowledge of radiologic physics, to prepare radiography students for the certification examination by the ARRT, and to provide a base of knowledge from which practicing radiographers can make informed decisions about technical factors, diagnostic image quality, and radiation management for both patients and personnel.

This textbook provides a solid presentation of radiologic science, including the fundamentals of radiologic physics, imaging, radiobiology, and radiation protection. Special topics include mammography, fluoroscopy, interventional procedures, multislice spiral computed tomography, and the various emerging modes of digital imaging.

The fundamentals of radiologic science cannot be divorced from mathematics, but this textbook does not assume a mathematics background for the readers. Mathematical equations are always followed by sample problems with direct clinical application. As a further aid to learning, all mathematical formulas are highlighted with their own icon in a colorful box:

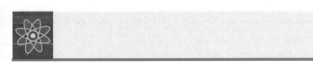

Likewise, the most important ideas under discussion are presented with their own colorful penguin icon and box:

The use of the penguin icon is described early in Chapter 1.

The eighth edition improves this popular feature of information bullets by including even more key concepts and definitions in each chapter. This edition also presents learning objectives, chapter overviews, and chapter summaries that encourage students and make the text user-friendly for all the readers. Challenge Questions at the end of each chapter include definition exercises, short-answer questions, and calculations. These questions can be used for homework assignments, review sessions, or self-directed testing and practice. Answers to all questions are provided on the Evolve site.

HISTORICAL PERSPECTIVE

For seven decades after Roentgen's discovery of x-rays in 1895, diagnostic radiology remained a relatively stable field of study and practice. Truly great changes during that time can be counted on one hand: the Crookes tube, the radiographic grid, radiographic intensifying screens, and image intensification.

Since the publication of the first edition of this textbook in 1975, however, more and more innovative types of medical imaging have come into routine use in medical imaging: computed tomography, computed radiography, digital radiography and fluoroscopy, and multislice spiral computed tomography. Truly spectacular advances in computer technology and x-ray tube and image receptor design have made these innovations possible, and they continue to transform the imaging sciences.

NEW TO THIS EDITION

The eighth edition presents many updates in the areas of special imaging, where the greatest advances in radiologic technology have occurred. There is an important new section on multislice spiral computed tomography. Another recent innovation described in this textbook is digital radiography and the imaging characteristics associated with the use of amorphous silicon and amorphous selenium. There is a new discussion of charge-coupled devices and the advantages for interventional procedures. Also discussed are advances in target composition, compression, and digital imaging for mammography.

The eighth edition also includes more in-text definitions and chapter cross-references. All boldface terms are defined when first introduced and are collected in an expanded glossary. New radiographs and line drawings keep this text fresh and fun.

ANCILLARIES
Student Workbook and Laboratory Manual

This three-part resource has been updated to reflect the changes in the text and the rapid advancements in the field of radiologic science. Part I offers a complete selection of worksheets organized by textbook chapter. Part II, the Math Tutor, provides an outstanding refresher for any student. Part III, Laboratory Experiments, collects experiments designed to demonstrate important concepts in radiologic science.

Mosby's Radiography Online

Instructional materials to support teaching and learning online, radiologic physics, radiographic imaging, radiobiology, and radiation protection have been developed by Mosby and may be obtained by contacting the publisher directly.

A NOTE ON THE TEXT

Although the United States has not formally adopted the International System of Units (SI units), they are presented in this textbook. With this system come the corresponding units of radiation and radioactivity. The roentgen, the rad, and the rem are being replaced by the coulomb/kilogram (C/kg), the gray (Gy), and the sievert (Sv), respectively. A summary of special quantities and units in radiologic science can be found on the inside front cover of the text.

Radiation in air may be quantified in terms of exposure, measured in SI units of C/kg, or in terms of air kerma, measured in mGy. Because mGy is also a unit of dose, a measurement of air kerma is distinguished from tissue dose by applying a subscript a or t to mGy, according to the recommendations of Archer and Wagner (*Minimizing Risk from Fluoroscopic X-rays*, PRM, 1999). Therefore, when the SI is used, air kerma is measured in mGy_a and tissue dose in mGy_t.

ACKNOWLEDGMENTS

For the preparation of the edition, I am indebted to the many readers of the earlier editions who submitted suggestions, criticisms, corrections, and compliments. And for this edition, I am particularly indebted to the following radiologic science educators and students for their suggestions for change and clarification. Many supplied radiographic illustrations, and they are additionally acknowledged with the illustration.

Pam Lee, Tacoma Community College; *Steve Strickland,* Aiken Technical College; *Glen Mitchell,* Laughlin Memorial Hospital; *Rita McLaughlin,* British Columbia Institute of Technology; *Don Summers,* Athens Technical College; *Richard Bayless,* University of Montana; *Tim Gienapp,* Apollo College; *Dorothy Saia,* Stamford Hospital; *Deborah Schroth,* St. Anthony Hospitals; *Robert Morrison,* Frank Barker Associates; *Kurt Loveland,* Drexel University; *Euclid Seeram,* British Columbia Institute of Technology; *Kyle Thornton,* City College of San Francisco; *Tammy Bauman,* Banner Thunderbird Medical Center; *Gene Frank,* Riverland Community College; *Ronald Bresell,* University of Wisconsin; *Daisy Dacara,* Stevens County Hospital; *Barry Chenkin,* Montgomery College; *Darrell Wakley,* Keiser College; *Andrew Woodward,* Wor-Wic Community College; *Robert Luke,* Boise State University; *Quinn Carroll,* Midland College; *Phil Ballinger,* Ohio State University; *Ryan Minic,* Pima Medical Institute; *David Ludema,* Delaware Technical and Community College; *Roger Freimark,* Oregon Imaging Center; *William Faulkner,* Faulkner and Associates; *Rune Sylvarnes,* Tromso College; *Mike Emery,* Sandhills Community College.

Special thanks to my colleagues *Benjamin Archer,* Baylor College of Medicine and *Louis Wagner,* University of Texas Health Science Center, for their introduction of the radiologic terms mGy_a and mGy_t.

I am deeply indebted to my associates *Sharon Glaze, David Hearne, P.S. Philip, Nasir Bhuiyan, Ishtiaq Hussain,* and *Ian Hamilton* who have assisted me with this revision. The illustrations are the product of many people who worked exceptionally hard to render all illustrations in full color, especially *Kraig Emmert.* His cartoons help ease any pain associated with medical physics.

I am also particularly indebted to *Yvonne Young* for the many times she had to struggle through my handwritten notes and unfamiliar symbols and equations. I appreciate her hard work and conscientious approach to preparing the manuscript.

As you, student or educator, use this text and have questions or comments, I hope you will email me at sbushong@bcm.tmc.edu so that together we can strive to make this very difficult material easier to learn.

"Physics is fun" is the motto of my radiologic science courses, and I believe this text will help make physics enjoyable for the student radiologic technologist.

Stewart C. Bushong

Contents

PART I

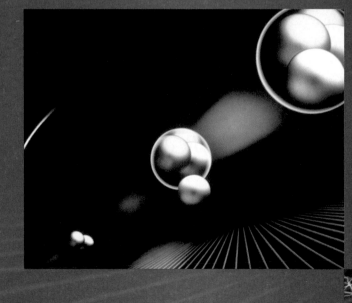

RADIOLOGIC PHYSICS

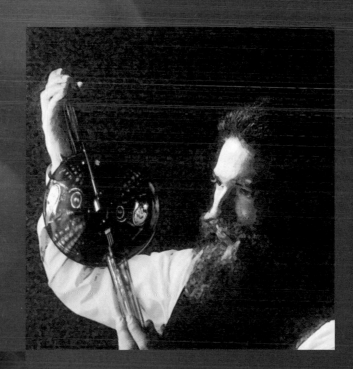

Concepts of Radiologic Science

OBJECTIVES

At the completion of this chapter, the student should be able to do the following:

1. Describe the characteristics of matter and energy
2. Identify the various forms of energy
3. Define electromagnetic radiation and specifically ionizing radiation
4. State the relative intensity of ionizing radiation from various sources
5. Relate the accidental discovery of x-rays by Roentgen
6. Discuss examples of human injury caused by radiation
7. List the concepts of basic radiation protection

OUTLINE

Nature of Our Surroundings
Matter and Energy
Sources of Ionizing Radiation
Discovery of X-rays
Development of Modern Radiology
Reports of Radiation Injury
Basic Radiation Protection
The Diagnostic Imaging Team

THIS CHAPTER explores the basic concepts of the science and technology of x-ray imaging. These include the study of matter, energy, the electromagnetic spectrum, and ionizing radiation. The production and use of ionizing radiation as a diagnostic tool are the bases of radiography. Radiologic technologists who deal specifically with x-ray imaging are radiographers. Radiographers have a great responsibility in performing x-ray examinations using established radiation protection standards for the safety of patients and medical personnel. Radiography is a career choice with great, yet diverse opportunities. Welcome to the field of medical imaging.

NATURE OF OUR SURROUNDINGS

In a physical analysis, all things in our physical environment can be classified as matter or energy. Matter is anything that occupies space and has mass. It is the material substance of which physical objects are composed. All matter is composed of fundamental building blocks called atoms, which are arranged in various complex ways. These atomic arrangements are considered at great length in Chapter 4.

A primary, distinguishing characteristic of matter is **mass,** the quantity of matter contained in any physical object. We generally use the term *weight* when describing the mass of an object, and for our purposes we may consider mass and weight to be the same. Remember, however, that in the strictest sense they are not the same. Mass is actually described by its energy equivalence, whereas weight is the force exerted on a body under the influence of gravity.

 Mass is the quantity of matter described by its energy equivalence.

Mass is measured in kilograms (kg). For example, on earth a 200-lb (91-kg) man weighs more than a 120-lb (55-kg) woman. This occurs because of the mutual attraction, called *gravity,* between the earth's mass and the mass of the man or woman. On the moon the man and woman would weigh only about one-sixth what they weigh on earth because the mass of the moon is much less than that of the earth. However, the mass of the man and woman remains unchanged at 91 kg and 55 kg, respectively.

MATTER AND ENERGY

Matter is anything that occupies space. It is the material substance with mass of which physical objects are

---

A Penguin Tale

BY BENJAMIN ARCHER

In the vast and beautiful expanse of the Arctic region, there was once a great, isolated iceberg floating in the serene sea. Because of its location and accessibility, the great iceberg became a Mecca for penguins from the entire area. As more and more penguins flocked to their new home and began to cover the slopes of the ice field, the iceberg began to sink further and further into the sea. Penguins kept climbing on, forcing others that once were securely ensconced off the island and back into the ocean. Soon, the entire iceberg became submerged owing to the sheer number of penguins that attempted to take up residence there.

Moral: The **PENGUIN** represents an important fact or bit of information that we must learn to understand a subject. The brain, like the iceberg, can retain only so much information before it becomes overloaded. When this happens, concepts begin to become dislodged like penguins from the sinking iceberg. So, the key to learning is to reserve space for true "penguins" to fill the valuable and limited confines of our brains. Thus, key points in this book are highlighted and referred to as **"PENGUINS."**

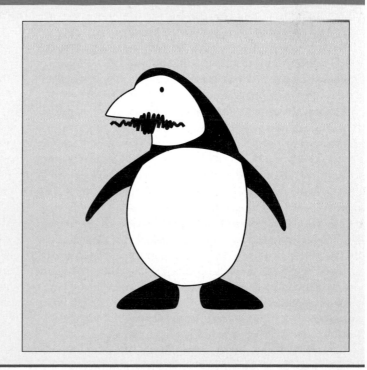

composed. The fundamental, complex building blocks of matter are **atoms** and **molecules.** The kilogram is the scientific unit of mass and is unrelated to gravitational effects. The prefix kilo stands for 1000; a kilogram (kg) is equal to 1000 grams (g).

Although mass, the quantity of matter, remains unchanged regardless of its state, it can be transformed from one size, shape, and form to another. Consider a 1-kg block of ice, where shape changes as the block of ice melts into a puddle of water. If the puddle is allowed to dry, the water apparently disappears entirely. We know, however, that the ice is transformed from a solid state to a liquid state and that liquid water becomes water vapor suspended in the air. If we could gather all the molecules making up the ice, the water, and the water vapor and measure their masses, we would find that each form has the same mass.

 Energy is the ability to do work.

Like matter, energy can exist in several forms. In the International System (SI), energy is measured in joules (J). In radiology, the unit electron volt (eV) is often used.

Potential energy is the ability to do work by virtue of position. A guillotine blade held aloft by a rope and pulley is an example of an object that possesses potential energy (Figure 1-1). If the rope is cut, the blade will descend and do its ghastly task. Work was required to get the blade to its high position and because of this position the blade is said to possess potential energy. Other examples of objects that possess potential energy include a roller coaster on top of the incline and the stretched spring of an open screen door.

Kinetic energy is the energy of motion. It is possessed by all matter in motion: a moving automobile, a turning windmill wheel, a falling guillotine blade. These systems can all do work because of their motion.

Chemical energy is the energy released by a chemical reaction. An important example of this type of energy is that which is provided to our bodies through chemical reactions involving the food we eat. At the molecular level this area of science is called **biochemistry.** The energy released when dynamite explodes is a more dramatic example of chemical energy.

Electrical energy represents the work that can be done when an electron moves through an electric potential difference. The most familiar form of electrical energy is normal household electricity, which involves the movement of electrons through a copper wire by an electric potential difference of 110 volts (V). All electric apparatus, such as motors, heaters, and blowers, function through the use of electrical energy.

Thermal energy (**heat**) is the energy of motion at the atomic and molecular level. It is the kinetic energy of molecules and is closely related to temperature. The

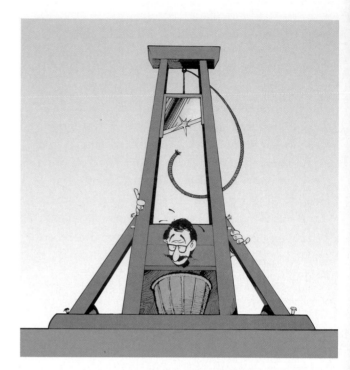

FIGURE 1-1 The blade of a guillotine offers a dramatic example of both potential and kinetic energy. When the blade is pulled to its maximum height and locked in place, it has potential energy. When the blade is allowed to fall, the potential energy is released as kinetic energy.

faster the molecules of a substance are vibrating, the more thermal energy the substance contains and the higher its temperature.

Nuclear energy is the energy contained in the nucleus of an atom. We control the release and use of this type of energy in nuclear electric power plants. An example of the uncontrolled release of nuclear energy is the atomic bomb.

Electromagnetic energy is perhaps the least familiar form of energy. It is the most important for our purposes, however, because it is the type of energy in an x-ray. In addition to x-rays, electromagnetic energy includes radio waves, microwaves, and ultraviolet, infrared, and visible light.

Just as matter can be transformed from one size, shape, and form to another, so energy can be transformed from one type to another. In radiology, for example, electrical energy in the x-ray imaging system is used to produce electromagnetic energy (the x-ray), which then is converted to chemical energy in the radiographic film.

Reconsider now the statement that all things can be classified as matter or energy. Look around you and think of absolutely anything, and you should be convinced of this statement. You should be able to classify anything as matter, energy, or both. Frequently, matter and energy exist side by side—a moving automobile has mass and kinetic energy, boiling water has mass and thermal energy, the Leaning Tower of Pisa has mass and potential energy.

Perhaps the strangest property associated with matter and energy is that they are interchangeable, a characteristic first described by Albert Einstein in his famous theory of relativity. Einstein's **mass-energy equivalence** equation is a cornerstone of that theory.

MASS-ENERGY
$E = mc^2$
E is energy, *m is* mass, *c* is the speed of light in a vacuum.

This mass-energy equivalence is the basis for the atomic bomb, nuclear power plants, and certain nuclear medicine imaging techniques.

Energy emitted and transferred through space is called **radiation.** When a piano string vibrates it is said to radiate sound; the sound is a form of radiation. Ripples or waves radiate from the point where a pebble is dropped into a still pond. Visible light, a form of electromagnetic energy, is radiated by the sun and often is called **electromagnetic radiation.** In fact, electromagnetic energy traveling through space is usually referred to as electromagnetic radiation or, simply, **radiation.**

Radiation is the transfer of energy.

Matter that intercepts radiation and absorbs part or all of it is said to be **exposed** or **irradiated.** Spending a day at the beach exposes you to ultraviolet light. Ultraviolet light is the kind of radiation that causes sunburn. During a radiographic examination, the patient is exposed to x-rays. **The patient is said to be irradiated.**

Ionizing radiation is a special type of radiation that includes x-rays. Ionizing radiation is any kind of radiation capable of removing an orbital electron from the atom with which it interacts (Figure 1-2). This type of interaction between radiation and matter is called **ionization.** Ionization occurs when an x-ray passes close to an orbital electron of an atom and transfers sufficient energy to the electron to remove it from the atom. The ionizing radiation may interact with and ionize additional atoms. The orbital electron and the atom from which it was separated are called an **ion pair.** The electron is a negative ion and the remaining atom is a positive ion.

Ionization is the removal of an electron from an atom.

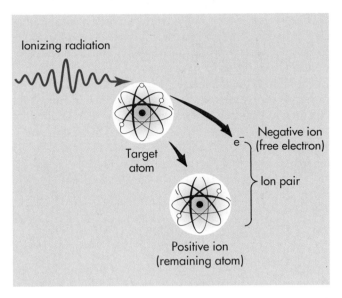

FIGURE 1-2 Ionization is the removal of an electron from an atom. The ejected electron and the resulting positively charged atom are called an *ion pair.*

Thus, any type of energy capable of ionizing matter is known as ionizing radiation. X-rays, gamma rays, and ultraviolet light are the only forms of electromagnetic radiation with sufficient energy to ionize. Some fast-moving particles (particles with high kinetic energy) are also capable of ionization. Examples of particle-type ionizing radiation are alpha and beta particles (see Chapter 4). Although alpha and beta particles are sometimes called rays, this designation is incorrect.

SOURCES OF IONIZING RADIATION

Many types of radiation are harmless, but ionizing radiation can injure humans. We are exposed to many sources of ionizing radiation (Figure 1-3). These sources can be divided into two main categories: **natural environmental radiation** and **man-made radiation.**

Natural radiation results in an annual dose of approximately 300 millirem (mrem). Man-made radiation results in approximately 60 mrem. A mrem is 1/1000 of a **rem.** The rem is the unit of radiation equivalent man. It is used to express radiation exposure of populations (see Chapter 2).

There are three components to natural environmental radiation: **cosmic rays, terrestrial radiation,** and **internally deposited radionuclides.** Cosmic rays are particulate and electromagnetic radiation emitted by the sun and stars. On earth, the intensity of cosmic radiation increases with altitude and latitude. Terrestrial radiation results from deposits of uranium, thorium, and other radionuclides in the earth. The intensity is very dependent on the geology of the local area. Internally deposited radionuclides, mainly potassium-40 (^{40}K), are natural metabolites. They have always been with us and contribute an equal dose to each of us.

The largest source of natural environmental radiation is **radon**. Radon is a radioactive gas produced by the natural decay of uranium, which is present in trace quantities in the earth. All earth-based materials, such as concrete, bricks, and gypsum wallboard, contain radon. Radon emits alpha particles, which are not penetrating, and therefore contributes a radiation dose only to the lung.

Collectively, these sources of natural environmental radiation result in approximately 2 to 10 microroentgens (μR)/hr at waist level in the United States (Figure 1-4). This equals an annual exposure of approximately 20 mR/yr along the Gulf Coast and Florida to 90 mR/yr and higher in the Rocky Mountain region.

Remember, however, that humans have existed for several hundred thousand years in the presence of this natural environmental radiation level. Human evolution has undoubtedly been influenced by this natural environmental radiation. Some geneticists contend that evolution is influenced primarily by ionizing radiation. If this is so, then we must indeed be concerned with control of unnecessary radiation exposure because over the last century, with the increasing medical applications of radiation, the average annual exposure of our population to radiation has increased significantly.

Diagnostic x-rays constitute the largest man-made source of ionizing radiation (39 mrem/yr). This estimate was made in 1990 by the National Council on Radiation Protection and Measurements (NCRP). More recent estimates put this source at nearly 50 mrem/yr, with the increase due principally to the increasing use of multislice spiral computed tomography (MSCT) and high-level fluoroscopy.

The benefits derived from the application of x-rays in medicine are indisputable; however, such applications must be made with prudence and with care taken to reducing unnecessary exposure of patients and personnel. This responsibility falls primarily on the radiologic technologist because the technologist usually controls the

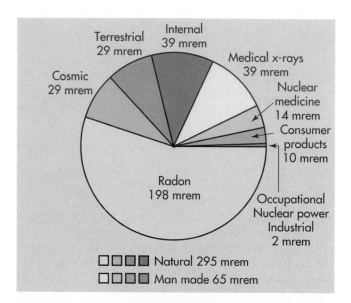

FIGURE 1-3 The contribution of various sources to the average United States population radiation dose.

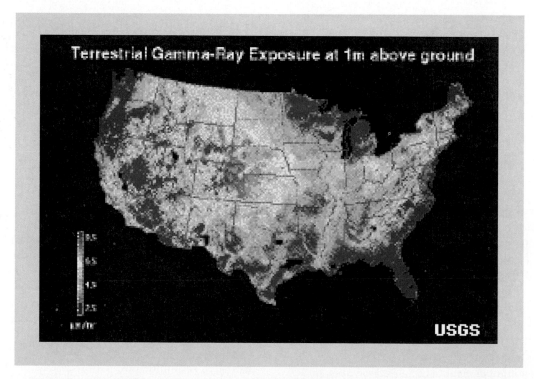

FIGURE 1-4 Radiation exposure at waist level throughout the United States. (Courtesy United States Geological Survey.)

operation of the x-ray imaging system during a radiologic examination.

The approximate annual dose resulting from medical applications of ionizing radiation is 50 mrem. Unlike the natural environmental radiation dose, this level takes into account people not receiving a radiologic examination and those receiving several in a year.

The medical radiation exposure for some in our population will be zero, but for others it may be quite high. Although this average level is comparable with natural environmental radiation levels, it is actually a rather small amount of radiation. One could question, therefore, why it is necessary to be concerned with radiation control and radiation safety in radiology.

Question: What percentage of our annual average radiation dose is due to diagnostic x-rays? (See Figure 1-3)

Answer: $\dfrac{39 \text{ mrad}}{360 \text{ mrad}} = 0.108 \cong 11\%$

Other sources of man-made radiation include nuclear power generation, research applications, industrial sources, and consumer items. Nuclear power stations and other industrial applications contribute very little to our radiation dose. Consumer products such as watch dials, exit signs, smoke detectors, camping lantern mantles, and airport surveillance systems contribute a few millirem to our annual radiation dose.

DISCOVERY OF X-RAYS

X-rays were not developed; they were discovered, and quite by accident. During the 1870s and 1880s, many university physics laboratories were investigating the conduction of **cathode rays,** or electrons, through a large, partially evacuated glass tube known as a **Crookes tube.** Sir William Crookes was an Englishman from a rather humble background who was a self-taught genius.

The tube that bears his name was the forerunner of modern fluorescent lamps and x-ray tubes. There were many different types of Crookes tubes; most of them were capable of producing x-rays. Wilhelm Roentgen was experimenting with a type of Crookes tube when he discovered x-rays (Figure 1-5).

On November 8, 1895, Roentgen was working in his physics laboratory at Würzburg University in Germany. He had darkened his laboratory and completely enclosed his Crookes tube with black photographic paper so that he could better visualize the effects of the cathode rays in the tube. A plate coated with **barium platinocyanide,** a fluorescent material, happened to be lying on a bench top several feet from the Crookes tube.

No visible light escaped from the Crookes tube because of the black paper enclosing it, but Roentgen noted that the barium platinocyanide glowed regardless of its distance from the Crookes tube. The intensity of the glow increased as the plate was brought closer to the tube; consequently, there was little doubt about the origin of the stimulus of the glow. This glow is called **fluorescence.**

Roentgen's immediate approach to investigating this "X-light," as he called it, was to interpose various materials—wood, aluminum, his hand!—between the Crookes tube and the fluorescing plate. The "X" was for unknown! He feverishly continued these investigations for several weeks.

Roentgen's initial investigations were extremely thorough and he was able to report his experimental results to the scientific community before the end of 1895. For this work, in 1901 he received the first Nobel Prize in physics. Roentgen recognized the value of his discovery to medicine. He produced and published the first medical x-ray image in early 1896. It was an image of his wife's hand (Figure 1-6). Figure 1-7 is a photograph of what is reported to be the first x-ray examination in the United States, conducted in early February, 1896 in the physics laboratory at Dartmouth College.

There are many amazing features about the discovery of x-rays that cause it to rank high in the events of human history. First, the discovery was accidental. Second, probably no fewer than a dozen contemporaries of Roentgen had previously observed x-radiation, but none of these other physicists had recognized its significance or investigated it. Third, Roentgen followed his discovery with such scientific vigor that within little more than a month he had described x radiation with nearly all the properties we recognize today.

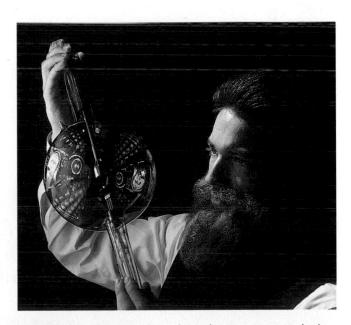

FIGURE 1-5 The type of Crookes tube Roentgen used when he discovered x-rays. Cathode rays (electrons) leaving the cathode are attracted to the anode by the high voltage, where they produced x-rays and fluorescent light. (Courtesy Gary Leach.)

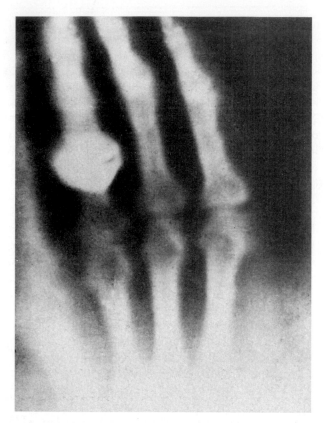

FIGURE 1-6 The hand shown in this radiograph is Mrs. Roentgen's. This was the first indication of the possible medical applications of x-rays and was made within a few days of the discovery. (Courtesy Deutsches Roentgen Museum.)

DEVELOPMENT OF MODERN RADIOLOGY

There are two general types of x-ray examinations: **radiography** and **fluoroscopy**. Radiography uses x-ray film and usually an x-ray tube mounted from the ceiling on a track that allows the tube to be moved in any direction. Such examinations provide the radiologist with fixed images.

Fluoroscopy is usually conducted with an x-ray tube located under the examination table. The radiologist is provided with moving images on a television monitor or flat panel display. There are many variations of these two basic types of examinations, but in general the x-ray equipment is similar.

 To provide an x-ray beam satisfactory for imaging, you must supply the x-ray tube with a high voltage and a sufficient electric current.

X-ray voltages are measured in kilovolt peak (**kVp**). One kilovolt (**kV**) is equal to 1000 V of electric potential. X-ray currents are measured in milliampere (**mA**), where the ampere (A) is a measure of electric current. The prefix **milli** stands for 1/1000 or 0.001.

Question: The usual x-ray source-to-image receptor distance (SID) is 1 meter. How many millimeters is that?

Answer: 1 mm = 1/1000 m or 10^{-3}, therefore 1000 mm = 1 m.

FIGURE 1-7 This photograph records the first medical x-ray examination in the United States. A young patient, Eddie McCarthy of Hanover, New Hampshire, broke his wrist while skating on the Connecticut River and submitted to having it photographed by the "X-light." With him are *(left to right)* Professor E. B. Frost, Dartmouth College and his brother, Dr. G. D. Frost, Medical Director, Mary Hitchcock Hospital. The apparatus was assembled by Professor F. G. Austin in his physics laboratory in Reed Hall, Dartmouth College, on February 3, 1896. (Courtesy Mary Hitchcock Hospital.)

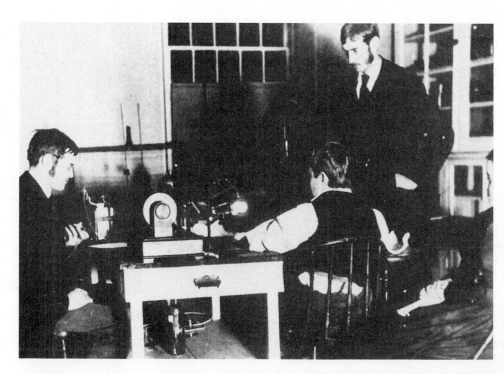

Today, voltage and current are supplied to an x-ray tube through rather complicated electric circuits, but in Roentgen's time only simple static generators were available. These units could provide currents of only a few milliamperes and voltages to 50 kVp. Today, 1000 mA and 150 kVp are common.

Radiographic procedures using equipment with these limitations of electric current and potential often required exposure times of 30 minutes or more for a satisfactory examination. Long exposure time results in image blur. One development that helped reduce this exposure time was the use of a fluorescent **intensifying screen** in conjunction with the glass photographic plates.

Michael Pupin is said to have demonstrated the use of a radiographic intensifying screen in 1896, but only many years later did it receive adequate recognition and use. Radiographs during Roentgen's time were made by exposing a glass plate with a layer of photographic emulsion coated on one side.

Charles L. Leonard found that by exposing two glass x-ray plates with the emulsion surfaces together, exposure time was halved and the image was considerably enhanced. This demonstration of double-emulsion radiography was conducted in 1904, but **double-emulsion film** did not become commercially available until 1918.

During World War I, radiologists began to make use of film rather than glass plates. Much of the high-quality glass used in radiography came from Belgium and other European countries. This supply was interrupted during World War I.

The demands of the army for increased radiologic services made a substitute for the glass plate necessary. The substitute was **cellulose nitrate,** and it quickly became apparent that the substitute was better than the original glass plate.

The **fluoroscope** was developed in 1898 by the American inventor Thomas A. Edison (Figure 1-8). Edison's original fluorescent material was barium platinocyanide, a widely used laboratory material. He investigated the fluorescent properties of over 1800 other materials, including **zinc cadmium sulfide** and **calcium tungstate,** two materials in use today.

There is no telling what further inventions Edison might have developed had he continued his x-ray research, but he abandoned it when his assistant and long-time friend, Clarence Dally, suffered a severe x-ray burn that eventually required amputation of both arms. Dally died in 1904 and is counted as the first x-ray fatality in the United States.

Two devices designed to reduce the exposure of patients to x-rays and thereby minimize the possibility of x-ray burn were introduced before the turn of the 20th century by a Boston dentist, William Rollins. Rollins used x-rays to image teeth and found that restricting the x-ray beam with a sheet of lead having a

hole in the center, a **diaphragm,** and inserting a leather or aluminum filter improved the diagnostic quality of his radiographs.

This first application of **collimation** and **filtration** was followed very slowly by general adoption of these techniques. It was later recognized that these devices reduce the hazard associated with x-rays.

Two developments that occurred at approximately the same time transformed the use of x-rays from a novelty in the hands of a few physicists into a valuable, large-scale medical specialty. In 1907, H. C. Snook introduced a substitute high-voltage power supply, an interrupterless **transformer,** for the static machines and induction coils then in use.

Although the Snook transformer was far superior to these other devices, its capability greatly exceeded the capability of the Crookes tube. It was not until the introduction of the Coolidge tube that the Snook transformer was widely adopted.

 Radiology emerged as a medical specialty because of the Snook transformer and the Coolidge x-ray tube.

The type of Crookes tube that Roentgen used in 1895 had existed for a number of years. Although some modifications were made by x-ray workers, it remained essentially unchanged into the second decade of the twentieth century.

After considerable clinical testing, William D. Coolidge unveiled his hot-cathode x-ray tube to the medical community in 1913. It was immediately recognized

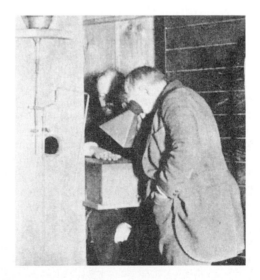

FIGURE 1-8 Thomas Edison is seen viewing the hand of his unfortunate assistant, Clarence Dally, through a fluoroscope of his own design. Dally's hand rests on the box containing the x-ray tube.

BOX 1-1 Some Important Dates in the Development of Modern Radiology

DATE	EVENT
1895	Roentgen discovers x-rays.
1896	First medical applications of x-rays in diagnosis and therapy are made.
1900	The American Roentgen Society, the first American radiology organization, is founded.
1901	Roentgen receives the first Nobel Prize in physics.
1905	Einstein introduces his theory of relativity and the famous equation $E = mc^2$.
1907	The Snook interrupterless transformer is introduced.
1913	Bohr theorizes his model of the atom, featuring a nucleus and planetary electrons.
1913	The Coolidge hot-filament x-ray tube is developed.
1917	Cellulose nitrate film base is widely adopted.
1920	Several investigators demonstrate the use of soluble iodine compounds as contrast media.
1920	The American Society of Radiologic Technologists (ASRT) is founded.
1921	The Potter-Bucky grid is introduced.
1922	Compton describes the scattering of x-rays.
1923	Cellulose acetate "safety" x-ray film is introduced (Eastman Kodak).
1925	The First International Congress of Radiology is convened in London.
1928	The roentgen is defined as the unit of x-ray intensity.
1929	Forssmann demonstrates cardiac catheterization . . . on himself!
1929	The rotating anode tube is introduced.
1930	Tomographic devices are shown by several independent investigators.
1932	Blue tint is added to x-ray film (Dupont).
1932	The U.S. Committee on X-ray and Radium Protection (now the NCRP) issues first dose limits.
1942	Morgan exhibits an electronic phototiming device.
1942	First automatic film processor (Pako) is introduced.
1948	Coltman develops the first fluoroscopic image intensifier.
1951	Multidirectional tomography (polytomography) is introduced.
1953	The rad is officially adopted as the unit of absorbed dose.
1956	Xeroradiography is demonstrated.
1956	First automatic roller transport film processing (Eastman Kodak) is introduced.
1960	Polyester base film is introduced (Dupont).
1963	Kuhl and Edwards demonstrate single-photon emission computed tomography (SPECT).
1965	Ninety-second rapid processor is introduced (Eastman Kodak).
1966	Diagnostic ultrasound enters routine use.
1972	Single-emulsion film and one-screen mammography became available (Dupont).
1973	Hounsfield completes development of first computed tomography imaging system (EMI, Ltd.).
1973	Damadian and Lauterbur produce first magnetic resonance images (MRI).
1974	Rare-earth radiographic intensifying screens are introduced.
1979	Mistretta demonstrates digital fluoroscopy.
1980	First commercial superconducting MRI system is introduced.
1981	The International System of Units (SI) is adopted by the International Commission on Radiation Units and Measurements (ICRU).
1982	Picture archiving and communications systems (PACS) become available.
1983	First tabular grain film emulsion (Eastman Kodak) is developed.
1984	Laser-stimulable phosphors for computed radiography appear (Fuji).
1988	First use of a superconducting quantum interference device (SQUID) for magnetoencephalography (MEG).
1990	Last xeromammography system is produced.
1990	Spiral CT is introduced (Toshiba).
1991	Twin-slice CT is developed (Elscint).
1992	Mammography Quality Standard Acts (MQSA) is passed.
1996	Direct digital radiography developed using thin-film transistors (TFT).
1998	Multislice CT is introduced (General Electric).
1998	Amorphous silicon and amorphous selenium are demonstrated for digital radiography.
2000	The first direct digital mammographic imaging system is made available (General Electric).
2002	Sixteen-slice spiral CT is introduced.
2002	Positron emission tomography (PET) is placed into routine clinical service.

as far superior to the Crookes tube. It was a vacuum tube and allowed x-ray intensity and energy to be selected separately and with great accuracy. This had not been possible with gas-filled tubes, which made standards for techniques difficult to obtain. X-ray tubes in use today are refinements of the **Coolidge tube.**

The era of modern radiography is dated from the matching of the Coolidge tube with the Snook transformer; only then did acceptable kilovolt peak and milliampere levels become possible. Few developments since that time have had such a major influence on diagnostic radiology.

In 1921, the Potter-Bucky grid, which greatly improved image contrast, was developed. In 1946, the light amplifier tube was demonstrated at Bell Telephone Laboratories. This device was adapted for fluoroscopy by 1950. Today, image-intensified fluoroscopy is universal.

Each recent decade has seen remarkable improvements in medical imaging. Diagnostic ultrasound appeared in the 1960s as well as the gamma camera; positron emission tomography (PET) and x-ray computed tomography (CT) were developed in the 1970s. Magnetic resonance imaging (MRI) became an accepted modality in the 1980s, and now magnetoencephalography (MEG) is being investigated. Box 1-1 chronologically summarizes some of the more important developments.

REPORTS OF RADIATION INJURY

The first x-ray fatality in the United States occurred in 1904. Unfortunately, radiation injuries occurred rather frequently in the early years. These injuries usually took the form of skin damage (sometimes severe), loss of hair, and anemia. Physicians and, more commonly, patients were injured, primarily because the low energy of radiation then available resulted in the necessity for long exposure times to obtain an acceptable radiograph.

By about 1910, these acute injuries began to be controlled as the biologic effects of x-rays were scientifically investigated and reported. With the introduction of the Coolidge tube and the Snook transformer, the frequency of reports of injuries to superficial tissues decreased.

Years later, it was discovered that blood disorders such as aplastic anemia and leukemia were developing in radiologists at a much higher rate than in others. Because of these observations, protective devices and apparel, such as lead gloves and aprons, were developed for use by radiologists. X-ray workers were routinely observed for any effects of their occupational exposure and were provided with personnel radiation monitoring devices. This attention to radiation safety in radiology has been effective.

Because of effective radiation protection practices, radiology is now considered a safe occupation.

BASIC RADIATION PROTECTION

Today the emphasis on radiation control in diagnostic radiology has shifted back to protection of the patient. Current studies suggest that even the low doses of x-radiation used in routine diagnostic procedures may result in a small incidence of latent harmful effects. It is also well established that the human fetus is sensitive to x-radiation early in pregnancy.

It is hoped that this introduction has emphasized the importance of providing adequate protection for both radiologic technologist and patient. As you progress through your training in radiologic technology, you will quickly learn how to operate your x-ray imaging systems safely, with minimal radiation exposures, by following standard radiation protection procedures.

One caution is in order early in your training—after having worked with x-ray imaging systems, you will become so familiar with your work environment that you may become complacent about radiation control. Do not allow yourself to develop this attitude because it can lead to unnecessary radiation exposure. Radiation protection must be an important consideration during each x-ray procedure. Box 1-2 reports the Ten Commandments of Radiation Protection.

Always practice ALARA: Keep radiation exposures *As Low As Reasonably Achievable.*

BOX 1-2   The Ten Commandments of Radiation Protection

1. Understand and apply the cardinal principles of radiation control: time, distance, and shielding.
2. Do not allow familiarity to result in false security.
3. Never stand in the primary beam.
4. Always wear protective apparel when not behind a protective barrier.
5. Always wear a radiation monitor and position it outside the protective apron at the collar.
6. Never hold a patient during radiographic examination. Use mechanical restraining devices when possible. Otherwise, have parents or friends hold the patient.
7. The person holding the patient must always wear a protective apron and, if possible, protective gloves.
8. Use gonadal shields on all people of childbearing age when such use will not interfere with the examination.
9. Examination of the pelvis and lower abdomen of a pregnant patient should be avoided whenever possible, especially during the first trimester.
10. Always collimate to the smallest field size appropriate for the examination.

Minimizing radiation exposure to technologist and patient is easy if the radiographic and fluoroscopic imaging systems designed for this purpose are recognized and understood (Figure 1-8). A brief description of some of the primary radiation protection devices follows:

Filtration. Metal filters, usually aluminum or copper, are inserted into the x-ray tube housing so that low-energy x-rays are absorbed before they reach the patient. These x-rays have little diagnostic value.

Collimation. Collimation restricts the useful x-ray beam to that part of the body to be imaged and thereby spares adjacent tissue from unnecessary exposure. Collimators take many different forms. Adjustable light-locating collimators are the most frequently used collimating devices. Collimation also reduces scatter radiation and thus improves image contrast.

Intensifying screens. Today, most x-ray films are exposed in a cassette with radiographic intensifying screens on both sides of the film. Examinations conducted with radiographic intensifying screens reduce the exposure of the patient to x-rays by more than 95% compared with examinations conducted without radiographic intensifying screens.

Protective apparel. Lead-impregnated material is used to make aprons and gloves worn by radiologists and radiologic technologists during fluoroscopy and some radiographic procedures.

Gonadal shielding. The same lead-impregnated material used in aprons and gloves is used to fabricate gonadal shields. Gonadal shields should be used with all persons of childbearing age when the gonads are in or near the useful x-ray beam and when use of such shielding will not interfere with the diagnostic value of the examination.

Protective barriers. The radiographic control console is always located behind a protective barrier. Often the barrier is lead-lined and equipped with a leaded-glass window. Under normal circumstances, personnel remain behind the barrier during radiographic examination. Figure 1-9 is a rendering of a radiographic/fluoroscopic examination room. Many of the radiation safety features are illustrated.

Other procedures should be followed. Abdominal x-ray examinations of expectant mothers should never be taken during the first trimester unless absolutely necessary. Every effort should be taken to ensure that an examination will not have to be repeated because of technical error. Repeat examinations subject the patient to twice the necessary radiation.

When shielding patients for x-ray examination, one should consider the medical management of the patient. Except for screening mammography, examination of asymptomatic patients is not indicated.

Patients who require assistance during examination should never be held by x-ray personnel. Mechanical restraining devices should be used. When necessary, a member of the patient's family should provide the necessary assistance.

THE DIAGNOSTIC IMAGING TEAM

To become part of this exciting profession, a student must complete the prescribed academic courses, obtain clinical experience, and pass the national certification examination given by the American Registry of Radiologic Technologists (ARRT). Both academic expertise and clinical skills are required of radiographers. Box 1-3 is a list of the clinical skills required by an individual who can put the RT(R) after his or her name. The requisite personal skills are shown in Box 1-4.

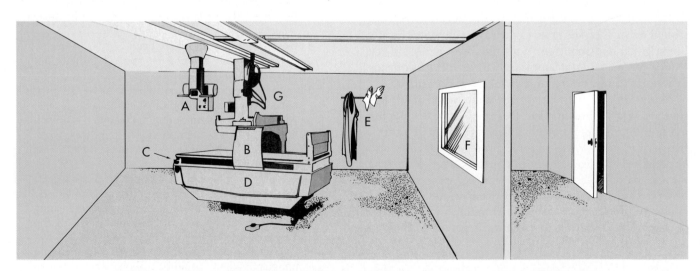

FIGURE 1-9 The general-purpose x-ray room usually includes an overhead radiographic tube (**A**) and a fluoroscopic examining table (**D**) with an x-ray tube under the table. Some of the more common radiation protection devices are lead curtain (**B**), Bucky slot cover (**C**), leaded apron and gloves (**E**), and protective viewing window (**F**). The location of the image intensifier (**G**) and associated imaging equipment is also shown.

BOX 1-3   Clinical Skills Required for Examination by the American Registry of Radiologic Technologists

Evaluate the need for and use of protective shielding.

Take appropriate precautions to minimize radiation exposure to patients.

Restrict beam to limit exposure area, improve image quality, and reduce radiation dose.

Set kilovolt peak level, milliamperage, and time or automated exposure system to achieve optimal image quality, safe operating conditions, and minimum radiation dose.

Prevent all unnecessary persons from remaining in area during x-ray exposure.

Take appropriate precautions to minimize occupational radiation exposure.

Wear a personnel radiation monitoring device while on duty.

Review and evaluate individual occupational exposure reports.

Warm up the x-ray tube according to manufacturer's recommendations.

Prepare and adjust radiographic imaging system and accessories.

Prepare and adjust the fluoroscopic imaging system and accessories.

Recognize and report malfunctions in the radiographic or fluoroscopic imaging system and accessories.

Perform basic evaluations of radiographic equipment and accessories (e.g., lead aprons, collimator accuracy).

Inspect and clean screens and cassettes.

Perform startup or shutdown procedures on automatic film processor.

Recognize and report malfunctions in the automatic processor.

Process exposed film.

Reload cassettes by selecting film of proper size and type.

Store film or cassette in a manner that will reduce the possibility of artifact production.

Select appropriate film—screen combination or grid.

Determine appropriate exposure factors using calipers, technique charts, and tube-rating charts.

Modify exposure factors for circumstances such as involuntary motion, casts and splints, pathologic conditions, or patient's inability to cooperate.

Use radiopaque markers to indicate anatomic side, position, or other relevant information.

Evaluate patient and radiographs to determine if additional projections or positions should be recommended.

Evaluate radiographs for diagnostic quality.

Determine corrective measures if radiograph is not of diagnostic quality and take appropriate action.

Select equipment and accessories for the examination requested.

Remove all radiopaque materials from patient or table that could interfere with the radiographic image.

BOX 1-4   Personal Skills Required for Examination by the American Registry of Radiologic Technologists

Explain breathing instructions before making the exposure.

Position patient to demonstrate the desired anatomy using body landmarks.

Explain patient preparation (e.g., diet restrictions, preparatory medications) before an imaging procedure.

Properly sequence radiograph procedures to avoid residual contrast material affecting future examinations.

Examine radiographic requisition to verify accuracy and completeness of information.

Use universal precautions.

Confirm patient's identity.

Question female patients of childbearing age about possible pregnancy.

Explain procedures to patient or patient's family.

Evaluate patient's ability to comply with positioning requirements for the requested examination.

Observe and monitor vital signs.

Use proper body mechanics or mechanical transfer devices when assisting patients.

Provide for patient comfort and modesty.

Select immobilization devices, when indicated, to prevent patient movement or ensure patient safety.

Verify accuracy of patient film identification.

Maintain confidentiality of patient information.

Use sterile or aseptic technique to prevent contamination of sterile trays, instruments, or fields.

Prepare contrast media for administration.

Before administration of contrast agent, gather information to determine if the patient is at increased risk for adverse reaction.

Perform venipuncture.

Observe patient after administration of contrast media to detect adverse reactions.

Recognize need for prompt medical attention and administer emergency care.

Document required information on patient's medical record.

Clean, disinfect, or sterilize facilities and equipment, and dispose of contaminated items in preparation for next examination.

Follow appropriate procedures when in contact with a patient in reverse/protective isolation.

Monitor medical equipment attached to the patient (e.g., intravenous lines, oxygen) during the radiographic procedure.

Position patient, x-ray tube, and image receptor to produce radiographs.

SUMMARY

Radiography offers a career in many areas of medical imaging and it requires a modest knowledge of medicine, biology, and physics(radiologic science. This first chapter weaves the history and development of radiography with an introduction to medical physics.

Medical physics includes the study of matter, energy, and the electromagnetic spectrum of which x-radiation is a part. It is the production of x-radiation and its safe, diagnostic use that is the basis of radiography. As well as emphasizing the importance of radiation safety, this chapter also presents a detailed list of clinical and patient care skills required of the radiographer.

CHALLENGE QUESTIONS

1. Define or otherwise identify:
   a. Energy
   b. Einstein's mass-energy equivalence equation
   c. Ionizing radiation
   d. The mrad
   e. The average level of natural environmental radiation
   f. The Coolidge tube
   g. Fluoroscopy
   h. Collimation
   i. The term applied to the chemistry of the body
   j. Barium platinocyanide
2. Match the following dates with the appropriate event:
   a. 1901   1. Roentgen discovers x-rays
   b. 1907   2. Roentgen wins first Nobel Prize in physics
   c. 1913   3. The Snook transformer is developed
   d. 1895   4. The Coolidge hot-cathode x-ray tube is introduced
3. Describe how weight is different from mass.
4. Name four examples of electromagnetic radiation.
5. How do x-rays interact differently from other electromagnetic radiation?
6. What is the purpose of x-ray beam filtration?
7. Describe the process that results in the formation of a negative ion and a positive ion.
8. What percentage of average radiation exposure to a human is due to medical x-rays?
9. Why was the discovery of x-rays an amazing event in human history?
10. Why is radiography now considered a radiation-safe occupation?
11. The acronym ALARA stands for what?
12. Name devices designed for minimizing radiation exposure to the patient and the operator.
13. Briefly describe the history of x-ray film.
14. What are the three sources of whole-body radiation exposure from natural sources?
15. What naturally occurring radiation source is responsible for dose to lung?
16. How would you describe the term "radiation?"
17. What are cathode rays?
18. Place the following in chronologic order of appearance:
    a. Digital fluoroscopy
    b. American Society of Radiologic Technologists (ASRT)
    c. Computed tomography (CT)
    d. Radiographic grids
    e. Automatic film processing
19. List five clinical skills required by the ASRT.
20. List five personal skills required by the ASRT.

Radiologic Quantities and Units

OBJECTIVES

At the completion of this chapter, the student should be able to do the following:

1. Calculate problems using fractions, decimals, exponents, and algebraic equations
2. Identify scientific exponential notation and the associated prefixes
3. List and define units of radiation and radioactivity

OUTLINE

THIS CHAPTER defines and illustrates the units of radiation and radioactivity used in medical imaging. To understand such units, a brief review of mathematics is offered. Emphasis is placed on basic mathematics that apply to x-ray imaging: number systems, algebra, exponents, and graphing.

MATHEMATICS FOR RADIOLOGY

Physics owes a great deal of its certainty to the use of mathematics, and accordingly most of the concepts of physics can be expressed mathematically. It is therefore important in the study of radiologic science to have a solid foundation in the basic concept of mathematics. The following sections review fundamental mathematics. You should become proficient at working each type of problem presented in this review.

Fractions

A **fraction** is a numerical value expressed by dividing one number by another; it is also called the *quotient* of two numbers. A fraction has a numerator and a denominator.

FRACTION

$$\text{fraction} = \frac{x}{y} = \frac{\text{numerator}}{\text{denominator}}$$

If the quotient of the numerator divided by the denominator is less than one, the value is a **proper fraction.** **Improper factions** have values greater than one.

Question: Give examples of a proper fraction.

Answer: $\frac{1}{2}, \frac{3}{5}, \frac{5}{7}, \frac{9}{10}$

Question: Give examples of an improper fraction.

Answer: $\frac{3}{2}, \frac{6}{5}, \frac{10}{7}, \frac{13}{10}$

Addition and Subtraction. First, find a common denominator, then add or subtract.

ADDING FRACTIONS

$$\frac{x}{y} + \frac{a}{b} = \frac{xb}{yb} + \frac{ay}{yb} = \frac{xb + ay}{yb}$$

Question: What is the value of $\frac{2}{3} + \frac{4}{5}$?

Answer: $\frac{2}{3} + \frac{4}{5} = \frac{10}{15} + \frac{12}{15} = \frac{22}{15}$

an improper fraction

Question: What is the value of $\frac{4}{5} - \frac{2}{3}$?

Answer: $\frac{4}{5} - \frac{2}{3} = \frac{12}{15} - \frac{10}{15} = \frac{2}{15}$

a proper fraction

Multiplication. To multiply fractions, simply multiply numerators and denominators.

MULTIPLYING FRACTIONS

$$\frac{x}{y} \times \frac{a}{b} = \frac{xa}{yb}$$

Question: What is the value of $\frac{2}{5} \times \frac{7}{4}$?

Answer: $\frac{2}{5} \times \frac{7}{4} = \frac{14}{20} = \frac{7}{10}$

a proper fraction

Question: What is the value of $\frac{9}{8} \times \frac{12}{7}$?

Answer: $\frac{9}{8} \times \frac{12}{7} = \frac{108}{56} = \frac{27}{14}$

an improper fraction

Division. To divide fractions, invert the second fraction and multiply.

DIVIDING FRACTIONS

$$\frac{x}{y} \div \frac{a}{b} = \frac{x}{y} \times \frac{b}{a} = \frac{xb}{ya}$$

Question: What is the value of $\frac{5}{2} \div \frac{7}{4}$?

Answer: $\frac{5}{2} \div \frac{7}{4} = \frac{5}{2} \times \frac{4}{7} = \frac{20}{14} = \frac{10}{7}$

an improper fraction

Question: What is the value of $\frac{3}{10} \div \frac{7}{2}$?

Answer: $\frac{3}{10} \div \frac{7}{2} = \frac{3}{10} \times \frac{2}{7} = \frac{6}{70} = \frac{3}{35}$

a proper fraction

A special application of fractions to radiology is the **ratio.** Ratios express the mathematical relationship between similar quantities, such as feet to the mile or pounds to the kilogram.

Question: What is the ratio of feet to a mile?

Answer: There are 5280 feet in a mile; therefore, the ratio is $\dfrac{5280 \text{ ft}}{1 \text{ mile}}$

Question: What is the ratio of kilograms to the pound?

Answer: There are 2.2 pounds in a kilogram; therefore, the ratio is $\dfrac{2.2 \text{ lb}}{\text{kg}}$

Decimals

Fractions in which the denominator is a power of 10 may easily be converted to decimals.

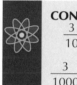

CONVERTING FRACTIONS TO DECIMALS	
$\dfrac{3}{10} = 0.3$	$\dfrac{161}{10,000} = 0.0161$
$\dfrac{3}{1000} = 0.003$	$\dfrac{1527}{10,000} = 0.1527$

If the denominator is not a power of 10, the decimal equivalent can be found by division or with a calculator.

$$\frac{5}{12} = \text{(long division equation)}$$

$$
\begin{array}{r}
0.41\overline{6} \\
12\overline{)5.000} \\
\underline{48} \\
20 \\
\underline{12} \\
80 \\
\underline{72} \\
8
\end{array}
$$

The bar above the 6 indicates that this digit is repeating. When one divides 5 by 12, the answer is 0.416666.

Rarely do we convert fractions to decimals without a hand calculator or computer. Depending on the calculator, it is simply a matter of keying numbers in the proper sequence.

Question: What is the decimal equivalent of the proper fraction $\dfrac{3}{7}$?

Answer: $\dfrac{3}{7} = 0.429$

Question: What is the decimal equivalent of the improper fraction $\dfrac{123}{69}$?

Answer: $\dfrac{123}{69} = 1.78$

Significant Figures

Students often wonder how many decimal places to report in an answer. For example, suppose you were asked to find the area of a circle.

Question: What is the area of a circle with a radius of 1.25 cm?

Answer: $A = \pi r^2$
$= (3.14)(1.25 \text{ cm})^2$
$= (3.14)(1.5625 \text{ cm}^2)$
$= 4.90625 \text{ cm}^2$

This answer is unsuitable, however, because it implies much greater precision in the measurement of the area than we actually have. This result must be rounded off according to specific rules.

 In addition and subtraction, round to the same number of decimal places as the entry with the least number of decimal places to the right of the decimal place.

Question: Add 5.0631, 117.2, and 21.42 and round off the answer.

Answer:
$$
\begin{array}{r}
5.0631 \\
117.2 \\
+\ 21.42 \\
\hline
143.6831
\end{array}
$$

Since 117.2 has one digit, 2, to the right of the decimal point, the answer is 143.7.

Question: Solve the following and round off the answer: 42.83 − 7.6147.

Answer:
$$
\begin{array}{r}
42.83 \\
-7.6147 \\
\hline
35.2153
\end{array}
$$

Because 42.83 has two digits, 83, to the right of the decimal point, the answer is 35.22.

 In multiplication and division, round to the same number of digits as the entry with the least number of significant figures.

Question: What is the product of 17.24 and 0.382?

Answer:
$$
\begin{array}{r}
17.24 \\
\times\ 0.382 \\
\hline
6.58568
\end{array}
$$

Since 0.382 has three significant figures (the zero is not significant) and 17.24 has four, the answer must have three digits. The answer is 6.59.

Question: How would you report the area of the circle discussed previously?

Answer: 4.91 cm²

Question: What is the quotient of 3.1416 by 1.05?

Answer: $\dfrac{3.1416}{1.05} = 2.992$

Because 1.05 has three significant digits (in this case, the zero is significant because it is followed by a number greater than zero) and 3.1416 five significant digits, the answer must have three digits. The answer is 2.99.

Algebra

Rules of algebra provide definite ways to manipulate fractions and equations to solve for unknown quantities. Usually, the unknowns are designed by an alphabetic symbol such as x, y, or z. Three principal rules of algebra are used in the solutions of problems of diagnostic radiology.

When an unknown, x, is multiplied by a number, divide both sides of the equation by that number.

$$ax = c$$

$$\frac{ax}{a} = \frac{c}{a}$$

$$x = \frac{c}{a}$$

Question: Solve the equation $5x = 10$ for x.

Answer: $5x = 10$

$$\frac{5x}{5} = \frac{10}{5}$$

$$x = 2$$

When numbers are added to an unknown, x, subtract that number from both sides of the equation.

$$x + a = b$$
$$x + a - a = b - a$$
$$x = b - a$$

Question: Solve the equation $x + 7 = 10$.

Answer: $x + 7 - 7 = 10 - 7$

$$x = 3$$

When an equation is presented in the form of a proportion, cross-multiply and then solve for the unknown, x.

$$\frac{x}{a} = \frac{b}{c}$$

$$\frac{x}{a} \diagdown \diagup \frac{b}{c}$$

$$cx = ab$$

$$x = \frac{ab}{c}$$

The crossed arrows show the direction of cross-multiplication.

Question: Solve the equation $\dfrac{x}{5} = \dfrac{3}{8}$ for x.

Answer: $\dfrac{x}{5} = \dfrac{3}{8}$

$$8x = 3 \times 5$$
$$8x = 15$$
$$\frac{8x}{8} = \frac{15}{8}$$
$$x = 1\frac{7}{8}$$

Often, all three rules may be necessary to solve a particular problem.

Question: Solve $6x + 3 = 15$ for the value of x.

Answer: $6x + 3 = 15$

$$6x + 3 - 3 = 15 - 3$$
$$6x = 12$$
$$\frac{6x}{6} = \frac{12}{6}$$
$$x = 2$$

Question: Solve $\dfrac{4}{x} = \left(\dfrac{3}{4}\right)^2$ for the value of x.

Answer: $\dfrac{4}{x} = \left(\dfrac{3}{4}\right)^2$

$$\frac{4}{x} = \frac{9}{16}$$
$$64 = 9x$$
$$\frac{64}{9} = \frac{9x}{9}$$
$$7.1 = x$$

Question: Solve $ABx + C = D$ for x.

Answer: $ABx + C = D$

$$ABx + C - C = D - C$$
$$ABx = D - C$$
$$\frac{ABx}{AB} = \frac{D - C}{AB}$$
$$x = \frac{D - C}{AB}$$

Note that the first and third of the previous examples are nearly identical in form. Symbols are often used in physics equations instead of numbers.

A special application of fractions and rules of algebra to radiology is the **proportion**. A proportion expresses the relationship of one ratio to another ratio. The ratio of a radiographic grid is directly proportional to the quotient of the height to the interspace between grid lines.

Question: If the grid height is 800 μm and the interspace 80 μm, what is the grid ratio?

Answer: $\dfrac{800 \ \mu m}{80 \ \mu m} = \dfrac{10}{1}$ the grid ratio

Sometimes this is written 10:1 and expressed as "10 to 1 ratio."

The statement "gas mileage is inversely proportional to automobile weight" can be used as a numerical proportion to solve for an unknown quantity.

Question: A 1650-pound compact car gets 34 miles per gallon of gas. What is the expected mileage for a 3600-pound luxury car?
Answer: Set up the inverse proportion as follows

$$\frac{x}{1650 \text{ lb}} = \frac{34 \text{ mpg}}{3600 \text{ lb}}$$

and use the rules of algebra to solve for x

$$x = \frac{(34 \text{ mpg})(1650 \text{ lb})}{3600 \text{ lb}}$$

$$x = 15.6 \text{ mpg}$$

Radiation output is directly proportional to the mAs of an x-ray imaging system.

Question: At 50 milliampere-seconds (mAs), the entrance skin exposure (ESE) is 240 mR. What will be the ESE if the technique is increased to 60 mAs?

Answer: $$\frac{x}{60 \text{mAs}} = \frac{240 \text{ mR}}{50 \text{ mAs}}$$

$$x = \frac{(240 \text{ mR})(60 \text{ mAs})}{50 \text{ mAs}}$$

$$x = 288 \text{ mR}$$

Number Systems

We use a system of numbers that is based on multiples of 10, called the **decimal system.** The origin of this system is unknown, but there are theories (Figure 2-1).

Numbers in this system can be represented in various ways, four of which are shown in Table 2-1. The logarithmic form, although particularly useful in some area of physics and mathematics, has little application in radiology except in the description of some characteristics of radiographic film.

The superscript on "10" in the exponential form column of Table 2-1 is called the **exponent.** The **exponential form,** also referred to as **power-of-ten notation** or **scientific notation,** is particularly useful in radiology.

Note that very large and very small numbers are difficult to write in decimal and fractional form. In radiology, many numbers are either very large or very small. Scientific notation allows these numbers to be written and manipulated with relative ease.

To express a number in scientific notation, first write the number in decimal form. If there are digits to the left of the decimal point, the exponent will be positive.

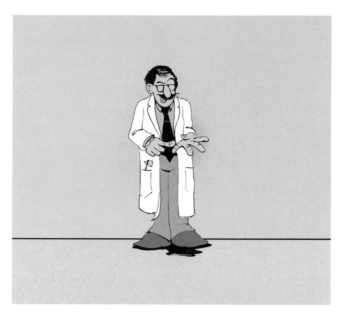

FIGURE 2-1 The probable origin of the decimal number system.

To determine the value of this positive exponent, position the decimal point after the first digit and count the number of digits the decimal point was moved. For example, the national debt of the United States was approximately 7 trillion dollars on January 1, 2004. To express this in scientific notation, we must position the decimal point after the first 7 and count the number of digits that was moved. This indicates that the exponent will be + 12.

 United States National Debt = \$7,327,644,102,329 = \$7.3 \times 10^{12}

If there are no nonzero digits to the left of the decimal point, the exponent will be negative. The value of this negative exponent is found by positioning the decimal point to the right of the first nonzero digit and counting the number of digits the decimal point was moved.

A string on Robert Earle Keene's guitar has a diameter of 0.00075 m. What is its diameter in scientific notation? First, position the decimal point between the 7 and the 5. Next, count the number of digits the decimal point has moved and express this quantity as the negative exponent.

 0.00075 m - 7.5×10^{-4} m

Another example from physics is a number called **Planck's constant,** symbolized by **h.** Planck's constant is related to the energy of an x-ray. Its decimal form is:

h = 0.00000000000000000000000000000000663 J s

Obviously this form is too cumbersome to write each time. Thus, Planck's constant is always written in scientific notation:

$$h = 6.63 \times 10^{-34} \text{ J s}$$

Question: Express 4050 in scientific notation.
Answer: $4050 = 4.05 \times 10^3$

Question: Express $\dfrac{1}{2000}$ in scientific notation.

Answer: First convert $\dfrac{1}{2000}$ to decimal form

$$\frac{1}{2000} = 0.0005$$
$$0.0005 = 5 \times 10^{-4}$$

Question: X-rays have a velocity of 300,000,000 m/s. Express this in scientific notation.
Answer: $300{,}000{,}000 = 3 \times 10^8$ m/s

Question: Dedicated chest x-ray imaging systems used to be installed with a 10-ft source-to-image receptor distance (SID). Express this in centimeters in scientific notation.

Answer: $10 \text{ ft } \times \dfrac{12 \text{ in}}{\text{ft}} = \dfrac{2.54 \text{ cm}}{\text{in}}$ 304.8 cm

$$304.8 \text{ cm} = 3.048 \times 10^2 \text{ cm}$$

Actually, today's dedicated chest units are installed at a 3-m SID.

Rules for Exponents

Another advantage of handling numbers in exponential form is evident in operations other than addition and subtraction. The general rules for these types of numerical operations are shown in Table 2-2.

The following examples should sufficiently emphasize the principles involved.

Multiplication: Add the exponents.

Question: Simplify $10^6 \times 10^8$.
Answer: $10^6 \times 10^8 = 10^{6+8} = 10^{14}$

Question: Simplify $2^8 \times 2^{12}$.
Answer: $2^8 \times 2^{12} = 2^{8+12} = 2^{20}$

Division: Subtract the exponents.

Question: $10^{10} \div 10^2$.
Answer: $10^{10} \div 10^2 = 10^{10-2} = 10^8$

Question: Simplify $\dfrac{2^3}{2^5}$.

Answer: $\dfrac{2^3}{2^5} = 2^{3-5} = 2^{-2} = \dfrac{1}{2^2} = \dfrac{1}{4}$

Raising to a Power: Multiply the exponents.

Question: Simplify $(3 \times 10^{10})^2$
Answer: $(3 \times 10^{10})^2 = 3^2 \times (10^{10})^2$
$$= 9 \times 10^{20}$$

TABLE 2-1	Various Ways to Represent Numbers in the Decimal System		
Fractional Form	**Decimal Form**	**Exponential Form**	**Logarithmic Form**
10,000	10,000	10^4	4.000
1000	1000	10^3	3.000
100	100	10^2	2.000
10	10	10^1	1.000
1	1	10^0	0.000
1/10	0.1	10^{-1}	−1.000
1/100	0.01	10^{-2}	−2.000
1/1000	0.001	10^{-3}	−3.000
1/10,000	0.0001	10^{-4}	−4.000

TABLE 2-2	Rules for Handling Numbers in Exponential Form	
Operation	**Rule**	**Example**
Multiplication	$10^x \times 10^y = 10^{x+y}$	$10^2 \times 10^3 = 10^{2+3} = 10^5$
Division	$10^x \div 10^y = 10^{x-y}$	$10^6 \div 10^4 = 10^{6-4} = 10^2$
Raising to a power	$(10^x)^y = 10^{xy}$	$(10^5)^3 = 10^{5 \cdot 3} = 10^{15}$
Inverse	$10^{-x} = 1/10^x$	$10^{-3} = 1/10^3 = 1/1000$
Unity	$10^0 = 1$	$3.7 \times 10^0 = 3.7$

Question: Simplify $(2.718 \times 10^{-4})^3$
Answer: $(2.718 \times 10^{-4})^3 = (2.718)^3 \times (10^{-4})^3$
$= 20.08 \times 10^{-12}$
$= 2.008 \times 10^{-11}$

Note that the rules for exponents apply only when the numbers raised to a power are the same.

Question: Given $a = 6.62 \times 10^{-27}$, $b = 3.766 \times 10^{12}$, what is $a \times b$?
Answer: $a \times b = 6.62 \times 10^{-27} \times 3.766 \times 10^{12}$
$= (6.62 \times 3.766) \times 10^{-27} \times 10^{12}$
$= 24.931 \times 10^{-27+12}$
$= 24.93 \times 10^{-15}$
$= 2.49 \times 10^{-14}$

Graphing

Knowledge of graphing is essential to the study of radiologic science. It is important not only to be able to read information from graphs but to graph data obtained from measurements or observations.

Most graphs are based on two **axes**: a horizontal or **x-axis** and a vertical or **y-axis**. The point where the two axes meet is called the **origin** (labeled 0 in Figure 2-2). Coordinates have the form of **ordered pairs** (x,y), where the first number of the pair represents a distance along the x-axis and the second number indicates a distance up the y-axis.

The ordered pair (3,2) represents a point three units over on the x-axis and two units up on the y-axis. This point is plotted in Figure 2-2. How does it differ from the point (2,3)? If the value of one additional ordered pair is known [e.g. (9,10)], a straight-line graph can be constructed.

In radiologic science the axes of graphs are not usually labeled x and y. Usually, the relationship between two specific quantities is desired. Suppose, for example, that you were asked to graph the effect of milliampere-seconds on optical density (OD), the darkening of a radiograph.

mAs VS. OD	
mAs	OD
0	0.20
10	0.25
20	0.46
30	0.70
40	0.91
60	1.24
80	1.45
100	1.60

The first step is to draw the axes. In this example, the data are recorded in ordered pairs, where mAs represents the x-value and OD represents the y-value.

Next, note the range of each quantity and choose a convenient scale that allows the data adequately to fill the graph. Very small graphs should usually be avoided. Then label the axes and carefully plot each point. Finally, draw the best smooth curve through the points. The curve need not touch each of the plotted points. A completed graph of the preceding data is shown in Figure 2-3.

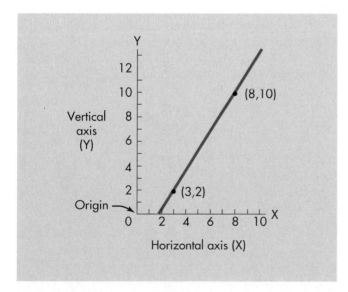

FIGURE 2-2 The principal features of any graph are x- and y-axes that intersect at the origin. Points of data are entered as ordered pairs.

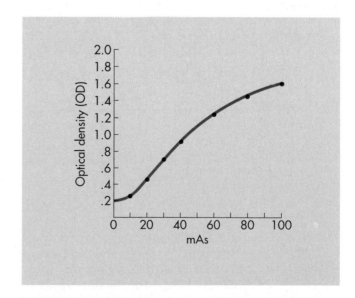

FIGURE 2-3 Relationship of optical density and milliampere seconds from the data presented in the text.

Question: The following data were obtained from an experiment to determine how much x-radiation it takes to kill 50% of irradiated mice in 30 days ($LD_{50/30}$). Plot these data and estimate the $LD_{50/30}$.

Radiation dose (rad)	Number of mice irradiated	Number of mice dead within 30 days	Percentage lethality
700	36	0	0
750	36	2	6
800	46	5	11
850	36	13	36
900	46	29	63
950	36	31	86
1000	40	37	93

Answer: The columns of data to be plotted are the first and the last. Label the axes so that the range of data is covered. Now, plot the ordered pairs of data and connect them with a smooth curve.

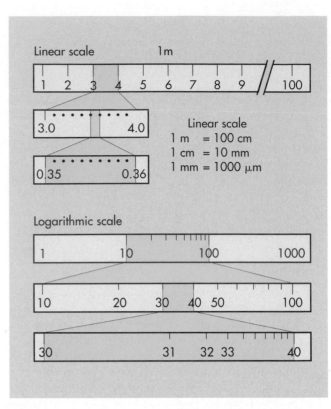

FIGURE 2-4 Equal lengths of linear scale have equal value. The logarithm scale allows a large range of values to be plotted.

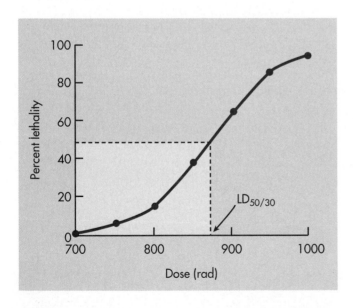

Finally, draw a horizontal line at the 50% lethality level and, when it intersects the smooth curve, drop to the dose axis. This is the $LD_{50/30}$ for the mice in this experiment (approximately 880 rad). The $LD_{50/30}$ for humans is approximately 350 rad.

Often the data to be plotted are in scientific notation and therefore extend over a very large range of values. In these situations a linear scale is not adequate, and a logarithmic scale must be used (Figure 2-4).

Radiologic data frequently require a graph using a semilogarithmic scale on one axis (Figure 2-5). The y-axis on semilog paper is a logarithmic scale used to accommodate a wide range of values. The x-axis is a linear scale.

Question: The following data were obtained to determine how much lead would be required to reduce x-ray intensity from 330 mR to 10 mR.

Lead thickness (mm)	0	2	4	6	8
X-ray intensity (mR)	330	140	58	25	11

Plot these data on linear and semilog graph paper and estimate the thickness of lead required.

Answer: From the semilog plot it is easy to see that the answer is 8.2 mm Pb. The linear plot is not so easy to read.

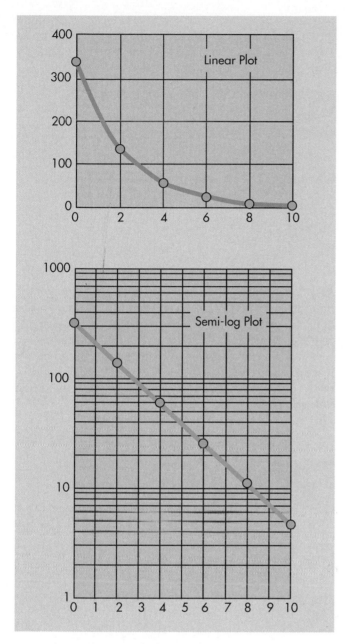

FIGURE 2-5 Semilogarithmic paper is often used for plotting radiologic data.

★ KNOW THESE ★

TABLE 2-3	Standard Scientific and Engineering Prefixes	
Multiple	**Prefix**	**Symbol**
10^{18}	exa-	E
10^{15}	peta-	P
10^{12}	tera-	T
10^{9}	giga-	G
10^{6}	**mega-**	**M**
10^{3}	**kilo-**	**k**
10^{2}	hecto-	h
10	deka-	da
10^{-1}	deci-	d
10^{-2}	**centi-**	**c**
10^{-3}	**milli-**	**m**
10^{-6}	**micro-**	**μ**
10^{-9}	nano-	n
10^{-12}	pico-	p
10^{-15}	femto-	f
10^{-18}	atto-	a

Boldfaced prefixes are those most frequently used in radiologic science.

already been discussed. By writing 70 kVp instead of 70,000 volt peak, we can understandably express the same quantity with fewer characters. For such economy of expression, scientists have devised a system of prefixes and symbols (Table 2-3).

Question: How many kilovolts equal 37,000 volts?
Answer: $37,000 \text{ V} = 37 \times 10^{3} \text{ V}$
                $= 37 \text{ kV}$

Question: The diameter of a blood cell is approximately 10 micrometers (μ). How many meters is that?
Answer: $10 \text{ μ} = 10 \times 10^{-6} \text{ m}$
                $= 10^{-5} \text{ m}$
                $= 0.00001 \text{ m}$

Radiologic Units

The four units used to measure radiation should become a familiar part of your vocabulary. Figure 2-6 relates them to a hypothetical situation in which they would be used. Table 2-4 shows the relationship of the customary radiology units to their International System (SI) equivalents.

In 1981, the International Commission on Radiation Units and Measurements (ICRU) issued standard units based on SI that have since been adopted by all countries except the United States. Most U.S. scientific journals and societies have adopted Le Système International d'Unités (The International System, SI), but regulatory agencies and the American Registry of Radiologic Technologists (ARRT) have not. Consequently, this book uses the customary radiologic units followed by the SI equivalent in parentheses throughout.

TERMINOLOGY FOR RADIOLOGY

Every profession has its own language. Radiologic technology is no exception. Several words and phrases characteristic of radiologic technology already have been identified; many more will be defined and used throughout this book. For now, an introduction to this terminology should be sufficient.

Numeric Prefixes

Often in radiologic technology, we must describe very large or very small multiples of standard units. Two units, milliampere (mA) and kilovolt peak (kVp), have

Roentgen (R) (Gya). The roentgen is equal to the radiation intensity that will create 2.08×10^8 ion pairs in a cubic centimeter of air; that is, $1\ R = 2.08 \times 10^9$ ip/cm³. The official definition, however, is in terms of electric charge per unit mass of air ($1\ R = 2.58 \times 10^{-4}$ C/kg). The charge refers to the electrons liberated by ionization.

The roentgen was first defined as a unit of radiation quantity in 1928. Since then, the definition has been revised many times. Radiation monitors usually are calibrated in roentgens. The output of x-ray imaging systems is usually specified in milliroentgens (mR). The roentgen applies only to x-rays and gamma rays and their interactions with air. In keeping with the adoption of the Wagner/Archer method described in the preface, the SI unit of air kerma (mGy$_a$) is used.

 The roentgen is the unit of radiation exposure or intensity.

Question: The output intensity of an x-ray imaging system is 100 mR. What is this value in SI units?
Answer: 100 R = Gy$_a$
    100 mR = .001 Gy$_a$
    100 mR = 1 mGy$_a$

Rad (Gyt). Biologic effects usually are related to the radiation absorbed dose, and therefore the rad is the unit most often used when describing the quantity of radiation received by a patient. The rad is used for any type of ionizing radiation and any exposed matter, not just air. One rad is equal to 100 erg/g (10^{-2} Gyt), where the **erg (joule)** is a unit of energy and the **gram (kilogram)** is a unit of mass. The units Gy$_a$ and Gy$_t$ refer to radiation dose in air or tissue.

 The rad is the unit of *radiation* absorbed *dose.*

Rem (Sv). Occupational radiation monitoring devices are analyzed in terms of rem (**r**adiation **e**quivalent **m**an). The rem is used to express the quantity of radiation received by radiation workers and populations.

$$100\ mrem = 1\ mSv$$

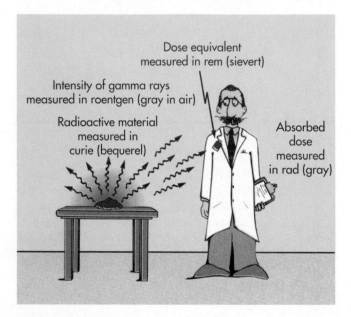

FIGURE 2-6 Radiation is emitted by radioactive material. The quantity of radioactive material is measured in curies. Radiation quantity is measured in roentgens, rads, or rems, depending on precise use. In diagnostic imaging, we may consider 1 R = 1 rad = 1 rem.

TABLE 2-4	Special Quantities of Radiologic Science and Their Associated Special Units				
	CUSTOMARY UNIT			**SI UNIT**	
Quantity	**Name**		**Symbol**	**Name**	**Symbol**
Exposure	roentgen		R	air kerma	Gy$_a$
Absorbed dose	rad		rad	gray	Gy$_t$
Effective dose	rem		rem	seivert	Sv
Radioactivity	curie		Ci	becquerel	Bq
Multiply	R	by	0.01	to obtain	Gy$_a$
Multiply	rad	by	0.01	to obtain	Gy$_t$
Multiply	rem	by	0.01	to obtain	Sv
Multiply	Ci	by	3.7×10^{10}	to obtain	Bq

Some types of radiation produce more damage than x-rays. The rem accounts for these differences in biologic effectiveness. This is particularly important to persons working near nuclear reactors or particle accelerators or with x-rays.

 The rem is the unit of occupational radiation exposure expressed as effective dose (E).

Curie (Ci) (Bq). The curie is the unit of the quantity of radioactive material and not the radiation emitted by that material. One curie is that quantity of radioactivity in which 3.7×10^{10} nuclei disintegrate every second (3.7×10^{10} becquerels [Bq]). The millicurie (mCi) and microcurie (μCi) are common quantities of radioactive material. Radioactivity and the curie have nothing to do with x-rays.

 The curie is a unit of radioactivity.

Question: 0.05 μCi iodine-125 is used for radioimmunoassay. What is this radioactivity in becquerels?

Answer: 0.05 μCi $= 0.05 \times 10^{-6}$ Ci
$= (0.05 \times 10^{-6}$ Ci$) (3.7 \times 10^{10}$ Bq/Ci$)$
$= 0.185 \times 10^{4}$ Bq $= 1850$ Bq

Diagnostic radiology is concerned primarily with x-rays. We may consider 1 R is equal to 1 rad is equal to 1 rem (1 mGy$_a$ = 1 mGy$_t$ = 1 mSv). With other types of ionizing radiation, this generalization is not true.

SUMMARY

The technical aspects of radiography are complex. A basic knowledge of mathematics is required, as well as identification and proper use of the units of radiation measurements.

As you review this chapter, consider again the fraction/decimal conversion, algebraic relations, numeric prefixes/exponents, and graphing. All are important to understanding the principles of radiologic science related to x-ray imaging. Figure 2-7 summarizes the conversion from conventional units of radiation exposure to SI units.

CHALLENGE QUESTIONS

1. Define or otherwise identify the following:
   a. Linear scale
   b. Significant figure
   c. Radiologic unit
   d. Ordered pair
   e. Units of Planck's constant
   f. Ratio
   g. Logarithmic scale
   h. x/y is a fraction. What is y called?
   i. Scientific notation
   j. Radiation equivalent man
2. Determine your height in the SI system.
3. Simplify the fraction $\dfrac{2^2}{2^5}$.
4. Evaluate the following:
   a. $\dfrac{7}{8} + \dfrac{5}{32} =$

   b. $\dfrac{4}{9} \times \dfrac{3}{8} =$

   c. $\dfrac{16}{2} \div \dfrac{4}{9} =$

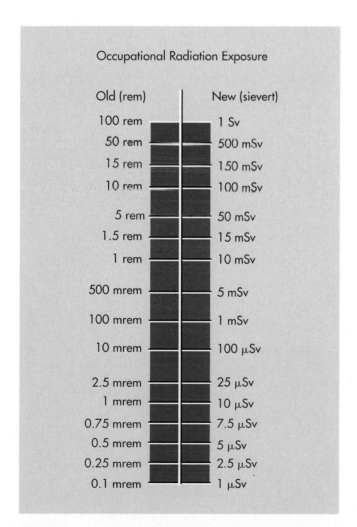

Occupational Radiation Exposure	
Old (rem)	New (sievert)
100 rem	1 Sv
50 rem	500 mSv
15 rem	150 mSv
10 rem	100 mSv
5 rem	50 mSv
1.5 rem	15 mSv
1 rem	10 mSv
500 mrem	5 mSv
100 mrem	1 mSv
10 mrem	100 μSv
2.5 mrem	25 μSv
1 mrem	10 μSv
0.75 mrem	7.5 μSv
0.5 mrem	5 μSv
0.25 mrem	2.5 μSv
0.1 mrem	1 μSv

FIGURE 2-7 Equivalent scales for radiation dose equivalent.

5. Write the following as decimals:

   a. $\dfrac{7}{10} =$

   b. $\dfrac{81}{1000} =$

   c. $\dfrac{7}{15} =$

6. Write the following in scientific notation:
   a. 1,480,000
   b. 711,000
7. Write the following in scientific notation:
   a. 0.0042
   b. 0.01067
8. Solve the following:
   a. $(2 \times 10^6) \times (4 \times 10^4) =$
   b. $(8 \times 10^{15}) \div (2 \times 10^5) =$
9. Solve the following:
   a. $3x - 9 = 12; x =$

   b. $\dfrac{x}{3} = \dfrac{5}{7}; x =$

10. Given $a = 6.62 \times 10^{-27}$ and $b = 3.766 \times 10^{12}$, what is $a \times b$?

11. Find the decimal equivalent of $\dfrac{3}{1000}$.

12. What is the decimal equivalent of $\dfrac{5}{12}$?

13. What is the first step when adding or subtracting fractions?
14. What sequence of steps should be taken when dividing fractions?
15. What does the phrase "directly proportional to" mean?
16. Which number system is easiest for you to understand?
17. What is the product of 17.24 and 0.382? Round off to the appropriate decimal places.

18. In the equation $\dfrac{x}{5} = \dfrac{3}{8}$, $x =$

19. If gas mileage were inversely proportional to automobile weight, what would be the expected mileage for a 1600-kg car if a 750-kg car gets 14 km/l?
20. Radiation exposure is directly proportional to the technical factor, milliampere seconds. At 50 mAs, the entrance skin exposure (ESE) is 240 mR. What will be the ESE if the x-ray tube current is increased to 60 mAs.

Fundamentals of Physics

OBJECTIVES

At the completion of this chapter, the student should be able to do the following:

1. Discuss the derivation of scientific systems of measurement
2. List the three systems of measurement
3. Identify nine categories of mechanics

OUTLINE

Standard Units of Measurement
    Length
    Mass
    Time
    Units
Mechanics
    Velocity
    Acceleration
    Newton's Laws of Motion
    Weight
    Momentum
    Work
    Power
    Energy
    Heat

N CHAPTER 1, matter and energy were defined. **Mechanics,** which involves matter in motion, is discussed in this chapter. However, when dealing with matter, energy, or mechanics, standards of measurement are required. This chapter also deals with such standards.

The instant an x-ray tube produces x-rays, all the laws of physics and mechanics introduced in this text are evident. The projectile electron from the **cathode** hits the target of the anode, producing x-rays. Some x-rays interact with tissue and other x-rays interact with the image receptor, forming an image. The physics of radiography deals with the interaction of x-rays with matter.

Physics is traditionally grouped into fields such as **thermodynamics, optics, acoustics, mechanics, electromagnetism,** and **atomic** and **nuclear** physics. In radiography, however, physics is limited principally to mechanics and electromagnetism.

Before the discussion of mechanics, the units of measurement in physics and their derivation is introduced. All scientists strive for exactness in describing physical phenomena. They try to remove the uncertainties by eliminating subjective descriptions of events. To do so, scientists use measurements that can ultimately be represented by numbers. The following discussion describes the building blocks of physics.

STANDARD UNITS OF MEASUREMENT

Physics is the study of interactions of matter and energy in all their diverse forms. Like all scientists, physicists strive for exactness or certainty in describing these interactions.

Consider, for example, the act of kicking a football. If several observers were asked to describe this event, each would give a description based on his or her perception. One might describe the stature of the kicker and the kicking stance. Another might simply conclude that "a football was kicked about 30 yards" or "the kick was wide left." There could be as many different descriptions as observers.

Physicists, however, try to remove uncertainty by eliminating subjective descriptions such as these. A physicist describing this event might determine quanti-

ties such as the mass of the football, the initial velocity of the ball, the wind velocity, and the exact distance the football travels.

Each of these requires a measurement and ultimately can be represented by a number. Assuming that all measurements are correctly made, each observer using the methods of physics will obtain exactly the same results.

In addition to seeking certainty, physicists strive for simplicity. For mechanics, only three measurable quantities are considered basic. These base quantities are **mass, length,** and **time,** and they are the building blocks of all other quantities. Figure 3-1 indicates the role these base quantities play in supporting some of the other quantities used in radiologic science.

The secondary quantities are called **derived quantities** because they are derived from a combination of one or more of the three base quantities. For example, volume is length cubed (l^3), mass density is mass divided by volume (m/l^3), and velocity is length divided by time (l/t).

Additional quantities are designed to support measurement in specialized areas of science and technology. These additional quantities are called **special quantities;** in radiology, the special quantities are those of **exposure, dose, effective dose,** and **radioactivity,** which are discussed in Chapter 2.

Whether a physicist is studying something large, such as the universe, or something small, such as an atom, meaningful measurements must be reproducible. Therefore, once the fundamental quantities are established, it is essential that they be related to a well-defined and invariable standard. Standards are normally defined by international organizations and usually redefined when the progress of science requires greater precision.

Length

For many years the standard unit of length was accepted to be the distance between two lines engraved on a platinum–iridium bar kept at the International Bureau of Weights and Measures in Paris, France. This distance was defined to be exactly 1 meter (m).

The English-speaking countries also base their standards of length on the meter:

$$1 \text{ yd} = 0.9144 \text{ m}$$
$$1 \text{ in} = 2.54 \text{ cm} = 0.0254 \text{ m}$$

In 1960, the need for a more accurate standard of length led to the redefinition of the meter in terms of the wavelength of orange light emitted from an isotope of krypton (krypton-86). One meter is now defined as the distance traveled by light in 1/299,792,468 second.

The meter is based on the speed of light.

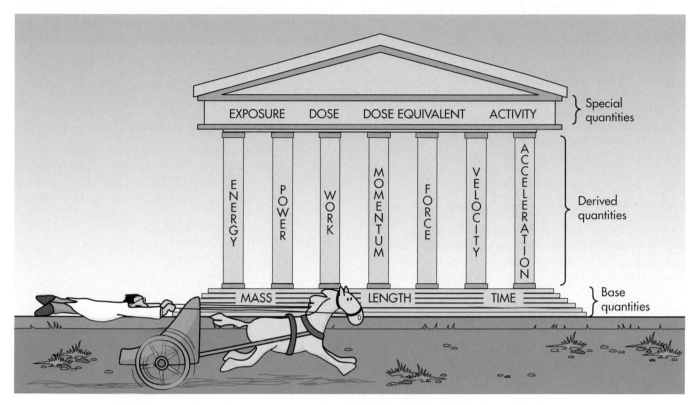

FIGURE 3-1 Base quantities support derived quantities, which in turn support the special quantities of radiologic science.

Mass

The kilogram was originally defined to be the mass of 1000 cm³ of water at 4° Celsius (°C). In the same vault in Paris where the standard meter was kept, there is a platinum–iridium cylinder that represents the standard unit of mass—the **kilogram (kg)**, which has the same mass as 1000 cm³ of water. As discussed in Chapter 1, mass is not the same quantity as weight. The kilogram is a unit of mass, whereas the **newton** or the **pound**, a British unit, are units of weight.

 The kilogram (kg) is the mass of 1000 cm³ of water at 4°C.

Time

The standard unit of time is the **second (s)**. Originally, the second was defined in terms of the rotation of the earth on its axis—the mean solar day. In 1956, it was redefined to be a certain fraction of the tropical year 1900. In 1964, the need for a better standard of time led to another redefinition.

Now, time is measured by an atomic clock and is based on the vibration of cesium atoms. The atomic clock is capable of keeping time correctly to about 1 second in 5000 years. The accuracy of future hydrogen maser clocks promises to be even greater—perhaps to 1 second in several million years.

 The second (s) is based on the vibration of atoms of cesium.

Units

Every measurement has two parts: a **magnitude** and a **unit**. For example, the standard source-to-image-receptor distance (SID) is 100 cm. The magnitude, 100, is not meaningful unless a unit is also designated. Here the unit of measurement is the centimeter.

Table 3-1 shows that there are four **systems of units** to represent the base quantities. The MKS (meters, kilograms, seconds) and the CGS (centimeters, grams, and seconds) systems are more widely used in science and in most countries of the world than is the British system.

The International System (Le Système International d'Unités, SI) is an extension of the MKS system and represents the current state of units. SI includes the three base units of the MKS system plus an additional four. There are **derived units** and **special units** of the SI to

TABLE 3-1	System of Units			
	SI*	**MKS**	**CGS**	**British**
Length	Meter (m)	Meter (m)	Centimeter (cm)	Foot (ft)
Mass	Kilogram (kg)	Kilogram (kg)	Gram (g)	Pound (lb)†
Time	Second (s)	Second (s)	Second (s)	Second (s)

*The SI includes four additional base units.
†The pound is actually a unit of force but is related to mass.

TABLE 3-2	Special Quantities of Radiologic Science and Their Units	
Radiographic Quantities	**Special Units**	**SI Units**
Exposure dose	C/kg	Air Kerma (Gy$_a$)
Dose	J/kg	Gray$_t$ (Gy$_t$)
Effective dose	J/kg	Sievert (Sv)
Radioactivity	s^{-1}	Becquerel (Bq)

represent **derived quantities** and **special quantities** of radiologic science (Table 3-2).

 The same system of units must always be used when working on problems or reporting answers.

The following would be unacceptable because of inconsistent units: mass density = 8.1 g/ft^3 and pressure = 700 lb/cm^2.

Mass density should be reported with units of grams per cubic centimeter (g/cm^3), kilograms per cubic meter (kg/m^3), or pounds per cubic foot (lbs/ft^3). Pressure should be given in pounds per square inch (lbs/in^2) or newtons per square meter (N/m^2).

Question: The dimensions of a box are 30 cm × 86 cm × 4.2 m. Find the volume.

Answer: The formula for the volume of a rectangle is given by
V = length × width × height
or
V = lwh

Because the dimensions are given in different systems of units, however, we must choose only one system. Therefore,
V = (0.30 m)(0.86 m)(4.2m)
  = 1.1 m^3

Note that the units are multiplied also: m × m × m = m^3.

Question: Find the mass density of a ball with a volume of 200 cm^3 and a mass of 0.4 kg.

Answer: D = mass/volume   (change 0.4 kg
  = 400 g/200 cm^3 to 400 g)
  = 2 g/cm^3

or

$$D = \frac{0.4 \text{ kg}}{200 \text{ cm}^3 \times \frac{1 \text{m}^3}{10^6 \text{ cm}^3}}$$ (change 200 cm^3 to 2 × 10^{-4} m^3)

$$= \frac{0.4 \text{ kg}}{2 \times 10^{-4} \text{m}^3}$$

$$= \frac{0.4 \text{ kg}}{2 \text{m}^3} \times 10^4$$

= 4000 kg/2 m^3
= 2000 kg/m^3

Question: A 9-inch-thick patient has a coin placed on the skin. The SID is 100 cm. What will be the magnification of the coin? (See Figure 21-11.)

Answer: The formula for magnification is

$$M = \frac{SID}{SOD} = \frac{\text{source-to-image receptor distance}}{\text{source-to-object distance}}$$

$$M = \frac{SID}{SOD} = \frac{100 \text{ cm}}{100 \text{ cm} - 9 \text{ inches}}$$

The 9 inches must be converted to centimeters so the units are consistent.

$$M = \frac{SID}{SOD} = \frac{100 \text{ cmn}}{100 \text{ cm} - (9 \text{ inches} \times 2.54 \text{ cm/in})}$$

$$= \frac{100 \text{ cm}}{100 \text{ cm} - (23 \text{ cm})}$$

$$= \frac{100 \text{ cm}}{77 \text{ cm}}$$

= 1.3 cm

MECHANICS

Mechanics is a segment of physics that deals with objects at rest (statics) and objects in motion (dynamics).

Velocity

The motion of an object can be described by the use of two terms: **velocity** and **acceleration.** Velocity, sometimes called **speed,** is a measure of how fast something is moving or, more precisely, the rate of change of its position with time.

The velocity of a car is measured in miles per hour (kilometers per hour). Units of velocity in SI are meters per second (m/s). The equation for velocity (v) is:

VELOCITY

$$v = \frac{d}{t}$$

where d represents the distance traveled in time t.

Question: What is the velocity of a ball that travels 60 m in 4 s?

Answer: $v = \dfrac{d}{t}$

$= 60 \text{ m}/4 \text{ s}$

$= 15 \text{ m/s}$

Question: Light is capable of traveling 669 million miles in 1 hour. What is its velocity in SI units?

Answer: $v = \dfrac{d}{t}$

$= \dfrac{6.69 \times 10^8 \text{ miles}}{\text{hour}} \times \dfrac{1609 \text{ m/mile}}{3600 \text{ s/hr}}$

$= 2.99 \times 10^8 \text{ m/s}$

The velocity of light is constant and symbolized by c: $c = 3 \times 10^8$ m/s.   *speed of light*

Often the velocity of an object changes as its position changes. For example, a dragster running a race starts from rest and finishes with a velocity of 80 m/s. The **initial velocity,** designated by v_o, is 0 (Figure 3-2). The **final velocity,** represented by v_f, is 80 m/s. The **average velocity** can be calculated from the expression:

AVERAGE VELOCITY

$$\bar{v} = \frac{v_o + v_f}{2}$$

where the bar over the "v" represents average velocity.

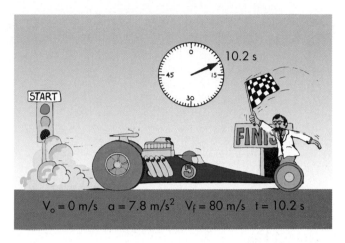

$V_o = 0$ m/s $a = 7.8$ m/s^2 $V_f = 80$ m/s $t = 10.2$ s

FIGURE 3-2 Drag racing provides a familiar example for the relationships among initial velocity, final velocity, acceleration, and time.

Question: What is the average velocity of the dragster?

Answer: $\bar{v} = \dfrac{0 \text{ m/s} + 80 \text{ m/s}}{2}$

$= 40 \text{ m/s}$

Question: A Corvette can reach a velocity of 88 mph in one quarter of a mile. What is its average velocity?

Answer: $\bar{v} = \dfrac{v_o + v_f}{2}$

$v = \dfrac{0 \text{ mph} + 88 \text{ mph}}{2}$

$v - 44 \text{ mph}$

Acceleration

The rate of change of velocity with time is **acceleration.** It is how "quickly or slowly" the velocity is changing. Because acceleration is velocity divided by time, the unit is meters per second squared (m/s^2).

If velocity is constant, the acceleration is zero. On the other hand, a constant acceleration of 2 m/s^2 means that the velocity of an object increased by 2 m/s each second. The defining equation for acceleration is given by:

ACCELERATION

$$a = \frac{v_f - v_o}{t}$$

Question: What is the acceleration of the dragster?

Answer: $a = \dfrac{80 \text{ m/s} - 0 \text{ m/s}}{10.2 \text{ s}}$

$= 7.8 \text{ m/s}^2$

Question: A 5L Mustang can accelerate to 60 mph in 5.9 s. What is the acceleration in SI units?

Answer: $a = \dfrac{v_f - v_o}{t}$

$$v_f = (60 \text{ mph} \times \frac{1609 \text{ m}}{\text{mi}}) \div \frac{3600 \text{ s}}{\text{hr}}$$

$$= 26.8 \text{ m/s}$$

$$a = \frac{26.8 \text{ m/s} - 0 \text{ m/s}}{5.9\text{s}}$$

$$= 4.5 \text{ m/s}^2$$

Newton's Laws of Motion

In 1686 the English scientist Isaac Newton presented three principles that even today are recognized as **fundamental laws of motion.**

Newton's First Law: Inertia—A body will remain at rest or continue to move with constant velocity in a straight line unless acted on by an external force.

Newton's first law states that if no force acts on an object, there will be no acceleration. The property of matter that acts to resist a change in its state of motion is called **inertia.** Newton's first law is thus often referred to as the **Law of Inertia** (Figure 3-3). A portable x-ray imaging system obviously will not move until forced by a push. Once in motion, however, it will continue to move forever, even when the pushing force is removed, unless an opposing force is present—friction.

Newton's Second Law: Force—The force (F) acting on an object with acceleration (a) is equal to the mass (m) multiplied by the acceleration.

Newton's second law is a definition of the concept of **force.** Force can be thought of as a push or pull on an object. If a body of mass *m* has an acceleration *a*, then **the force on it is given by the mass times the acceleration.** Newton's second law is illustrated in Figure 3-4. Mathematically, this law can be expressed as:

FORCE
F = ma

The SI unit of force is the **newton (N).**

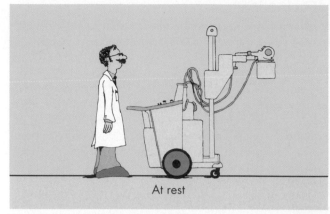
At rest

In motion

FIGURE 3-3 Newton's first law states that a body at rest will remain at rest and a body in motion will continue in motion until acted on by an outside force.

Question: Find the force on a 55-kg mass accelerated at 14 m/s².

Answer: F = ma
= (55 kg)(14 m/s²)
= 770 N

Question: For a 3600-lb (1636-kg) Ford Explorer to accelerate at 15 m/s², what force is required?

Answer: F = ma
= (1636 kg)(15 m/s²)
= 24,540 N

Newton's Third Law: Action/reaction—For every action there is an equal and opposite reaction.

Newton's third law of motion states that **to every action there is an equal and opposite reaction.** "Action" was Newton's word for "force." According to this law, if you push on a heavy block, the block will push back on you with the same force that you apply. On the other hand, if you were the physics professor illustrated in

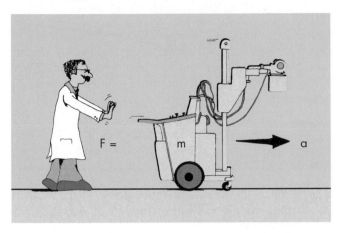

FIGURE 3-4 Newton's second law states that the force applied to move an object is equal to the mass of the object multiplied by the acceleration.

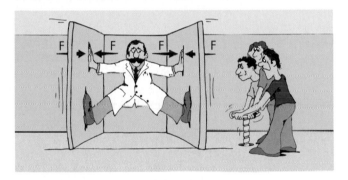

FIGURE 3-5 Crazed student technologists performing a routine physics experiment to prove Newton's third law.

Figure 3-5, whose crazed students had tricked him into the clamp room, no matter how hard you pushed, the walls would continue to close.

Weight

Weight (Wt) is a **force** on a body caused by the downward pull of gravity on it. Experiments have shown that objects falling to earth accelerate at a constant rate. This rate, termed the **acceleration due to gravity** and represented by the symbol **g,** has the following values on earth:

$$g = 9.8 \text{ m/s}^2 \text{ in SI units}$$
$$g = 32 \text{ ft/s}^2 \text{ in British units}$$

The value of acceleration due to gravity on the moon is only about one-sixth that on the earth. "Weightlessness" observed in outer space is due to the absence of gravity. Thus, the value of gravity in outer space is

zero. The weight of an object is equal to the product of its mass and the acceleration of gravity.

WEIGHT

$$Wt = mg$$

The units of weight are the same as those for force: newtons and pounds.

Weight is the product of mass and the acceleration of gravity on earth; 1 lb = 4.5 N.

Question: A student has a mass of 75 kg. What is her weight on the earth? On the moon?
Answer: Earth: g = 9.8 m/s²
            Wt = mg
               = 75 kg (9.8 m/s²)
               = 735 N
          Moon: g = 1.6 m/s²
            Wt = mg
               = 75 kg (1.6 m/s²)
               = 120 N

This example displays an important concept. The weight of an object can vary according to the value of gravity acting on it. Note, however, that the mass of an object does not change, regardless of its location. The student's 75 kg mass remains the same on earth, on the moon, or in space.

Momentum

The product of the mass of an object and its velocity is called **momentum,** represented by **p.**

MOMENTUM

$$p = mv$$

The greater the velocity of an object, the more momentum the object possesses. A truck accelerating down a hill, for example, gains momentum as its velocity increases.

Momentum is the product of mass and velocity.

The total momentum before any interaction is equal to the total momentum after the interaction. Imagine a billiard ball colliding with two other balls at rest (Figure 3-6). The total momentum before the collision is the

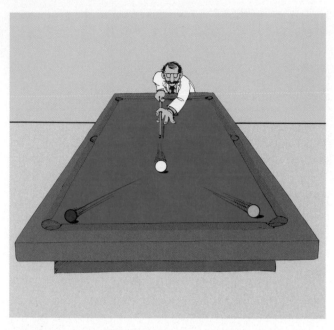

FIGURE 3-6 The conservation of momentum occurs with every billiard shot.

mass times the velocity of the cue ball. After the collision this, momentum is shared by the three balls. Thus, the original momentum of the cue ball is conserved after the interaction.

Work

Work, as used in physics has specific meaning. The work done on an object is the force applied times the distance over which it is applied. In mathematical terms:

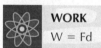

WORK

W = Fd

The unit of work is the joule (J). When you lift a cassette, you are doing work. When the cassette is merely held motionless, however, no work (in the physics sense) is being performed, even though considerable effort is being expended.

   Work is the product of force and distance.

Question: Find the work done in lifting an infant patient weighting 90 N (20 lbs) to a height of 1.5 m.

Answer: Work = Fd
             = (90 N) (1.5 m)
             = 135 J

Power

Power is the rate of doing work. The same amount of work is required to lift a cassette to a given height, whether it takes 1 second or 1 minute to do so. Power gives us a way to include the time required to perform the work.

POWER

P = Work/t = Fd/t

The SI unit of power is the joule/second (J/s), which is called the **watt (W)**. The British unit of power is the **horsepower (hp)**.

1 hp = 746 W
1000 W = 1 kilowatt (kW)

   Power is the quotient of work by time.

Question: A radiographer lifts a 0.8-kg cassette from the floor to the top of a 1.5-m table with an acceleration of 3 m/s². What is the power exerted if it takes 1.2 s?

Answer: This is a multistep problem. We know that P = work/t; however, the value of work is not given in the problem. Recall that work = Fd and F = ma. First, find F.
             F = ma
               = (0.8 kg)(3 m/s²)
               = 2.4 N
             Next, find work:
             Work = Fd
                  = (2.4 N)(1.5 m)
                  = 3.6 J
             Now, P can be determined:
             P = Work/t
               = 3.6 J/1.2 s
               = 3 W

Question: A hurried radiographer pushes a 35-kg portable down a 25-m hall in 9 s with a final velocity of 3 m/s. How much power did this require?

Answer: $a = \dfrac{v_f - v_o}{t}$

             $a = \dfrac{3 - 0}{9}$

             = 0.33 m/s²
             F = ma
               = 35 kg × 0.33 m/s²
               = 11.6 N

$$\begin{aligned} \text{Work} &= \text{Fd} \\ &= 11.6 \text{ N} \times 25 \text{ m} \\ &= 290 \text{ J} \\ \text{P} &= 290 \text{ J}/9 \text{ s} \\ &= 32 \text{ W} \end{aligned}$$

Energy

There are many forms of energy, as discussed in Chapter 1. The law of conservation of energy states that **energy may be transformed from one form to another but it cannot be created or destroyed**; the total amount of energy is constant. For example, electrical energy is converted into light energy and heat energy in an electric light bulb. The unit of energy and work is the same, the joule.

 Energy is the ability to do work.

There are two forms of **mechanical energy** that are often used in radiologic science: kinetic energy and potential energy. **Kinetic energy (KE)** is the energy associated with the motion of an object as expressed by:

KINETIC ENERGY
$$KE = \frac{1}{2} mv^2$$

It is apparent that kinetic energy depends on the mass of the object and on the **square** of its velocity.

Question: Consider two rodeo chuck wagons, A and B, with the same mass. If B has twice the velocity of A, verify that the KE of chuck wagon B is four times that of chuck wagon A.

Answer: Chuck wagon A: $KE_A = \frac{1}{2} mv_A^2$

Chuck wagon B: $KE_B = \frac{1}{2} mv_B^2$

However, $m_A = m_B$, $v_B = 2v_A$

therefore, $KE_B = \frac{1}{2} m_A (2v_A)^2$

$$= \frac{1}{2} m_A (4v_A^2)$$

$KE_B = 2 mv_A^2$

$$= 4 (\frac{1}{2} mv_A^2)$$

$$= 4 KE_A$$

Potential energy (PE) is the stored energy of position or configuration. A textbook on a desk has PE because of its height above the floor ... and the potential for a

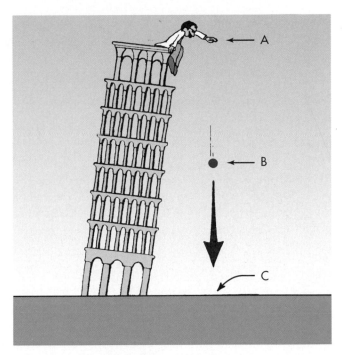

FIGURE 3-7 Potential energy results from the position of an object. Kinetic energy is the energy of motion. **A,** Maximum potential energy, no kinetic energy. **B,** Potential energy and kinetic energy. **C,** Maximum kinetic energy, no potential energy.

better job if it is read? It has the ability to do work by falling to the ground. Gravitational potential energy is given by:

POTENTIAL ENERGY
PE = mgh
where *h* is the distance above the earth's surface.

A skier at the top of a jump, a coiled spring, and a stretched rubber band are examples of other systems that have PE because of their position or configuration.

If a scientist held a ball in the air atop the Leaning Tower of Pisa (Figure 3-7), the ball would have only PE, no KE. When it is released and begins to fall, the PE decreases as the height decreases. At the same time the KE is increasing as the ball accelerates. Just before impact the KE of the ball becomes maximum as its velocity reaches maximum. Because it now has no height, the PE becomes zero. All the initial PE of the ball has been converted into KE during the fall.

Question: A radiographer holds a 6-kg x-ray tube 1.5 m above the ground. What is its potential energy?

Answer: PE = mgh
               = 6 kg × 9.8 m/s² × 1.5 m
               = 88 kg m²/s²
               = 88 J

Table 3-3 presents a summary of the quantities and units in mechanics.

Heat

Heat is a form of energy that is very important to the radiologic technologist. Excessive heat is a deadly enemy of an x-ray tube and can cause permanent damage. For this reason, the technologist should be aware of the properties of heat.

 Heat is the kinetic energy of the random motion of molecules.

The more rapid and disordered the motion of molecules, the more heat an object contains. The unit of heat, the **calorie,** is defined as the heat necessary to raise the temperature of 1 g of water through 1°C. The same amount of heat will have different effects on different materials. For example, the heat required to change the temperature of 1 g of silver by 1°C is approximately 0.05 calorie, or only ¹⁄₂₀ that required for a similar temperature change in water.

Heat is transferred by conduction, convection, and radiation.

HEAT TRANSFER

CONDUCTION   CONVECTION   RADIATION

Conduction is the transfer of heat through a material or by touching. Molecular motion from a high-temperature object touching a lower-temperature object equalizes the temperature of both.

Conduction is easily observed when a hot object and cold object are placed in contact. After a short time, heat conducted to the cooler object results in equal temperatures of the two objects. Heat is conducted from an x-ray tube anode through the rotor to insulating oil.

Convection is the mechanical transfer of "hot" molecules in a gas or liquid from one place to another. A steam radiator or forced-air furnace warms a room by convection. The air around the radiator is heated, causing it to rise, while cooler air circulates in and takes its place.

A forced-air furnace blows heated air into the room, providing forced circulation to complement the natural convection. Heat is convected from the housing of an x-ray tube to air.

Thermal radiation is the transfer of heat by the emission of **infrared radiation.** The reddish glow emitted by hot objects is evidence of heat transfer by radiation. **An x-ray tube cools primarily by radiation.**

Temperature is normally measured with a reproducible scale called a **thermometer.** A thermometer is usually calibrated at two reference points—the freezing and boiling points of water. The three scales that have been developed to measure temperature are Celsius (°C), Fahrenheit (°F), and Kelvin (K) (Figure 3-8).

These scales are interrelated as follows:

TEMPERATURE SCALES

$T_c = 5/9 \, (T_f - 32)$

$T_f = 9/5 \, T_c + 32$

$T_k = T_c + 273$

The subscripts c, f, and k refer to Celsius, Fahrenheit, and Kelvin, respectively.

| TABLE 3-3 | Summary of Quantities, Equations, and Units Used in Mechanics | | | |

Quantity	Symbol	Defining Equation	UNITS SI	British
Velocity	v	$v = d/t$	m/s	ft/s
Average velocity	$\bar{v}$	$v = \dfrac{v_0 + v_1}{2}$	m/s	ft/s
Acceleration	a	$a = \dfrac{v_1 - v_0}{t}$	m/s²	ft/s²
Force	F	$F = ma$	N	lb
Weight	Wt	$Wt = mg$	N	lb
Momentum	p	$p = mv$	kg-m/s	ft-lb/s
Work	W	$✳W = Fd$	J	ft-lb
Power	P	$P = W/t$	W	hp
Kinetic energy	KE	$KE = 1/2 \, mv^2$	J	ft-lb
Potential energy	PE	$PE = mgh$	J	ft-lb

— Know work equation

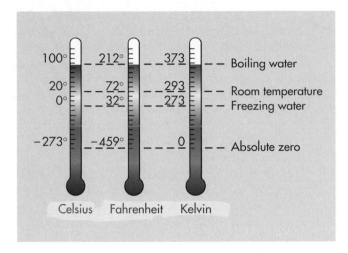

FIGURE 3-8 Three scales used to represent temperature. Celsius is the adopted scale for weather reporting everywhere except the United States. Kelvin is the scientific scale.

Question: Convert 77° F to degrees Celsius.

Answer: $T_c = \dfrac{5}{9}(T_f - 32)$

$= \dfrac{5}{9}(77 - 32) = \dfrac{5}{9}(45) = 25°C$

One can use the following for easy, approximate conversion:

APPROXIMATE TEMPERATURE CONVERSION
From °F to °C, subtract 30 and divide by 2
From °C to °F, double, then add 30

Magnetic resonance imaging (MRI) with a superconducting magnet requires extremely cold liquids called *cryogens*. Liquid nitrogen, which boils at 77 K and liquid helium, which boils at 4 K, are the two cryogens used.

Question: Liquid helium is used to cool superconducting wire in MRI systems. What is its temperature in degrees Fahrenheit?

Answer: $T_k = T_c + 273$
$T_c = T_k - 273$
$T_c = 4 - 273$
$T_c = -269°C$
$T_f = \dfrac{9}{5}(-269) + 32$
$T_f = -452°F$

The relationship between temperature and energy is often represented by an energy thermometer (Figure 3-9). We consider x-rays to be energetic, although on the cosmic scale they are rather ordinary.

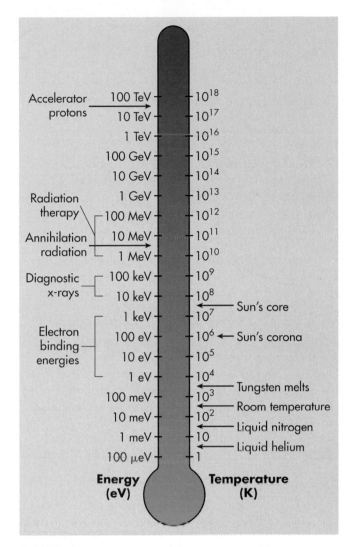

FIGURE 3-9 The energy thermometer scales temperature and energy together.

SUMMARY

This chapter introduces the various standards of measurement and applies them to concepts associated with mechanics and several areas that impact radiology. Table 3-3 summarizes the concepts addressed in this chapter. Practice the Challenge Questions using that table as a reference.

CHALLENGE QUESTIONS

1. Define or otherwise identify:
   a. Base quantity
   b. Derived quantity
   c. Special quantity
   d. Inertia
   e. Acceleration

f. Convection
g. Work
h. Velocity
i. Scalar versus vector quantity
j. Newton's Second Law of Motion

2. The dimensions of a radiographic cassette are 27 cm × 36 cm × 3 cm. Find the volume using the formula v (volume) = l (length) = w (width) = h (height).

3. What is the volume of a rectangular radiographic positioning sponge that measure 5 inches by 5 inches by 10 inches?

4. What is the velocity of a ball that travels 50 meters in 4 seconds?

5. What is the velocity of the mobile x-ray imaging system in the hospital elevator if the elevator travels 20 meters to the next floor in 30 seconds?

6. A Corvette can reach a velocity of 88 mph in ¼ mile. What is the average velocity?

7. Moving down a ramp, the C-arm fluoroscope reaches a velocity of 1 ft/s after 5 seconds. What is the average velocity?

8. A 5L Mustang can accelerate to 60 mph in 5.9 seconds. What is its acceleration in SI units?

9. Find the force on a 55-kg object accelerated at 14 m/s².

10. For a 2500-pound (1136-kg) car to accelerate at 12 m/s², what force is required?

11. A professor has a mass of 90 kg. What is his weight on the earth? On the moon?

12. Find the work done lifting an infant patient weighing 60 N to a height of 2.0 meters.

13. A radiographer lifts a 1.0-kg cassette from the floor to the top of a 1.5-meter table with an acceleration of 2 m/s². What is the power exerted if it takes 2.0 seconds?

14. A rushed radiographer pushes a 25-kg portable down a 50-meter hall in 10 seconds with a final velocity of 2 m/s. How much power did this require?

15. A radiographer holds a 3-kg x-ray tube 2.0 meters above the ground. What is its potential energy?

16. Liquid hydrogen with a boiling point of 77 K is used to cool some superconducting magnets. What is its temperature in degrees Fahrenheit?

17. Convert 77° F to degrees Celsius.

18. Convert 80° F to degrees Celsius.

19. What are the four special quantities of radiation measurement?

20. What are the three units common to both the SI and MKS systems?

CHAPTER

4

The Atom

OBJECTIVES

At the completion of this chapter, the student should be able to do the following:

1. Relate the history of the atom
2. Identify the structure of the atom
3. Describe electron shells and instability within atomic structure
4. Discuss radioactivity and the characteristics of alpha and beta particles
5. Explain the difference between two forms of ionizing radiation: particulate and electromagnetic

OUTLINE

THIS CHAPTER diverges from the study of energy and force to return to the basis of matter itself. What composes matter? What is the magnitude of matter?

From the inner space of the atom to the outer space of the universe, there is an enormous range in the size of matter. Over 40 orders of magnitude are needed to identify objects as small as the atom and as large as the universe. Because matter spans such a large magnitude, scientific notation is used to express the measurement of objects. Figure 4-1 shows the orders of magnitude and how matter in our surroundings varies in size.

The atom, as the smallest unit of matter, is the building block of the radiographer's understanding of the interaction between ionizing radiation and matter. This chapter explains what happens when energy in the form of an x-ray interacts with tissue. Although tissue has an extremely complex structure, it is made up of atoms and combinations of atoms. Examining the structure of atoms helps explain what happens when the structure is changed.

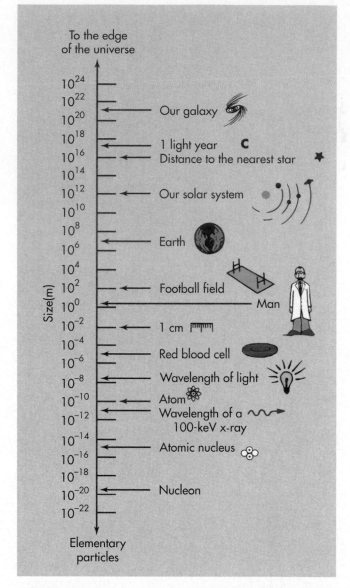

FIGURE 4-1 The size of objects varies enormously. The range of sizes in nature requires that scientific notation be used because over 40 orders of magnitude are necessary.

 An atom is the smallest particle that has all the properties of an element.

CENTURIES OF DISCOVERY
Greek Atom

One of civilization's most pronounced, continuing scientific investigation has been to determine precisely the structure of matter. The earliest recorded reference to this investigation comes from the Greeks, several hundred years B.C. They thought all matter was composed of four **substances:** earth, water, air, and fire. According to them, all matter could be described as combinations of these four basic substances in various proportions, modified by four basic **essences:** wet, dry, hot, and cold. Figure 4-2 shows how this theory of matter was represented at that time.

The Greeks used the term **atom,** meaning "indivisible" [*a* (not) + *temon* (cut)] to describe the smallest part of the four substances of matter. Each type of atom was represented by a symbol (Figure 4-3, *A*). Today, 112 substances or **elements** have been identified; 92 are naturally occurring and the additional 20 have been artificially produced in high-energy particle accelerators. We now know that the atom is the smallest particle of matter that has the properties of an element. Many particles are much smaller than the atom; these are called **subatomic particles.**

Dalton Atom

The Greek description of the structure of matter persisted for hundreds of years. In fact, it was the theoretical basis for the vain efforts by medieval alchemists to transform lead into gold. It was not until the nineteenth century that the foundation for modern atomic theory was laid. In 1808, John Dalton, an English schoolteacher, published a book summarizing his experiments,

200 B.C.

40

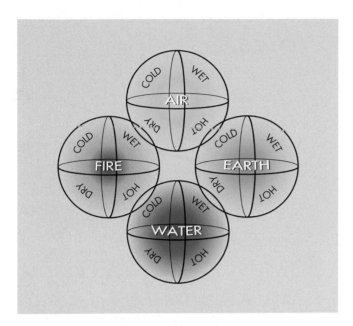

FIGURE 4-2 Symbolic representation of the substances and essences of matter as viewed by the ancient Greeks.

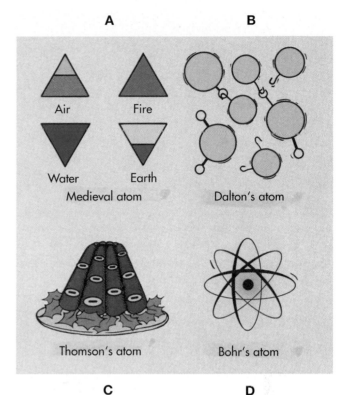

FIGURE 4-3 Through the years the atom has been represented by many symbols. **A,** The Greeks envisioned four different atoms, representing air, fire, earth, and water. These triangular symbols were adopted by medieval alchemists. **B,** Dalton's atoms had hooks and eyes to account for chemical combination. **C,** Thomson's model of the atom has been described as a plum pudding, with the plums representing the electrons. **D,** The Bohr atom has a small, dense, positively charged nucleus surrounded by electrons in precise energy levels.

which showed that the elements could be classified according to integral values of atomic mass.

According to Dalton, an element was composed of identical atoms that reacted the same way chemically. For example, all oxygen atoms were alike. They looked alike, they were constructed alike, and they reacted alike. They were, however, very different from atoms of any other element. The physical combination of one type of atom with another was visualized as being an eye-and-hook affair (Figure 4-3, *B*). The size and number of the eyes and hooks were different for each element.

Some 50 years after Dalton's work, a Russian scholar, Dmitri Mendeleev, showed that if the elements were arranged in order of increasing atomic mass, a periodic repetition of similar chemical properties occurred. At that time, about 65 elements had been identified. Mendeleev's work resulted in the first **periodic table of the elements.** Although there were many holes in Mendeleev's table, it showed that all the then-known elements could be placed in one of eight groups.

Figure 4-4 is a rendering of the periodic table of elements. Each block represents an element. The superscript is the atomic number. The subscript is the elemental mass.

All elements in the same group (i.e., column) react chemically in a similar fashion and have similar physical properties. Except for hydrogen, the elements of group I, called the *alkali metals*, are all soft metals that combine readily with oxygen and react violently with water. The elements of group VII, called *halogens*, are easily vaporized and combine with metals to form water-soluble salts. Group VIII elements, called

the *noble gases*, are highly resistant to reaction with other elements.

These elemental groupings are determined by the placement of electrons in each atom. This is considered more fully later.

Thomson Atom

After the publication of Mendeleev's periodic table, additional elements were separated and identified and the periodic table slowly became filled. Knowledge of the structure of the atom, however, remained scanty.

Before the turn of the twentieth century, atoms were considered indivisible. The only difference between the atoms of one element and the atoms of another was their mass. Through the efforts of many scientists, it slowly became apparent that there was an electrical nature to the structure of an atom.

In the late 1890s, while investigating the physical properties of **cathode rays (electrons),** J. J. Thomson concluded that electrons were an integral part of all

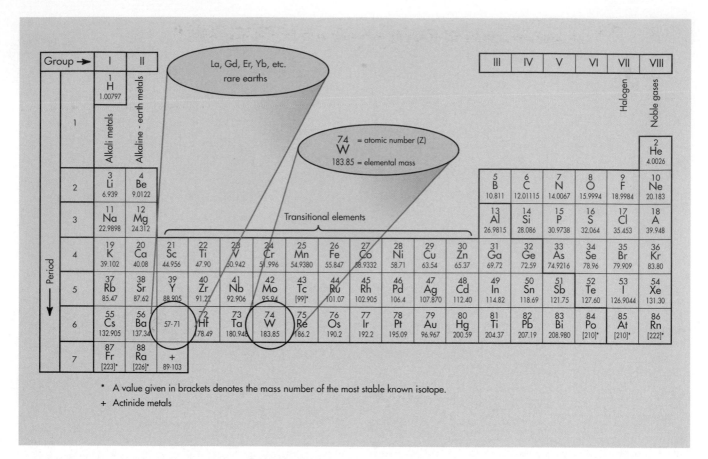

FIGURE 4-4 Periodic table of elements.

atoms. He described the atom as looking something like a plum pudding, where the plums represented negative electric charges (electrons) and the pudding was a shapeless mass of uniform positive electrification (Figure 4-3, *C*). The number of electrons was thought to equal the quantity of positive electrification because the atom was known to be electrically neutral.

Through a series of ingenious experiments, Ernest Rutherford in 1911 disproved Thomson's model of the atom. Rutherford introduced the nuclear model, which described the atom as containing a small, dense, positively charged center surrounded by a negative cloud of electrons. He called the center of the atom the **nucleus.**

Bohr Atom

In 1913, Niels Bohr improved Rutherford's description of the atom. Bohr's model was a miniature solar system in which the electrons revolved about the nucleus in prescribed orbits or **energy levels.** For our purposes, the Bohr atom (Figure 4-3, *D*) represents the best way to picture the atom, although the details of atomic structure are more accurately described by a newer model, called **quantum mechanics.**

Simply put, the Bohr atom contains a small, dense, positively charged nucleus surrounded by negatively

charged electrons that revolve in fixed, well-defined orbits about the nucleus. In the normal atom, the number of electrons is equal to the number of positive charges in the nucleus.

FUNDAMENTAL PARTICLES

Our understanding of the atom today is essentially that which Bohr presented nearly a century ago. With the development of high-energy **particle accelerators,** or "atom smashers," as some call them, the structure of the atomic nucleus is slowly being mapped and identified. Nearly 100 subatomic particles have been detected and described by physicists working with accelerators.

Nuclear structure is now well defined (Figure 4-5). Nucleons—protons and neutrons—are composed of quarks that are held together by gluons. These particles, however, are of little consequence to radiology. Only the three primary constituents of an atom, the **electron,** the **proton,** and the **neutron,** are considered here. They are the **fundamental particles** (Table 4-1).

 The fundamental particles of an atom are the electron, the proton, and the neutron.

| | | MASS | | | | | |
Particle	Location	Relative	Kilograms	amu	Number	Charge	Symbol
Electron	Shells	1	9.109×10^{-31}	0.000549	0	-1	$\ominus$
Proton	Nucleus	1836	1.673×10^{-27}	1.00728	1	$+1$	$\oplus$
Neutron	Nucleus	1838	1.675×10^{-27}	1.00867	1	0	O

TABLE 4-1   Important Characteristics of the Fundamental Particles

amu, atomic mass units.

The atom can be viewed as a miniature solar system whose sun is the nucleus and whose planets are the electrons. The arrangement of the electrons around the nucleus determines the manner in which atoms interact.

Electrons are very small particles carrying one unit of negative electric charge. Their mass is only 9.1×10^{-31} kg. They can be pictured as revolving about the nucleus in precisely fixed orbits, like the planets in our solar system revolve around the sun.

Because an atomic particle is extremely small, its mass is expressed in **atomic mass units (amu)** for convenience. One atomic mass unit is equal to $\frac{1}{12}$ the mass of a carbon-12 atom. The electron mass is 0.000549 amu. When precision is not necessary, a system of whole numbers called **atomic mass numbers** is used. The atomic mass number of an electron is zero.

The nucleus contains particles called **nucleons,** of which there are two types: protons and neutrons. Both have nearly 2000 times the mass of an electron. The mass of a proton is 1.673×10^{-27} kg and the neutron is just slightly heavier, at 1.675×10^{-27} kg. The atomic mass number of each is one. The primary difference between a proton and a neutron is electric charge. The proton carries one unit of positive electric charge. The neutron carries no charge; it is electrically neutral.

ATOMIC STRUCTURE

You might be tempted to visualize the atom as a beehive of subatomic activity because classical representations of it usually appear like that shown in Figure 4-3, *D*. Because of the space limitations of the printed page, Figure 4-3, *D* is greatly oversimplified. In fact, the atom is mostly empty space, like our solar system. The nucleus of an atom is very small but contains nearly all the mass of the atom.

 The atom is essentially empty space.

If a basketball, whose diameter is 9.6 in (0.23 m), represented the size of the uranium nucleus, the largest naturally occurring atom, the path of the orbital elec-

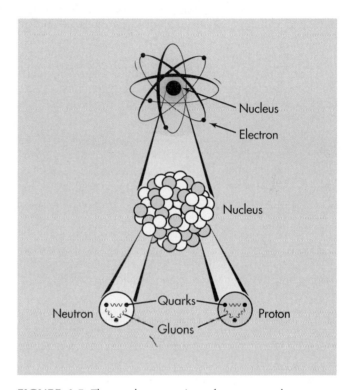

FIGURE 4-5 The nucleus consists of protons and neutrons, which are made of quarks bound together by gluons.

trons would take them over 8 miles (12.8 km) away. Because it contains all the neutrons and protons, the nucleus of the atom contains most of its mass. For example, the nucleus of an uranium atom contains 99.998% of the entire mass of the atom.

The possible electron orbits are grouped into different "shells." The arrangement of these shells helps determine how an atom reacts chemically, that is, how it combines with other atoms to form molecules. Because a neutral atom has the same number of electrons in orbits as protons in the nucleus, the number of protons ultimately determines the chemical behavior of an atom.

The number of protons determines the **chemical element.** Atoms that have the same number of protons but differ in the number of neutrons are called **isotopes** and behave in the same way in chemical reaction.

The periodic table of the elements (Figure 4-4) lists matter in order of increasing complexity, beginning with hydrogen (H). An atom of hydrogen contains one proton in its nucleus and one electron outside the nucleus. Helium (He), the second atom in the table, contains two protons, two neutrons, and two electrons.

The third atom, lithium (Li), contains three protons, four neutrons, and three electrons. Two of these electrons are in the same orbital shell, the K shell, as are the electrons of hydrogen and helium. The third electron is in the next farther orbital shell from the nucleus, the L shell.

Electrons can exist only in certain **shells,** which represent different **electron binding energies** or **energy levels.** For identification purposes, the electron orbital shells are given the code K, L, M, N, and so forth to represent the relative binding energies of electrons from closest to the nucleus to farthest from the nucleus. The closer an electron is to the nucleus, the higher is its binding energy.

The next atom on the periodic table, beryllium (Be), has four protons and five neutrons in the nucleus. Two electrons are in the K shell and two are in the L shell.

The complexity of the electron configuration of atoms increases as one progresses through the periodic table to the most complex naturally occurring element, uranium (U). Uranium has 92 protons and 146 neutrons. The electron distribution is as follows: 2 in the K shell, 8 in the L shell, 18 in the M shell, 32 in the N shell, 21 in the O shell, 9 in the P shell, and 2 in the Q shell.

Figure 4-6 is a schematic representation of four atoms. Although these atoms are mostly empty space, they have been diagrammed on one page. If the actual size of the helium nucleus were that in Figure 4-6, the K-shell electrons would be several city blocks away.

 In their normal state, *atoms are electrically neutral;* the electric charge on the atom is zero.

The total number of electrons in the orbital shells is exactly equal to the number of protons in the nucleus. If an atom has an extra electron or has had an electron removed, it is said to be **ionized.** An ionized atom is not electrically neutral but carries a charge equal in magnitude to the difference between the number of electrons and protons.

You might assume that atoms can be ionized by changing the number of positive charges as well as number of negative charges. Atoms, however, cannot be ionized by the addition or subtraction of protons because they are bound very strongly together and that would change the type of atom. An alteration in the number of neutrons does not ionize an atom because the neutron is electrically neutral.

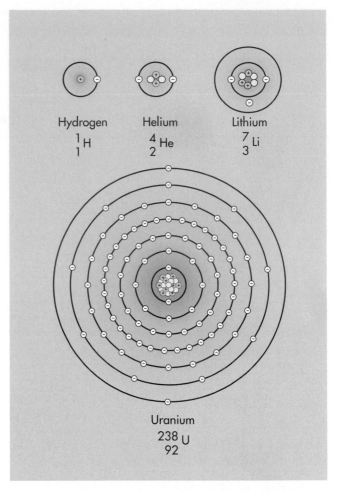

FIGURE 4-6 Atoms are composed of neutrons and protons in the nucleus and electrons in specific orbits surrounding the nucleus. Shown here are the three smaller atoms and the largest naturally occurring atom, uranium.

Figure 4-7 represents the interaction between an x-ray and a carbon atom, a primary constituent of tissue. The x-ray transfers its energy to an orbital electron and ejects that electron from the atom. This process requires approximately 34 eV of energy. The x-ray may cease to exist and an ion pair is formed. The remaining atom is now a positive ion because it contains one more positive charge than negative charge.

 Ionization is the removal of an orbital electron from an atom.

In all except the lightest atoms, the number of neutrons is always greater than the number of protons. The larger the atom, the greater the abundance of neutrons over protons.

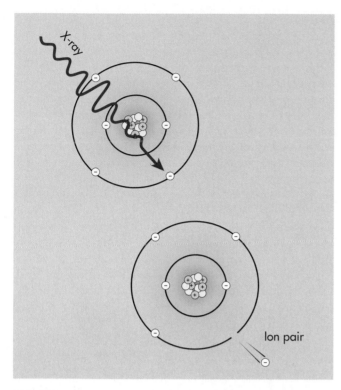

FIGURE 4-7 Ionization of a carbon atom by an x-ray leaves the atom with a net electric charge of +1. The ionized atom and the released electron are called an *ion pair*.

Electron Arrangement

The maximum number of electrons that can exist in each shell (Table 4-2) increases with the distance of the shell from the nucleus. These numbers need not be memorized because the electron limit per shell can be calculated from the expression:

MAXIMUM ELECTRONS PER SHELL

$2n^2$

where n is the shell number.

Question: What is the maximum number of electrons that can exist in the O shell?

Answer: The O shell is the fifth shell from the nucleus, therefore:
$$n = 5$$
$$2n^2 = 2(5)^2$$
$$= 2(25)$$
$$= 50 \text{ electrons}$$

This answer, 50 electrons, is a theoretical value. Even the largest atom does not completely fill shell O or higher.

TABLE 4-2	Maximum Number of Electrons That Can Occupy Each Electron Shell	
Shell Number	**Shell Symbol**	**Number of Electrons**
1	K	2
2	L	8
3	M	18
4	N	32
5	O	50
6	P	72
7	Q	98

Physicists call the shell number n the **principal quantum number.** Every electron in every atom can be precisely identified by four quantum numbers, the most important of which is the principal quantum number. The other three quantum numbers represent the existence of subshells, which are not important to radiology.

The observant reader may have noticed a relationship between the number of shells in an atom and its position in the periodic table of the elements. Oxygen has eight electrons; two occupy the K shell and six occupy the L shell. Oxygen is in the second period and the sixth group of the periodic table (Figure 4-4).

Aluminum has the following electron configuration: K shell, two electrons; L shell, eight electrons; M shell, three electrons. Therefore, aluminum is in the third period (M shell) and third group (three electrons) of the periodic table.

Electron Arrangement

The number of electrons in the outermost shell of an atom is equal to its group in the periodic table. The number of electrons in the outermost shell determines the valence of an atom. The number of the outermost electron shell of an atom is equal to its period in the periodic table.

Question: What are the period and group for the gastrointestinal contrast agent, barium (refer to Figure 4-4)?

Answer: Period 6 and group II.

No outer shell can contain more than eight electrons.

Why does the periodic table show elements repeating similar chemical properties in groups of eight? In addition to the limitation on the maximum number of electrons allowed in any shell, the outer shell is always limited to eight electrons.

All atoms having one electron in the outer shell lie in group I of the periodic table; atoms with two electrons in the outer shell fall in group II, and so on. When eight electrons are in the outer shell, the shell is filled. Atoms with filled outer shells lie in group VIII, the noble gases, and are very stable.

The orderly scheme of atomic progression from smallest to largest atom is interrupted in the fourth period. Instead of simply adding electrons to the next outer shell, electrons are added to an inner shell.

The atoms associated with this phenomenon are called the **transitional elements.** Even in these elements, no outer shell ever contains more than eight electrons. The chemical properties of the transitional elements depend on the number of electrons in the two outermost shells.

The shell notation of the electron arrangement of an atom not only identifies the relative distance of an electron from the nucleus but indicates the relative energy by which the electron is attached to the nucleus. You might expect that an electron would spontaneously fly off from the nucleus, just as a ball twirling on the end of a string would if the string was cut. The type of force that prevents this from happening is called **centripetal force** or "center-seeking" force, and results from a basic law of electricity that states that opposite charges attract one another and like charges repel.

 The force that keeps an electron in orbit is the centripetal force.

You might therefore expect the electrons would drop into the nucleus because of the strong electrostatic attraction. In the normal atom the centripetal force just balances the force created by the electron velocity, the **centrifugal force** or flying-out-from-the-center force, so that the electrons maintain their distance from the nucleus traveling in a circular or elliptical path.

Figure 4-8 is a representation of this state of affairs for a small atom. In more complex atoms, the same balance of force exists and each electron can be considered separately.

Electron Binding Energy

The strength of attachment of an electron to the nucleus is called the **electron binding energy,** designated E_b. The closer an electron is to the nucleus, the more tightly it is bound. K-shell electrons have higher binding energies than L-shell electrons, L-shell electrons are more tightly bound to the nucleus than M-shell electrons, and so on.

Not all K-shell electrons of all atoms are bound with the same binding energy. The greater the total number of electrons in an atom, the more tightly each is bound.

To put it differently, the larger and more complex the atom, the higher the E_b for electrons in any given shell. Because electrons of atoms with many protons are more tightly bound to the nucleus than those of small atoms, it generally takes more energy to ionize a large atom than a small atom.

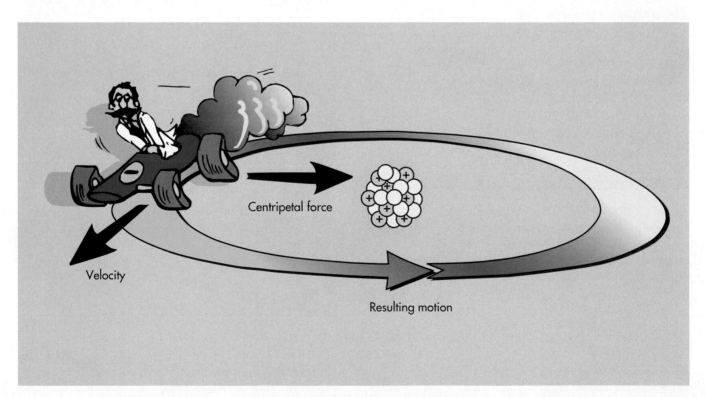

FIGURE 4-8 Electrons revolve about the nucleus in fixed orbits or shells. Electrostatic attraction results in a specific electron path about the nucleus.

Figure 4-9 represents the binding energy of electrons of several atoms of radiologic importance. The metals tungsten (W) and molybdenum (Mo) are the primary constituents of the target of an x-ray tube. Barium (Ba) and iodine (I) are used extensively in radiographic and fluoroscopic contrast agents.

Question: How much energy is required to ionize tungsten by removal of a K-shell electron?

Answer: The minimum energy must equal E_b or 70 keV—less than that and the atom cannot be ionized.

Carbon (C) is an important component of human tissue. As with other tissue atoms, E_b for the outer shell electrons is only approximately 10 eV. Yet approximately 34 eV is necessary to ionize tissue atoms. The value, 34 eV, is called the **ionization potential.** The difference, 24 eV, causes multiple electron excitations, which ultimately result in heat. The concept of ionization potential is important to the description of linear energy transfer (LET), which is discussed in Chapter 34.

Question: How much more energy is necessary to ionize barium than to ionize carbon by removal of K-shell electrons?

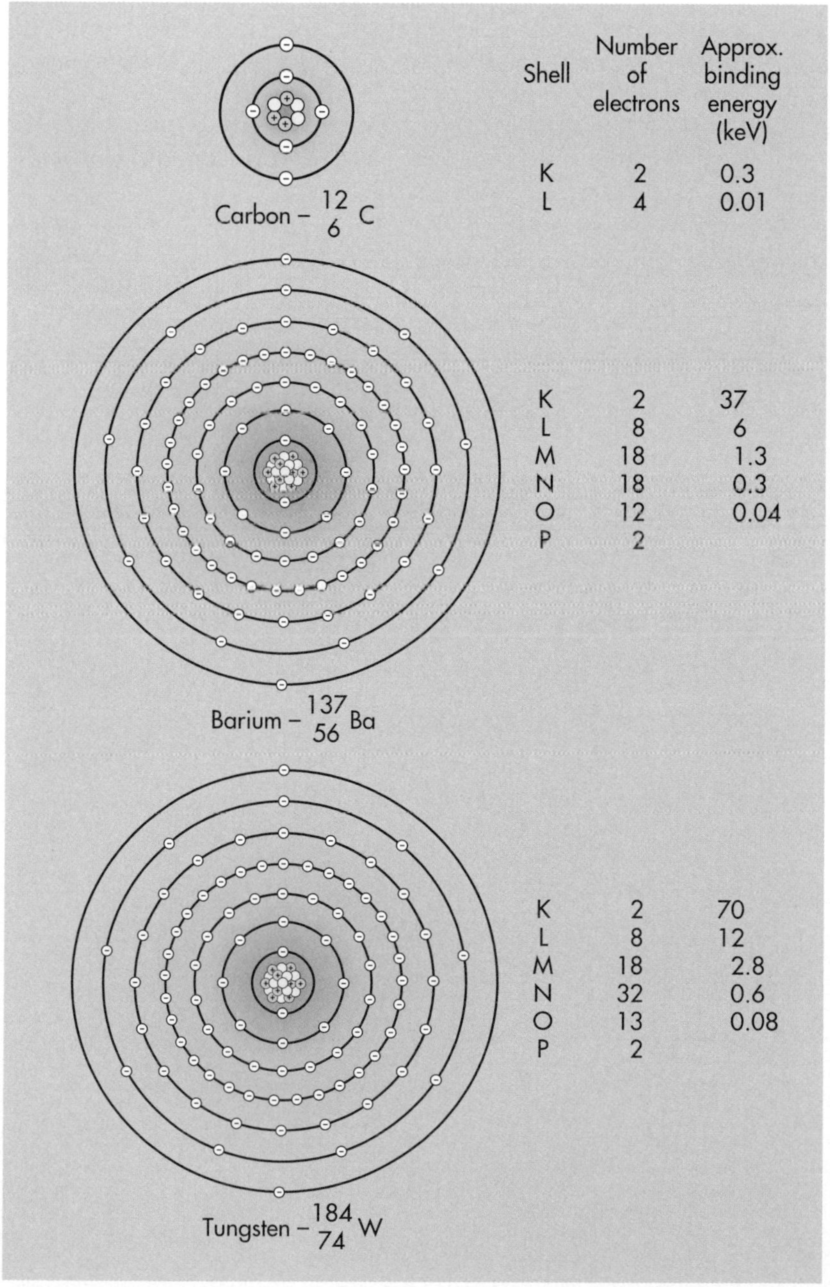

Shell	Number of electrons	Approx. binding energy (keV)
K	2	0.3
L	4	0.01

Carbon – $^{12}_{6}$C

Shell	Number of electrons	Approx. binding energy (keV)
K	2	37
L	8	6
M	18	1.3
N	18	0.3
O	12	0.04
P	2	

Barium – $^{137}_{56}$Ba

Shell	Number of electrons	Approx. binding energy (keV)
K	2	70
L	8	12
M	18	2.8
N	32	0.6
O	13	0.08
P	2	

Tungsten – $^{184}_{74}$W

FIGURE 4-9 Atomic configurations and approximate electron binding energies for three radiologically important atoms. As atoms get bigger, electrons in a given shell become more tightly bound.

Answer: E_b (Ba) = 37,400 eV
     E_b (C) = <u>300 eV</u>
     Difference = 36,100 eV
          = 37.1 keV

ATOMIC NOMENCLATURE

Often an element is indicated by an alphabetic abbreviation. Such abbreviations are called **chemical symbols.** Table 4-3 lists some of the important elements and their chemical symbols.

The chemical properties of an element are determined by the number and arrangement of electrons. In the neutral atom the number of electrons equals the number of protons. The number of protons is called the **atomic number,** represented by Z. Table 4-3 shows that the atomic number of barium is 56, thus indicating 56 protons are in the barium nucleus.

The number of protons plus the number of neutrons in the nucleus of an atom is called the **atomic mass number,** symbolized by A. The atomic mass number is always a whole number. The use of atomic mass numbers is helpful in many areas of radiologic science.

  The atomic mass number and the precise mass of an atom are not equal.

An atom's atomic mass number is a whole number equal to the number nucleons in the atom. The actual atomic mass of an atom is determined by measurement and rarely is a whole number. ^{135}Ba has A = 135 because its nucleus contains 56 protons and 79 neutrons. The atomic mass of ^{135}Ba is 134.91 amu.

Only one atom, ^{12}C, has an atomic mass equal to its atomic mass number. This occurs because the ^{12}C atom is the arbitrary standard for atomic measure.

Many elements in their natural state are composed of atoms with different atomic mass numbers and different atomic masses but identical atomic numbers. The characteristic mass of an element, the **elemental mass,** is determined by the relative abundance of isotopes and their respective atomic masses.

Barium, for example, has an atomic number of 56. The atomic mass number of its most abundant isotope is 138. Natural barium, however, consists of seven different isotopes with atomic mass numbers of 130, 132, 134, 135, 136, 137, and 138; the elemental mass is determined by the average weight of all these isotopes.

With the protocol described in Figure 4-10, the atoms of Figure 4-6 would have the following symbolic representation:

$$^1_1H, \; ^4_2He, \; ^7_3Li, \; ^{238}_{92}U$$

Because the chemical symbol also indicates the atomic number, the subscript is often omitted.

$$^1H, \; ^4He, \; ^7Li, \; ^{238}U$$

TABLE 4-3	Characteristics of Some Radiographically Important Elements					
Element	Chemical Symbol	Atomic Number (Z)	Atomic Mass Number (A)*	Number of Naturally Occurring Isotopes	Elemental Mass (amu)†	K-Shell Electron Binding Energy (keV)
Beryllium	Be	4	9	1	9.012	0.11
Carbon	C	6	12	3	12.01	0.28
Oxygen	O	8	16	3	15.00	0.53
Aluminum	Al	13	27	1	26.98	1.56
Calcium	Ca	20	40	6	40.08	4.04
Iron	Fe	26	56	4	55.84	7.11
Copper	Cu	29	63	2	63.54	8.98
Molybdenum	Mo	42	98	7	95.94	20.0
Ruthenium	Ru	44	102	7	101.0	22.1
Silver	Ag	47	107	2	107.9	25.7
Tin	Sn	50	120	10	118.6	29.2
Iodine	I	53	127	1	126.9	33.2
Barium	Ba	56	138	7	137.3	37.4
Tungsten	W	74	184	5	183.8	69.5
Gold	Au	79	197	1	196.9	80.7
Lead	Pb	82	208	4	207.1	88.0
Uranium	U	92	238	3	238.0	116.0

amu, atomic mass units.
*Most abundant isotope.
†Average of naturally occurring isotopes.

Isotopes

Atoms that have the same atomic number but different atomic mass numbers are isotopes.

Isotopes of a given element contain the same number of protons but varying numbers of neutrons. Most elements have more than one stable isotope. The seven natural isotopes of barium are:

$$^{130}Ba, {}^{132}Ba, {}^{134}Ba, {}^{135}Ba, {}^{136}Ba, {}^{137}Ba, {}^{138}Ba$$

The term *isotope* describes all atoms of a given element. Such atoms have different nuclear configurations but nevertheless react the same chemically.

Question: How many protons and neutrons are in each of the seven naturally occurring isotopes of barium?

Answer: The number of protons in each isotope is 56. The number of neutrons is equal to A − Z. Therefore,
^{130}Ba: 130 − 56 = 74 neutrons
^{132}Ba: 132 − 56 = 76 neutrons
^{134}Ba: 134 − 56 = 78 neutrons
and so on.

Isobar

Atomic nuclei that have the same atomic mass number but different atomic numbers are isobars.

Isobars are atoms that have different numbers of protons and different numbers of neutrons but the same total number of nucleons. Isobaric radioactive transitions from parent atom to daughter atom result from the release of a beta particle or positron. The parent and daughter are atoms of different elements.

Isotone

Atoms that have the same number of neutrons but different numbers of protons are isotones.

Isotones are atoms with different atomic numbers and different mass numbers but a constant value for the quantity A − Z. Consequently, isotones are atoms with the same number of neutrons in the nucleus.

The final category of atomic configuration is the **isomer.**

Isomer

Isomers have the same atomic number and the same atomic mass number.

In fact, isomers are identical atoms except that they exist at different energy states because of differences in nucleon arrangement. Technetium-99m decays to technetium-99 with the emission of a 140-keV gamma ray, which is very useful in nuclear medicine. Table 4-4 is a summary of the characteristics of these nuclear arrangements.

Question: From the following list of atoms, pick out those that are isotopes, isobars, and isotones.

$$^{131}_{54}Xe, {}^{130}_{53}I, {}^{132}_{55}Cs, {}^{131}_{53}I$$

Answer: ^{130}I and ^{131}I are isotopes. ^{131}I and ^{131}Xe are isobars. ^{130}I, ^{131}Xe, and ^{132}Cs are isotones.

COMBINATIONS OF ATOMS

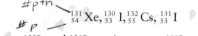

Molecule

Atoms of various elements may combine to form structures called *molecules.*

Four atoms of hydrogen (H_2) and two atoms of oxygen (O_2) can combine to form two molecules of water (2 H_2O). The following equation represents this atomic combination:

$$2 H_2 + O_2 \rightarrow 2 H_2O$$

TABLE 4-4	Characteristics of Various Nuclear Arrangements		
Arrangement	Atomic Number	Atomic Mass Number	Neutron Number
Isotope	Same	Different	Different
Isobar	Different	Same	Different
Isotone	Different	Different	Same
Isomer	Same	Same	Same

An atom of sodium (Na) can combine with an atom of chlorine (Cl) to form a molecule of sodium chloride (NaCl), which is common table salt:

$$Na + Cl \rightarrow NaCl$$

Both of these molecules are common in the human body. Molecules, in turn, may combine to form even larger structures: cells and tissues.

> **Compound**
> A *chemical compound* is any quantity of one type of molecule.

Although over 100 different elements are known, most elements are rare. Approximately 95% of the earth and its atmosphere consists of only a dozen elements. Similarly, hydrogen, oxygen, carbon, and nitrogen compose over 95% of the human body. Water molecules make up approximately 80% of the human body.

There is an organized scheme for representing elements in a molecule (Figure 4-10). This shorthand notation that incorporates the chemical symbol with subscripts and superscripts is used to identify atoms.

The chemical symbol (X) is positioned between two subscripts and two superscripts. The subscript and superscript to the left of the chemical symbol represent the atomic number and atomic mass number, respectively. The subscript and superscript to the right are values for the number of atoms per molecule and the valence state of the atom, respectively. We are concerned only with the scripts to the left of X.

The formula NaCl represents one molecule of the compound sodium chloride. Sodium chloride has properties that are different from either sodium or chlorine. Atoms combine with each other to form compounds (chemical bonding) in two main ways. The examples of H_2O and NaCl can be used to describe these two types of chemical bonds.

Oxygen and hydrogen combine into water through **covalent bonds.** Oxygen has six electrons in its outermost shell. It has room for two more electrons, so in a water molecule two hydrogen atoms share their single electrons with the oxygen. The hydrogen electrons orbit both the H and O, thus binding the atoms together. This covalent bonding is characterized by the sharing of electrons.

Sodium and chlorine combine into salt through **ionic bonds.** Sodium has one electron in its outermost shell. Chlorine has space for one more electron in its outermost shell. The sodium atom will give up its electron to the chlorine. When it does, it becomes ionized because it has lost an electron and now has an imbalance of electrical charges.

The chlorine atom also becomes ionized because it has gained an electron and then has more electrons than protons. The two atoms are attracted to each other, resulting in an ionic bond because they have opposite electrostatic charges.

Sodium, hydrogen, carbon, and oxygen atoms can combine to form a molecule of sodium bicarbonate ($NaHCO_3$). A measurable quantity of sodium bicarbonate constitutes a chemical compound commonly called **baking soda.**

> The smallest particle of an element is an atom; the smallest particle of a compound is a molecule.

The interrelations between atoms, elements, molecules, and compounds are orderly. This organizational scheme is what the ancient Greeks were trying to describe by their substances and essences. Figure 4-11 is a diagram of this current scheme of matter.

RADIOACTIVITY

Some atoms exist in an abnormally excited state characterized by an unstable nucleus. To reach stability, the nucleus spontaneously emits particles and energy and transforms itself into another atom. This process is called **radioactive disintegration** or **radioactive decay.** The atoms involved are **radionuclides.** Any nuclear arrangement is called a **nuclide;** only nuclei that undergo radioactive decay are radionuclides.

> **Radioactivity**
> Radioactivity is the emission of particles and energy in order to become stable.

Radioisotopes

Many factors affect nuclear stability. Perhaps the most important is the number of neutrons. When a nucleus contains either too few or too many neutrons, the atom

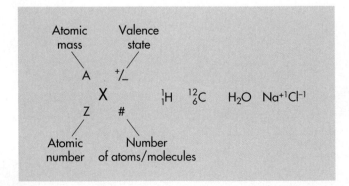

FIGURE 4-10 Protocol for representing elements in a molecule.

can disintegrate radioactively, bringing the number of neutrons and protons into a stable and proper ratio.

In addition to stable isotopes, many elements have radioactive isotopes or **radioisotopes.** These may be artificially produced in machines such as particle accelerators or nuclear reactors. Seven radioisotopes of barium have been discovered, all of which are artificially produced. In the following list of barium isotopes, the radioisotopes are larger and in boldface:

^{127}**Ba**, ^{128}**Ba**, ^{129}**Ba**, ^{130}Ba, ^{131}**Ba**, ^{132}Ba, ^{133}**Ba**,

^{134}Ba, ^{135}Ba, ^{136}Ba, ^{137}Ba, ^{138}Ba, ^{139}**Ba**, ^{140}**Ba**

Artificially produced radioisotopes have been identified for nearly all elements. A few elements have naturally occurring radioisotopes as well.

There are two primary sources of naturally occurring radioisotopes. Some originated at the time of the earth's formation and are still decaying very slowly. An example is uranium, which ultimately decays to radium, which, in turn, decays to radon. These and other decay products of uranium are also radioactive. Others, such as ^{14}C, are continuously produced in the upper atmosphere by the action of cosmic radiation.

Radioisotopes can decay to stability in many ways, but only two, **beta emission** and **alpha emission,** are of particular importance here.

During beta emission, an electron created in the nucleus is ejected from the nucleus with considerable kinetic energy and escapes from the atom. The result is the loss of a small quantity of mass and one unit of negative electric charge from the nucleus of the atom. Simultaneously, a neutron undergoes conversion to a proton.

The result of beta emission therefore is to increase the atomic number by one (Z → Z + 1), while the atomic mass number remains the same (A = constant). This nuclear transformation therefore results in an atom changing from one type of element to another (Figure 4-12).

Radioactivity decay by alpha emission is a much more violent process. The alpha particle consists of two protons and two neutrons bound together; its atomic mass number is 4. A nucleus must be extremely unstable to emit an alpha particle, but when it does, it loses two units of positive charge and four units of mass. The transformation is significant because the resulting atom is not only chemically different but is also lighter by 4 amu (Figure 4-13).

Radioactive decay results in emission of alpha particles, beta particles, and usually gamma rays.

Beta emission occurs much more frequently than alpha emission. Virtually all radioisotopes are capable of

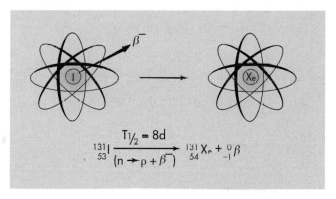

FIGURE 4-12 ^{131}I decays to ^{131}Xe with the emission of a beta particle.

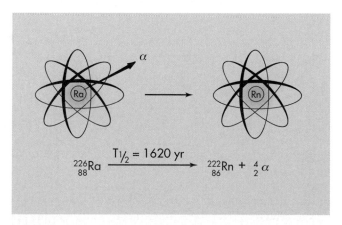

FIGURE 4-13 The decay of ^{226}Ra to ^{222}Rn is accompanied by alpha emission.

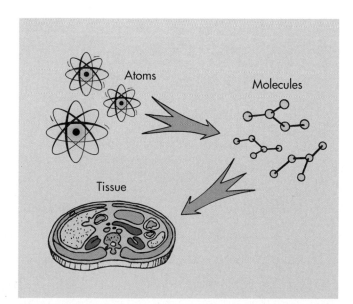

FIGURE 4-11 Matter has many levels of organization. Atoms combine to make molecules and molecules combine to make tissues.

transformation by beta emission, but only heavy radioisotopes are capable of alpha emission. Some radioisotopes are pure beta emitters or pure alpha emitters, and most emit gamma rays simultaneously with the particle emission.

Question: $_{56}^{139}$Ba is a radioisotope that decays by beta emission. What will be the values of A and Z for the atom that results from this emission?

Answer: In beta emission a neutron is converted to a proton and a beta particle: $n \rightarrow p + \beta$, therefore $_{56}^{139}$Ba $\rightarrow$ $_{57}^{139}$? Lanthanum is the element with Z = 57; thus, $_{57}^{139}$La is the result of the beta decay of $_{56}^{139}$Ba.

Radioactive Half-Life

Radioactive matter is not here one day and gone the next. Rather, radioisotopes disintegrate into stable isotopes of different elements at a decreasing rate, so that the quantity of radioactive material never quite reaches zero. Remember from Chapter 2 that radioactive material is measured in curies (Ci) and that 1 Ci is equal to 3.7×10^{10} atoms disintegrating each second (3.7×10^{10} Bq).

The rate of radioactive decay and the quantity of material present at any given time are described mathematically by a formula known as the **radioactive decay law**. From this formula we obtain a quantity known as **half-life ($T_{1/2}$)**. Half-lives of radioisotopes vary from less than a second to many years. Each radioisotope has a unique, characteristic half-life.

Half-Life
The half-life of a radioisotope is the time required for a quantity of radioactivity to be reduced to one-half its original value.

The half-life of ^{131}I is 8 days (Figure 4-14). If 100 mCi (3.7×10^9 Bq) of ^{131}I were present on January 1 at noon, then at noon on January 9 only 50 mCi (1.85×10^9 Bq) would remain. On January 17, 25 mCi (9.25×10^8 Bq) would remain, and on January 25, 12.5 mCi (4.63×10^8 Bq) would remain. A plot of the radioactive decay of ^{131}I allows one to determine the amount of radioactivity remaining after any given time (Figure 4-14).

After approximately 24 days, or three half-lives, the linear-linear plot of the decay of ^{131}I becomes very difficult to read and interpret. Consequently, such graphs are usually presented in semilogarithmic form (Figure 4-15). With a presentation such as this, one can estimate radioactivity after a very long time.

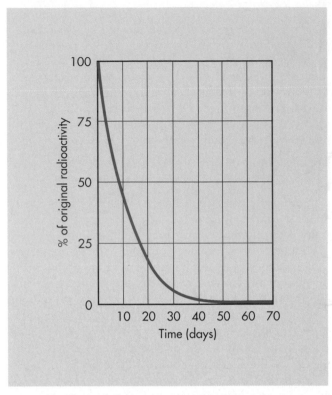

FIGURE 4-14 ^{131}I decays with a half-life of 8 days. This linear graph allows estimation of radioactivity only for a short time.

ON REGISTRY
* Half-life on semilog paper = straight line
* Half-life on regular graph = curve

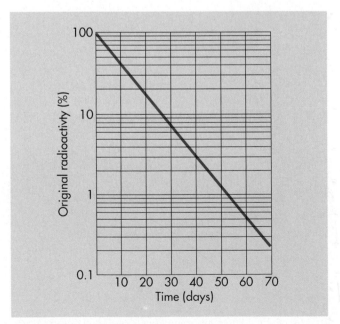

FIGURE 4-15 This semilog graph is useful for estimating the radioactivity of ^{131}I at any time.

Question: On Monday at 8 A.M., 100 (CI (3.7×10^6 Bq) of ^{131}I is present. How much will remain on Friday at 5 P.M.?

Answer: The time of decay is $4\frac{1}{3}$ days. According to Figure 4-15, at $4\frac{1}{3}$ days approximately 63% of the original activity will remain. Therefore, 63 μCI (2.33×10^6 Bq) will be present on Friday at 5 PM

Theoretically, all the radioactivity of a radioisotope never disappears. After each period of time equivalent to one half-life, one-half the activity present at the beginning of that time will remain. Therefore, although the quantity of radioisotope progressively decreases, it never quite reaches zero.

Figure 4-16 shows two similar graphs used to estimate the quantity of any radioisotope remaining after any time. In these graphs the percentage of original radioactivity remaining is plotted against time, measured in units of half-life. To use these graphs, one must express the initial radioactivity as 100% and convert the time of interest into units of half-life. For decay times exceeding three half-lives, the semilog form is easier to use.

Question: 65 mCi (2.4×10^9 Bq) of ^{131}I are present at noon on Wednesday. How much will remain 1 week later?

Answer: 7 days $= \frac{7}{8}$ $T_{1/2} = 0.875$ $T_{1/2}$. Figure 4-16 shows that at 0.875 $T_{1/2}$ approximately 55% of the initial radioactivity will remain; 55% $\times$ 65 mCi (2.4×10^9 Bq) = 0.55 $\times$ 65 = 35.8 mCi (1.32×10^9 Bq).

^{14}C is a naturally occurring radioisotope with $T_{1/2}$ = 5730 years. The concentration of ^{14}C in the environment is constant and ^{14}C is incorporated into living material at a constant rate. Trees of the Petrified Forest contain less ^{14}C than living trees because the ^{14}C of living trees is in equilibrium with the atmosphere; the carbon in a petrified tree was fixed many thousands of years ago, and the fixed ^{14}C is reduced with time by radioactive decay (Figure 4-17).

Question: If a piece of petrified wood contains 25% of the ^{14}C that a tree living today contains, how old is the petrified wood?

Answer: The ^{14}C in living matter remains constant as long as the matter is alive because it is constantly exchanged with the environment. In this case, the petrified wood has been dead long enough for the ^{14}C to decay to 25% of its original value. That time period represents two half-lives. Consequently, we can estimate that the petrified wood sample is approximately 2 $\times$ 5730 = 11,460 years old.

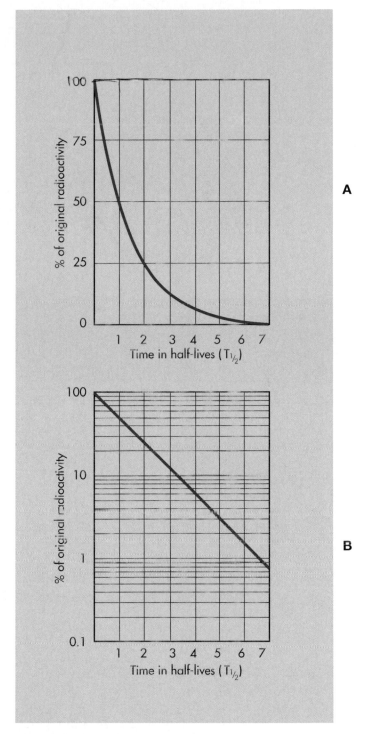

FIGURE 4-16 The radioactivity after any period can be estimated from either the linear **(A)** or the semilog **(B)** graph. The original quantity is assigned a value of 100% and the time of decay is expressed in units of half-life.

Question: How many half-lives are required before a quantity of radioactive material has decayed to less than 1% of its original value?

Answer: A simple approach to this type of problem is to count half-lives.

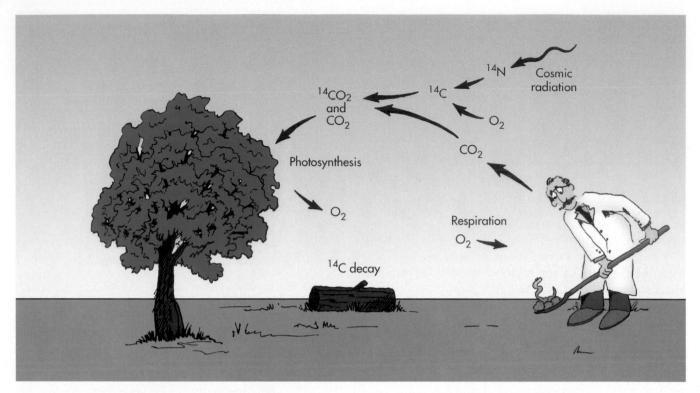

FIGURE 4-17 Carbon is a biologically active element. A small fraction of all carbon is the radioisotope ^{14}C. As a tree grows, ^{14}C is incorporated into the wood in proportion to the amount of ^{14}C in the atmosphere. When the tree dies, further exchange of ^{14}C with the atmosphere does not take place. If the dead wood is preserved by petrification, the ^{14}C content diminishes as it radioactively decays. This phenomenon is the basis for radiocarbon dating.

Half-life number	Radioactivity remaining
1	50%
2	25%
3	12.5%
4	6.25%
5	3.12%
6	1.56%
7	0.78%

A simpler approach finds the answer more precisely on Figure 4-16: 6.5 half-lives.

Another approach is to use the following relationship:

RADIOACTIVE DECAY

Activity Remaining = Original Activity $(0.5)^n$
where n = number of half-lives.

The concept of half-life is essential to radiology. It is used daily in nuclear medicine and has an exact parallel in x-ray terminology, the **half-value layer.** The better you understand half-life now, the better you will understand the meaning of half-value layer later.

TYPES OF IONIZING RADIATION

All ionizing radiation can be conveniently classified into only two categories: **particulate radiation** and **electromagnetic radiation** (Table 4-5). The types of radiation used in diagnostic ultrasound and in magnetic resonance imaging are **nonionizing radiation.**

Although all ionizing radiation acts on biologic tissue in the same manner, there are fundamental differences between various types of radiation. These differences can be analyzed according to five physical characteristics: mass, energy, velocity, charge, and origin.

Particulate Radiation

Many subatomic particles are capable of causing ionization. Consequently, electrons, protons, and even rare nuclear fragments can all be classified as particulate ionizing radiation if they are in motion and possess sufficient kinetic energy. At rest, they cannot cause ionization.

There are two main types of particulate radiation: **alpha particles** and **beta particles.** Both are associated with radioactive decay.

The alpha particle is equivalent to a helium nucleus. It contains two protons and two neutrons. Its mass is approximately 4 amu, and it carries two units of posi-

TABLE 4-5	General Classification of Ionizing Radiation				
Type of Radiation	Symbol	Atomic Mass Number	Charge	Origin	
PARTICULATE					
Alpha radiation	α	4	+2	Nucleus	
Beta radiation	β⁻	0	−1	Nucleus	
	β⁺	0	+1	Nucleus	
ELECTROMAGNETIC					
Gamma rays	γ	0	0	Nucleus	
X-rays	X	0	0	Electron cloud	

tive electric charge. Compared with an electron, the alpha particle is large and exerts a great electrostatic force. Alpha particles are emitted only from the nuclei of heavy elements. Light elements cannot emit alpha particles because they do not have enough excess mass (excess energy).

ALPHA PARTICLE
An alpha particle is a helium nucleus containing two protons and two neutrons.

Once emitted from a radioactive atom, the alpha particle travels with high velocity through matter. Because of its great mass and charge, however, it easily transfers this kinetic energy to orbital electrons of other atoms.

Ionization accompanies alpha radiation. The average alpha particle possesses 4 to 7 MeV of kinetic energy and ionizes approximately 40,000 atoms for every centimeter of travel through air.

Because of this amount of ionization, the energy of an alpha particle is quickly lost. It has a very short range in matter. In air, alpha particles can travel approximately 5 cm, whereas in soft tissue the range may be less than 100 μm. Consequently, alpha radiation from an external source is nearly harmless because the radiation energy is deposited in the superficial layers of the skin.

With an internal source of radiation, just the opposite is true. If an alpha-emitting radioisotope is deposited in the body, it can intensely irradiate the local tissue.

Beta particles differ from alpha particles in both mass and charge. They are light particles with an atomic mass number of 0 and carry one unit of negative or positive charge. The only difference between electrons and beta minus particles is their origin. Beta particles originate in the nuclei of radioactive atoms and electrons exist in shells outside the nuclei of all atoms. Beta plus particles are positrons. They have the same mass as electrons and

are considered to be antimatter. We will see positrons again when we discuss pair-production.

BETA PARTICLE
A beta particle is an electron emitted from the nucleus of a radioactive atom.

Once emitted from a radioisotope, beta particles traverse air, ionizing several hundred atoms per centimeter. The beta particle range is longer than that for the alpha particle. Depending on its energy, a beta particle may traverse 10 to 100 cm of air and approximately 1 to 2 cm of soft tissue.

Electromagnetic Radiation

X-rays and gamma rays are forms of electromagnetic ionizing radiation. This type of radiation is covered more completely in the next chapter; the discussion here is necessarily brief.

X-rays and gamma rays are often called **photons.** Photons have no mass and no charge. They travel at the speed of light ($c = 3 \times 10^8$ m/s) and are considered energy disturbances in space.

X-rays and gamma rays are the only forms of ionizing electromagnetic radiation of radiologic interest.

Just as the only difference between beta particles and electrons is their origin, so the only difference between x-rays and gamma rays is their origin. Gamma rays are emitted from the nucleus of a radioisotope and are usually associated with alpha or beta emission. X-rays are produced outside the nucleus in the electron shells.

X-rays and gamma rays exist either at the speed of light or not at all. Once emitted, they have an ionization rate in air of approximately 100 ion pairs/cm, about

TABLE 4-6	Characteristics of Several Types of Ionizing Radiation				
		APPROXIMATE RANGE			
Type of Radiation	Approximate Energy	In Air	In Soft Tissue	Origin	
PARTICULATE					
Alpha particles	4-7 MeV	1-10 cm	Up to 0.1 mm	Heavy radioactive nuclei	
Beta particles	0-7 MeV	0-10 m	0-2 cm	Radioactive nuclei	
ELECTROMAGNETIC					
X-rays	0-10 MeV	0-100 m	0-30 cm	Electron cloud	
Gamma rays	0-5 MeV	0-100 m	0-30 cm	Radioactive nuclei	

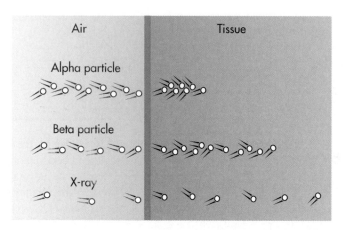

FIGURE 4-18 Different types of radiation ionized matter with different degrees of efficiency. Alpha particles are highly ionizing radiation with a very short range in matter. Beta particles do not ionize so readily and have a longer range. X-rays have low ionization rate and a very long range.

equal to that for beta particles. Unlike beta particles, however, x-rays and gamma rays have an unlimited range in matter.

Photon radiation loses intensity with distance but theoretically never reaches zero. Particulate radiation, on the other hand, has a finite range in matter, and that range depends on the particle's energy.

Table 4-6 summarizes the more important characteristics of each of these types of ionizing radiation. In nuclear medicine, beta and gamma radiation are most important. In radiography, only x-rays are important. The penetrability and low ionization rate of x-rays make them particularly useful for medical imaging (Figure 4-18).

SUMMARY

As a miniature solar system, the Bohr atom set the stage for the modern interpretation of the structure of matter. An atom is the smallest part of an element, and a molecule is the smallest part of a compound.

The three fundamental particles of the atom are the electron, proton, and neutron. Electrons are negatively charged particles orbiting the nucleus in configurations or shells held in place by electrostatic forces. Chemical reactions occur when outermost orbital electrons are shared or given up to other atoms. Nucleons, neutrons and protons, are each nearly 2000 times the mass of electrons. Protons are positively charged and neutrons have no charge.

Elements are grouped in a periodic table in order of increasing complexity. The groups on the table indicate the number of electrons in the outermost shell. The elements in the periods on the periodic table have the same number of orbital shells.

Some atoms have the same number of protons and electrons as other elements but a different number of neutrons, giving the element a different atomic mass. These are isotopes.

Some atoms, which contain too many or too few neutrons in the nucleus, can disintegrate. This is called *radioactivity*. Two types of particulate emission following radioactive disintegration are alpha and beta particles. The half-life of a radioactive element or a radioisotope is the time required for the quantity of radioactivity to be reduced to one-half its original value.

Ionizing radiation is either particulate or electromagnetic radiation. Alpha and beta particles are particulate radiation. Alpha particles have four atomic mass units, are positive in charge, and originate from the nucleus of heavy elements. Beta particles have an atomic mass number of zero and have one unit of negative charge. Beta particles originate in the nucleus of radioactive atoms.

X-rays and gamma rays are forms of electromagnetic radiation called *photons*. These rays have no mass and no charge. X-rays are produced in the electron shells and gamma rays are emitted from the nucleus of a radioisotope.

CHALLENGE QUESTIONS

1. Define or otherwise identify:
   a. Photon
   b. The Rutherford atom
   c. Positron
   d. Nucleons
   e. The arrangement of the periodic table of the elements
   f. Radioactive half-life
   g. W (chemical symbol for what element?)
   h. Alpha particle
   i. K shell
   j. Chemical compound
2. Figure 4-1 shows the following approximate sizes: an atom, 10^{-10} m; the earth, 10^7 m. By how many orders of magnitude do these objects differ?
3. How many protons, neutrons, electrons, and nucleons are in the following?

$$^{17}_{8}O, \quad ^{27}_{13}Al, \quad ^{60}_{27}Co, \quad ^{226}_{88}Ra$$

4. Using the data in Table 4-1, determine the mass of $^{99}_{43}Tc$ in atomic mass units and in grams.
5. Diagram the expected electron configuration of $^{40}_{20}Ca$.
6. If atoms large enough to have electrons in the *T*-shell existed, what would be the maximum number allowed in that shell?
7. How much more tightly bound are K-shell electrons in tungsten than (a) L-shell electrons, (b) M-shell electrons, (c) free electrons? (Refer to Figure 4-9.)

8. From the following list of nuclides, identify sets of isotopes, isobars, and isotones.

   $^{60}_{28}Ni$ $^{61}_{28}Ni$ $^{62}_{28}Ni$

   $^{59}_{27}Co$ $^{60}_{27}Co$ $^{61}_{27}Co$

   $^{58}_{26}Fe$ $^{59}_{28}Fe$ $^{60}_{28}Fe$

9. $^{90}_{38}Sr$ has a half-life of 29 years. If 10 Ci (3.7×10^{11} Bq) were present in 1950, approximately how much would remain in 2010?
10. Complete the following table with relative values.

Type of radiation	Mass	Energy	Charge	Origin
α				
β				
β+				
γ				
X				

11. For what is Mendeleev remembered?
12. Who developed the concept of the atom as a miniature solar system?
13. List the fundamental particles within an atom.
14. What property of an atom does binding energy describe?
15. Can atoms be ionized by changing the number of positive charges?
16. Describe how ion pairs are formed.
17. What determines the chemical properties of an element?
18. Why doesn't an electron spontaneously fly away from the nucleus of an atom?
19. Describe the difference between alpha and beta emission.
20. How does carbon-14 dating determine the age of petrified wood?

Electromagnetic Radiation

OBJECTIVES

At the completion of this chapter, the student should be able to do the following:

1. Identify the properties of photons
2. Explain the inverse square law
3. Define wave theory and quantum theory
4. Discuss the electromagnetic spectrum

OUTLINE

PHOTONS WERE first described by the ancient Greeks. Today photons are known as electromagnetic energy; however, these words are commonly used interchangeably. Electromagnetic energy is present everywhere and exists over a wide energy range. X-rays and light are examples of electromagnetic photons.

The properties of photons include frequency, wavelength, velocity, and amplitude. In this chapter, discussions of visible light, radiofrequency, and ionizing radiation highlight these properties and the importance of electromagnetic radiation in radiography. The **wave equation** and the **inverse square law** are mathematical formulas that further describe how photons behave.

The wave-particle duality of electromagnetic radiation is introduced as **wave theory** and **quantum theory**. Matter and energy, as well as their importance to x-ray imaging, are summarized.

PHOTONS

Ever present all around us is a field or state of energy called **electromagnetic energy**. This energy exists over a wide range called an energy **continuum**. A continuum is an uninterrupted (continuous) ordered sequence. Examples of continuums are free-flowing rivers and sidewalks. If the river is dammed or the sidewalk curbed, then the continuum is interrupted. Only an extremely small segment of the electromagnetic energy continuum—the visible light segment—is naturally apparent to us.

The ancient Greeks recognized the unique nature of light. It was not one of their four basic essences, but light was given entirely separate status. They called an atom of light a **photon**. Today many types of electromagnetic radiation in addition to visible light are recognized, but the term *photon* is still used.

A photon is the smallest quantity of any type of electromagnetic radiation, just as an atom is the smallest quantity of an element. A photon may be pictured as a small bundle of energy, sometimes called a **quantum**, traveling through space at the speed of light. We speak of x-ray photons, light photons, and other types of electromagnetic radiation as photon radiation.

 An x-ray photon is a quantum of electromagnetic energy.

The physics of visible light has always been a subject of investigation quite apart from other areas of science.

Nearly all the classical laws of optics were described hundreds of years ago. Late in the nineteenth century, James Clerk Maxwell showed that visible light has both electric and magnetic properties, hence the term **electromagnetic radiation.**

By the beginning of the twentieth century, other types of electromagnetic radiation had been described and a uniform theory evolved. Electromagnetic radiation is best explained by reference to a model, in much the same way that the atom is best described by the Bohr model.

Velocity and Amplitude

Photons are energy disturbances moving through space at the speed of light *(c)*. Some sources give the speed of light as 186,000 miles per second, but in the SI system of units it is 3×10^8 m/s.

Question: What is the value of c in miles per second, given c = 3×10^8 m/s?

Answer:
$$c = \frac{3 \times 10^8 \text{ m}}{s} \times \frac{\text{mile}}{5280 \text{ ft}} \times \frac{3.2808 \text{ ft}}{m}$$

$$= \frac{3 \times 3.2808 \times 10^8 \text{ m - mile - ft}}{5.280 \times 10^3 \text{ s - ft - m}}$$

$$= 1.864 \times 10^5 \text{ miles/s}$$

$$= 186,400 \text{ miles/s}$$

 The velocity of all electromagnetic radiation is 3×10^8 m/s.

Although photons have no mass and therefore no identifiable form, they do have electric and magnetic fields that are continuously changing in a **sinusoidal** fashion. Physicists use the term **field** to describe interactions among different energies, forces, or masses that can otherwise be described only mathematically. For instance, we can understand the gravitational field even though we cannot see it. We know the gravitational field exists because we are held to the earth by it.

The gravitational field governs the interaction of different masses. Similarly, the electric field governs the interaction of electrostatic charges and the magnetic field, the interaction of magnetic poles.

Figure 5-1 shows three examples of a sinusoidal variation. This type of variation is usually called a **sine wave**. Sine waves can be described by a mathematical formula and therefore have many applications in physics.

Sine waves also exist in nature and are associated with many familiar objects (Figure 5-2). Simplistically, sine waves are variations of amplitude over time.

Alternating electric current consists of electrons moving back and forth sinusoidally through a conductor. A long rope fastened at one end vibrates as a sine wave if

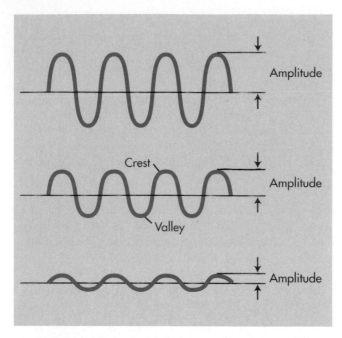

FIGURE 5-1 These three sine waves are identical except for their amplitudes.

the free end is moved up and down in whiplike fashion. The arms of a tuning fork vibrate sinusoidally after being struck with a hard object. The weight on the end of a coil spring varies sinusoidally up and down after the spring has been stretched.

The sine waves in Figure 5-1 are identical except for their amplitude; sine wave *A* has the largest amplitude and sine wave *C* has the smallest. Sine wave amplitude is discussed later in connection with high-voltage generation and rectification in an x-ray machine.

> *Amplitude* is one half the range from crest to valley over which the sine wave varies.

Frequency and Wavelength

The sine wave model of electromagnetic radiation describes the variations of the electric and magnetic fields as the photon travels with velocity *c*. The important properties of this model are **frequency,** represented by f, and **wavelength,** represented by the Greek letter *lambda* (λ).

Another interpretation of the vibrating rope in Figure 5-2 is the Texas roadside critter observing the motion of the rope from a point midway between the fastened end and the scientist (Figure 5-3).

What does the critter see? If he moves his field of view along the rope, he will observe the crest of the sine wave traveling along the rope to the end. If he fixes his attention on one segment of the rope such as point *A*, he will see the rope rise and fall harmonically as the waves pass. The more rapidly the scientist holding the

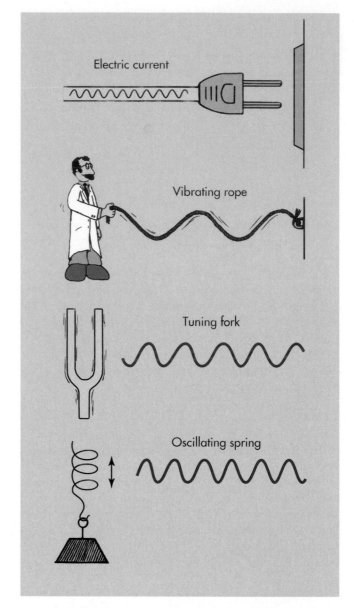

FIGURE 5-2 Sine waves are associated with many naturally occurring phenomena in addition to electromagnetic radiation.

loose end moves the rope up and down, the faster the sequence of rise and fall.

The rate of rise and fall is frequency. It is usually identified as oscillations per second or cycles per second. The unit of measurement is the **hertz (Hz).** One hertz is equal to 1 cycle per second. The frequency is equal to the number of crests or the number of valleys that pass the point of an observer per unit of time. If the critter used a stopwatch and counted 20 crests passing in 10 s, then the frequency would be 20 cycles in 10 s, or 2 Hz. If the scientist doubles the rate at which he moves the rope up and down, the critter would count 40 crests passing in 10 s and the frequency would be 4 Hz.

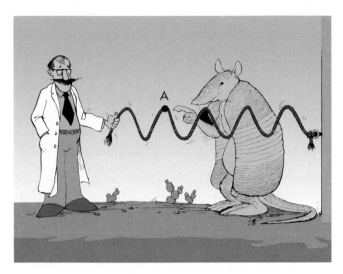

FIGURE 5-3 Moving one end of a rope in a whiplike fashion will set into motion sine waves that travel down the rope to the fastened end. An observer, midway, can determine the frequency of oscillation by counting the crests or valleys that pass a point (A) per unit time.

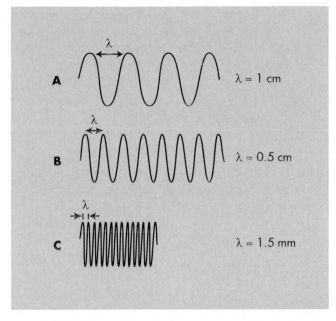

FIGURE 5-4 These three sine waves have different wavelengths. The shorter the wavelength (λ), the higher the frequency.

 Frequency is the number of wavelengths passing a point of observation per second.

The **wavelength** is the distance from one crest to another, from one valley to another, or from any point on the sine wave to the next corresponding point. Figure 5-4 shows sine waves of three different wavelengths. With a meter rule, you can verify that wave *A* repeats every 1 cm and therefore has a wavelength of 1 cm. Similarly, wave *B* has a wavelength of 0.5 cm and wave *C* has a wavelength of 1.5 mm. Clearly, then, as the frequency is increased, the wavelength is reduced. The wave amplitude is not related to wavelength or frequency.

Three wave parameters—velocity, frequency, and wavelength—are needed to describe electromagnetic radiation. The relationships among these parameters is important. A change in one affects the value of the other. Velocity is constant.

Suppose a radiologic technologist is positioned to observe the flight of the sine wave arrows to determine their frequency (Figure 5-5). The first sine wave is measured and found to have a frequency of 60 Hz, which is 60 oscillations (wavelengths) of the sine wave every second.

The unknown archer now puts an identical sine wave arrow into his bow and shoots it with less force so that this second arrow has only half the velocity of the first arrow. The observer correctly measures the frequency at 30 Hz, even though the wavelength of the second arrow was the same as that of the first arrow. In other words, as the velocity decreases, the frequency decreases proportionately.

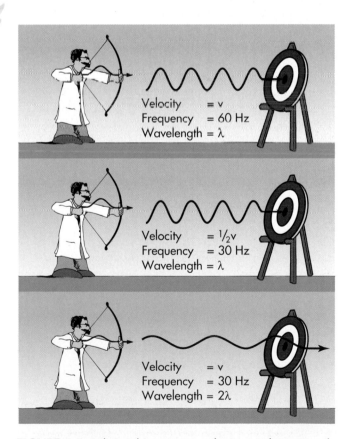

FIGURE 5-5 Relationships among velocity (v), frequency (f), and wavelength for any sine wave.

Now the archer shoots a third sine wave arrow with precisely the same velocity as the first but with a wavelength twice as long as that of the first. What should be the observed frequency? The correct answer is 30 Hz.

 At a given velocity, wavelength, and frequency are inversely proportional.

This brief analogy demonstrates how the three parameters associated with a sine wave are interrelated. A simple mathematical formula, called the **wave equation**, expresses this interrelationship:

 THE WAVE EQUATION

Velocity = Frequency × Wavelength

or

$v = f\lambda$

The wave equation is used for both sound and electromagnetic radiation. However, keep in mind that sound waves are very different from electromagnetic photons. The sources of sound are different, they are propagated in different ways, and their velocities vary greatly. The velocity of sound waves depends on the density of the material through which it passes. Sound cannot travel through a vacuum.

Question: The speed of sound in air is approximately 340 m/s. The highest treble tone that a person can hear is about 20 kHz. What is the wavelength of this sound?

Answer: $v = f\lambda$

$$\lambda = \frac{v}{f}$$

$$= \frac{340 \text{ m/s}}{20 \text{ kHz}}$$

$$= \frac{3.40 \times 10^2 \text{ m}}{s} \times \frac{s}{2 \times 10^4 \text{ cycle}}$$

$$= 1.7 \times 10^{-2} \text{ m}$$

$$= 1.7 \text{ cm}$$

When dealing with electromagnetic radiation, we can simplify the wave equation because all such radiation travels with the same velocity.

 ELECTROMAGNETIC WAVE EQUATION

$c = f\lambda$

The product of frequency and wavelength always equals the velocity of light for electromagnetic radiation.

Stated differently, **for electromagnetic radiation, frequency and wavelength are inversely proportional.** The following are alternative forms of the electromagnetic wave equation.

 ELECTROMAGNETIC WAVE EQUATION

$f = \dfrac{c}{\lambda}$ and $\lambda = \dfrac{c}{f}$

As the frequency of electromagnetic radiation increases, the wavelength decreases, and vice versa.

Question: Yellow light has a wavelength of 580 nm. What is the frequency of a photon of yellow light?

Answer: $f = \dfrac{c}{\lambda}$

$$= \frac{3 \times 10^8 \text{ m/s}}{580 \text{ nm}}$$

$$= \frac{3 \times 10^8 \text{ m}}{s} \times \frac{1}{580 \times 10^{-9} \text{ m}}$$

$$= \frac{3 \times 10^8 \text{ m}}{s} \times \frac{1}{5.8 \times 10^{-7} \text{ m}}$$

$$= 0.517 \times 10^{15} \text{ cycles/s}$$

$$= 5.17 \times 10^{14} \text{ Hz}$$

Question: The highest energy x-ray produced at 100 kVp (100 keV) has a frequency of 2.42×10^{19} Hz. What is its wavelength?

Answer: $x = \dfrac{c}{f}$

$$= \frac{3 \times 10^8 \text{ m}}{s} \times \frac{s}{2.42 \times 10^{19} \text{ cycle}}$$

$$= 1.24 \times 10^{-11} \text{ m}$$

$$= 12.4 \text{ pm}$$

ELECTROMAGNETIC SPECTRUM

The frequency range of electromagnetic radiation extends from approximately 10^2 to 10^{24} Hz. The photon wavelengths associated with these radiations are approximately 10^7 to 10^{-16} m, respectively. This wide range of values covers many types of electromagnetic radiation, most of which are familiar to us. Grouped together, these radiations make up the **electromagnetic spectrum**.

 The electromagnetic spectrum includes the entire range of electromagnetic radiation.

The known electromagnetic spectrum has three regions most important to radiologic technology: visible light, x-radiation, and radiofrequency. Other portions of the spectrum include ultraviolet radiation, infrared light, and microwave radiation.

With each of these various radiations, photons are essentially the same. Each can be represented as a bundle of energy consisting of varying electric and magnetic fields traveling at the speed of light. The photons of these various portions of the electromagnetic spectrum differ only in frequency and wavelength.

Ultrasound is not produced in photon form and does not have a constant velocity. Ultrasound is a wave of moving molecules. Ultrasound requires matter; electromagnetic radiation can exist in a vacuum.

 Diagnostic ultrasound is not a part of the electromagnetic spectrum.

Measurement of the Electromagnetic Spectrum

The electromagnetic spectrum shown in Figure 5-6 contains three different scales, one each for energy, frequency, and wavelength. Since the velocity of all electromagnetic radiation is constant, the wavelength and frequency are inversely related.

Although segments of the electromagnetic spectrum are often given precise ranges, these ranges actually overlap because of production methods and detection techniques. For example, by definition ultraviolet light

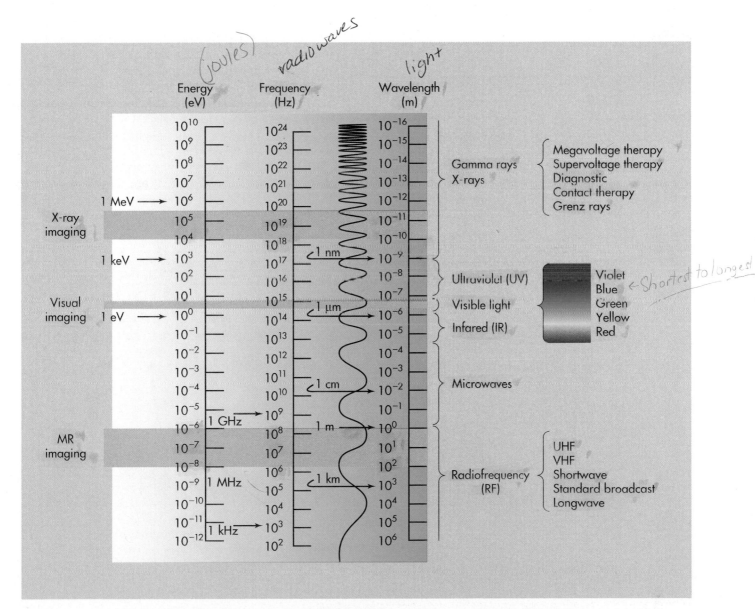

FIGURE 5-6 The electromagnetic spectrum extends over more than 25 orders of magnitude. This chart shows the values of energy, frequency, and wavelength and identifies the three imaging windows.

has a shorter wavelength than violet light and cannot be sensed by the eye. What is visible violet light to one observer, however, may be ultraviolet light to another. Similarly, microwaves and infrared radiation are indistinguishable in their common region of the spectrum.

The earliest investigations concerned visible light. Studies of reflection, refraction, and diffraction showed light to be wavelike. Consequently, visible light is described by wavelength, measured in meters.

In the 1880s some scientists began experimenting with the radio, which required the oscillation of electrons in a conductor. Consequently, the unit of frequency, the hertz, is used to describe radio waves.

Finally, in 1895 Roentgen discovered x-rays by applying an electric potential (kilovolts) across a Crookes tube. Consequently, x-rays are described using a unit of energy, the electron volt (eV).

 The energy of a photon is directly proportional to its frequency.

It should be clear that these three scales are directly related mathematically. If you know the value of electromagnetic radiation of one scale, you can easily compute its value on the other two.

The electromagnetic spectrum has been scientifically investigated for more than a century. Scientists working with radiation in one portion of the spectrum were often unaware of others investigating another portion. Consequently, there is no generally accepted, single dimension for measuring electromagnetic radiation.

Visible Light

An optical physicist describes visible light in terms of wavelength. When sunlight passes through a prism (Figure 5-7), it emerges not as white sunlight but as the colors of the rainbow.

Although photons of visible light travel in straight lines, their course can be deviated when they pass from one transparent medium to another. This deviation in line of travel, called **refraction,** is the cause of many peculiar but familiar phenomena, such as a rainbow or the apparent bending of a straw in a glass of water.

White light is composed of photons of a range of wavelengths, and the prism acts to separate and group the emerging light into colors because different wavelengths are refracted through different angles. The component colors of white light have wavelength values ranging from approximately 400 nm for violet to 700 nm for red.

Visible light occupies the smallest segment of the electromagnetic spectrum, and yet it is the only portion that we can sense directly. Sunlight also contains two types of invisible light: infrared and ultraviolet.

Infrared light consists of photons with wavelengths longer than those of visible light but shorter than those of microwaves. Infrared light heats any substance on which it shines. It may be considered radiant heat.

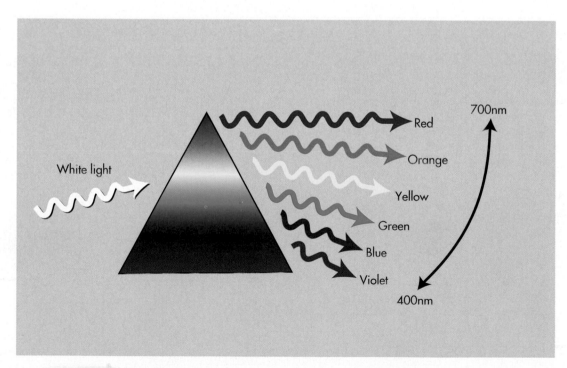

FIGURE 5-7 When it passes through a prism, white light is refracted into its component colors. These colors have wavelengths extending from approximately 400 to 700 nm.

Ultraviolet light is located in the electromagnetic spectrum between visible light and ionizing radiation. It is responsible for molecular interactions that can result in sunburn.

Radiofrequency

A radio or television engineer describes radio waves in terms of their frequency. For example, radio station WIMP might broadcast at 960 kHz and its associated television station WIMP-TV might broadcast at 63.7 MHz. Communication broadcasts are usually identified by their frequency of transmission and are called **radiofrequency (RF)** emissions.

RF covers a considerable portion of the electromagnetic spectrum. RF waves have very low energy and very long wavelength. Ham operators speak of broadcasting on the 10 m band or the 30 m band; these numbers refer to the approximate wavelength of emission.

Standard AM radio broadcasts have a wavelength of about 100 m. Television and FM broadcasting occur at a much shorter wavelength. Because microwaves are also used for communication, RF and microwave emissions overlap considerably.

Very-short-wavelength RF is **microwave** radiation. Microwave frequencies vary according to use but are always higher than broadcast RF and lower than infrared. Microwaves have many uses, such as cellular telephone communication, highway speed monitoring, medical diathermy, and hot dog preparation.

Ionizing Radiation

Unlike RF or visible light, ionizing electromagnetic radiation is usually characterized by the energy contained in a photon. When an x-ray imaging system is operated at 80 kVp, the x-rays it produces contain energies varying from 0 to 80 keV.

An x-ray photon contains considerably more energy than a visible light photon or an RF photon. The frequency of x-radiation is much higher and the wavelength much shorter than for other types of electromagnetic radiation.

It is sometimes said that gamma rays have higher energy than x-rays. In the early days of radiology this was true because of the limited capacity of available x-ray imaging systems. Today, linear accelerators make it is possible to produce x-rays of considerably higher energies than gamma-ray emissions. Consequently, the distinction by energy is not appropriate.

 The only difference between x-rays and gamma rays is their origin.

X-rays are emitted from the electron cloud of an atom that has been artificially stimulated (Figure 5-8).

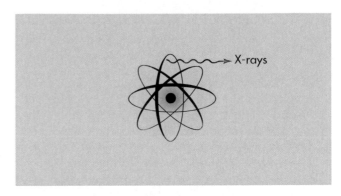

FIGURE 5-8   X-rays are produced outside the nucleus of excited atoms.

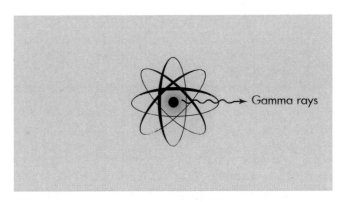

FIGURE 5-9   Gamma rays are produced inside the nucleus of radioactive atoms.

Gamma rays, on the other hand, come from inside the nucleus of a radioactive atom (Figure 5-9).

X-rays are produced in electrical imaging systems, whereas gamma rays are emitted spontaneously from radioactive material. Nevertheless, given an x-ray and a gamma ray of equal energy, one could not tell them apart.

This situation is analogous to the difference between beta particles and electrons. These particles are the same except that beta particles come from the nucleus and electrons come from outside the nucleus.

 Visible light is identified by wavelength, RF is identified by frequency, and x-rays are identified by energy.

Once again, three regions of the electromagnetic spectrum are particularly important to radiologic technology. Naturally, the x-ray region is fundamental to producing a high-quality radiograph. The visible light region is also important because the viewing conditions of a radiographic or fluoroscopic image are critical to diagnosis. With the introduction of magnetic resonance imaging (MRI), the radiofrequency region has become more important to medical imaging.

WAVE-PARTICLE DUALITY

A photon of x-radiation and a photon of visible light are fundamentally the same, except that x-radiation has much higher frequency, and hence a shorter wavelength, than visible light. These differences result in differences in the way these photons interact with matter.

Visible-light photons tend to behave more like waves than particles. The opposite is true of x-ray photons, which behave more like particles than waves. In fact, both types of photons exhibit both types of behavior, a phenomenon known as the **wave-particle duality** of radiation.

Photons interact with matter most easily when the matter is approximately the same size as the photon wavelength.

Another general way to consider the interaction of electromagnetic radiation with matter is as a function of wavelength. Radio and TV waves, whose wavelengths are measured in meters, interact with metal rods or wires called *antennas*.

Microwaves, whose wavelengths are measured in centimeters, interact most easily with objects of the same size, such as hot dogs and hamburgers.

The wavelength of visible light is measured in nanometers (nm); visible light interacts with living cells, such as the rods and cones of the eye. Ultraviolet light

interacts with molecules, and x-rays interact with atoms and subatomic particles. All radiation with wavelengths longer than that of x-radiation interacts primarily as a wave phenomenon.

X-rays behave as though they are particles.

Wave Model: Visible Light

One of the unique features of animal life is the sense of vision. It is interesting that we have developed organs that sense only a very narrow portion of the enormous spread of the electromagnetic spectrum. This narrow portion is called **visible light**.

The visible-light spectrum extends from short-wavelength violet radiation through green and yellow to long-wavelength red radiation. On either side of the visible-light spectrum are ultraviolet and infrared radiation. Neither can be detected by the human eye but they can be detected by other means, such as a photographic emulsion.

Visible light interacts with matter very differently from x-rays. When a photon of light strikes an object, it sets the object's molecules into vibration. The orbital electrons of some atoms of certain molecules are excited to an energy level that is higher than normal. This energy is immediately re-emitted as another photon of light; it is reflected.

The atomic and molecular structures of any object determine which wavelengths of light are reflected. A leaf in the sunlight appears green because all the visible-

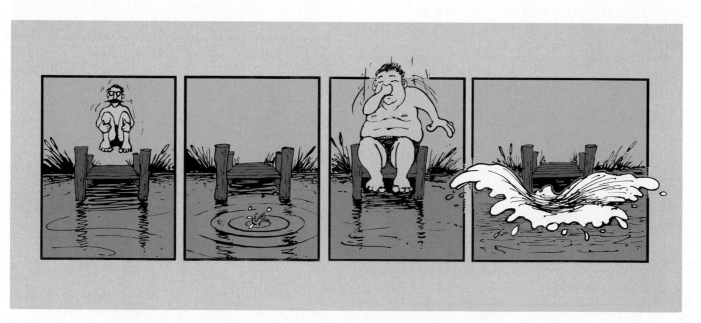
FIGURE 5-10 A small object dropped into a smooth pond creates waves of short wavelength. A large object creates waves of much longer wavelength.

light photons are absorbed by the leaf but only photons with wavelengths in the green region are reflected. Similarly, a balloon may appear red by absorbing all visible photons and reflecting only the long-wavelength red photons.

Many familiar phenomena of light, such as reflection, absorption, and transmission, are most easily explained by using the wave model of electromagnetic radiation. When a pebble is dropped into a still pond, ripples radiate from the center of the disturbance like miniature waves.

This situation is similar to the wave nature of visible light. Figure 5-10 shows the difference in the water waves between an initial disturbance caused by a small object and one caused by a large object. The distance between the crests of waves is much greater with the large object than with the small object.

Visible light behaves like a wave.

With these water waves, the difference in wavelength is proportional to the energy introduced into the system. With light, the opposite is true: the shorter the photon wavelength, the higher the photon energy.

If the analogy of the pebble in the pond is extended to a continuous succession of pebbles dropped into a smooth ocean, then at the edge of the ocean the waves will appear straight rather than circular. Light waves behave as though they were straight rather than circular because the distance from the source is great. The manner in which light is reflected from or transmitted through a surface is a consequence of this straight wave-like motion.

When the waves of the ocean crash into a vertical bulkhead (Figure 5-11), the reflected waves scatter from the bulkhead at the same angle at which the incident waves struck it. When the bulkhead is removed and replaced with a beach, the water waves simply crash onto the beach, dissipate their energy, and are absorbed. When an intermediate condition exists in which the bulkhead has been replaced by a line of pilings, the energy of the waves is scattered and absorbed.

Radiation attenuation is the reduction in intensity resulting from scattering and absorption.

Visible light can similarly interact with matter. **Reflection** from the silvered surface of a mirror is common. Examples of **transmission, absorption,** and **attenuation** of light are equally easy to identify. When light waves are absorbed, the energy deposited in the absorber reappears as heat. A black asphalt road reflects very little visible light but absorbs a considerable amount. In so doing, the road surface can become quite hot.

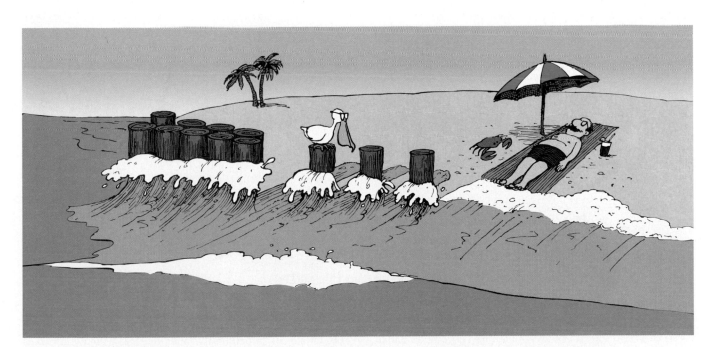

FIGURE 5-11 Energy is reflected when waves crash into a bulkhead. It is absorbed by a beach. It is partially absorbed or attenuated by a line of pilings. Light is also reflected, absorbed or attenuated, depending on the composition of the surface on which it is incident.

Just a slight modification can change how some materials transmit or absorb light. There are three degrees of interaction between light and an absorbing material: transparency, translucency, and opacity (Figure 5-12). Window glass is **transparent**; it allows light to be transmitted almost unaltered. One can see through glass because the surface is smooth and the molecular structure is tight and orderly. Incident light waves cause molecular and electronic vibrations within the glass. These vibrations are transmitted through the glass and re-irradiated almost without change.

When the surface of the glass is roughened with sandpaper, light is still transmitted through the glass but is greatly scattered and reduced in intensity. Instead of seeing through clearly, one sees only blurred forms. Such glass is **translucent**.

When the glass is painted black, the characteristics of the pigment in the paint are such that no light can pass through. Any incident light is totally absorbed in the paint. Such glass is **opaque** to visible light.

The terms *radiopaque* and *radiolucent* are used routinely in x-ray diagnosis to describe the visual appearance of anatomic structures. Structures that absorb x-rays are called **radiopaque**. Structures that attenuate x-rays are called **radiolucent** (Figure 5-13). Bone is radiopaque, whereas lung tissue and to some extent soft tissue are radiolucent.

Inverse Square Law

When light is emitted from a source such as the sun or a light bulb, the intensity decreases rapidly with the distance from the source. X-rays exhibit precisely the same property. Figure 5-14 shows that as a book is moved farther from a light source, the intensity of light falls.

This decrease in intensity is inversely proportional to the square of the distance of the object from the source. Mathematically, this is called the **inverse square law** and is expressed as:

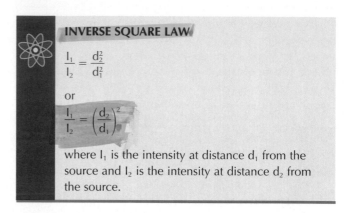

INVERSE SQUARE LAW

$$\frac{I_1}{I_2} = \frac{d_2^2}{d_1^2}$$

or

$$\frac{I_1}{I_2} = \left(\frac{d_2}{d_1}\right)^2$$

where I_1 is the intensity at distance d_1 from the source and I_2 is the intensity at distance d_2 from the source.

The reason for the rapid decrease in intensity with increasing distance is that the total light emitted is spread out over an increasingly larger area. The equivalent of

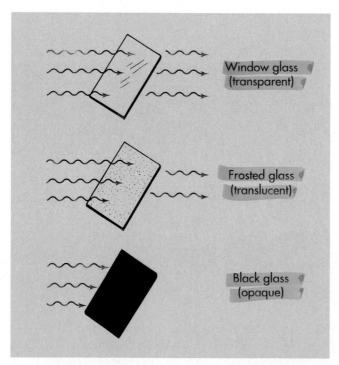

FIGURE 5-12 Objects absorb light in three degrees: not at all (transmission), partially (attenuation), and completely (absorption). The objects associated with these degrees of absorption are called transparent, translucent, and opaque, respectively.

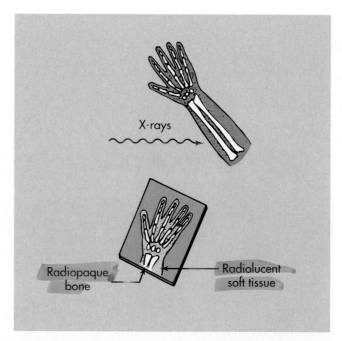

FIGURE 5-13 Structures that attenuate x-rays are described as radiolucent or radiopaque, depending on the relative degree of x-ray transmission or absorption, respectively.

this phenomenon in the water-wave analogy is the reduction of wave amplitude with distance from the source. The wavelength remains fixed.

 Radiation intensity is inversely related to the square of the distance from the source.

If the source of radiation is not a point but rather a line, such as a fluorescent lamp, the inverse square law does not hold at distances close to the source. At great distances from the source, the inverse square law can be applied.

 The inverse square law can be applied to distances greater than seven times the longest dimension of the source.

To apply the inverse square law, you must know three of the four parameters, which are *two distances* and *two intensities*. The usual situation involves a known intensity at a fixed distance from the source and an unknown intensity at a greater distance.

Question: The intensity of light from a reading lamp is 100 millilumens (mlm), I_2, at a distance of 1 m, d_2. (The lumen is a unit of light intensity.) What is the intensity, I_1, of this light at 3 m, d_1?

Answer:
$$\frac{I_1}{I_2} = \frac{d_2^2}{d_1^2}$$

$$\frac{I_1}{100 \text{ mlm}} = \frac{1 \text{ m}^2}{3 \text{ m}^2}$$

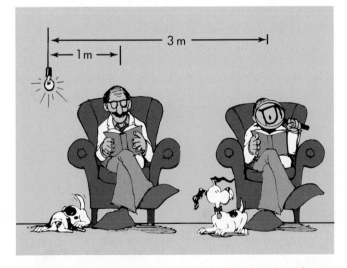

FIGURE 5-14 The inverse square law describes the relationship between radiation intensity and distance from the radiation source.

$$I_1 = (100 \text{ mlm})\left(\frac{1 \text{ m}}{3 \text{ m}}\right)^2$$

$$= (100 \text{ mlm})(\tfrac{1}{9})$$

$$= 11 \text{ mlm}$$

This relationship between radiation intensity and distance from the source applies equally well to x-ray intensity.

Question: The exposure from an x-ray tube operated at 70 kVp, 200 mAs is 400 mR (4 mGy$_a$), I_2, at 90 cm, d_2. What will the exposure be at 180 cm, d_1?

Answer:
$$\frac{I_1}{I_2} = \left(\frac{d_2}{d_1}\right)^2$$

$$I_1 = I_2\left(\frac{d_2}{d_1}\right)^2$$

$$= (400 \text{ mR})\frac{90 \text{ cm}}{180 \text{ cm}}^2$$

$$= (400 \text{ mR})(\tfrac{1}{2})^2$$

$$= (400 \text{ mR})(\tfrac{1}{4})$$

$$= 100 \text{ mR}$$

This example illustrates that when the distance from the source is doubled, the intensity of radiation is reduced by one fourth; conversely, when the distance is halved, the intensity is increased by a factor of four.

Question: For a given technique, the x-ray intensity at 1 m, d_2, is 450 mR (4.5 mGy$_a$), I_2. What is the intensity at the edge of the control booth, a distance of 3 m, d_1, if the useful beam is directed at the booth? (This, of course, should never be done!)

Answer:
$$\frac{I_1}{I_2} = \left(\frac{d_2}{d_1}\right)^2$$

$$I_1 = I_2\left(\frac{d_2}{d_1}\right)^2$$

$$= (450 \text{ mR})\left(\frac{1 \text{ m}}{3 \text{ m}}\right)^2$$

$$= 450 \text{ mR }(\tfrac{1}{3})^2$$

$$= 450 \text{ mR }(\tfrac{1}{9})$$

$$= 50 \text{ mR}$$

Often it is necessary to determine the distance from the source at which the radiation has a given intensity. This type of problem is common in designing radiologic facilities.

Question: A temporary chest radiographic imaging system is to be set up in a large hall. The

TABLE 5-1	Some of the Wide Range of X-rays Produced by Application in Medicine, Research, and Industry	
Type of X-ray	**Approximate Energy**	**Application**
Diffraction	Less than 10 kVp	Research: structural and molecular analysis
Grenz rays*	10 to 20 kVp	Medicine: dermatology
Superficial	50 to 100 kVp	Medicine: therapy of superficial tissues
Diagnostic	30 to 150 kVp	Medicine: imaging anatomic structures and tissues
Orthovoltage*	200 to 300 kVp	Medicine: therapy of deep-lying tissues
Supervoltage*	300 to 1000 kVp	Medicine: therapy of deep-lying tissues
Megavoltage	Greater than 1 MV	Medicine: therapy of deep-lying tissues
		Industry: checking integrity of welded metals

* These radiation therapy modalities are no longer in use.

technique used results in an exposure of 25 mR (0.25 mGy$_a$) at 180 cm. The area behind the chest stand in which the exposure intensity exceeds 1 mR is to be cordoned off. How far from the x-ray tube will this area extend?

Answer:

$$\frac{I_1}{I_2} = \frac{d_2^2}{d_1^1}$$

$$\frac{25 \text{ mR}}{1 \text{ mR}} = \frac{(d_2)^2}{(180 \text{ cm})^2}$$

$$(d_2)^2 = (180 \text{ cm})^2 \left(\frac{25 \text{ mR}}{1 \text{ mR}}\right)$$

$$d_2 = \left[(180^2)\left(\frac{25}{1}\right)\right]^{1/2}$$

$$= (180)(25)^{1/2}$$
$$= (180)(5)$$
$$= 900 \text{ cm}$$
$$= 9 \text{ m}$$

Particle Model: Quantum Theory

Unlike other portions of the electromagnetic spectrum, x-rays are usually identified by their energy, measured in electron volts (eV). X-ray energy ranges from approximately 10 keV to 50 MeV. The associated wavelength for this range of x-radiation is approximately 10^{-10} to 10^{-14} m. The frequency of these photons varies from approximately 10^{18} to 10^{22} Hz.

Table 5-1 describes the various types of x-rays produced and the general use made of each. We are interested primarily in the diagnostic range of x-radiation, though what is said for that range holds equally well for other types of x-radiation.

An x-ray photon can be thought of as containing an electric field and a magnetic field that vary sinusoidally

at right angles to each other with a beginning and end having diminishing amplitude (Figure 5-15). The wavelength of an x-ray photon is measured like that of any electromagnetic radiation: it is the distance from any position on the sine wave to the corresponding position of the next wave. The frequency of an x-ray photon is calculated like the frequency of any electromagnetic photon, by use of the Wave Equation.

 The x-ray photon is a discrete bundle of energy.

X-rays are created with the speed of light (c) and either exist with velocity **c** or do not exist at all. That is one of the substantive statements of **Planck's quantum theory.** Max Planck was a German physicist whose mathematical and physical theories synthesized our understanding of electromagnetic radiation into a uniform model; for this work he received the Nobel Prize in 1918.

Another important consequence of this theory is the relationship between energy and frequency: photon energy is directly proportional to photon frequency. The constant of proportionality, known as **Planck's constant** and symbolized by h, has a numerical value of 4.15×10^{-15} eVs or 6.63×10^{-34} Js. Mathematically, the relationship between energy and frequency is expressed as:

PLANCK'S QUANTUM EQUATION

$E = hf$

where E is the photon energy, h is Planck's constant, and f is the photon frequency in hertz.

 The energy of a photon is directly proportional to its frequency.

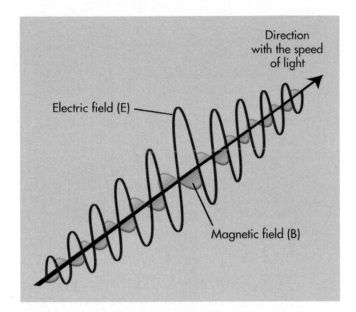

Direction with the speed of light

Electric field (E)

Magnetic field (B)

FIGURE 5-15 All electromagnetic radiation, including x-rays, can be visualized as two perpendicular sine waves traveling in a straight line at the speed of light. One of the sine waves represents an electric field and the other a magnetic field.

Question: What is the frequency of a 70 keV x-ray?
Answer: $E = hf$

$$f = \frac{E}{h}$$

$$= \frac{7 \times 10^4 \text{ eV}}{4.15 \times 10^{-15} \text{ eVs}}$$

$$= 1.69 \times 10^{19}/\text{s}$$

$$= 1.69 \times 10^{19} \text{ Hz}$$

Question: What is the energy contained in one photon of radiation from radio station WIMP-AM, which has a broadcast frequency of 960 kHz?
Answer: $E = hf$

$$= (4.15 \times 10^{-15} \text{ eVs})(9.6 \times 10^5/\text{s})$$

$$= 3.98 \times 10^{-9} \text{ eV}$$

An extension of Planck's equation is the relationship between photon energy and photon wavelength; this relationship is useful in computing equivalent wavelengths of x-rays and other types of radiation.

EQUIVALENT PLANCK EQUATION
$E = hf,\ f = E/h,\ E = \dfrac{hc}{\lambda}$

In other words, photon energy is inversely proportional to photon wavelength. In this relationship the constant of proportionality is a combination of two constants, Planck's constant and the speed of light. The longer the wavelength of radiation, the lower the energy of each photon.

Question: What is the energy in one photon of green light whose wavelength is 550 nm?

Answer: $E = \dfrac{hc}{\lambda}$

$$= \frac{(4.15 \times 10^{-15} \text{ eVs})(3 \times 10^8 \text{ m/s})}{550 \times 10^{-9} \text{ m}}$$

$$= \frac{12.45 \times 10^{-7} \text{ eVm}}{5.5 \times 10^{-7} \text{ m}}$$

$$= 2.26 \text{ eV}$$

MATTER AND ENERGY

We began Chapter 1 with the statement that everything in existence can be classified as matter or energy. We further stated that matter and energy are really manifestations of each other. According to classical physics, matter can be neither created nor destroyed, a law known as the **law of conservation of matter**. A similar law, the **law of conservation of energy**, states that energy can be neither created nor destroyed.

Planck and Einstein greatly extended these theories. According to quantum physics and the physics of relativity, matter can be transformed into energy and vice versa. Nuclear fission, the basis for generating electricity, is an example of converting matter into energy. In radiology, a process known as *pair production* (Chapter 12) is an example of the conversion of energy into mass.

A simple relationship introduced in Chapter 1 allows the calculation of energy equivalence of mass and the mass equivalence of energy. This equation is a consequence of Einstein's theory of relativity and is familiar to all.

RELATIVITY
$E = mc^2$
E in the equation is the energy measured in joules, *m* is the mass measured in kilograms, and *c* is the velocity of light measured in meters per second.

Like the electron volt, the joule (J) is a unit of energy. One joule is equal to 6.24×10^{18} eV.

Question: What is the energy equivalence of an electron (mass = 9.109×10^{-31} kg), measured in joules and in electron volts?

Answer: $E = mc^2$

$= (9.109 \times 10^{-31} \text{ kg})(3 \times 10^8 \text{ m/s})^2$

$= 81.972 \times 10^{-15} \text{ J}$

$= (8.1972 \times 10^{-14} \text{ J})\left(\dfrac{6.24 \times 10^{18} \text{ eV}}{\text{J}}\right)$

$= 51.15 \times 10^4 \text{ eV}$

$= 511.5 \text{ keV}$

multiply same level

The problem might be stated in the opposite direction as follows:

Question: What is the mass equivalent of a 70 keV x-ray?

Answer: $E = mc^2$

$$m = \frac{E}{c^2}$$

$$= \frac{(70 \times 10^3 \text{ eV})\left(\dfrac{\text{J}}{6.24 \times 10^{18} \text{ eV}}\right)}{(3 \times 10^8 \text{ m/s})^2}$$

$$= \frac{11.2 \times 10^{-15} \text{ J}}{9 \times 10^{16} \text{ m}^2/\text{s}^2}$$

$$= 1.25 \times 10^{-31} \text{ kg}$$

divide diff level

By using the relationships reported earlier, one can calculate the mass equivalence of a photon when only the photon wavelength or photon frequency is known.

Question: What is the mass equivalence of one photon of 1000 MHz microwave radiation?

Answer: $E = hf = mc^2$

$$m = \frac{hf}{c^2}$$

E=hf
← sub

hf=mc²
m = hf/c²

$$= \frac{(6.626 \times 10^{-34} \text{ Js})(1000 \times 10^6 \times \text{Hz})}{(3 \times 10^8 \text{ m/s})^2}$$

$$= 0.736 \times 10^{-41} \text{ kg}$$

$$= 7.36 \times 10^{-42} \text{ kg}$$

Question: What is the mass equivalence of a 330 nm photon of ultraviolet light?

Answer: $E = \dfrac{hc}{\lambda} = mc^2$

$$m = \left(\frac{hc}{\lambda}\right)\left(\frac{1}{c^2}\right) = \frac{h}{\lambda c}$$

$$= \frac{6.626 \times 10^{-34} \text{ Js}}{(330 \times 10^{-9} \text{ m})(3 \times 10^8 \text{ m/s})}$$

$$= 0.00669 \times 10^{-33} \text{ kg}$$

$$= 6.69 \times 10^{-36} \text{ kg}$$

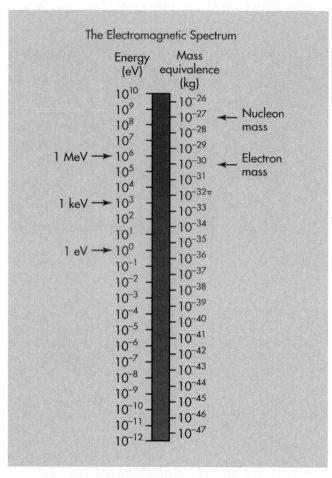

FIGURE 5-16 Mass and energy are two forms of the same medium. This scale shows the equivalence of mass measured in kilograms to energy measured in electron volts.

Calculations of this type can be used to set up a scale of mass equivalence for the electromagnetic spectrum (Figure 5-16). This scale can be used to check the answers to the above examples and to some of the problems in the companion *Workbook and Laboratory Manual*.

SUMMARY

Although matter and energy are interchangeable, x-ray imaging is based on energy in the form of x-ray photons interacting with tissue and an image receptor.

X-rays are one type of photon of electromagnetic radiation. Frequency, wavelength, velocity, and amplitude are used to describe the various imaging regions of the electromagnetic spectrum. These characteristics of electromagnetic radiation determine how such radiation interacts with matter.

CHALLENGE QUESTIONS

1. Define or otherwise identify:
   a. Photon
   b. Radiolucency
   c. The inverse square law
   d. Frequency
   e. The law of conservation of energy
   f. Gamma rays
   g. Electromagnetic spectrum
   h. Sinusoidal (sine) variation
   i. Quantum
   j. Visible light
2. Accurately diagram one photon of orange light ($\lambda = 620$ nm) and identify its velocity, electric field, magnetic field, and wavelength.
3. A thunder clap associated with lightning has a frequency of 800 Hz. If its wavelength is 50 cm, what is its velocity? How far away is the thunder if the time interval between seeing the lightning and hearing the thunder is 6 s?
4. What is the frequency associated with a photon of microwave radiation having a wavelength of 10^{-4} m?
5. Radio station WIMP-FM broadcasts at 104 MHz. What is the wavelength of this radiation?
6. In mammography, 28 keV x-rays are used. What is the frequency of this radiation?
7. Radiography of a barium-filled colon calls for high-kVp technique. These x-rays can have energy of 110 keV. What is the frequency and wavelength of this radiation?

$f = 2.7 \times 10^{9}$ hz
$\omega = 1.13 \times 10^{-11}$ m

8. What is the energy of the 110 keV x-ray of question 7 when expressed in joules? What is its mass equivalence?
9. The output intensity of a normal radiographic imaging system is 5 mR/mAs at 100 cm. What is the output intensity of such a system at 200 cm?
10. A mobile x-ray imaging system has an output intensity of 4 mR/mAs at 100 cm. Conditions require that a particular examination be conducted at 75 cm SID. What will be the output intensity at this distance?
11. Write the wave equation.
12. How are frequency and wavelength related?
13. Write the inverse square law and describe its meaning.
14. The intensity of light from a reading lamp is 200 millilumens (mlm) at a distance of 2 meters (m). What is the intensity of light at 3 m?
15. What are the three imaging windows of the electromagnetic spectrum and what unit of measure is applied to each?
16. What is the energy range of diagnostic x-rays?
17. What is the difference between x-rays and gamma rays?
18. Some regions of the electromagnetic spectrum behave like waves and some regions behave like particles in their interaction with matter. What is this phenomenon called?
19. Define attenuation.
20. What is the frequency of a 70 keV x-ray photon?

CHAPTER 6

Electricity and Magnetism

OBJECTIVES

At the completion of this chapter, the student should be able to do the following:

1. Define electrification and provide examples
2. List the laws of electrostatics
3. Define direct current and alternating current
4. Identify units of electric potential and electric power
5. Define magnetic dipole
6. Identify the interactions between matter and magnetic fields
7. Discuss the four laws of magnetism

OUTLINE

Electrostatics
  Electrification
  Electrostatic Charge
  Electrostatic Laws
  Electric Potential
Electrodynamics
  Conductors and Insulators
  Electric Circuits
  Direct Current and Alternating Current
  Electric Power
Nature of Magnetism
Classification of Magnets
Magnetic Laws
  Dipoles
  Attraction and Repulsion
  Magnetic Induction
  Magnetic Force

THIS CHAPTER on electricity and magnetism introduces the basic concepts needed for further study of the x-ray imaging system and its various components.

Because the primary function of the x-ray imaging system is to convert electric energy into electromagnetic energy—x-rays—the study of electricity and magnetism is particularly important.

This chapter begins by introducing some examples of familiar devices that convert electricity into other forms of energy. Electrostatics is the science of stationary electric charges. Electrodynamics is the science of electric charges in motion. This chapter presents the laws governing electrostatics and electrodynamics.

Magnetism has become increasingly important in diagnostic imaging with the application of magnetic resonance imaging (MRI) as a medical diagnostic tool. MRI physics is based on the angular momentum or precession of hydrogen nuclei within the body and the effect on these nuclei by the externally applied magnetic field. Magnetic field safety is an issue in the modern diagnostic imaging workplace.

This chapter describes the nature of magnetism by discussing the laws governing magnetic fields. These laws are similar to those governing the electric fields; knowing them is essential to understanding the function of several components of the x-ray imaging system, such as the transformer.

The primary function of an x-ray imaging system (Figure 6-1) is to convert electric energy into electromagnetic energy. Electric energy is supplied to the x-ray imaging system in the form of well-controlled electric current. A conversion takes place in the x-ray tube, where some of this electric energy is transformed into x-rays.

Figure 6-2 shows other, more familiar examples of electric energy conversion. When an automobile battery runs down, an electric charge restores the chemical energy of the battery. Electric energy is converted into mechanical energy with a device known as an *electric motor*, which can be used to drive a circular saw. A kitchen toaster or electric range converts

electric energy into thermal energy. There are, of course, many other examples of converting electric energy into other forms of energy.

ELECTROSTATICS

Matter has mass and energy equivalence. Matter may also have electric charge.

Electric charge comes in discrete units that are either **positive** or **negative**. Electrons and protons are the smallest units of electric charge. The electron has one unit of negative charge; the proton has one unit of positive charge. Thus, **the electric charges associated with an electron and a proton have the same magnitude but opposite signs.**

Electrostatics is the study of stationary electric charges.

Because of the way atoms are constructed, electrons often are free to travel from the outermost shell of one atom to the next. Protons, on the other hand, are fixed inside the nucleus of an atom and are not free to move. Consequently, nearly all discussions of electric charge deal with negative electric charges, those associated with the electron.

Electrification

On touching a metal doorknob after having walked across a deep-pile carpet in winter, you get a shock (contacts). Such a shock occurs because electrons are rubbed off the carpet into your shoes (friction), causing you to become electrified. An object is said to be **electrified** if it has too few or too many electrons.

Electrification can be created by contact, friction, or induction.

However, the outer shell electrons of some types of atoms are loosely bound and can easily be removed. Removal of these electrons electrifies the substances from which they were removed and results in static electricity.

Electrification is due to the movement of negative electric charges.

If you run a comb through your hair, electrons are removed from the hair and deposited on the comb. The comb becomes electrified with too many negative charges. An electrified comb can pick up tiny pieces of

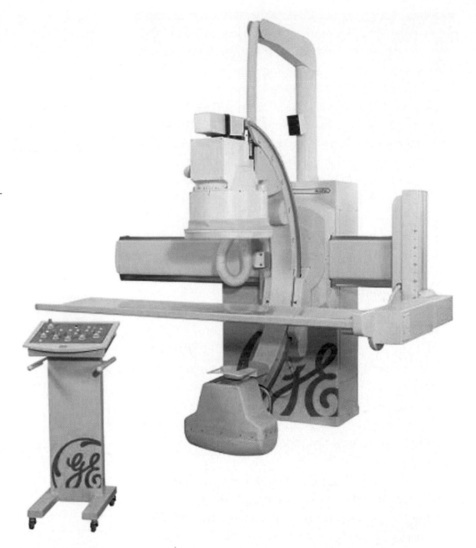

FIGURE 6-1 The x-ray imaging system converts electrical energy into electromagnetic energy. (Courtesy General Electric Medical Systems.)

paper as though the comb were a magnet (Figure 6-3). Because of its excess electrons, the comb repels some electrons in the paper, causing the closest end of the paper to become slightly positively charged. This results in a small electrostatic attractive force. Similarly, hair is electrified because it has an abnormally low number of electrons and may stand on end because of mutual repulsion.

Positive electric charges do not move. The transfer of electrons from one object to another causes the first to be positively electrified and the second to be negatively electrified.

One object always available to accept electric charges from an electrified object is the Earth. The Earth behaves as a huge reservoir for stray electric charges. In this capacity, it is called an **electric ground.**

During a thunderstorm, wind and cloud movement can remove electrons from one cloud and deposit them on another (induction). Both such clouds become electrified, one negatively and one positively.

If the electrification becomes intense enough, a discharge can occur between the clouds; in this case, electrons are rapidly transported back to the cloud that is deficient. This phenomenon is called **lightning.** Although lightning can occur between clouds, it most frequently occurs between an electrified cloud and the earth (Figure 6-4).

Another familiar example of electrification is seen in every Frankenstein movie. Usually Dr. Frankenstein's laboratory is filled with electric gadgets, wire, and large steel balls with sparks flying in every direction (Figure 6-5). The sparks are created because the various objects—wires, steel balls, and so on—are highly electrified.

Electrostatic Charge

The smallest unit of electric charge is the electron. This charge is much too small to be useful, so the fundamental unit of electric charge is considered the *coulomb (C):* $1 \text{ C} = 6.3 \times 10^{18}$ electron charges.

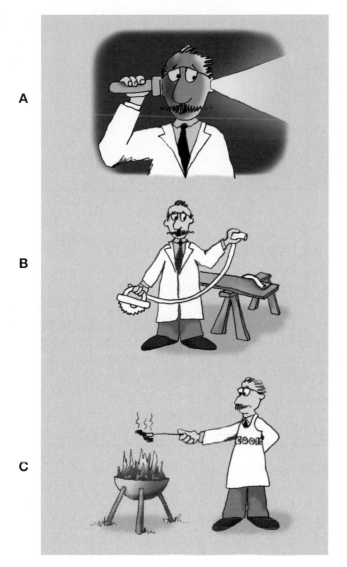

FIGURE 6-2 Electric energy can be converted from or to other forms by various devices, such as the battery **(A)** from chemical energy, the motor **(B)** to mechanical energy, and the barbeque **(C)** to thermal energy.

Question: What is the electrostatic charge of one electron?

Answer: One coulomb (C) is equivalent to 6.3×10^{18} electron charges; therefore,

$$\frac{1C}{6.3 \times 10^{18} \text{ electron charges}} =$$

$$1.6 \times 10^{-19} \text{ C/electron charge}$$

Question: The electrostatic charge transferred between two people after one has scuffed his feet across a nylon rug is one microcoulomb. How many electrons are transferred?

Answer: $1 \text{ C} = 6.3 \times 10^{18}$ electrons
$1 \mu\text{C} = 6.3 \times 10^{12}$ electrons transferred

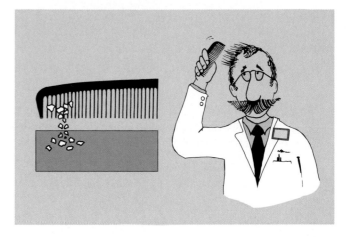

FIGURE 6-3 Running a comb briskly through your hair may cause both hair and comb to become electrified through the transfer of electrons from hair to comb. The electrified condition may make it possible to pick up small pieces of paper with the comb and may cause one's hair to stand on end.

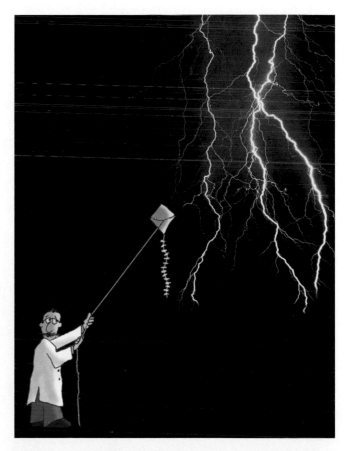

FIGURE 6-4 Electrified clouds are the source of lightning in a storm.

Question: "mAs" is a measure of what quantity?

Answer: $mAs = m\dfrac{C}{s}s = mC$, which is electrostatic charge

Electrostatic Laws

Four general laws of electrostatics describe how electric charges interact with each other and with neutral objects.

 Unlike charges attract; like charges repel.

Associated with each electric charge is an **electric field**. The electric field points outward from a positive charge and into a negative charge. Uncharged particles do not have an electric field. In Figure 6-6, lines associated with each charged particle illustrate the intensity of the electric field.

When two similar electric charges, negative and negative or positive and positive, are brought close together, their electric fields are in opposite directions and cause the electric charges to repel each other.

When unlike charges, one negative and one positive, are close to each other, the electric fields radiate in the same direction and cause the two charges to attract each other. The force of attraction between unlike charges or repulsion between like charges is due to the electric field. It is called an **electrostatic force.**

Coulomb's Law. The magnitude of the electrostatic force is given by Coulomb's law as follows:

COULOMB'S LAW

$$F = k\frac{Q_AQ_B}{d^2}$$

where *F* is the electrostatic force (newtons),
Q_A and Q_B are electrostatic charges (coulombs),
d is the distance between the charges (meters),
and *k* is a constant of proportionality.

 Coulomb's law: the electrostatic force is directly proportional to the product of the electrostatic charges and inversely proportional to the square of the distance between them.

The electrostatic force is very strong when objects are close but decreases rapidly as objects separate. This **inverse square** relationship for electrostatic force is the same as that for x-ray intensity (see Chapter 5).

 Electric charge distribution is uniform throughout or on the surface.

When a diffuse nonconductor such as a thunder cloud becomes electrified, the electric charges are distributed rather uniformly throughout. With electrified copper wire, excess electrons are distributed on the outer surface (Figure 6-7).

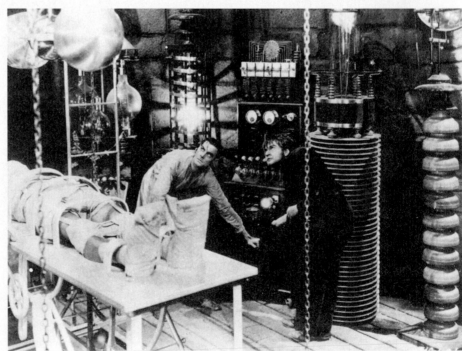

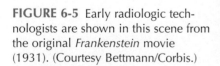
FIGURE 6-5 Early radiologic technologists are shown in this scene from the original *Frankenstein* movie (1931). (Courtesy Bettmann/Corbis.)

Electric charge of a conductor is concentrated along the sharpest curvature of the surface.

With an electrified cattle prod (Figure 6-8), electric charges are equally distributed on the surface of the two electrodes except at each tip, where electric charge is concentrated. "Our business is shocking" is the motto of the manufacturer of the cattle prod shown.

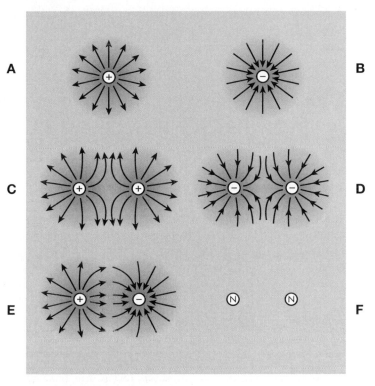

A **B**

C **D**

E **F**

FIGURE 6-6 Electric fields radiate out from a positive charge **(A)** and toward a negative charge **(B).** Like charges repel one another **(C** and **D).** Unlike charges attract one another **(E).** Uncharged particles do not have an electric field **(F).**

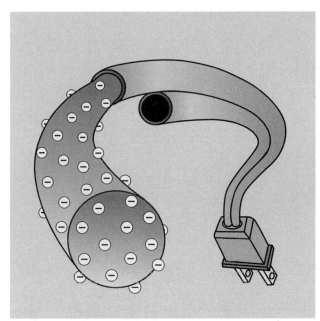

FIGURE 6-7 Cross-section of an electrified copper wire, showing that the surface of the wire has excess electrostatic charges.

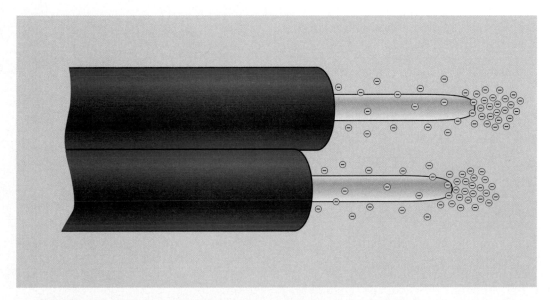

FIGURE 6-8 Electrostatic charges are concentrated on surfaces of sharpest curvature. The cattle prod is a device that takes advantage of this electrostatic law.

Electric Potential

The discussion of potential energy in Chapter 1 emphasized the relationship of such energy to work. A system possessing potential energy is a system with stored energy. Such a system has the ability to do work when this energy is released.

Electric charges have potential energy. When positioned close to each other, like electric charges have electric potential energy because they can do work when they fly apart. Electrons bunched up at one end of a wire create an electric potential because the electrostatic repulsive force will cause some electrons to move along the wire and work can be done.

The unit of electric potential is the volt (V).

Electric potential is sometimes called *voltage;* the higher the voltage, the greater the potential to do work. In the United States, the electric potential in homes and offices is 110 V. X-ray imaging systems usually require 220 V or higher. The volt is potential energy/unit charge, or a *joule/coulomb* (J/C).

ELECTRODYNAMICS

We recognized electrodynamic phenomena as electricity. If an electric potential is applied to objects, such as copper wires, then electrons move along the wire. This is called an **electric current,** or **electricity.**

Electric currents occur in many types of objects and range from the very small currents of the human body (such as those measured by electrocardiograms) to the very large currents of 440,000 V cross-country electrical transmission lines.

Electrodynamics is the study of electric charges in motion.

The direction of electric current is important. In his early classic experiments, Benjamin Franklin assumed that positive electric charges were conducted on his kite string. The unfortunate result is the convention that the direction of electric current is always opposite that of electron flow. Electrical engineers work with electric current, whereas physicists are usually concerned with electron flow.

Conductors and Insulators

A section of conventional household electric wire consists of a metal conducting wire, usually copper, coated with a rubber or plastic insulating material. The insulator confines the electron flow to the conductor. Touching the insulator does not result in a shock; touching the conductor does.

A conductor is any substance through which electrons flow easily.

Most metals are good electric conductors, copper being one of the best, although aluminum is also used. Water is also a good electric conductor because of the salts and other impurities it contains. That is why everyone should avoid water when operating power tools. Glass, clay, and other earthlike materials are usually good electric insulators.

An insulator is any material that does not allow electron flow.

Other materials exhibit two entirely different electric characteristics. In 1946, William Shockley demonstrated *semiconduction.* The principal semiconductor materials are silicon (Si) and germanium (Ge). This development led to microchips and hence the explosive rise of computer technology.

A semiconductor is a material that under some conditions behaves as an insulator and in other conditions behaves as a conductor.

At room temperature, all material resists the flow of electricity. Resistance decreases as the temperature of material is reduced (Figure 6-9). **Superconductivity** is the property of some materials to exhibit no resistance below a *critical temperature (Tc).*

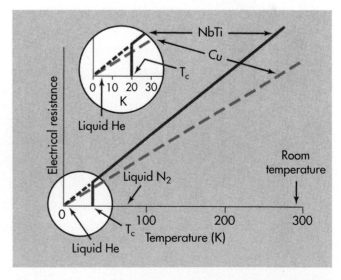

FIGURE 6-9 The electrical resistance of a conductor (Cu) and a superconductor (NbTi) as a function of temperature.

Superconductivity was discovered in 1911 but was not developed commercially until the early 1960s. Scientific investigation into superconductivity has grown in recent years and now focuses on high-temperature superconductivity (Figure 6-10).

Superconducting materials such as niobium and titanium allow electrons to flow without any resistance. Ohm's law, described in the next section, does not hold true for superconductors. A superconducting circuit can be viewed as one in perpetual motion because electric current exists without voltage. For material to behave as a superconductor, however, it must be made very cold, which requires energy.

Table 6-1 summarizes the four electrical states of matter.

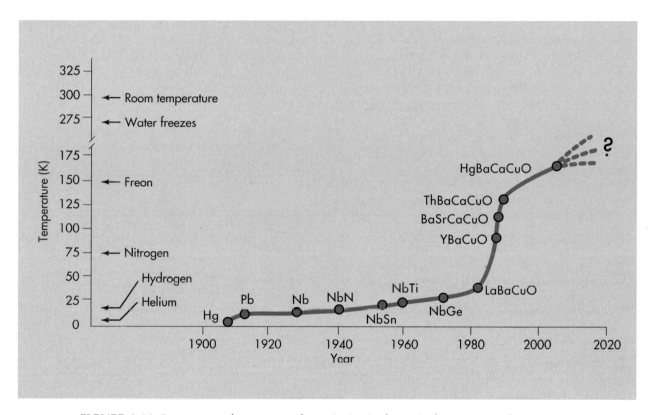

FIGURE 6-10 Recent years have seen a dramatic rise in the critical temperature for super-conducting materials.

TABLE 6-1	Four Electrical States of Matter	
State	**Material**	**Characteristics**
✳Superconductor	Niobium Titanium	✳No resistance to electron flow No electric potential required Must be very cold
✳Conductor	Copper Aluminum	✳Variable resistance Obeys Ohm's law Requires a voltage
✳Semiconductor	Silicon Germanium	✳Can be conductive Can be resistive Basis for computer technology
✳Insulator	Rubber Glass	✳Does not permit electron flow Extremely high resistance Necessary with high voltage

Electric Circuits

Electrons flow throughout a wire. Modifying the wire by reducing its diameter (wire gauge) or inserting different material (circuit elements) can increase its resistance. When this resistance is controlled and the conductor is made into a closed path, the result is an **electric circuit.**

 Increasing electric resistance results in a reduced electric current.

Electric current is measured in amperes (A). The ampere is proportional to the number of electrons flowing in the electric circuit. One ampere is equal to an electric charge of 1 C flowing through a conductor each second.

Electric potential is measured in volts (V), and electric resistance is measured in ohms (Ω). Electrons powered by high voltage have high potential energy and high capacity to do work. If electron flow is inhibited, the circuit resistance is high.

The manner in which electric currents behave in an electric circuit is described by a relationship known as Ohm's law.

 Ohm's law: the voltage across the total circuit or any portion of the circuit is equal to the current times the resistance.

 OHM'S LAW

$V = IR$

where V is the electric potential in volts, I is the electric current in amperes and R is the electric resistance in ohms. Variations of this relationship are:

$$R = \frac{V}{I}$$

and

$$I = \frac{V}{R}$$

Question: If there is a current of 0.5 A through a conductor that has a resistance of 6 Ω, what is the voltage across the conductor?

Answer: $V = IR$
$= (0.5 \text{ A})(6 \text{ Ω})$
$= 3 \text{ V}$

Question: A kitchen toaster draws a current of 2.5 A. If the household voltage is 110 V, what is the electric resistance of the toaster?

Answer: $R = \dfrac{V}{I}$
$= \dfrac{110 \text{ V}}{2.5 \text{ A}}$
$= 44 \text{ Ω}$

Most electric circuits, such as those used in radios, televisions, and other electronic devices, are very complicated. X-ray circuits are also complicated and contain a number of different types of circuit elements. Table 6-2 identifies some of the important types of circuit elements, the functions of each, and their symbols.

Usually electric circuits can be reduced to one of two basic kinds: a series circuit (Figure 6-11) or a parallel circuit (Figure 6-12).

 In a *series circuit,* all circuit elements are connected in a line along the same conductor.
If I burns out they all are out

 Rules for series circuits:
1. The total resistance is equal to the sum of the individual resistances.
2. The current through each circuit elements is the same and is equal to the total circuit current.
3. The sum of the voltages across each circuit element is equal to the total circuit voltage.

 A *parallel circuit* contains elements that are connected at their ends rather than lie in a line along a conductor.
separate lines so if I burns out the rest still work.

 The rules for a parallel circuit:
1. The sum of the currents through each circuit element is equal to the total circuit current.
2. The voltage across each circuit element is the same and is equal to the total circuit voltage.
3. The total resistance is the inverse of the sum of the reciprocals of each individual resistance.

Question: A series circuit contains three resistive elements having values of 8, 12, and 15 Ω. If the voltage is 110 V, what is the total resistance and current, the current through each resistor, and the voltage across each resistor?

TABLE 6-2   Symbol and Function of Electric Circuit Elements

Circuit Element	Symbol	Function
Resistor		Inhibits flow of electrons
Battery		Provides electrical potential
Capacitor (condenser)		Momentarily stores electric charge
Ammeter	(A)	Measures electric current
Voltmeter	(V)	Measures electric potential
Switch		Turns circuit on or off by providing infinite resistance
Transformer	*step-up transformer*	Increases or decreases voltage by fixed amount (AC only)
Rheostat		Variable resistor
Diode		Allows electrons to flow in only one direction

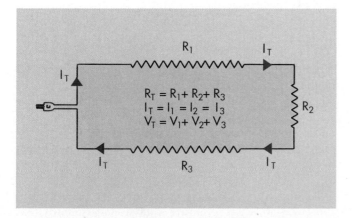

FIGURE 6-11 Series circuit and its basic rules.

$$R_T = R_1 + R_2 + R_3$$
$$I_T = I_1 = I_2 = I_3$$
$$V_T = V_1 + V_2 + V_3$$

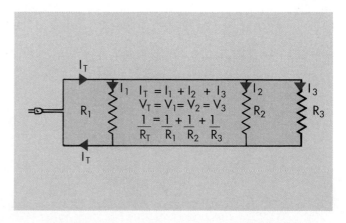

FIGURE 6-12 Parallel circuit and its basic rules.

$$I_T = I_1 + I_2 + I_3$$
$$V_T = V_1 = V_2 = V_3$$
$$\frac{1}{R_T} = \frac{1}{R_1} + \frac{1}{R_2} + \frac{1}{R_3}$$

Answer: Refer to Figure 6-11; let $R_1 = 8\ \Omega\ R_2$
$= 12\ \Omega$, and $R_3 = 15\Omega$

$R_T = 8\ \Omega + 12\ \Omega + 15\ \Omega = 35\ \Omega$

$I = \frac{U}{R}$ $I_T = I_1 = I_2 = I_3 = V/R = 110/35 = 3.14\ A$

$U = IR$ $V_1 = (3.14\ A)(8\ \Omega) = 25.12\ V$

$V_2 = (3.14\ A)(12\ \Omega) = 37.68\ V$

$V_3 = (3.14\ A)(15\ \Omega) = 47.10\ V$

Question: Suppose the previous example were a parallel circuit rather than a series circuit. What would be the correct values for total resistance and current, the current through each resistor, and the voltage across each resistor?

Answer: Refer to Figure 6-12.

$$\frac{1}{R_T} = \frac{1}{8\Omega} + \frac{1}{12\Omega} + \frac{1}{15\Omega} =$$

$$\frac{15}{120} + \frac{12}{120} + \frac{8}{120} = \frac{33}{120}$$

$$R_T = \frac{120}{33} = 3.6\Omega$$

$I = \frac{U}{R}$ $I_T = 110\ V/3.6\ \Omega = 30.2\ A$

$I_1 = 110\ V/8\ \Omega = 13.6\ A$

$I_2 = 110\ V/12\ \Omega = 9.2\ A$

$I_3 - 110\ V/15\ \Omega = 7.3\ A$

$V_1 = V_2 = V_3 = V_T = 110\ V$

Christmas lights are a good example of the difference between series and parallel circuits. Christmas lights wired in series have only one wire connecting each lamp; when one lamp burns out, the entire string of lights goes out. Christmas lights wired in parallel, on the other hand, have two wires connecting each lamp; when one lamp burns out, the rest remain lit.

Most electric circuits are much more complicated. For example, the television monitor in fluoroscopy has more than a thousand elements wired into a giant circuit consisting of many subcircuits, each of which is series, parallel, or a combination of both.

Direct Current and Alternating Current

Electric current, or electricity, is the flow of electrons through a conductor. These electrons can be made to flow in one direction along the conductor, in which case the electric current is called **direct current (DC)**.

Most applications of electricity require that the electrons be controlled so that they flow first in one direction and then in the other. Current in which electrons oscillate back and forth is called **alternating current (AC)**.

 Electrons flowing in only one direction constitute DC; Electrons flowing alternately in opposite directions constitute AC.

Figure 6-13 diagrams the phenomenon of DC and shows how it can be described by a graph called a wave-

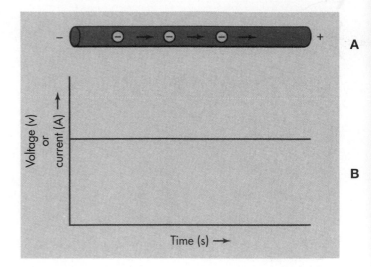

FIGURE 6-13 Representation of direct current. **A,** Electrons flow in one direction only. **B,** The graph of the associated electric waveform is a straight line.

form. The horizontal axis, or x-axis, of the electronic waveform represents time; the vertical axis, or y-axis, represents the amplitude of the electric current. For DC, the electrons always flow in the same direction; therefore, DC is represented by a horizontal line.

The vertical separation between this line and the time axis represents the magnitude of the current or the voltage. If the line representing the current is above the time axis, it represents the flow of electrons in one direction.

Electron flow in the opposite direction is shown by a current line below the time axis. When the current line coincides with the time axis, the magnitude of current is zero, indicating that no electrons flow.

The waveform for AC is a sine curve (Figure 6-14). Electrons flow first in a positive direction, then in a negative direction. At one instant in time (point 0 in Figure 6-14), all electrons are at rest. Then they move, first in the positive direction with increasing potential (segment A).

Once they reach maximum flow number, represented by the vertical distance from the time axis (point 1), the electron flow is reduced (segment B). They come to zero again momentarily (point 2) and then reverse motion and flow in the negative direction (segment C), increasing in flow number it is maximum in the negative direction (point 3). Next, the potential is reduced to zero (segment D).

This oscillation in electron direction occurs sinusoidally, with each requiring 1/60 s. Consequently, AC is identified as a 60 Hz current (50 Hz in Europe and much of the rest of the world).

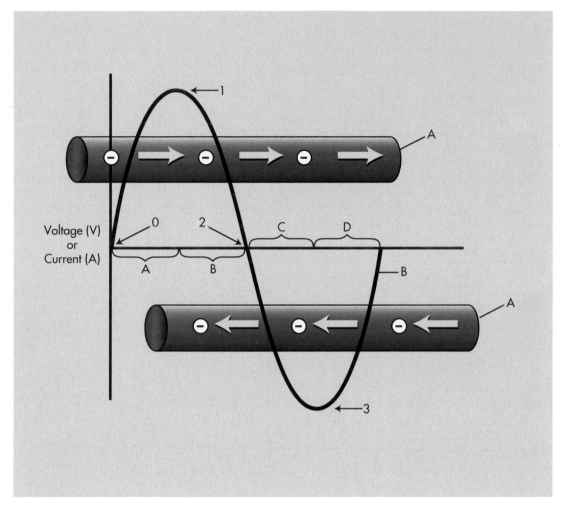

FIGURE 6-14 Representation of alternating current. **A,** Electrons flow alternately in one direction and then the other. **B,** Alternating current is represented graphically by a sinusoidal electric waveform.

Electric Power

Electric power is measured in **watts (W)**. Common household electric appliances, such as toasters, blenders, mixers, and radios generally require 500 to 1500 W of electric power. Light bulbs require 30 to 150 W of electric power. An x-ray imaging system requires 20 to 150 kW of electric power.

 One watt is equal to 1 A of current flowing through an electric potential of 1 V.

Question: If the cost of electric power is 10 cents per kilowatt hour, how much does it cost to operate a 100 W light bulb an average of 5 hours per day for 1 month?

Answer: Total on time = (30 days/mo) (5 hr/day)
= 150 hr/mo

Total power consumed = (150 hr/mo)
(100 W)
= 15,000 W-hr/mo
= 15 kW-hr/mo
Total cost = (15 kW-hr/mo)
(10 cents/kW-hr)
= $1.50/mo

ELECTRIC POWER

$P = IV$

where P is the power in watts, I is the current in amperes, and V is the electric potential in volts

alternatively,

$P = IV = IIR$

therefore,

$P = I^2R$

where R is resistance in ohms

Question: An x-ray imaging system that draws a current of 80 A is supplied with 220 V. What is the power consumed?

Answer: P = IV
= (80 A) (220 V)
= 17,600 W
= 17.6 kW

Question: The overall resistance of a mobile x-ray imaging system is 10 Ω. When plugged into a 110 V receptacle, how much current does it draw and how much power is consumed?

Answer: $I = \dfrac{V}{R} = \dfrac{110}{10} = 11A$

P = IV
= (11 A)(110 V)
= 1210 W
or P = I²R
= (11 A)² 10
= 1210 W

NATURE OF MAGNETISM

Around 1000 B.C. shepherds and dairy farmers near the village of Magnesia (what is now Western Turkey) discovered magnetite, a magnetic oxide of iron (Fe_3O_4). This rodlike stone, when suspended by a string, would rotate back and forth; when it came to rest, it pointed the way to water. It was called a **lodestone** or leading stone.

Of course, if you walk toward the north pole from any spot on earth, you will find water. So, the word **magnetism** comes from the name of that ancient village where the cows too were very curious. When milked, they produced Milk of Magnesia! Magnetites are a nat-

urally occurring magnet and were first used as a compass by the ancient Chinese.

Magnetism is a fundamental property of some forms of matter. Ancient observers knew that lodestones would attract iron filings. They also knew that rubbing an amber rod with fur caused it to attract small, light-weight objects such as paper. They considered both of these phenomena to be the same. We know them to be magnetism and electrostatics, respectively.

Magnetism is perhaps more difficult to understand than other characteristic properties of matter, such as mass, energy, and electric charge, because magnetism is difficult to detect and measure. We can feel mass, visualize energy, and be shocked by electricity but we cannot sense magnetism.

 Any charged particle in motion creates a magnetic field.

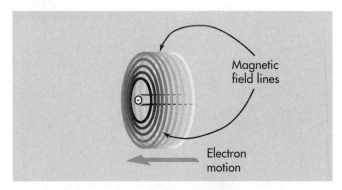

FIGURE 6-15 A moving charged particle induces a magnetic field in a plane perpendicular to its motion.

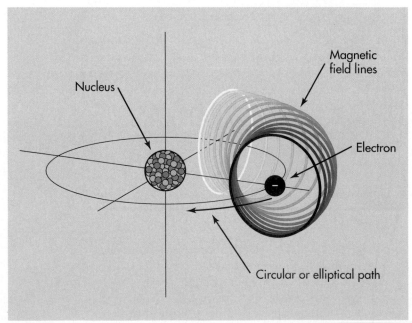

FIGURE 6-16 When a charged particle moves in a circular or elliptical path, the perpendicular magnetic field moves with the charged particle.

The magnetic field of a charged particle such as an electron in motion is perpendicular to the motion of that particle. The intensity of the magnetic field is represented by imaginary lines (Figure 6-15).

If the electron's motion is a closed loop, as with an electron circling a nucleus, the magnetic field lines will be perpendicular to the plane of motion (Figure 6-16).

Electrons rotate on an axis either clockwise or counterclockwise. This rotation creates a property called **electron spin**. The electron spin creates a magnetic field, which is neutralized in electron pairs. Therefore, atoms having an odd number of electrons in any shell exhibit a very small magnetic field.

 The lines of a magnetic field are always closed loops.

The lines of a magnetic field do not start or end as the lines of an electric field do. Such a field is called **bipolar** or **dipolar**; it always has a north and a south pole. The small magnet created by the electron orbit is called a **magnetic dipole**. An accumulation of many atomic magnets with their dipoles aligned creates a **magnetic domain**. If all the magnetic domains in an object are aligned, it acts like a magnet.

In a hydrogen atom the magnetic dipole is strong because of the unpaired electron, but in a hydrogen molecule (H_2) the magnetic dipoles of the two electrons cancel one another. Under normal circumstances, magnetic domains are randomly distributed (Figure 6-17, A).

When acted on by an external magnetic field, however, such as the earth in the case of naturally occurring ores or an electromagnet in the case of artificially induced magnetism, the randomly oriented dipoles align with the magnetic field (Figure 6-17, B). This is what happens when ferromagnetic material is made into a permanent magnet.

Spinning electric charges also induce a magnetic field (Figure 6-18). The proton in a hydrogen nucleus spins on its axis and creates a nuclear magnetic dipole called a **magnetic moment**. This is the basis of MRI.

The magnetic dipoles in a bar magnet can be thought of as generating imaginary lines of the magnetic field (Figure 6-19). If a nonmagnetic material is brought near such a magnet, these field lines are not disturbed. However, if ferromagnetic material such as soft iron is brought near the bar magnet, the magnetic field lines deviate and are concentrated into the ferromagnetic material.

 Magnetic permeability is the ability of a material to attract the lines of magnetic field intensity.

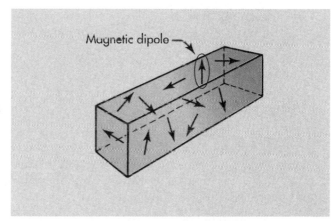

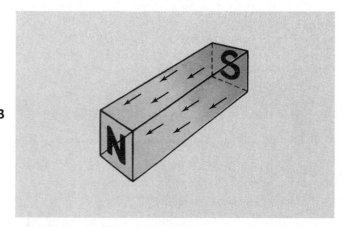

FIGURE 6-17 A, In ferromagnetic material, the magnetic dipoles are randomly oriented. **B,** This changes when the dipoles are brought under the influence of an external magnetic field.

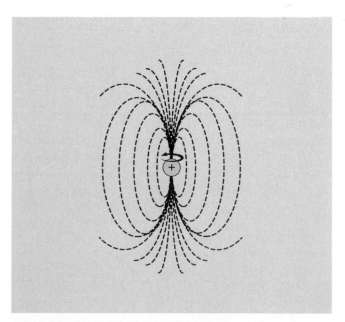

FIGURE 6-18 A spinning charged particle will induce a magnetic field along the axis of spin.

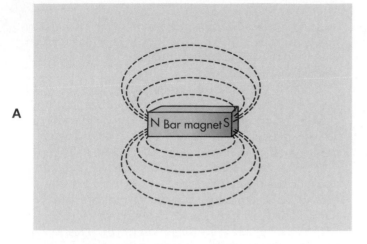

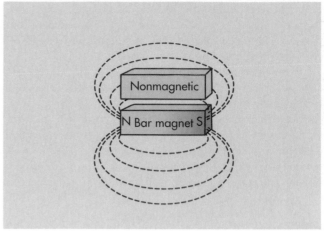

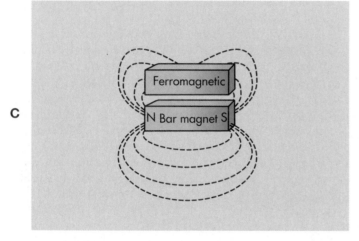

FIGURE 6-19 **A**, Imaginary lines of force. **B**, These lines of force are undisturbed by nonmagnetic material. **C**, They are deviated by ferromagnetic material.

CLASSIFICATION OF MAGNETS

There are three principal types of magnets: naturally occurring magnets, artificially induced permanent magnets, and electromagnets.

 Magnets are classified according to the *origin* of the magnetic property.

The best example of a **natural magnet** is the earth itself. The earth has a magnetic field because it spins on an axis. Lodestones in the earth exhibit strong magnetism presumably because they have remained undisturbed for a long time in the earth's magnetic field.

Artificially produced **permanent magnets** are available in many sizes and shapes but principally as bar or horseshoe-shaped magnets, usually made of iron. A compass is a prime example of an artificial permanent magnet. Permanent magnets are typically produced by aligning their domains in the field of an electromagnet (Figure 6-20).

Such permanent magnets do not necessarily stay permanent. One can destroy the magnetic property of a magnet by heating it or even by hitting it with a hammer. Either act causes the individual magnet domains to be jarred from their alignment. They thus again become randomly aligned, and magnetism is lost.

Electromagnets consist of wire wrapped around an iron core. When an electric current is conducted through the wire, a magnetic field is created. The intensity of the magnetic field is proportional to the electric current. The iron greatly increases its value.

 All matter can be classified according to the manner in which it interacts with an external magnetic field.

Many materials are unaffected when brought into a magnetic field. Such materials are nonmagnetic.

Diamagnetic materials are weakly repelled by either magnetic pole. They cannot be artificially magnetized and they are not attracted to a magnet. Examples of diamagnetic materials are wood, glass, and plastic.

Ferromagnetic materials are iron, cobalt, and nickel. These are strongly attracted by a magnet and can usu-

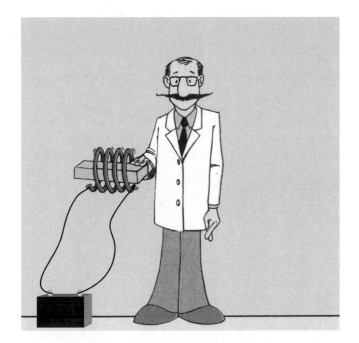

FIGURE 6-20 A method for using an electromagnet to render ceramic bricks magnetic.

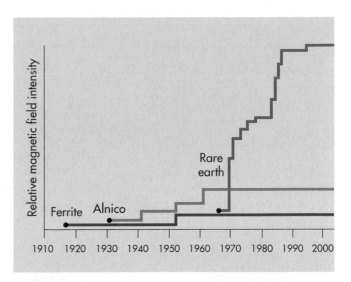

FIGURE 6-21 Developments in permanent magnet design have resulted in a great increase in magnetic field intensity.

TABLE 6-3	Five Magnetic States of Matter	
State	**Material**	**Characteristics**
Nonmagnetic	Wood, glass	Unaffected by a magnetic field
Diamagnetic	Water	Weakly repelled from both poles of a magnetic field
Paramagnetic	Gadolinium	Weakly attracted to both poles of a magnetic field
Ferromagnetic	Iron, nickel, cobalt	Can be strongly magnetized

ally be permanently magnetized by exposure to a magnetic field. An alloy of aluminum, nickel, and cobalt called **alnico** is one of the more useful magnets produced from ferromagnetic material. Rare earth ceramics have recently been developed and are considerably stronger magnets (Figure 6-21).

Paramagnetic materials lie somewhere between ferromagnetic and nonmagnetic. They are very slightly attracted to a magnet and loosely influenced by an external magnetic field. Contrast agents employed in MRI are paramagnetic.

 The degree to which a material can be magnetized is its *magnetic susceptibility.*

When wood is placed in a strong magnetic field, it does not increase the strength of the field: wood has low magnetic susceptibility. On the other hand, when iron is placed in a magnetic field, it greatly increases the strength of the field: iron has high magnetic susceptibility.

MAGNETIC LAWS

The physical laws of magnetism are similar to those of electrostatics and gravity. The forces associated with these three fields are fundamental (Table 6-3).

Note that the equations of force and the fields through which they act have the same form. Much work in theoretical physics involves the attempt to combine these fundamental forces with two others, the strong nuclear force and the weak interaction, to formulate a grand **unified field theory.**

Dipoles

Unlike the case with electricity, there is no smallest unit of magnetism. Dividing a magnet simply creates two smaller magnets, which when divided again and again make baby magnets (Figure 6-22).

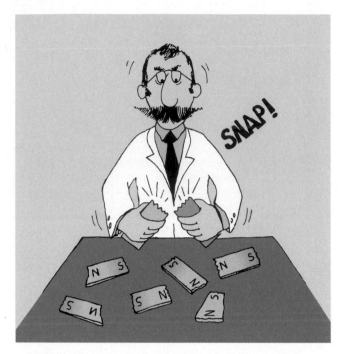

FIGURE 6-22 If a single magnet is broken into smaller and smaller pieces, baby magnets result.

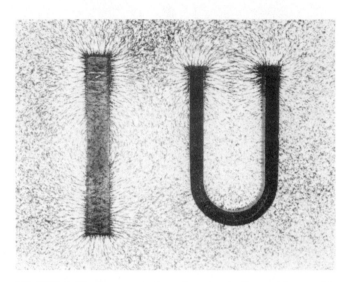

FIGURE 6-23 Demonstration of magnetic lines of force with iron filings.

How do we know that these imaginary lines of the magnetic field exist? They can be demonstrated by the action of iron fillings near a magnet (Figure 6-23).

If a magnet is placed on a surface with small iron fillings, the fillings attach most strongly and with greater concentration to the ends of the magnet. These ends are called **poles,** and every magnet has two poles. Magnetic poles exist in two forms, a **north pole** and a **south pole,** analogous to positive and negative electrostatic charges.

Attraction and Repulsion

As with electric charges, like magnetic poles repel, unlike magnetic poles attract. Also by convention, the imaginary lines of the magnetic field leave the north pole of a magnet and return to the south pole (Figure 6-24).

Magnetic Induction

Just as an electrostatic charge can be induced from one material to another, so some materials can be made magnetic by **induction.** The imaginary magnetic field lines just described are called *magnetic lines of induction,* and the density of the lines is proportional to the intensity of the magnetic field.

 Ferromagnetic objects can be made into magnets by induction.

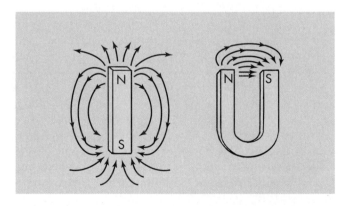

FIGURE 6-24 The imaginary lines of the magnetic field leave the north pole and enter the south pole.

When ferromagnetic material, such as a piece of soft iron, is brought into the vicinity of an intense magnetic field, the lines of induction are altered by attraction to the soft iron and the iron is made temporarily magnetic (Figure 6-25). If copper, a diamagnetic material, were to replace the soft iron, there would be no such effect.

This principle is employed with many MRI systems that use an iron magnetic shield to reduce the level of the fringe magnetic field. Ferromagnetic material acts as a magnetic sink by drawing the lines of the magnetic field into it. This also is the basis of antimagnetic

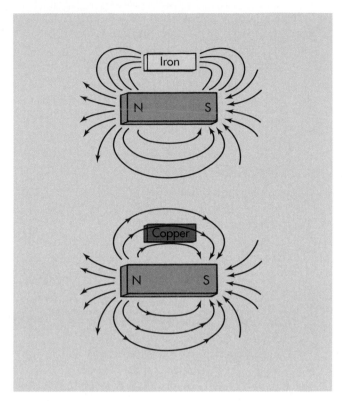

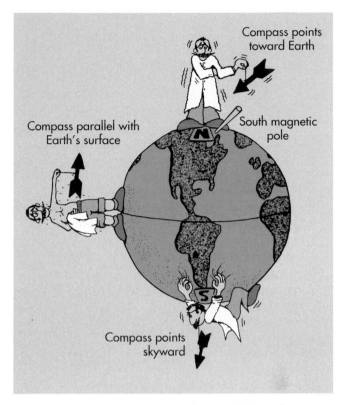

FIGURE 6-25 Ferromagnetic material such as iron attracts magnetic lines of induction, whereas nonmagnetic material such as copper does not.

FIGURE 6-26 A compass reacts with the earth as though it were a bar magnet.

watches, but do not believe it if you work near the strong field of an MRI system.

When ferromagnetic material is removed from the magnetic field, it usually does not retain its strong magnetic property. Soft iron, therefore, makes an excellent **temporary magnet.** It is a magnet only while its magnetism is being induced. If properly tempered by heat or exposed to an external field for a long period, however, some ferromagnetic materials retain their magnetism when removed from the external magnetic field and become **permanent magnets.**

Magnetic Force

The electric and magnetic forces were joined by Maxwell's field theory of electromagnetic radiation. The force created by a magnetic field and the force of the electric field behave similarly. This magnetic force is similar to electrostatic and gravitational forces that also are inversely proportional to the square of distance between the objects under consideration. If the distance between two bar magnets is halved, the magnetic force increases by four times.

 The magnetic force is proportional to the product of the magnetic pole strengths divided by the square of the distance between them.

The Earth behaves as though it has a large bar magnet embedded in it. The polar convention of magnetism actually has its origin in the compass. At the equator, the north pole of a compass points to the earth's North Pole (which is actually the earth's south magnetic pole).

As one travels toward the North Pole, the attraction of the compass becomes more intense until the compass needle points directly into the earth not at the geographic North Pole but at a region in northern Canada—the magnetic pole (Figure 6-26). The magnetic pole in the southern hemisphere is in Antarctica. There the north end of the compass would point to the sky.

 The SI unit of magnet field strength is the *tesla*. An older unit is the *gauss. One tesla (T) = 10,000 gauss (G).*

The use of a compass might suggest that the Earth has a strong magnetic field, but it does not. The Earth's magnetic field is approximately 50 μT at the equator and 100 μT at the poles. This is far less than the magnet on a cabinet door latch, which is approximately 100 mT.

SUMMARY

Electrons can flow from one object to another by contact, by friction, or by induction. The laws of electrostatics are:

Like charges repel.

Unlike charges attract.

Electrostatic force is directly proportional to the product of the charges and inversely proportional to the square of the distance between them.

Electric charges are distributed on the surface of a conductor.

Electric charges are concentrated along the sharpest curvature of the surface of the conductor.

Potential energy (Joules) is the ability do to work when energy is released. The related unit of electric potential is the volt (V).

Electrodynamics is the study of electrons in motion, otherwise known as *electricity*.

Conductors are materials through which electrons flow easily.

Insulators are materials that inhibit the flow of electrons.

Electric current is measured in amperes (A), electric potential is measured in volts (V), and electric resistance is measured in ohms (Ω).

Direct current is the flow of electrons in one direction along a conductor.

Alternating current is the flow of electrons back and forth along the conductor.

Electric power is energy produced or consumed per unit of time. One watt of power is equal to 1 A of electricity flowing through an electric potential of 1 V.

The magnetic properties of lodestone, or magnetite, were observed in the ancient world. Matter has magnetic properties because some atoms and molecules have an odd number of electrons in the outer shells. The unpaired spin of these electrons produces a magnetic field in the object.

One classification of magnets is the origin of their magnetism. Natural magnets get their magnetism from the Earth, permanent magnets are artificially induced magnets, and electromagnets are produced when electrified wire is wrapped around an iron core.

Another classification of magnets involves their interaction with an external magnetic field: ferromagnetic (easily magnetized), paramagnetic (magnetized with difficulty), and diamagnetic (cannot be magnetized). The laws of magnetism are:

Every magnet, no matter how small, has two poles: north and south.

Like magnetic poles repel and unlike magnetic poles attract.

Ferromagnetic material can be made magnetic when placed in an external magnetic field.

The force between poles is proportional to the product of the magnetic pole strengths divided by the square of the distance between them.

The increasing use of MRI as a medical diagnostic tool emphasizes the importance of magnetism as an area of study for radiologic technologists.

CHALLENGE QUESTIONS

1. Define or otherwise identify:
   a. Electric charge and its unit
   b. Electrodynamics
   c. Electric power
   d. Electrostatics
   e. Superconductor
   f. Dipole
   g. Induction
   h. Magnetic domain
   i. Magnetic susceptibility
   j. Gauss; Tesla
2. What is the total circuit resistance when resistive elements of 5, 10, 15, and 20 Ω are connected in (a) series and (b) parallel?
3. If the total current in the circuit in question 2 is 7 A, what is the voltage across the 10 Ω resistor for (a) series and (b) parallel operation?
4. A radiographic exposure requires 100 mAs. How many electrons is this?
5. What is the fundamental unit of electric charge? What is its value?
6. What are the three ways to electrify an object?
7. List the four laws of electrostatics.
8. Why is electrification easier in dry Phoenix than in humid Houston?
9. What is a semiconductor and how has it affected modern life?
10. What is the unit of electric power?
11. Magnetic fields in excess of 5 G can interfere with cardiac pacemakers. How many mT is this?
12. What is the role of magnetism in the study of x-ray imaging?
13. List the three principle types of magnets.
14. Describe an electromagnet.
15. Explain how a magnetic domain can cause an object to behave like a magnet.
16. Is a hydrogen atom a magnetic dipole? Explain.
17. What happens when a bar magnet is heated to a very high temperature?
18. List three diamagnetic materials.
19. Where does a compass point at the North Pole?
20. What is the range in intensity of the earth's magnetic field?

CHAPTER

7

Electromagnetism

OBJECTIVES

At the completion of this chapter, the student should be able to do the following:

1. Discuss the development of the battery as a reliable source of electric potential
2. Relate the experiments of Oersted, Lenz, and Faraday in defining the relationship between magnetism and electricity
3. Describe the solenoid and the electromagnet
4. Identify the laws of electromagnetic induction
5. Explain the design of the electric generator, the electric motor, and the transformer

OUTLINE

THIS CHAPTER combines information from the previous chapter on electricity and magnetism into a discussion of electromagnetism. Electromagnetism describes how electrons are given electric potential energy (voltage) and how electrons in motion create magnetism. Electromagnetic induction is a means of transferring electric potential energy from one position to another, as in a transformer.

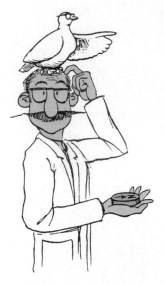

FIGURE 7-1 It has been shown that magnetic deposits in the head of the pigeon allow it to know which direction is north.

ELECTROMAGNETIC EFFECT

Electricity and magnetism are intimately connected. They are both different aspects of the same basic force: the electromagnetic force, one of the four fundamental forces of nature. The others are gravity, the strong nuclear force, and the weak interaction.

Until the nineteenth century, however, electricity and magnetism were viewed as separate effects. Although many scientists suspected that the two were connected, research was hampered by the lack of any convenient way of producing and controlling electricity.

As we saw in Chapter 6, magnetic fields could be generated and detected using various naturally occurring magnetic materials, such as the lodestone. Perhaps the earliest and most practical application of magnetism is the compass, which is simply a piece of magnetic metal used to detect the earth's magnetic field. The north pole of the magnetic needle always points to the North Pole (the south magnetic pole!).

European seafarers began using the compass as a navigational aid in the century before Columbus discovered America, but the compass was apparently known to Chinese navigators even earlier. The extensive migration of bees, birds, and turtles is thought to be controlled by an internal compass (Figure 7-1).

Thus, the early study of electricity was limited to the investigation of static electricity, which could be produced by friction (e.g., the effect produced by rubbing fur on a rubber rod). Charges could be induced to move but only in a sudden discharge, as with a spark jumping a gap.

The development of methods for producing a steady flow of charges (i.e., an electric current) during the nineteenth century stimulated investigations of both electricity and magnetism. These investigations led to an increased understanding of electromagnetic phenomena and ultimately led to the electronic revolution on which today's technology is largely based.

The Battery

In the late 1700s, an Italian anatomist, Luigi Galvani, made an accidental discovery. He observed that a dissected frog leg twitched when touched by two different metals, just as if it had been touched by an electrostatic charge. This prompted Alessandro Volta, an Italian physicist of the same era, to question whether an electric current might be produced when two different metals are brought into contact.

Using zinc and copper plates, Volta succeeded in producing a feeble electric current. To increase the current, he stacked the copper-zinc plates like a Dagwood sandwich to form what was called the **Voltaic pile,** a precursor of the modern battery. Each zinc-copper sandwich is called a **cell** of the battery.

Modern dry cells use a carbon rod as the positive electrode surrounded by an electrolytic paste housed in a negative zinc cylindrical can. Figure 7-2 shows the Voltaic pile, the modern battery, and the electronic symbol for the battery.

These devices are examples of sources of **electromotive force.** Any device that converts some form of energy directly into electric energy is said to be a source of electromotive force. Although still commonly used, this somewhat archaic term is a little misleading.

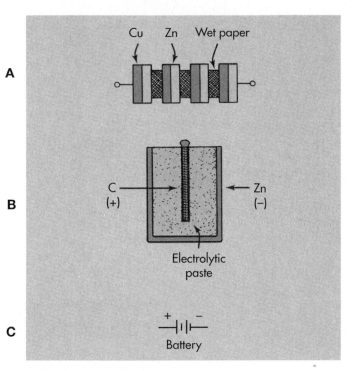

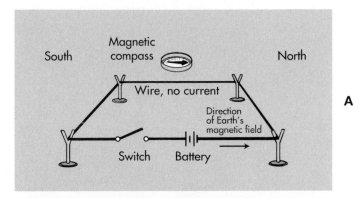

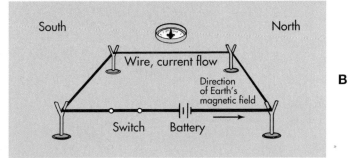

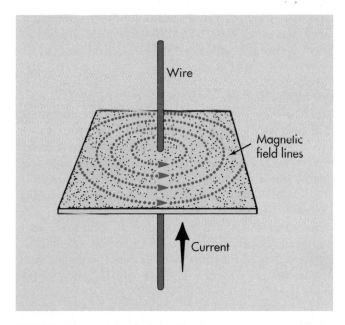

FIGURE 7-2 A, Original voltaic pile. **B,** A modern dry cell. **C,** Symbol for a battery.

FIGURE 7-3 Oersted's experiment. **A,** With no electric current in the wire, the compass points north. **B,** With electric current the compass points toward the wire.

Electromotive force is not really a force such as gravity; rather, the term refers to electric potential.

 Electric potential (energy) is measured in units of joule per coulomb, or volts.

Oersted's Experiment

Now that they finally had a source of constant electric current, scientists began extensive investigations into the possibility of a link between electric and magnetic forces. Hans Oersted, a Danish physicist, discovered the first such link in 1820.

Oersted fashioned a long straight wire, supported near a free-rotating magnetic compass (Figure 7-3). With no current in the wire, the magnetic compass pointed north as expected. When a current was passed through the wire, however, the compass needle swung to point straight at the wire. Here we have evidence of a direct link between electric and magnetic phenomena. The electric current evidently produced a magnetic field strong enough to overpower the earth's magnetic field and cause the magnetic compass to point toward the wire.

 Any charge in motion induces a magnetic field.

FIGURE 7-4 Magnetic field lines form concentric circles around the current-carrying wire.

A charge at rest produces no magnetic field. Electrons flowing through a wire produce a magnetic field about that wire. The magnetic field is represented by imaginary lines that form concentric circles centered on the wire (Figure 7-4).

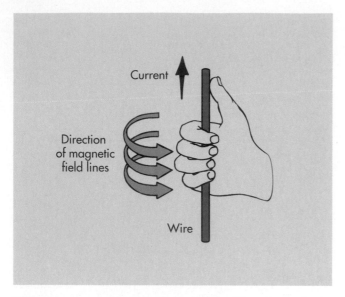

FIGURE 7-5 Determining the direction of the magnetic field around the wire using the right-hand rule.

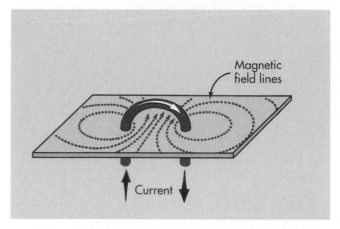

FIGURE 7-6 Magnetic field lines are concentrated on the inside of the loop.

The direction of the magnetic field lines can be determined by using the **right-hand rule.** Imagine gripping the wire with the right hand. If the thumb is pointed in the direction of the electric current, the fingers of your hand will then curl in the direction of the magnetic field lines (Figure 7-5). Similarly, the left hand is used if the thumb is pointed in the direction of electron flow, which is opposite to current.

The Solenoid

These same rules apply if the current is in a loop. Magnetic field lines form concentric circles around each tiny section of the wire. Because the wire is curved, however, these magnetic field lines overlap inside the loop. In particular, at the very center of the loop, all the field lines add together, making the magnetic field strong (Figure 7-6).

Stacking more loops on top of each other increases the intensity of the magnetic field running through the center or axis of the stack of loops. The magnetic field of a solenoid is concentrated through the center of the coil (Figure 7-7).

 A coil of wire is called a *solenoid.*

The magnetic field can further be intensified by wrapping the coil of wire around ferromagnetic material, such as iron. The iron core intensifies the magnetic field. In this case, almost all of the magnetic field lines are concentrated inside the iron core, escaping only near the ends of the coil. This type of device is called an **electromagnet** (Figure 7-8).

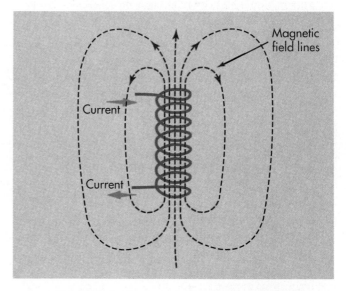

FIGURE 7-7 Magnetic field lines of a solenoid.

 An electromagnet is a current-carrying coil of wire wrapped around an iron core, which intensifies the magnetic field.

The magnetic field produced by an electromagnet is the same as that produced by a bar magnet. That is, if both were hidden from view behind a piece of paper, the pattern of magnetic field lines revealed by iron filings sprinkled on the paper surface would be the same. Of course, the advantage of the electromagnet is that its magnetic field can be adjusted or turned on and off simply by varying the current through its coil of wire.

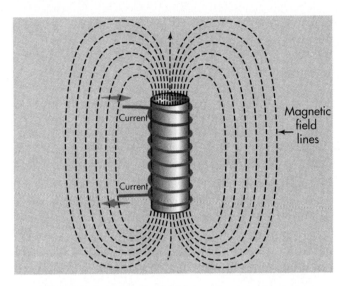

FIGURE 7-8 Magnetic field lines of an electromagnet.

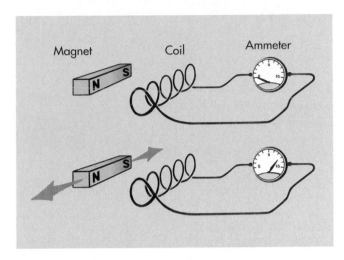

FIGURE 7-9 Schematic description of Faraday's experiment shows how a moving magnetic field induces an electric current.

ELECTROMAGNETIC INDUCTION

Oersted's experiment demonstrated that electricity can be used to generate magnetic fields. It is obvious, then, to wonder whether the reverse is true: can magnetic fields somehow be used to generate electricity? Michael Faraday, a self-educated British experimenter, found the answer to that question.

Faraday's Law

From a series of experiments, Faraday concluded that an electric current cannot be induced in a circuit merely by the presence of a magnetic field. For example, consider the situation illustrated in Figure 7-9. A coil of wire is connected to a current-measuring device called an **ammeter.** If a bar magnet were set next to the coil, the meter would indicate no current in the coil.

However, Faraday discovered that when the magnet is moved, the coiled wire does have a current as indicated by the ammeter. Therefore, to induce a current using a magnetic field, the magnetic field cannot be constant but must be changing.

 Electromagnetic induction: an electric current is induced in a circuit if some part of that circuit is in a changing magnetic field.

This observation is summarized in what is called Faraday's law, or the first law of electromagnetic induction.

The changing magnetic field can be produced in many ways. For example, a bar magnet or an electromagnet can be moved near a coil of wire. Conversely,

 Faraday's Law

The magnitude of the induced current depends on four factors:

1. The strength of the magnetic field
2. The velocity of the magnetic field as it moves past the conductor
3. The angle of the conductor to the magnetic field
4. The number of turns in the conductor

the magnet can be held stationary and the coil of wire moved near it.

Alternatively, there need be no physical motion. An electromagnet can be fixed near a coil of wire. If the current in the electromagnet is then either increased or decreased, its magnetic field will likewise change and induce a current in the coil.

A prime example of electromagnetic induction is radio reception (Figure 7-10). Radio emission consists of waves of electromagnetic radiation. Each wave has an oscillating electric field and an oscillating magnetic field. The oscillating magnetic field induces motion in electrons in the radio antennae, resulting in a radio signal. This signal is detected and decoded to produce sound.

The essential point in all these examples is that the intensity of the magnetic field at the wire must be changing to induce a current. If the magnetic field intensity is constant, there will be no induced current.

 Varying magnetic field intensity induces an electric current.

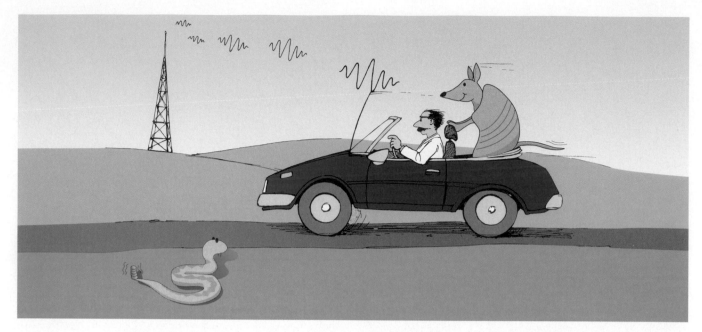

FIGURE 7-10 Radio reception is based on the principles of electromagnetic induction.

Lenz's Law

In 1834, a German scientist working in Russia, Heinrich Lenz, expanded on Faraday's work. He established the principle for determining the direction of the induced current. This principle is now known as the second law of electromagnetics.

 Lenz's law: the direction of induced electric current opposes the action that induces it.

This principle many seem a little confusing at first and is perhaps best illustrated by an example (Figure 7-11). Which direction is the current when the north pole of a magnet is pushed into a coil of wire? We know from the first law of electromagnetics that there is an induced current in the coil of wire.

We also know that a coil of wire with a current acts like a tiny magnet. One axis perpendicular to the coil will be a north pole and the other end will be a south pole, but which end will be which?

Lenz's law answers this question. The action that induces the current in the coil is the pushing of the north pole of the magnet into the coil. According to Lenz's law, to oppose this action, the coil of wire will induce a north magnetic field at the same end (since the coil's north pole repels, or *opposes,* the inward motion of the magnet's north pole). To induce a north magnetic pole at the same end of the coil of wire, the induced current must be as shown in Figure 7-11.

These electromagnetic laws govern the induction of electric currents by magnetic fields of changing intensity.

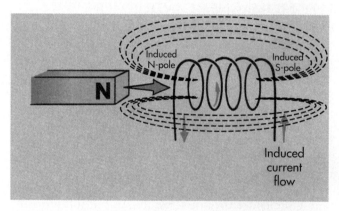

FIGURE 7-11 Demonstration of Lenz's law shows that the current induced in a coil by a moving magnet produces a magnetic field opposing the motion of the magnet.

There are two basic types of induction—**self-induction** and **mutual induction**—and these are fundamental to transformers, electric motors, and generators.

Self-Induction

If a constant voltage is supplied to a coil of wire, then a steady and relatively unimpeded current of electricity exists in the coil and the coil produces a constant magnetic field (Figure 7-12).

 A coil passes a steady and relatively unimpeded direct current but resists the passage of an alternating current because of self-induction in the coil.

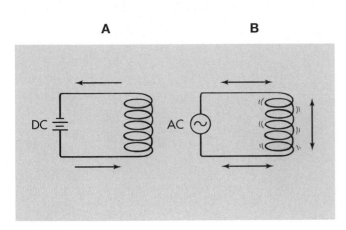

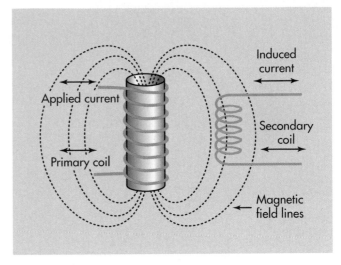

FIGURE 7-12 Demonstration of self-induction. **A,** A coil passes constant current unimpeded. **B,** It will resist the passage of a changing current because of self-induction.

FIGURE 7-13 Inducing a current in the secondary coil by mutual induction.

What will happen, however, if a varying source such as alternating current is connected to the coil? The current in the coil and the magnetic field produced by the coil will no longer be constant.

According to Lenz's law, this changing magnetic field induces an opposing action in the coil. In this case, the induced voltage will oppose the source voltage. If the source voltage increases, the induced-coil voltage opposes it by trying to reduce it. If, on the other hand, the source voltage is falling, then the induced-coil voltage will increase to oppose it.

This induction of an opposing voltage in a single coil by its own changing magnetic field is called *self induction.* The self-induction of AC circuit components such as **transformers** (read on!) is an important consideration in the design of x-ray imaging systems.

Mutual Induction

Faraday showed that it was not necessary to physically move a magnet near a coil to induce an electric current. All that is necessary is change in the intensity of the magnetic field. This can be accomplished by fixing an electromagnet near the coil and varying the current through the electromagnet (Figure 7-13).

 Mutual induction is the generation of an alternating current in a secondary coil by supplying an alternating current to the primary coil.

The varying current in the electromagnet creates a varying magnetic field, which induces a current in the coil when it passes through it. The first coil through which the varying current is passed is called the **primary coil.** The coil with the induced current is called the **secondary coil.**

The process of inducing a current through a secondary coil by passing a varying current through the primary coil is called **mutual induction.** Mutual induction is considered in more detail under the discussion of the transformer.

ELECTROMECHANICAL DEVICES

Electric motors and generators are practical applications of Oersted's and Faraday's experiments. In one experiment, an electric current produces a mechanical motion (the motion of the compass needle). This is the basis of the electric motor. In the other experiment, mechanical motion (the motion of a magnet near a coil of wire) induces electricity in a coil of wire. This is the principle on which the electric generator operates.

Electric Generator

Figure 7-14 shows the diagram of a simple electric generator. A coil of wire is placed in a strong magnetic field between two poles of a magnet. The coil is rotated by mechanical energy. The mechanical energy can be supplied by hand, by water flowing over a water wheel, or by steam flowing past the vanes of a turbine blade in an atomic power plant. Because the coil of wire is moving in the magnetic field, a current is induced in the coil of wire.

The induced current is not constant, however. It varies according to the orientation of the coil's wire in the magnetic field. The induced current flows first in one direction and then the other, following a sinusoidal pattern. Thus, this type of simple electric generator produces an **alternating current (AC).**

A **direct current (DC)** generator can be constructed by adding a simple device called a **commutator ring** (Figure 7-15). The commutator ring acts like a switch,

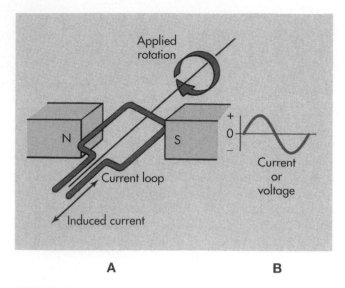

FIGURE 7-14 A, Simple electric generator. **B,** Its output waveform.

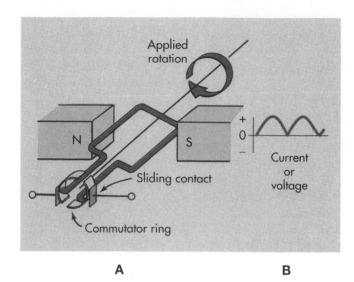

FIGURE 7-15 A, Direct current generator incorporates a commutator ring. **B,** Its output waveform.

changing the polarity of the contact on the loop of wire at precisely those contact points when the current through the loop is reversed. The resulting reversed current, out of the commutator ring assembly, varies in intensity but is always in the same direction.

The net effect of an electric generator is to convert mechanical energy into electrical energy. The conversion process is, of course, not 100% efficient because of frictional losses in the mechanical moving parts and heat losses caused by resistances in the electrical components.

Electric Motor

A simple electric motor has basically the same components as an electric generator (Figure 7-16). In this case, however, electric energy is supplied to the current loop to produce a mechanical motion—that is, a rotation of the loop in the magnetic field.

When a current is passed through the wire loop, a magnetic field is produced, making the loop behave like a tiny electromagnet. Being free to turn, the electromagnet-current loop rotates as it attempts to align itself with the stronger magnetic field produced by the external bar magnet.

Just as the current loop becomes aligned with the external magnetic field, the commutator ring switches the direction of current through the loop and therefore reverses the coil's required alignment.

Because of the reversal in current direction, the electromagnet is no longer aligned with the magnetic field of the bar magnet; it is now opposed to it. The electromagnet-current loop rotates 180° in an attempt to realign itself once again with the bar magnet field. As the electromagnet again nears alignment, the commutator

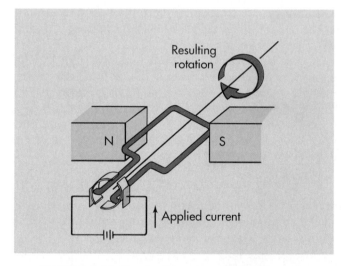

FIGURE 7-16 Simple direct current electric motor.

switches the direction of current and forces the loop to rotate again.

The electromagnet-current loop is never quite able to align itself with the magnetic field of the bar magnet. The net result is that the current loop rotates continuously.

A practical electric motor uses many turns of wire for the current loop and many bar magnets to create the external magnetic field. The principle of operation, however, is the same. This type of electric motor is called a **direct current motor.**

The type of motor used in x-ray tubes is an **induction motor** (Figure 7-17). In this type of motor the rotating **rotor** is still a series of wire loops; however, the external

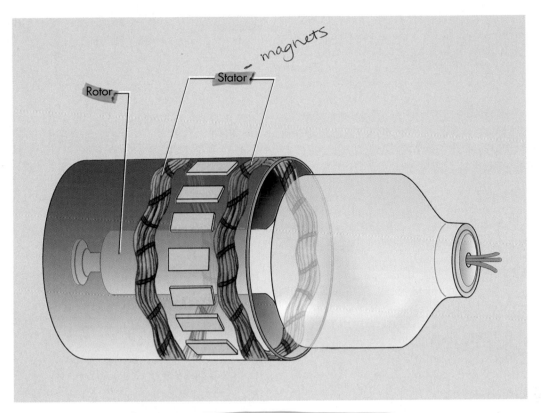

Rotor   Stator

FIGURE 7-17 Principal parts of an induction motor.

magnetic field is supplied by several fixed electromagnets called **stators**.

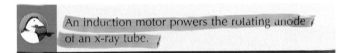

An induction motor powers the rotating anode of an x-ray tube.

No electric current is passed to the rotor. Instead, current is produced in the rotor windings by induction. The electromagnets surrounding the rotor are energized in sequence, producing a changing magnetic field. The induced current produced in the rotor windings generates a magnetic field.

Just as in a conventional electric motor, this magnetic field attempts to align itself with the magnetic field of the external electromagnets. Because these electromagnets are being energized in sequence, the rotor begins to rotate, trying to bring its magnetic field into alignment.

The result is the same as in a conventional electric motor; that is, the rotor rotates continuously. The difference, however, is that the electric energy is supplied to the external magnets rather than the rotor windings.

THE TRANSFORMER

Both electric motors and generators make use of interacting electromagnetic fields produced by electric currents. They convert mechanical energy to electrical energy (the generator) or electrical energy to mechanical energy (the motor).

Another device that uses the interacting magnetic fields produced by changing electric currents is the transformer. However, the transformer does not convert one form of energy to another but rather transforms electric potential and current into higher or lower intensity.

Recall from the discussion of mutual induction that if two coils are placed near each other and a changing current is applied to one of them (the primary), then a current will be induced in the other coil (the secondary). Recall also that placing a core of magnetic material in the center of the coil greatly increases the strength of the magnetic field passing through its center. The magnetic field lines tend to be concentrated in the ferromagnetic material of the core.

A transformer changes the intensity of alternating voltage and current by mutual induction.

Imagine, however, that this ferromagnetic core is bent around so that it forms a continuous loop (Figure 7-18). There are no end surfaces from which the ferromagnetic field lines can escape. Therefore, the magnetic field tends to be confined to the loop of magnetic core material.

If the secondary coil is then wound around the other side of this loop of core material, almost all the magnetic field produced by the primary coil will also pass through the center of the secondary coil. Thus, there is a good **coupling** between the magnetic field produced by the primary coil and the secondary coil. A changing current in the primary coil induces a changing current in the secondary coil. This type of device is called a transformer.

Because a transformer operates on the principle of mutual induction, it will only operate with a changing electric current (AC). A direct current applied to the primary coil will induce no current in the secondary coil.

The Transformer Law

The transformer is used to change the magnitude of voltage and current in an AC circuit. This change is *directly proportional* to the ratio of the number of turns (windings) of the secondary coil (N_s) to the number of turns in the primary coil (N_p). If there are 10 turns on the secondary coil for every turn on the primary coil, then the voltage generated in the secondary circuit (V_s) will be 10 times the voltage supplied to the primary circuit (V_p). Mathematically, the transformer law is represented as follows:

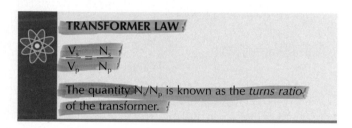

TRANSFORMER LAW

$$\frac{V_s}{V_p} = \frac{N_s}{N_p}$$

The quantity N_s/N_p is known as the *turns ratio* of the transformer.

Question: The secondary side of a transformer has 300,000 turns; the primary side has 600 turns. What is the turns ratio?

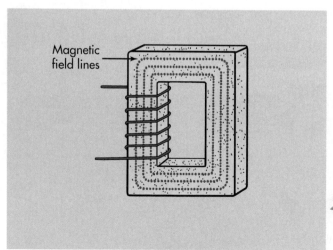

FIGURE 7-18 An electromagnet that incorporates a closed iron core produces a closed magnetic field primarily confined to the core.

Answer: $N_s = 300,000$ $N_p = 600$

$$\text{Turns ratio} = \frac{N_s}{N_p}$$
$$= 300,000/600$$
$$= 500:1$$

The voltage change across the transformer is proportional to the turns ratio. A transformer with a turns ratio greater than 1 is **a step-up transformer** because the voltage is increased or stepped up from the primary side to the secondary side. When the turns ratio is less than 1, the transformer is a step-down transformer.

As the voltage changes across a transformer, the current (I) changes also; the transformer law may also be written:

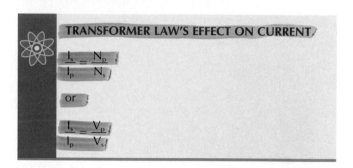

TRANSFORMER LAW'S EFFECT ON CURRENT

$$\frac{I_s}{I_p} = \frac{N_p}{N_s}$$

or

$$\frac{I_s}{I_p} = \frac{V_p}{V_s}$$

Question: The turns ratio of a filament transformer is 0.125. What is the filament current if the current through the primary winding is 0.8 A?

Answer:
$$\frac{I_s}{I_p} = \frac{N_p}{N_s}$$

$$I_s = I_p \left(\frac{N_p}{N_s} \right)$$

$$= (0.8\ A) \left(\frac{1}{0.125} \right)$$

$$= 6.4\ A$$
$$= 6400\ mA$$

The change in current across a transformer is in the opposite direction from the voltage change but in the same proportion: an inverse relationship. For example, if the voltage is doubled, the current is halved.

In a step-up transformer, the current on the secondary side (I_s) is smaller than the current on the primary side (I_p). In a step-down transformer, the secondary current is larger than the primary current.

The three main causes of transformer inefficiency are resistance, hysteresis, and eddy currents.

The transformer is not 100% efficient. However, losses in power from the primary side to the secondary side are considered negligible. Nevertheless, such losses have three principal causes.

Electric current in the copper wire experiences **resistance** that results in heat generation. The alternate reversal of the magnetic field caused by the alternating current causes an additional resistance known as **hysteresis.** Finally, **eddy currents** can be formed within the magnet as predicted by Lenz's law. These currents oppose the magnetic field that induced them, creating a loss of transformer efficiency.

Question: There are 125 turns on the primary side of a transformer and 90,000 turns on the secondary side. If 110 V AC is supplied to the primary winding, what is the voltage induced in the secondary winding?

Answer: $\dfrac{V_s}{V_p} = \dfrac{N_s}{N_p}$

$$V_s = V_p \left(\frac{N_s}{N_p} \right)$$

$$= (110 \text{ V}) \left(\frac{90,000}{125} \right)$$

$$= (110)(720) \text{ V}$$

$$= 79,200 \text{ V}$$

$$= 79.2 \text{ kV}$$

Types of Transformers

There are many ways to construct a transformer (Figure 7-19). The type of transformer discussed thus far, built about a square core of ferromagnetic material, is called a **closed-core transformer** (Figure 7-19, *A*).

The ferromagnetic core is not a single piece but rather is built up of laminated layers of iron. This layering helps reduce energy losses caused by eddy currents in the core produced by the transformer's changing magnetic field.

Another type of transformer is the **autotransformer** (Figure 7-19, *B*). It consists of an iron core with only one winding of wire about it. This single winding acts as both the primary and the secondary winding.

The autotransformer is based on self-induction rather than mutual induction. Connections are made at different points on the coil for both the primary and the secondary sides.

The autotransformer has one winding and varies voltage and current by self-induction.

An autotransformer is generally smaller and because both the primary and the secondary sides are connected to the same wire, its use is generally restricted to cases in which only a small step-up or step-down in voltage is required. Thus, an autotransformer would not be suitable for use as the high-voltage transformer in an x-ray imaging system.

The third type of transformer is the **shell-type transformer** (Figure 7-19, *C*). This type of transformer confines even more of the magnet field lines of the primary winding because the secondary is wrapped around it and there are essentially two closed cores. This type is more efficient than the closed-core transformer. Most currently used transformers are shell-type.

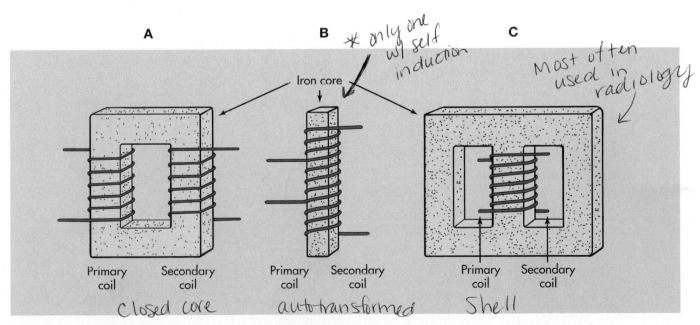

FIGURE 7-19 Type of transformers. **A,** Closed-core transformer. **B,** Autotransformer. **C,** Shell-type transformer.

SUMMARY

Alessandro Volta's development of the battery as a source of electric potential energy prompted further investigations of electric and magnetic fields. Hans Oersted demonstrated that electricity can be used to generate magnetic fields. It was Michael Faraday who observed the current in a changing magnetic field and described the first law of electromagnetics (Faraday's law). Heinrich Lenz expanded on Faraday's experiments. The second law of electromagnetics is Lenz's law, which states that the induced current is opposite to the action that causes it.

If current through a wire is steady or direct, a constant magnetic field is created around the wire. If, however, the current changes direction as in alternating current (AC), the magnetic field oscillates. Self-induction and mutual induction are the two forms of electromagnetic induction.

The practical applications of the laws of electromagnetism appear in the electric motor (electric current produces mechanical motion), the electric generator (mechanical motion produces electric current), and the transformer (alternating electric current and electric potential are transformed in intensity). The transformer law describes how electric current and voltage change from the primary coil to the secondary coil.

CHALLENGE QUESTIONS

1. Define or otherwise identify:
   a. Insulator
   b. Electromotive force
   c. Solenoid
   d. Mutual induction
   e. Commutator ring
   f. Autotransformer
   g. Ammeter
   h. Turns ratio
   i. Shell-type transformer
   j. Electric potential
2. State the two principal laws of electromagnetics.
3. A transformer has 220,000 turns on the secondary winding and 200 turns on the primary winding. If 220 V are supplied to the primary side, what is the voltage on the secondary side?
4. If 30 A are supplied to the primary side of the transformer in question 4, what is the secondary current?
5. What is the electric power resulting from the 220 V and 30 A supplied to the transformer in question 4? From the information given, will the power be the same on the secondary side?
6. A portable x-ray imager is designed to operate on conventional 110 V AC power. Its maximum capacity is 110 kV and 100 mA. What is the turns ratio of the high-voltage transformer?
7. What should be the primary current in question 6 to produce a secondary current of 100 mA?
8. What is the current supplied to an x-ray tube connected to a filament transformer with a turns ratio of 1:15 when the current supplied to the filament transformer is 30 A?
9. What is the difference between the right-hand rule and the left-hand rule?
10. What is a semiconductor and how has it affected modern life?
11. State Ohm's law and describe how it is used.
12. A kitchen toaster draws a current of 2.5 A. If the household voltage is 110 V, what is the electric resistance of the toaster?
13. An x-ray imager draws a current of 80 A and is supplied with 220 V. How much power does it consume?
14. What are the characteristics of a solenoid?
15. Where might one find an electromagnet in everyday life?
16. Describe the process of mutual induction.
17. Draw and label the parts of an electric motor.
18. Explain how an electric generator works.
19. List the components of an induction motor and describe how they work.
20. Describe three types of transformers.

PART II

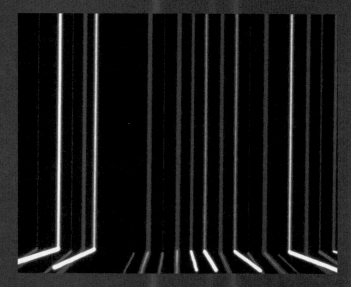

THE
X-RAY BEAM

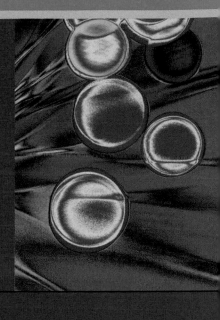

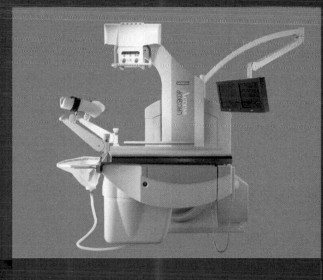

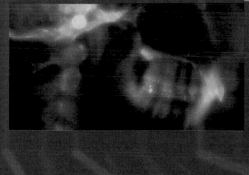

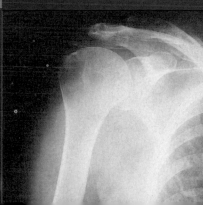

CHAPTER

8

The X-Ray Imaging System

OBJECTIVES

At the completion of this chapter, the student should be able to do the following:

1. Identify the components of the operating console positioned outside the x-ray examination room
2. Explain the operation of the high-voltage generator, including the filament transformer and the rectifiers
3. Relate the important differences among single-phase, three-phase, and high-frequency power
4. Identify the voltage ripple associated with various high-voltage generators
5. Discuss the importance of voltage ripple to x-ray quantity and quality
6. Define the power rating of an x-ray imaging system

OUTLINE

WHEN FAST-MOVING electrons slam into a metal object, x-rays are produced. The kinetic energy of the electrons is transformed into electromagnetic energy. The function of the x-ray imaging system is to provide a controlled flow of electrons intense enough to produce an x-ray beam appropriate for imaging.

The three main components of an x-ray imaging system are (1) the x-ray tube, (2) the operating console, and (3) the high-voltage generator. The x-ray tube is discussed in Chapter 9. This chapter describes the components of the operating console. The operating console is used to control the voltage applied to the x-ray tube, the current through the x-ray tube, and the exposure time.

This chapter also discusses the high-voltage generator in its many forms. The high-voltage generator contains the high-voltage step-up transformer and the rectification circuit. The final section of this chapter combines all components into a single complete circuit diagram.

The many different types of x-ray imaging systems are usually identified according to either the energy of the x-rays they produce or the purpose for which those x-rays are intended. Diagnostic x-ray imaging systems come in many different shapes and sizes, some of which are shown in Figure 8-1. These systems are usually operated at voltages of 25 to 150 kVp and at tube currents of 100 to 1200 mA.

The general purpose x-ray examination room usually contains a radiographic imaging system and a fluoroscopic imaging system with an image intensifier. The fluoroscopic x-ray tube is usually located under the examining table; the radiographic x-ray tube is attached to an overhead movable crane assembly that permits easy positioning of the tube and aiming of the x-ray beam. Refer back to Chapter 1, Figure 1-9.

This type of equipment can be used for nearly all radiographic and fluoroscopic examinations. Rooms with a fluoroscope and two or more overhead radiographic tubes are used for special angiointerventional applications.

Regardless of the type of x-ray imaging system, a patient-supporting examination table is required (Figure 8-2). The examination table may be flat or curved but must be uniform in thickness and as transparent to x-rays as possible. Carbon fiber tabletops are strong and absorb little x-radiation. This contributes to reduced patient dose.

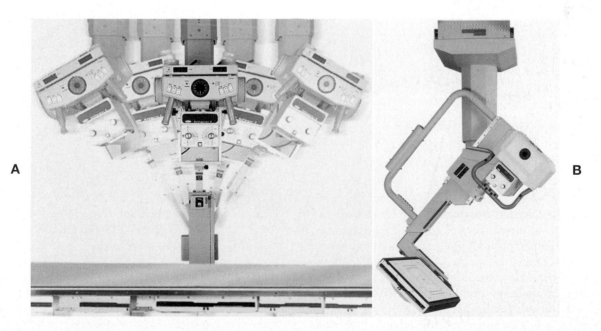

A   B

FIGURE 8-1 Types of diagnostic x-ray imaging systems. **A,** Tomographic. (Courtesy Fischer Imaging.) **B,** Trauma. (Courtesy Fischer Imaging.)

Continued

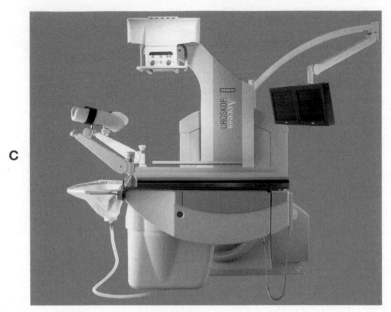

C

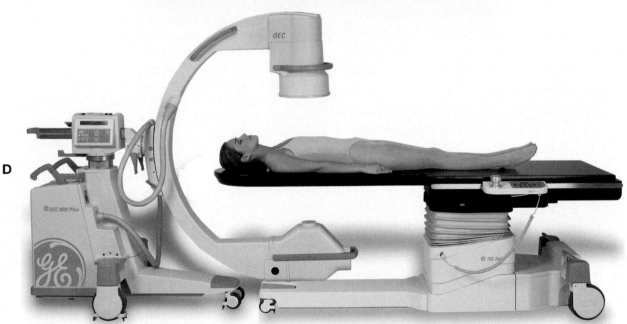

D

FIGURE 8-1, cont'd Types of diagnostic x-ray imaging systems. **C,** Urologic. (Courtesy Siemens Medical Systems.) **D,** Mobile. (Courtesy General Electric Medical Systems.)

Most tabletops are **floating**—easily unlocked and moved by the radiologic technologist—or motor-driven. Just under the tabletop is an opening to hold a thin tray for a cassette and grid. If the table is used for fluoroscopy, the tray must move to the foot of the table and the opening must be automatically shielded for radiation protection with a **Bucky slot cover** (see Chapter 39). Fluoroscopic tables tilt and are identified by their degree of tilt. For example, a 90/30 table would tilt 90° to the foot side and 30° to the head side (Figure 8-3).

Question: How far below horizontal will a patient's head go on a 90/15 fluoroscopic table?

Answer: 15° below horizontal

Regardless of its design, every x-ray imaging system has three principal parts: the **x-ray tube** (see Chapter 9), the **operating console,** and the **high-voltage generator.** In some types of x-ray imaging systems, such as dental and portable machines, these three components are housed compactly. With most systems, however, the x-ray tube

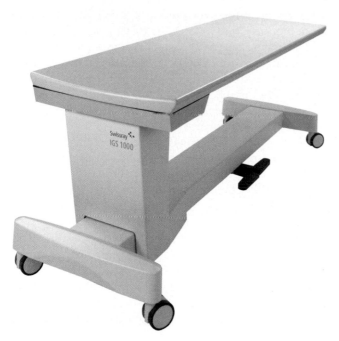

FIGURE 8-2 Flexible and mobile patient examination table. (Courtesy Swissray.)

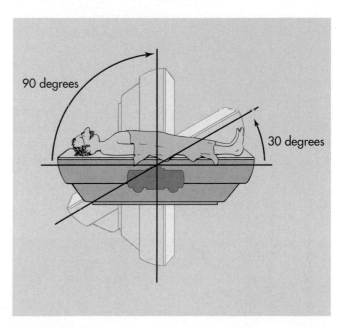

FIGURE 8-3 A fluoroscopic table is identified by its head and foot tilt.

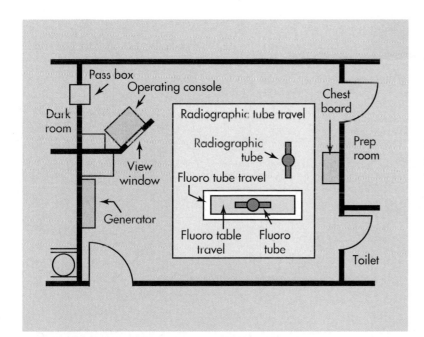

FIGURE 8-4 Plan drawing of a general-purpose x-ray examination room, showing locations of the various x-ray apparatus. Chapter 39 considers the layout of such rooms in greater detail.

is located in the examination room and the operating console is located in an adjoining room, with a protective barrier separating the two. The protective barrier must have a window for viewing the patient during the examination.

The high-voltage generator may be housed in an equipment cabinet positioned against a wall. The high-voltage generator is always close to the x-ray tube, usually in the examination room. A few installations take advantage of false ceilings and place these generators out of sight above the examination room.

Newer generator designs that use high-frequency circuits require even less space. Figure 8-4 is a plan drawing of a conventional, general-purpose x-ray examination room.

OPERATING CONSOLE

The part of the x-ray imaging system most familiar to the radiologic technologist is the operating console. The operating console allows the radiologic technologist to control the x-ray tube current and voltage so that the useful x-ray beam is of proper quantity and quality (Figure 8-5).

Quantity refers to the number of x-rays or the intensity of the x-ray beam. Quantity is usually expressed in milliroentgens (mR) or milliroentgens/milliampere-second (mR/mAs). Quality refers to the penetrability of the x-ray beam and is expressed in kilovolt peak (kVp) or, more precisely, half value layer (HVL) (see Chapter 11).

The operating console usually provides for control of line compensation, kVp, mA, and exposure time. Meters are provided for monitoring kVp, mA, and exposure time. Some consoles also provide a meter for mAs. Imaging systems that incorporate AEC may have separate controls for mAs.

All the electric circuits connecting the meters and controls on the operating console are at low voltage to minimize the possibility of hazardous shock. Figure 8-6 is a simplified schematic diagram for a typical operating console. A look inside an operating console will indicate how simplified this schematic drawing is!

Most operating consoles are based on computer technology. Controls and meters are digital, and techniques are selected with a touch screen. Numerical technique selection is sometimes replaced by icons indicating body part, size, and shape. Many of the features are automatic, but the radiologic technologist must know their purpose and proper use.

Line Compensation

Most x-ray imaging systems are designed to operate on 220 V power, although some can operate on 110 V or 440 V. Unfortunately, electric power companies are not capable of providing 220 V accurately and continuously.

Because of variations in power distribution to the hospital and in power consumption by the various sections of the hospital, the voltage provided to an x-ray unit may easily vary by as much as 5%. Such variation

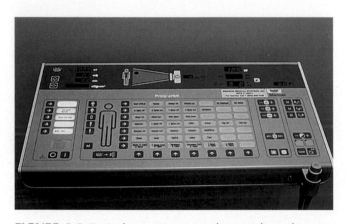

FIGURE 8-5 Typical operating console. Number of meters and controls depends on the complexity of the console.

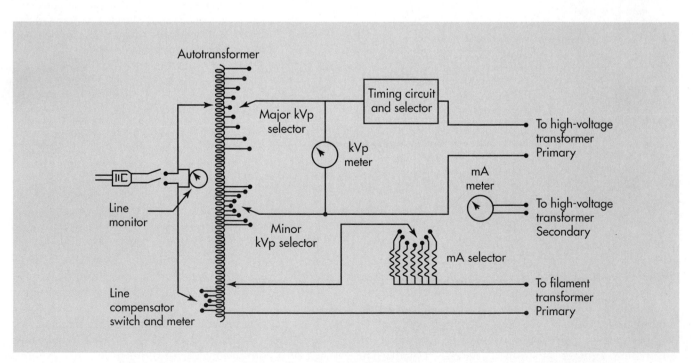

FIGURE 8-6 Circuit diagram of the operating console, identifying the controls and meters.

in supply voltage results in a large variation in the x-ray beam, which does not permit consistent production of high-quality images.

The line compensator incorporates a meter to measure the voltage provided to the x-ray imaging system and a control to adjust that voltage to precisely 220 V. The control is usually multistation and wired to the autotransformer. Older units required technologists to adjust the supply voltage while observing a line voltage meter. Today's x-ray imaging systems have automatic line compensation and hence have no meter.

AUTOTRANSFORMER

The power supplied to the x-ray imaging system is delivered first to the autotransformer. The voltage supplied from the autotransformer to the high-voltage transformer is controlled but variable. It is much safer and easier to select a low voltage and then increase it than to increase a low voltage to the kilovolt level and then vary its magnitude.

The autotransformer has a single winding and is designed to supply a precise voltage to the filament circuit and to the high-voltage circuit of the x-ray imaging system.

The autotransformer works on the principle of electromagnetic induction but is very different from the conventional transformer. It has only one winding and one core. This single winding has a number of connec-

tions along its length (Figure 8-7). Two of the connections, A and A' as shown in the figure, conduct the input power to the autotransformer and are called primary connections.

Some of the secondary connections, such as C in the figure, are located closer to one end of the winding than the primary connections. This allows the autotransformer to increase voltage. Other connections, such as E in the figure, allow a decrease in voltage. The autotransformer can be designed to step up voltage to approximately twice the input voltage value.

Because the autotransformer operates as an induction device, the voltage it receives (the primary voltage) and the voltage it provides (the secondary voltage) are related directly to the number of turns of the transformer enclosed by the respective connections. The **autotransformer law** is the same as the transformer law.

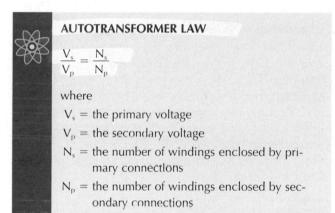

AUTOTRANSFORMER LAW

$$\frac{V_s}{V_p} = \frac{N_s}{N_p}$$

where

V_s = the primary voltage

V_p = the secondary voltage

N_s = the number of windings enclosed by primary connections

N_p = the number of windings enclosed by secondary connections

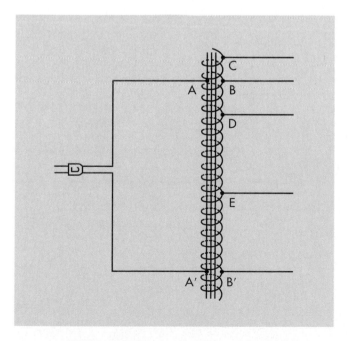

FIGURE 8-7 Simplified view of an autotransformer.

Question: If the autotransformer in Figure 8-7 is supplied with 220 V to the primary connections AA', which enclose 500 windings, what is the secondary voltage across BB' (500 windings), CB' (700 windings), and DE (200 windings)?

Answer: $BB' V_s = V_p \left(\frac{N_s}{N_p}\right)$

$= (220 \text{ V})\left(\frac{500}{500}\right) = (220 \text{ V})$

$CB': V_s = (220 \text{ V})\left(\frac{700}{500}\right)$

$= (220 \text{ V})(1.4) = 308 \text{ V}$

$DE: V_s = (220 \text{ V})\left(\frac{200}{500}\right)$

$= (220 \text{ V})(0.4) = 88 \text{ V}$

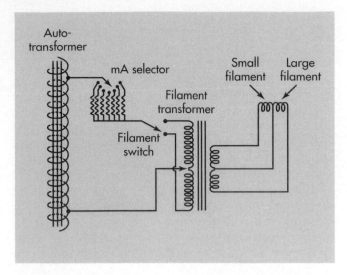

FIGURE 8-8 Filament circuit for dual-filament x-ray tube.

Adjustment of Kilovolt Peak (kVp)

Some older x-ray operating consoles have adjustment controls labeled **major kVp** and **minor kVp;** by selecting a combination of these controls, the radiologic technologist can provide precisely the required peak kilovoltage. The minor peak kilovoltage adjustment "fine tunes" the selected technique. The major peak kilovoltage adjustment and the minor peak kilovoltage adjustment represent two separate series of connections on the autotransformer.

 kVp determines the quality of the x-ray beam.

Appropriate connections can be selected with an adjustment knob, a push button, or a touch screen. If the primary voltage to the autotransformer is 220 V, the output of the autotransformer is usually controllable from about 100 to 400 V, depending on the design of the autotransformer. This low voltage from the autotransformer becomes the input to the high-voltage step-up transformer that increases the voltage to the chosen kilovoltage.

Question: An autotransformer connected to a 440 V supply contains 4000 turns, all of which are enclosed by the primary connections. If 2300 turns are enclosed by secondary connections, what is the voltage supplied to the high-voltage generator?

Answer: $V_s = V_p \left(\dfrac{N_s}{N_p} \right)$

$= (400 \text{ V}) \left(\dfrac{2300}{4000} \right)$

$= (440 \text{ V})(0.575)$

$= 253 \text{ V}$

The kVp meter is placed across the output terminals of the autotransformer and therefore actually reads voltage, not kVp. The scale of the kVp meter, however, registers kilovolts because of the known multiplication factor of the turns ratio.

On most operating consoles the kVp meter registers even though no exposure is being made and the circuit has no current. This type of meter is known as a **prereading kVp meter.** It allows the voltage to be monitored before an exposure.

Control of Milliamperage (mA)

The x-ray tube current, crossing from cathode to anode, is measured in milliamperes (mA). The number of electrons emitted by the filament is determined by the temperature of the filament.

The filament temperature is in turn controlled by the filament current, which is measured in amperes (A). As filament current increases, the filament becomes hotter and more electrons are released by thermionic emission. Filaments normally operate at currents of 3 to 6 A.

 Thermionic emission is the release of electrons from a heated filament.

X-ray tube current is controlled through a separate circuit called the filament circuit (Figure 8-8). Connections on the autotransformer provide voltage for the filament circuit. Precision resistors are used to reduce this voltage to a value corresponding to the selected milliamperage.

X-ray tube current normally is not continuously variable. The precision resistors result in fixed stations that provide tube currents of 100, 200, 300 mA, and higher.

The falling load generator constitutes an exception (see Chapter 18). In a falling load generator, the exposure begins at maximum mA, which drops as the anode heats. The result is minimum exposure time.

 The product of x-ray tube current (mA) and exposure (s) is mAs, which is also electrostatic charge (C).

Question: An image is made at 400 mA and an exposure time of 100 ms. Express this in mAs and as the total number of electrons.

Answer: 100 ms = 0.1 s

(400 mA)(0.1 s) = 40 mAs

40 mAs = (40 mC/s)(s) [remember,

1 A = 1 C/s]

$= 40 \text{ mC}$

$= (40 \times 10^{-3} \text{ C})(6.3 \times 10^{18} \text{ e}^- / \text{C})$

$= 252 \times 10^{15} \text{ e}^-$

$= 2.52 \times 10^{17} \text{ electrons}$

The voltage from the mA selector switch is then delivered to the filament transformer. The filament transformer is a step-down transformer; therefore, the voltage supplied to the filament is lower (by a factor equal to the turns ratio) than the voltage supplied to the filament transformer. Similarly, the current is increased across the filament transformer in proportion to the turns ratio.

Question: A filament transformer with a turns ratio of 1/10 provides 6.2 A to the filament. What is the current through the primary coil of the filament transformer?

Answer: $\dfrac{I_p}{I_s} = \dfrac{N_s}{N_p}$ where I_p = primary current,

I_s = secondary current and $\dfrac{N_s}{N_p}$ = turns ratio

$I_p = I\left(\dfrac{N_s}{N_p}\right)$

$= (6.2)\left(\dfrac{1}{10}\right)$

$= 0.62$ A

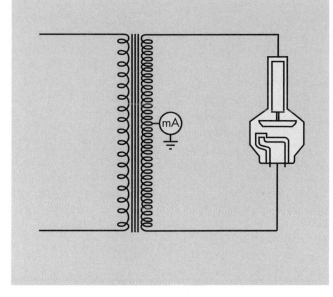

FIGURE 8-9 The mA meter is in the x-ray tube circuit at a center tap of the output of the high-voltage step-up transformer. This ensures electrical safety.

X-ray tube current is monitored with an mA meter that must be placed in the tube circuit. The mA meter is connected at the center of the secondary winding of the high-voltage step-up transformer. The secondary voltage is alternating at 60 Hz such that the center of this winding is always at zero volts (Figure 8-9).

In this way, no part of the meter is in contact with the high voltage and the meter may be safely put on the operating console. Sometimes this meter allows for variations such that mAs can be monitored in addition to mA.

EXPOSURE TIMERS

For any given radiographic examination, the number of x-rays reaching the image receptor is directly related to both the x-ray tube current and the time that the tube is energized. X-ray operating consoles provide a wide selection of x-ray beam-on times and, when used in conjunction with the appropriate mA station, provide an even wider selection of values for mAs.

Question: A KUB examination (radiography of the *k*idneys, *u*reters, and *b*ladder) calls for 62 kVp, 80 mAs. If the radiologic technologist selects the 200 mA station, what exposure time should be used?

Answer: $\dfrac{80 \text{ mAs}}{200 \text{ mA}} = 0.4$ s or 2/5 s or 400 ms

Question: A lateral cerebral angiogram calls for 92 kVp, 90 mAs. If the generator has a 1000 mA capacity, what is the shortest exposure time possible?

Answer: $\dfrac{90 \text{ mAs}}{1000 \text{ mA}} = 0.09$ s or 90 ms

The timer circuit is separate from the other main circuits of the x-ray imaging system. It consists of a mechanical or electronic device whose action is to "make" and "break" the high voltage across the x-ray tube. This is nearly always done on the **primary side** of the high-voltage transformer, where the voltage is lower.

There are five types of timing circuits. Four are controlled by the radiologic technologist and one is automatic. After studying this section, try to identify the types of timers on the equipment you use.

Mechanical Timers. Mechanical timers are very simple devices that are no longer used. The mechanical timer operates by clockwork. A preset exposure time is dialed by turning a knob that winds a spring. When the exposure button is depressed, the spring is released and unwinds. *shortest time 200 ms.*

Synchronous Timers. In the United States, electric current is supplied at a frequency of 60 Hz. In Europe, Latin America, and other parts of the world, the frequency is 50 Hz. A special type of electric motor, known as a synchronous motor, is a precision device designed to drive a shaft at precisely 60 revolutions per second (rps). In some x-ray imaging systems, synchronous motors are used as timing mechanisms.

X-ray imaging systems with synchronous timers are recognizable because the minimum exposure time possible is 1/60 s (17 ms) and timing intervals increase by multiples thereof, such as 1/30, 1/20, and so on. Synchronous timers cannot be used for serial exposures because they must be reset after each exposure, which even when done automatically requires too much time.

Electronic Timers. Electronic timers are the most sophisticated, most complicated, and most accurate of the x-ray exposure timers. Electronic timers consist of rather complex circuitry based on the time required to charge a capacitor through a variable resistance.

Electronic timers allow a wide range of time intervals to be selected and are accurate to intervals as small as 1 ms. Because they can be used for rapid serial exposures, they are particularly suitable for angiointerventional procedures.

 Most exposure timers are electronic and controlled by a microprocessor.

mAs Timers. Most x-ray apparatus are designed for accurate control of tube current and exposure time. However, the product of mA and time—mAs—determines the number of x-rays emitted and, therefore, the optical density of the image. A special kind of electronic timer, called an mAs timer, monitors the product of mA and exposure time and terminates the exposure when the desired mAs value is attained.

The mAs timer is usually designed to provide the highest safe tube current for the shortest exposure for any mAs selected. Since the mAs timer must monitor the actual tube current, it is located on the secondary side of the high-voltage transformer.

 mAs timers are used on falling-load and capacitor discharge imaging systems.

Automatic Exposure Control. The automatic exposure control (AEC) requires a special understanding on the part of the radiologic technologist. The AEC is a device that measures the quantity of radiation reaching the image receptor. It automatically terminates the exposure when the image receptor has received enough radiation to provide the required optical density. Figure 8-10 shows two types of AEC design.

The type of AEC used by most manufacturers incorporates a flat, parallel plate ionization chamber positioned between the patient and the image receptor. The chamber is made radiolucent so that it will not interfere with the radiographic image. Ionization within the chamber creates a charge calibrated to produce a given optical density on the radiograph. When the appropriate charge has been reached, the exposure is terminated.

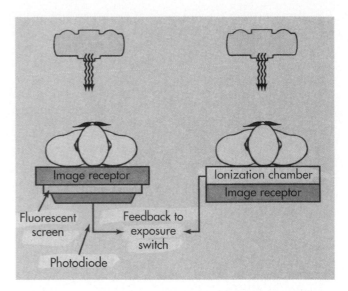

FIGURE 8-10 Automatic exposure control (AEC) terminates the x-ray exposure at the desired film optical density. This is done with an ionization chamber or photodiode detector assembly.

When an AEC x-ray imaging system is installed, it must be calibrated. This calls for making exposures of a phantom and adjusting the AEC for the range of diagnostic optical densities required for a quality image. The service engineer usually takes care of this calibration.

Once the AEC is in clinical operation, the radiologic technologist selects the desired optical density, which then sets the appropriate mA and kVp. At the same time, the exposure timer is set to the backup time. When the electric charge from the ionization chamber reaches a preset level, a signal is returned to the operating console, where the exposure is terminated.

The AEC is now widely used and often is provided in addition to an electronic timer. The AEC mode requires particular care, especially in examinations using low kVp such as mammography. Because of varying tissue thickness and composition, the AEC may not respond properly at low kVp, which can result in varying optical density.

When radiographs are taken in the AEC mode, the electronic timer should be set to 1.5 times the expected exposure time as a backup timer in case the AEC fails to terminate. This precaution should be followed for the protection of the patient and the x-ray tube. Many units automatically set this precaution.

Exposure timers on x-ray imaging systems must function properly and accurately. Inaccurate or malfunctioning exposure timers result in poor images, retakes, and unnecessary patient exposure.

Solid-state radiation detectors are now used for exposure-timer checks (Figure 8-11). These devices operate with a very accurate internal clock based on a

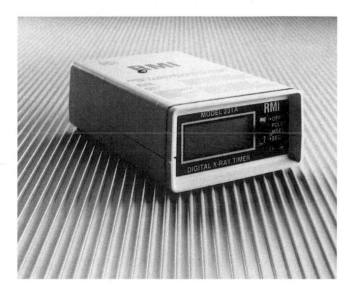

FIGURE 8-11 Solid-state radiation detectors are used to check timer accuracy. (Courtesy Gammex RMI.)

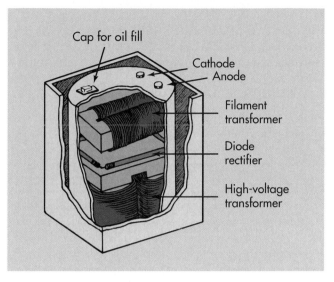

FIGURE 8-12 Cutaway view of a typical high-voltage generator, showing oil-immersed diodes and transformers.

quartz-crystal oscillator. They can measure exposure times as short as 1 ms and, when used with an oscilloscope, can display the radiation waveform.

HIGH-VOLTAGE GENERATOR

The high-voltage generator of an x-ray imaging system is responsible for increasing the output voltage from the autotransformer to the kVp necessary for x-ray production. A cutaway view of a typical high-voltage generator is shown in Figure 8-12. Although some heat is generated in the high-voltage section and is conducted to oil, the oil is used primarily for electrical insulation.

 The high-voltage generator contains three primary parts: the *high-voltage transformer,* the *filament transformer* (discussed previously), and *rectifiers.*

High-Voltage Transformer

The high voltage transformer is a step-up transformer; that is, the secondary voltage is higher than the primary voltage because the number of secondary windings is higher than the number of primary windings. The ratio of the number of secondary windings to the number of primary windings is called the **turns ratio** (see Chapter 7). The voltage increase is proportional to the turns ratio, according to the transformer law (also discussed in Chapter 7). Also, the current is reduced proportionately.

The turns ratio of a high-voltage transformer is usually between 500:1 and 1000:1. Since **transformers operate only on alternating current,** the voltage waveform on both sides of a high-voltage transformer is sinusoidal

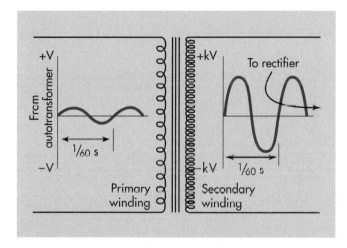

FIGURE 8-13 Voltage induced in the secondary winding of a high-voltage step-up transformer is alternating like the primary voltage but has a higher value.

(Figure 8-13). The only difference between the primary and secondary waveforms is their **amplitude.** The primary voltage is measured in volts (V), and the secondary voltage is measured in kilovolt peak (kVp). The primary current is measured in amperes (A), and the secondary current is measured in milliamperes (mA).

Question: The turns ratio of a high-voltage transformer is 700:1 and the supply voltage is peaked at 120 V. What is the secondary voltage supplied to the x-ray tube?

Answer: (120 Vp)(700:1) = 84,000 Vp
                    = 84 kVp

Voltage Rectification

The current from a common wall plug is 60 Hz AC. The current changes direction 120 times each second. However, an x-ray tube requires a DC current, that is, electron flow in only one direction. Therefore, some means must be provided for converting AC to DC.

 Rectification is the process of converting AC to DC.

The electronic device that allows current flow in only one direction is a **rectifier.** Although transformers operate with alternating current, x-ray tubes must be provided with direct current. X-rays are produced by the acceleration of electrons from the cathode to the anode and cannot be produced by electrons flowing in the reverse direction, from anode to cathode.

Reversal of electron flow would be disastrous for the x-ray tube. The construction of the cathode assembly is such that it could not withstand the tremendous heat generated by such operation even if the anode could emit electrons thermionically. If the electron flow is to be only in the cathode-to-anode direction, the secondary voltage of the high-voltage transformer must be **rectified.**

 Voltage rectification is required to ensure that electrons flow from cathode to anode only.

Rectification is accomplished with diodes. A diode is an electronic device containing two electrodes. Originally, all diode rectifiers were vacuum tubes called **valve tubes;** these have been replaced by solid-state rectifiers made of silicon (Figure 8-14).

Vacuum Tube Rectifiers. Consider an evacuated glass tube with a small coil of wire, the filament, at one end (Figure 8-15). If a large current is passed through this filament, it heats up and "boils" electrons off its surface. This process is called **thermionic emission.** *Therm* refers to heat, *ion* refers to a charged particle, and *emission,* of course, means to give off; thus, thermionic emission is the process of giving off electrons from a heated surface.

A simple vacuum tube conducts electrons in only one direction, from the cathode to the anode and not from the anode to the cathode. This type of vacuum tube, sometimes called a *diode* because it has two (di-) electrodes, is therefore a rectifier. Vacuum tube rectifiers are found in older x-ray imaging systems; solid-state rectifiers are components of modern imaging systems.

Solid-State Rectifiers. It has long been known that metals are good conductors of electricity and that some other materials, such as glass and plastic, are poor conductors of electricity or insulators.

A third class of materials, called **semiconductors,** lie between the range of insulators and conductors in their ability to conduct electricity. Tiny crystals of these semiconductors have some useful electrical properties and allow semiconductors to serve as the basis for today's solid-state microchip marvels.

Semiconductors are classed into two types: **n-type** and **p-type.** N-type semiconductors have loosely bound electrons that are relatively free to move. P-type semiconductors have spaces, called **holes,** where there are no

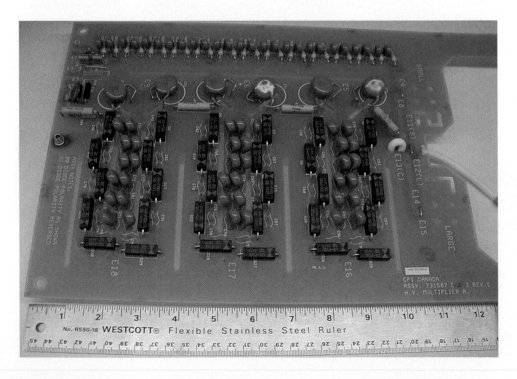

FIGURE 8-14 Rectifiers in most modern x-ray generators are the silicon, semiconductor type. The multiple black components on this 75 kVp high voltage multiplier board are rectifiers. (Courtesy of CMP/CPII, Inc.)

electrons. These holes are like the space between cars in heavy traffic. Holes are as mobile as electrons.

Consider a tiny crystal of n-type material placed in contact with a p-type crystal to form what is called an **n-p junction** (Figure 8-16). If a higher potential is placed on the p side of the junction, then the electrons and holes will both migrate toward the junction and wander across it. This flow of electrons and holes constitutes an electric current.

If, however, a positive potential is placed on the n side of the junction, both the electrons and holes will be swept away from the junction and no electrons will be available at the junction surface to form a current.

Thus, in this case, no electric current passes through the p-n junction.

Therefore, a solid-state p-n junction tends to conduct electricity in only one direction. This type of p-n junction is called a **solid-state diode.** Solid-state diodes are rectifiers because they conduct electric current in only one direction. The arrowhead in the symbol for a diode indicates the direction of conventional electric current, which is opposite to the flow of the electrons (Figure 8-17).

Rectification is essential for the safe and efficient operation of the x-ray tube. Rectifiers are located in the high-voltage section.

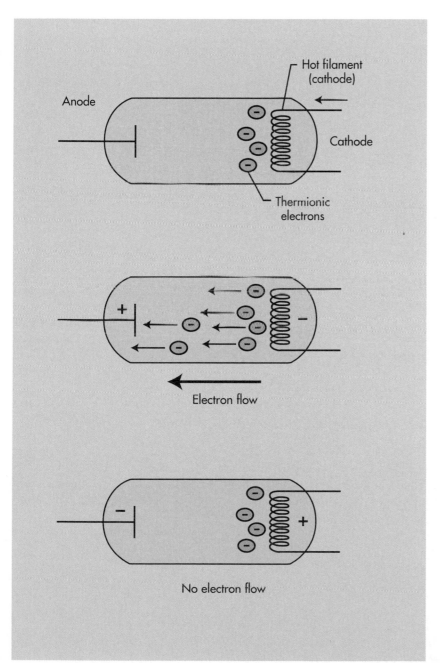

FIGURE 8-15 Schematic diagram of a valve tube-type diode, which conducts electrons in only one direction, from cathode to anode.

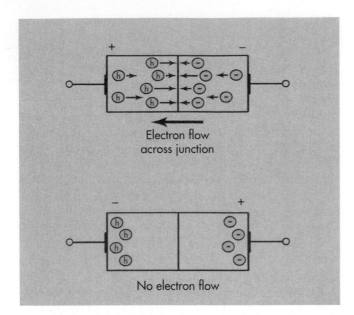

FIGURE 8-16 A p-n junction semiconductor shown as a solid-state diode.

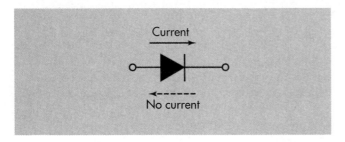

FIGURE 8-17 The electronic symbol for a solid-state diode.

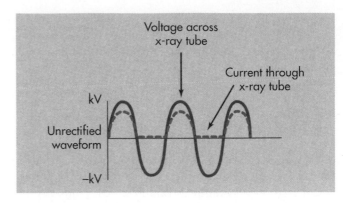

FIGURE 8-18 Unrectified voltage and current waveforms on the secondary side.

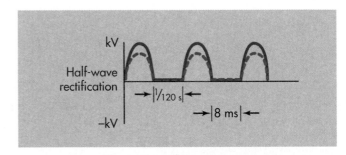

FIGURE 8-19 Half-wave rectification.

Unrectified Voltage. Figure 8-18 shows the unrectified voltage at the secondary side of the high-voltage step-up transformer. This voltage waveform appears as the voltage waveform supplied to the primary side of the high-voltage transformer, except its amplitude is much greater.

The current passing through the x-ray tube, however, exists only during the positive half of the cycle, when the anode is positive and the cathode is negative. During the negative half of the cycle, current can flow only from anode to cathode, but this does not occur because the anode is not constructed to emit electrons.

Half-Wave Rectification. The inverse voltage is removed from the supply to the x-ray tube by rectification. Half-wave rectification (Figure 8-19) is a condition in which the voltage is not allowed to swing negatively during the negative half of its cycle.

Rectifiers are assembled into electronic circuits to convert alternating current into the direct current necessary for the operation of an x-ray tube (Figure 8-20). During the positive portion of the AC wave-

form, the rectifier allows electric current to pass through the x-ray tube.

During the negative portion of the AC waveform, however, the rectifier does not conduct, and thus no electric current is allowed. The resulting electric current is a series of positive pulses separated by gaps when the negative current is not conducted.

This resulting electric current is a rectified current because electrons flow in only one direction. This form of rectification is called **half-wave rectification** because only one half of the AC waveform appears in the output.

In some portable and dental x-ray imaging systems, the x-ray tube serves as the vacuum tube rectifier. Such a system is said to be **self-rectified,** and the resulting waveform is the same as that of half-wave rectification.

Half-wave–rectified circuits contain zero, one, or two diodes. The x-ray output from a half-wave high-voltage generator pulsates, producing 60 x-ray pulses each second.

Full-Wave Rectification. One shortcoming of half-wave rectification is that it wastes half the supply of power. It also requires twice the exposure time. It is possible, however, to devise a circuit that rectifies the entire AC waveform. This form of voltage rectification is called full-wave rectification.

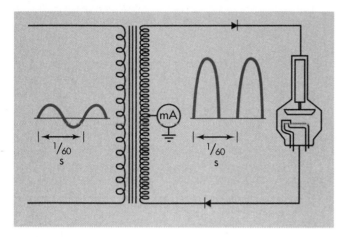

FIGURE 8-20 A half-wave–rectified circuit usually contains two diodes, although some contain one or more.

Full-wave–rectified x-ray imaging systems contain at least four diodes in the high-voltage circuit, usually arranged as in Figure 8-21. In a full-wave–rectified circuit, the negative half-cycle corresponding to the inverse voltage is reversed so that the anode is always positive (Figure 8-22).

The current through the circuit is shown during both the positive and the negative phases of the input waveform. Note that in both cases the output voltage across the x-ray tube is positive. Also, there are no gaps in the output waveform. All of the input waveform is rectified into usable output.

Figure 8-23 helps explain full-wave rectification. During the positive half-cycle of the secondary voltage waveform, electrons flow from the negative side to diodes C and D. Diode C is unable to conduct electrons in that direction, but diode D can. The electrons flow through diode D and the x-ray tube.

The electrons then butt into diodes A and B. Only diode A is positioned to conduct them, and they flow to the positive side of the transformer, thus completing the circuit.

During the negative half-cycle, diodes B and C are pressed into service while diodes A and D block electron flow. Note that the **polarity** of the x-ray tube remains unchanged. The cathode is always negative and the anode always positive, even though the induced secondary voltage alternates between positive and negative.

The main advantage to full-wave rectification is that the exposure time for any given technique is cut in half. The half-wave–rectified x-ray tube emits x-rays only half of the time. The pulsed x-ray output of a full-wave–rectified machine occurs 120 times each second instead of 60 times per second as with half-wave rectification.

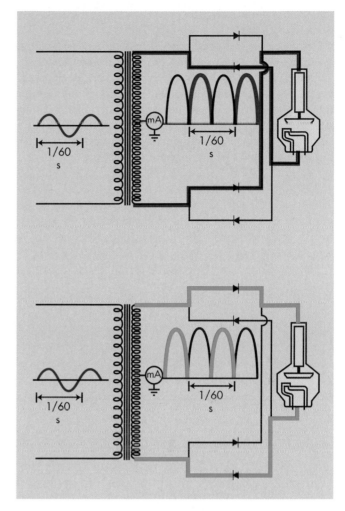

FIGURE 8-21 A full-wave–rectified circuit contains at least four diodes. Current is passed through the tube at 120 pulses per second.

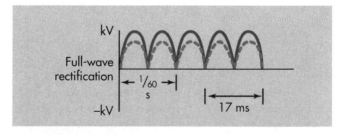

FIGURE 8-22 Voltage across a full-wave–rectified circuit is always positive.

Single-Phase Power

All of the voltage waveforms discussed so far are produced by single-phase electric power. Single-phase power results in a pulsating x-ray beam. This is caused by the alternate swing in voltage from zero to maximum potential 120 times each second under full-wave rectification.

The x-rays produced when the single-phase voltage waveform has a value near zero are of little diagnostic value because of their low energy, and therefore these x-rays have low penetrability. One method of overcoming this deficiency is to use some sophisticated electrical engineering principles to generate three simultaneous voltage waveforms out of step with one another. Such a manipulation results in **three-phase electric power.**

Three-Phase Power

The engineering required to produce three-phase power involves the manner in which the high-voltage step-up transformer is wired into the circuit, the details of which are beyond the scope of this discussion. Figure 8-24 shows the voltage waveforms for single-phase power, for three-phase power, and for full-wave–rectified three-phase power.

With three-phase power, multiple voltage waveforms are superimposed on one another, resulting in a waveform that maintains a nearly constant high voltage. There are six pulses per 1/60 s, compared to the two pulses characteristic of single-phase power.

With three-phase power, the voltage impressed across the x-ray tube is nearly constant, never dropping to zero during exposure.

There are limitations to the speed of starting an exposure—**initiation time**—and ending an exposure—**extinction time.** Additional electronic circuits and hardware are necessary to correct this deficiency, which adds to the additional size and cost of the three-phase generator.

High-Frequency Generator

High-frequency circuits are finding increasing application in generating high voltage for many x-ray imaging systems. Full-wave–rectified power at 60 Hz is converted to a higher frequency, usually 500 to 25,000 Hz, and then transferred to high voltage (Figure 8-25).

One advantage to the high-frequency generator is size. They are very much smaller than 60 Hz high-voltage generators. High-frequency generators produce a nearly constant potential voltage waveform, improving image quality at lower patient dose.

This technology was first used with portable x-ray imaging systems. Now, nearly all mammography and spiral computed tomography systems use high-frequency circuits.

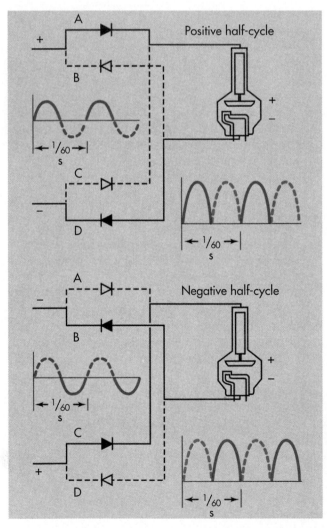

FIGURE 8-23 In a full-wave–rectified circuit, two diodes (A and D) conduct during the positive half-cycle and two (B and C) conduct during the negative half-cycle.

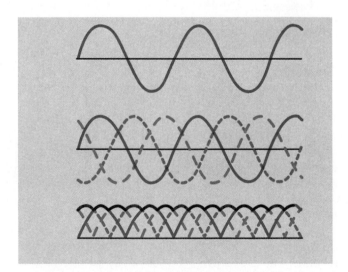

FIGURE 8-24 Three-phase power is a more efficient way to produce x-rays than is single-phase power. Shown are the voltage waveforms for unrectified single-phase power, three-phase power, and rectified three-phase power.

High-frequency voltage generation uses **inverter** circuits (Figure 8-26). Inverter circuits are high-speed switches, or *choppers*, which convert DC into a series of square pulses.

Many portable x-ray high-voltage generators use storage batteries and silicon-controlled rectifiers (SCRs) to generate square waves at 500 Hz, which becomes the input to the high-voltage step-up transformer. The high-voltage step-up transformer operating at 500 Hz is about 1/10 the size of a 60 Hz transformer, which is rather large and heavy. At 500 Hz, one can sometimes hear the transformer "sing" during exposure.

High-frequency x-ray generators are sometimes grouped by frequency (Table 8-1). The principal differences are in the electrical components designed as the inverter module. The real advantage to such circuits is that they are much smaller, less costly, and more efficient than 60 Hz high-voltage generators.

 Full-wave rectification or high-frequency voltage generation is used in almost all stationary x-ray imaging systems.

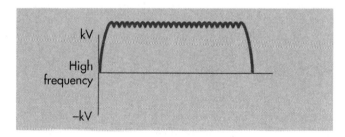

FIGURE 8-25 High-frequency voltage waveform.

Capacitor Discharge Generator

Some portable x-ray imaging systems still use a high-voltage generator, which operates by charging a series of SCRs from the DC voltage of a nickel-cadmium (NiCd) battery. By stacking (in an electrical sense) the SCRs, the charge is stored at very high voltage. During exposure, the charge is released (discharged) to form the x-ray tube current to produce x-rays (Figure 8-27).

 During capacitor discharge, the voltage falls approximately 1 kV/mAs.

This falling voltage limits the available x-ray tube current and causes kVp to fall during exposure. The result is the need for precise radiographic technique charts.

Following a given exposure time the capacitor bank continues to discharge, which could cause continued x-ray emission. Such x-ray emission is stopped by a grid-controlled x-ray tube, an automatic lead beam stopper, or both. A grid-controlled x-ray tube has a specially designed cathode to control x-ray tube current.

TABLE 8-1	Characteristics of High-Frequency X-Ray Generators	
Frequency Range	**Inverter Features**
Up to 1 kHz	Thyristers
1–10 kHz	Large silicon-controlled rectifier
10–100 kHz	Power field effect transistors

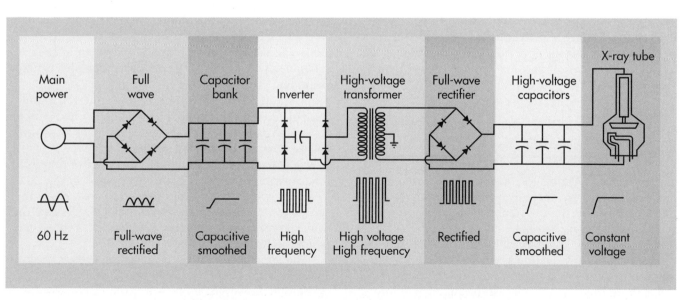

FIGURE 8-26 Inverter circuit of a high-voltage generator.

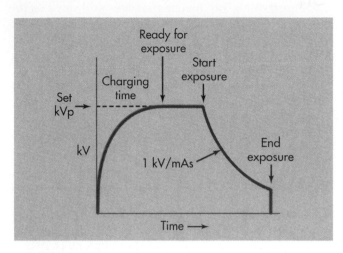

FIGURE 8-27 Tube voltage falls during exposure using a capacitor discharge generator.

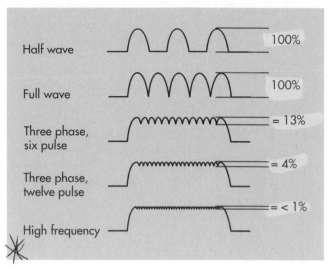

FIGURE 8-28 Voltage waveforms resulting from various power supplies. The ripple of the kilovoltage is indicated as a percentage for each waveform.

Voltage Ripple

Another way to characterize these voltage waveforms is by **voltage ripple.** Single-phase power has **100% voltage ripple:** the voltage varies from zero to its maximum value. Three-phase, six-pulse power produces voltage with only approximately **13% ripple;** consequently, the voltage supplied to the x-ray tube never falls below 86% of the maximum value.

A further improvement in three-phase power results in twelve pulses per cycle rather than six. Three-phase, twelve-pulse power results in only **4% ripple,** and therefore the voltage supplied to the x-ray tube does not fall below 96% of the maximum value. High-frequency generators have approximately **1% ripple** and therefore higher x-ray quantity and quality.

Figure 8-28 shows these various power sources and the resulting voltage waveforms they provide to the x-ray tube, as well as the approximate voltage ripple. The most efficient method of x-ray production also has the waveform with the lowest voltage ripple.

 Less voltage ripple results in higher radiation quantity and quality.

There are many advantages to an x-ray tube voltage with less ripple. The principal advantage is the higher radiation quantity and quality resulting from the more constant voltage supplied to the x-ray tube (Figure 8-29).

The radiation quantity is higher because the efficiency of x-ray production is higher when x-ray tube voltage is high. Stated differently, for any projectile electron emitted by the x-ray tube filament, more x-rays are produced when the electron energy is high than when it is low.

Low-voltage ripple increases radiation quality because fewer low-energy projectile electrons pass from cathode to anode to produce low-energy x-rays. Consequently, the average x-ray energy is higher than that resulting from high-voltage ripple modes.

Because the x-ray beam intensity and penetrability are greater for less voltage ripple than for single-phase power, technique charts developed for one cannot be used on the other. New technique charts are needed with three-phase or high-frequency x-ray imaging systems.

Three-phase operation may require as much as a 10 kVp reduction to produce the same radiographic optical density when operated at the same mAs as single phase. A high-frequency generator may require a 12 kVp reduction.

Three-phase radiographic equipment is manufactured with tube currents as high as 1200 mA, and therefore exceedingly short, high-intensity exposures are possible. This capacity is particularly helpful in interventional procedures.

When three-phase power is provided for a radiographic/fluoroscopic room or for an angiointerventional room, all radiographic exposures are made with three-phase power. The fluoroscopic mode, however, usually remains single-phase and takes advantage of the electrical capacitance of the x-ray tube cables.

Fluoroscopic mA is very low compared with radiographic mA. Because the x-ray cables are long, they have considerable capacitance, which results in a smoother voltage waveform (Figure 8-30).

The principal disadvantage of a three-phase x-ray apparatus is its initial cost. The cost of installation and operation, however, can be lower than those associated with single-phase equipment. The cost of high-frequency generators is moderate. Low-ripple genera-

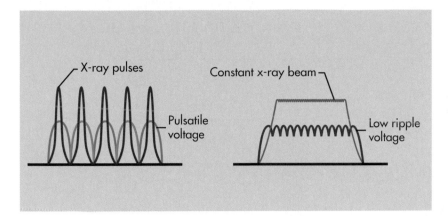

FIGURE 8-29 Both the number of x-rays and x-ray energy increases as the voltage waveform increases.

tors have greater overall capacity and flexibility than single-phase equipment.

Power Rating

Transformers and high-voltage generators are usually identified by their power rating in kilowatts (kW). Electrical power for any device is specified in watts, as was shown in the following equation from Chapter 6:

Power = Current × Potential

Watts = Amperes × Volts

A high-voltage generator for a basic radiographic unit is rated at 30 to 50 kW. Generators for angiointerventional suites have power ratings up to approximately 150 kW.

For specifying high-voltage generators, the industry standard is to use the maximum tube current (mA) possible at 100 kVp for an exposure of 100 ms. That generally results in the maximum available power.

High-voltage generator power (kW) = maximum x-ray tube current (mA) at 100 kVp and 100 ms.

Power is the product of amperes and volts. This assumes constant current and voltage, which does not exist in single-phase x-ray imaging systems. However, the actual power is close enough to the low-ripple power of three-phase and high-frequency generators that the equation holds.

Question: When a system with low voltage ripple is energized at 100 kVp, 100 ms, the maximum possible tube current is 800 mA. What is the power rating?

Answer: Power rating = Current (A) × Potential (V)
= 800 mA × 100 kVp
= 80,000 mA × kVp
= 80,000 W
= 80 kW

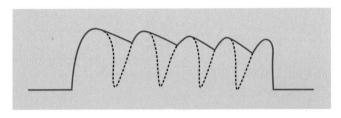

FIGURE 8-30 Voltage waveform is smoothed by the capacitance of long high-voltage cables.

Since the product of amperes × volts = watts, the product of milliamperes × kilovolts = watts. However, power rating is expressed in kilowatts, and so the defining equation for three-phase and high-frequency power is as follows:

$$\text{Power rating (kW)} = \frac{\text{mA} \times \text{kVp}}{1000}$$

Question: An interventional system is capable of 1200 mA when operated in 100 kVp, 100 ms. What is the power rating?

Answer: $$\text{Power rating (kW)} = \frac{1200 \text{ mA} \times 100 \text{ kVp}}{1000}$$
$$= 120 \text{ kW}$$

Single-phase generators have 100% voltage ripple and are less efficient x-ray generators. Consequently, the single-phase expression of power rating is:

$$\text{Power rating (kW)} = (0.7)\frac{\text{mA} \times \text{kVp}}{1000}$$

Question: A single-phase radiographic unit installed in a private office reaches maximum capacity

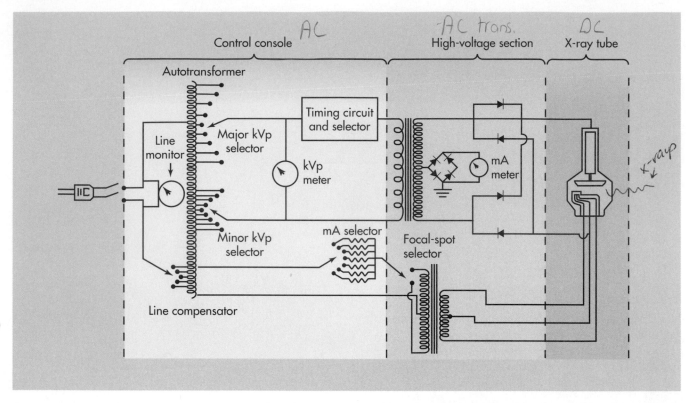

FIGURE 8-31 The schematic circuit of an x-ray imaging system.

at 100 ms of 120 kVp and 500 mA. What is its power rating?

Answer: Power rating $= (0.7)\dfrac{(500\,mA)(120\ kVp)}{1000}$

$$= 42\ kW$$

X-Ray Circuit

Figure 8-31 is a simplified schematic diagram of the three main sections of the x-ray imaging system: the x-ray tube, the operating console, and the high-voltage generator. The figure also shows the location of all meters, controls, and important components.

SUMMARY

The x-ray imaging system has three principal sections: (1) the x-ray tube, (2) the operating console, and (3) the high-voltage generator. The design and operation of the x-ray tube are discussed in Chapter 9.

The operating console consists of an on/off control and controls to select kVp, mA, and time or mAs. The AECs are also on the operating console.

The high-voltage generator provides power to the x-ray tube in three possible ways: single-phase power, three-phase power, and high-frequency power. The difference between single- and three-phase power involves the manner in which the high-voltage step-up trans-

former is electrically positioned. The waveforms for single-phase, three-phase, and three-phase fully rectified power were shown in Figure 8-24. With three-phase power, the voltage across the x-ray tube is nearly constant during exposure and never drops to zero as does the voltage for single-phase power.

The components of an x-ray imaging system are sometimes identified by their power rating in kilowatts (kW). Maximum available power for high-voltage generators equals the maximum tube current (mA) at 100 kVp for an exposure of 100 ms.

CHALLENGE QUESTIONS

1. Define or otherwise identify:
   a. Semiconductor
   b. Automatic exposure control (AEC)
   c. Line compensation
   d. Capacitor
   e. mA meter location
   f. Diode
   g. Voltage ripple
   h. Rectification
   i. Autotransformer
   j. Power
2. 220 V is supplied across 1200 windings of the primary coil of the autotransformer. If 1650 windings are tapped, what voltage will be

supplied to the primary coil of the high-voltage transformer?

3. A kVp meter reads 86 kVp and the turns ratio of the high-voltage step-up transformer is 1200. What is the true voltage across the meter?
4. The supply voltage from the autotransformer to the filament transformer is 60 V. If the turns ratio of the filament transformer is 1/12, what is the filament voltage?
5. If the current in the primary of the filament transformer in question 4 were 0.5 A, what would be the filament current?
6. The supply to a high-voltage step-up transformer with a turns ratio of 550 is 190 V. What is the voltage across the x-ray tube?
7. Locate the various meters and controls shown in Figure 8-31 on an x-ray imaging system you operate.
8. The radiographic table must be radiolucent. Define *radiolucent*.
9. Describe the movements of a 90/20 table.
10. List the five major controls on the operator's console.
11. What is the purpose of the autotransformer?

12. How does primary voltage relate to secondary voltage in an autotransformer?
13. What does the prereading kVp meter allow?
14. Operating console controls are set at 200 mA with an exposure time of 1/60 s. What is the milliamperage per second (mAs)?
15. In an examination of a pediatric patient, the operating console controls are set at 600 mA/30 ms. What is the mAs?
16. What is the difference between a high-voltage generator and a high-voltage transformer?
17. Why does the x-ray circuit require rectification?
18. Match the power source with the voltage ripple.

POWER	% VOLTAGE RIPPLE
Single-phase	4%
Three-phase, twelve-pulse	100%
Three-phase, six-pulse	14%
High-frequency	1%

19. What is the only type of high-voltage generator that can be positioned in or on the x-ray tube housing?
20. State the equations for computing single-phase and high-frequency power rating.

The X-Ray Tube

OBJECTIVES

At the completion of this chapter, the student should be able to do the following:

1. Describe the general design of an x-ray tube
2. List the external components that house and protect the x-ray tube
3. Identify the purpose of the glass or metal enclosure
4. Discuss the cathode and filament currents
5. Describe the parts of the anode and the induction motor
6. Define the line-focus principle and the heel effect
7. Identify the three causes of x-ray tube failure
8. Explain and interpret x-ray tube rating charts

OUTLINE

THE X-RAY tube is a component of the x-ray imaging system rarely seen by the radiologic technologist. It is contained in a protective housing, and therefore is inaccessible. Figure 9-1 is a schematic diagram of a rotating anode diagnostic x-ray tube. Its components are considered separately, but it should be clear that there are two primary parts: the **cathode** and the **anode.** Each of these is an **electrode,** and any tube with two electrodes is a **diode.** An x-ray tube is a special type of diode.

The external structure of the x-ray tube consists of three parts: the support structure, the protective housing, and the glass or metal enclosure. The internal structures of the x-ray tube are the anode and the cathode.

An explanation of the external components of the x-ray tube and the internal structure of the x-ray tube follows. The causes and prevention of x-ray tube failure are discussed. With proper use, x-ray tubes should last many years.

EXTERNAL COMPONENTS
X-Ray Tube Support

The x-ray tube and housing assembly are quite heavy, and therefore require a support mechanism so that the radiologic technologist can position it. Figure 9-2 illustrates the three main methods of x-ray tube support.

Ceiling Support System. The **ceiling support** system is probably the most frequently used. It consists of two perpendicular sets of ceiling-mounted rails. This allows for both longitudinal and transverse travel of the x-ray tube.

A telescoping column attaches the x-ray tube housing to the rails, allowing for variable source-to-image receptor distance (SID). When the x-ray tube is centered above the examination table at the standard SID, the x-ray tube is in a **preferred detent** position. Other positions can be chosen and locked by the radiologic technologist.

Floor-to-Ceiling Support System. The **floor-to-ceiling** support system has a single column with rollers at each end, one attached to a ceiling-mounted rail and the other attached to a floor-mounted rail. The x-ray tube slides up and down the column as the column rotates. A variation of this type of support system has the column positioned on a single **floor support system** using one or two floor-mounted rails.

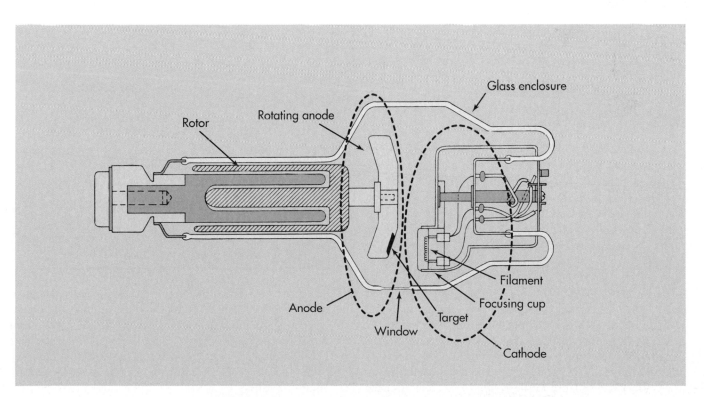

FIGURE 9-1 Principal parts of a rotating anode x-ray tube.

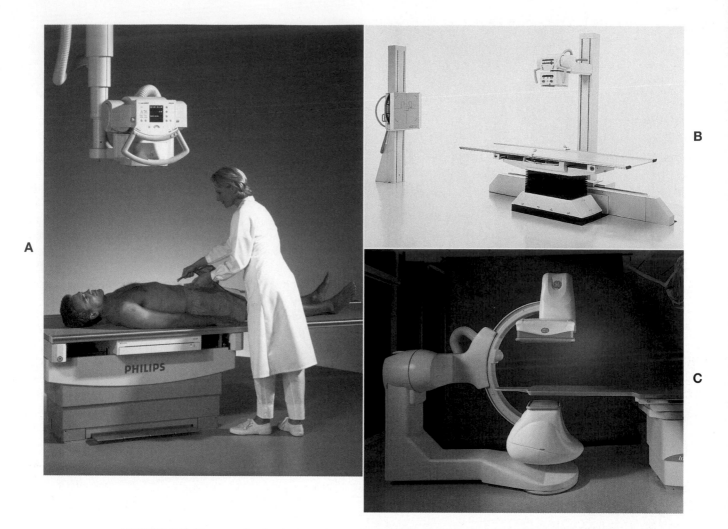

FIGURE 9-2 Three methods of supporting an x-ray tube. **A,** Ceiling support. **B,** Floor support. **C,** C-arm support. (**A,** Courtesy Philips Medical Systems. **B,** Courtesy Toshiba Corp. **C,** Courtesy General Electric Medical Systems.)

C-arm Support System. Interventional radiology suites often are equipped with C-arm support systems, so called because the system is shaped like a "C." These systems are ceiling mounted and provide for very flexible x-ray tube positioning. The image receptor is attached to the other end of the C-arm from the x-ray tube. Variations called L-arm or U-arm support are also common.

Protective Housing

When x-rays are produced, they are emitted **isotropically**, that is, with equal intensity in all directions. We use only those emitted through the special section of the x-ray tube called the **window** (Figure 9-3). Those x-rays emitted through the window are called the **useful beam.**

X-rays that escape through the protective housing are **leakage radiation;** they contribute nothing in the way of diagnostic information and result in unnecessary exposure of the patient and radiologic technologist. A properly designed protective housing reduces the level of leakage radiation to less than **100 mR/hr at 1 m** when operated at maximum conditions.

  The protective housing guards against excessive radiation exposure and electrical shock.

The protective housing incorporates specially designed high-voltage receptacles to protect against accidental electric shock. Death by electrocution was a very real hazard to early radiologic technologists. The protective housing also provides **mechanical support** for the x-ray tube and protects the tube from damage caused by rough handling.

The protective housing around some x-ray tubes contains oil that serves as both an **insulator** against electric

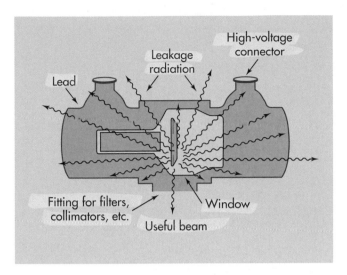

FIGURE 9-3 Protective housing reduces the intensity of leakage radiation to less than 100 mR/hr at 1 m.

shock and as a **thermal cushion** to dissipate heat. Some protective housings have a cooling fan to air-cool the tube or the oil in which the x-ray tube is immersed. A bellows-like device allows the oil to expand when heated. If the expansion is too great, a microswitch is activated so that the tube cannot be used until it cools.

Glass or Metal Exposure

An x-ray tube is an electronic vacuum tube with components contained within a glass or **metal enclosure.** The x-ray tube, however, is a special kind of vacuum tube containing two electrodes: the cathode and the anode. It is relatively large, perhaps 30 to 50 cm long and 20 cm in diameter. The glass enclosure is made of Pyrex glass to enable it to withstand the tremendous heat generated.

The enclosure maintains a vacuum inside the tube. This vacuum allows for more efficient x-ray production and longer tube life. When just a little gas is in the enclosure, the electron flow from cathode to anode is reduced, fewer x-rays are produced, and more heat is generated.

Early x-ray tubes, modifications of the Crookes tube, were not vacuum tubes but rather contained controlled quantities of gas within the enclosure. The modern x-ray tube, the Coolidge tube, is a vacuum tube. If it becomes gassy, x-ray production falls off and the tube can fail.

An improvement in tube design incorporates metal rather than glass as part or all of the enclosure. As a glass enclosure tube ages, some tungsten vaporizes and coats the inside of the glass enclosure. This alters the electrical properties of the tube, allowing tube current to stray and interact with the glass enclosure; the result is arcing and tube failure.

Metal enclosure tubes maintain a constant electric potential between the electrons of the tube current and the enclosure. Therefore, they have longer life and are less likely to fail. Virtually all current high-capacity x-ray tubes use metal enclosures.

 X-ray tubes are designed with either a glass enclosure or metal enclosure.

The x-ray tube window is an area of the glass or metal enclosure, approximately 5 cm², that is thin and through which the useful beam of x-rays is emitted. Such a window allows maximum emission of x-rays with minimum absorption.

INTERNAL COMPONENTS
Cathode

Figure 9-4 shows a photograph of a dual-filament cathode and a schematic drawing of its electrical supply. The two filaments supply separate electron beams to produce two focal spots.

 The cathode is the negative side of the x-ray tube and has two primary parts: a filament and a focusing cup.

Filament. The filament is a coil of wire similar to that in a kitchen toaster, except much smaller. The filament is usually approximately 2 mm in diameter and 1 or 2 cm long. In the kitchen toaster, an electric current is conducted through the coil, causing it to glow and emit a large quantity of heat.

An x-ray tube filament emits electrons when it is heated. When the current through the filament is sufficiently high, the outer-shell electrons of the filament atoms are "boiled off" and ejected from the filament. This phenomenon is known as **thermionic emission.**

Filaments are usually made of **thoriated tungsten.** Tungsten provides for higher thermionic emission than other metals. Its melting point is 3410°C, and therefore it is not likely to burn out like the filament of a light bulb. Also, tungsten does not vaporize easily. If it did, the tube would quickly become gassy and its internal parts coated with tungsten. The addition of 1% to 2% thorium to the tungsten filament increases efficiency of thermionic emission and prolongs tube life.

 Tungsten vaporization with deposition on the inside of the glass enclosure is the most common cause of tube failure.

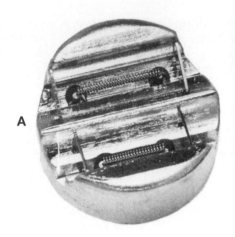

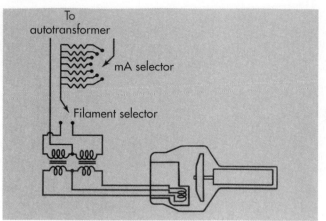

FIGURE 9-4 **A,** Dual-filament cathode designed to provide focal spots of 0.5 mm and 1.5 mm. **B,** Schematic for dual-filament cathode. (**A,** Courtesy The Machlett Laboratories, Inc.)

Ultimately, however, tungsten metal does vaporize and is deposited on internal components. This upsets some of the electrical characteristics of the tube and can cause arcing and lead to tube failure. Such malfunction is usually abrupt.

Focusing Cup. The filament is embedded in a metal cup called the **focusing cup** (Figure 9-5). Because all the electrons accelerated from cathode to anode are electrically negative, the electron beam tends to spread out owing to electrostatic repulsion. Some electrons can even miss the anode completely.

The focusing cup is negatively charged so that it electrostatically confines the electron beam to a small area of the anode (Figure 9-6). The effectiveness of the focusing cup is determined by its size and shape, its charge, the filament size and shape, and the position of the filament in the focusing cup.

Certain types of x-ray tubes called **grid-controlled** tubes are designed to be turned on and off very rapidly. Grid-controlled tubes are used in portable capacitor discharge imaging systems and in digital subtraction angiography, digital radiography, and cineradiography, all of which require multiple exposures each for precise exposure time.

The term **grid** is borrowed from vacuum tube electronics and refers to an element in the tube that acts as the switch. In a **grid-controlled x-ray tube** the focusing cup is the grid and, therefore, the exposure switch.

Filament Current. When the x-ray imaging system is first turned on, a low current passes through the filament to warm it and prepare it for the thermal jolt necessary for x-ray production. At low filament current, there is no tube current because the filament does not get hot enough for thermionic emission. Once the filament current is high enough for thermionic emission, a small rise in filament current results in a large rise in tube current.

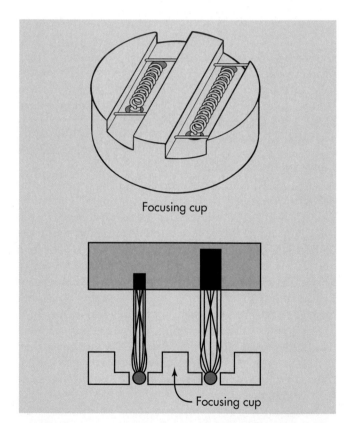

FIGURE 9-5 The focusing cup is a metal shroud surrounding the filament.

 The x-ray tube current is adjusted by controlling the filament current.

This relationship between filament current and tube current depends on the tube voltage (Figure 9-7). Fixed stations of 100, 200, 300 mA, and so on, usually corre-

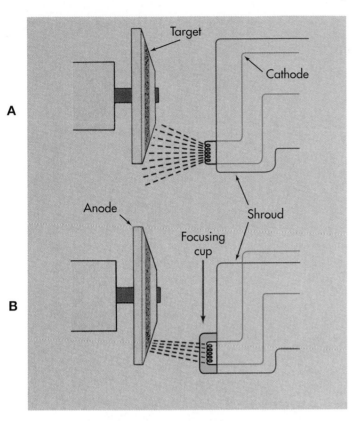

FIGURE 9-6 **A,** Without a focusing cup, the electron beam is spread beyond the anode because of mutual electrostatic repulsion among the electrons. **B,** With a focusing cup, which is negatively charged, the electron beam is condensed and directed to the target.

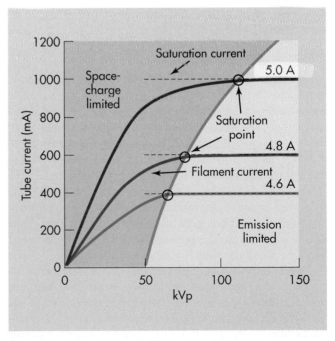

FIGURE 9-7 X-ray tube current is actually controlled by changing the filament current. Because of thermionic emission, a small change in filament current results in a large change in tube current.

spond to discrete connections on the filament transformer or to precision resistors.

When emitted from the filament, electrons are in the vicinity of the filament before being accelerated to the anode. Because these electrons carry negative charges, they repel one another and tend to form a cloud around the filament.

This cloud of electrons, called a **space charge**, makes it difficult for subsequent electrons to be emitted by the filament because of the electrostatic repulsion. This phenomenon is called the **space-charge effect.** A major obstacle in producing x-ray tubes with currents exceeding 1000 mA is the design of adequate space-charge–compensating devices.

 Thermionic emission at low kVp and high mA can be space-charge limited.

At any given filament current, say, 5.2 A (Figure 9-8), the x-ray tube current rises with increasing voltage to a maximum value. A further increase in kVp does not

FIGURE 9-8 At a given filament current, tube current reaches a maximum level called *saturation current.*

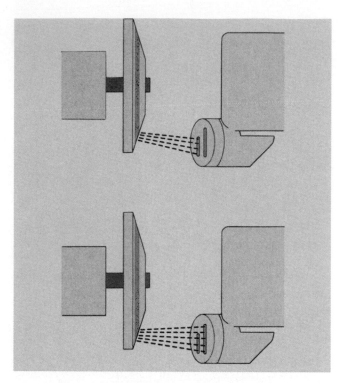

FIGURE 9-9 In a dual-focus x-ray tube, focal spot size is controlled by heating one of the two filaments.

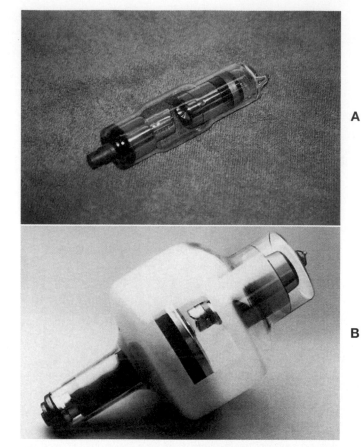

FIGURE 9-10 All diagnostic x-ray tubes can be classified according to their type of anode. **A,** Stationary anode. **B,** Rotating anode. (Courtesy Philips Medical Systems.)

result in a higher mA because all of the available electrons have been used. This is the **saturation current.**

Saturation current is not reached at a lower kVp because of space-charge limitation. When an x-ray tube is operated at the saturation current, it is said to be *emission limited.*

Dual-Focus

Most diagnostic x-ray tubes have two focal spots, one large and the other small. The small focal spot is used when better spatial resolution is required. The large focal spot is used when large body parts are imaged and when other techniques that produce high heat are required.

The selection of one or the other focal spot is usually made with the mA station selector on the operating console. Normally, either filament can be used with the lower mA station, approximately 300 mA or less. At approximately 400 mA and up, only the larger focal spot is allowed because the heat capacity of the anode could be exceeded if the small focal spot were used.

Small focal spots range from 0.1 to 1 mm; large focal spots usually range from 0.3 to 2 mm. Each filament of a dual-filament cathode assembly is embedded in the focusing cup (Figure 9-9). The small focal spot size is associated with the small filament and the large focal spot size with the large filament. There is an electric current through the appropriate filament.

Anode

The anode is the positive side of the x-ray tube. There are two types of anodes—**stationary** and **rotating** (Figure 9-10). Stationary anode x-ray tubes are used in dental x-ray imaging systems, some portable imaging systems, and other special-purpose units in which high tube current and power are not required. General-purpose x-ray tubes use the rotating anode because they must be capable of producing high-intensity x-ray beams in a short time.

 The anode is the positive side of the x-ray tube; it conducts electricity and radiates heat and contains the target.

The anode serves three functions in an x-ray tube. The anode tube is an **electrical conductor.** It receives electrons emitted by the cathode and conducts them through the tube to the connecting cables and back to the high-voltage generator. The anode also provides **mechanical support** for the target.

The anode must also be a good **thermal dissipator**. When the projectile electrons from the cathode interact with the anode, more than 99% of their kinetic energy is converted into heat. This heat must be dissipated quickly. Copper, molybdenum, and graphite are the most common anode materials. Adequate heat dissipation is the major engineering hurdle in designing higher-capacity x-ray tubes.

Target. The **target** is the area of the anode struck by the electrons from the cathode. In stationary anode tubes, the target consists of a tungsten alloy embedded in the copper anode (Figure 9-11, *A*). In rotating anode tubes, the entire rotating disc is the target (Figure 9-11, *B*).

Alloying the tungsten (usually with rhenium) gives it added mechanical strength to withstand the stresses of high-speed rotation. High-capacity x-ray tubes have molybdenum or graphite layered under the tungsten target (Figure 9-12). Both molybdenum and graphite have lower mass density than tungsten, making the anode easier to rotate.

3400 RPMs

Tungsten is the material of choice for the target for general radiography for three main reasons:
1. **Atomic number**—tungsten's high atomic number, 74, results in high-efficiency x-ray production and in high-energy x-rays. The reason for this is discussed more fully in Chapter 11.
2. **Thermal conductivity**—tungsten has a thermal conductivity nearly equal to that of copper. It is therefore an efficient metal for dissipating the heat produced.
3. **High melting point**—any material, if heated sufficiently, will melt and become liquid. Tungsten has a high melting point (3400° C, compared with 1100° C for copper) and therefore can stand up under high tube current without pitting or bubbling.

Specialty x-ray tubes for mammography have molybdenum or rhodium targets principally because of their low atomic number and low K-characteristic x-ray energy. Table 9-1 summarizes the properties of these target materials, all of which have excellent heat conduction.

Rotating Anode. The rotating anode x-ray tube allows the electron beam to interact with a much larger target area, and therefore the heating of the anode is not confined to one small spot as in a stationary anode tube. Figure 9-13 compares the target areas of typical stationary anode and rotating anode x-ray tubes with 1-mm focal spots.

The actual target for the stationary tube is 1 mm × 4 mm = 4 mm². If the rotating anode diameter is 15 cm, then the radius of the target area is approximately 14 cm (140 mm). The total target area of the rotating anode is $2\pi(140) \times 4$ mm = 3519 mm². Thus, the ro-

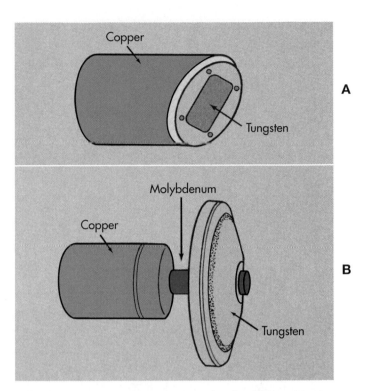

FIGURE 9-11 A, In a stationary anode tube the target is embedded in the anode. **B,** In a rotating anode tube the target is the rotating disc.

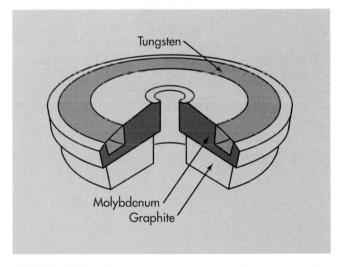

FIGURE 9-12 A layered anode consists of a target surface backed by one or more layers to increase heat capacity.

tating anode tube provides nearly 1000 times more area to interact with the electron beam than a stationary anode tube.

Higher tube currents and shorter exposure times are possible with the rotating anode.

TABLE 9-1	Characteristics of X-ray Targets			
Element	Chemical Symbol	Atomic Number	K X-ray Energy*	Melting Temperature
Tungsten	W	74	69 keV	3400°C
Molybdenum	Mo	42	20 keV	2600°C
Rhodium	Rh	45	23 keV	3200°C

*X-rays resulting from electron transitions into the K shell.

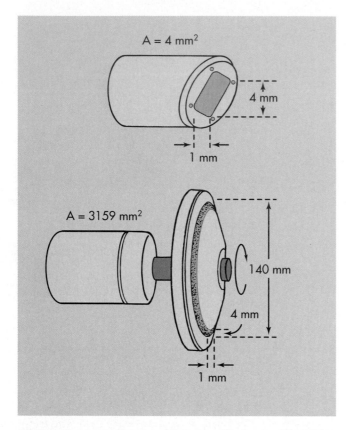

FIGURE 9-13 Stationary anode tube with a 1-mm focal spot may have a target area of 4 mm². A comparable 15-cm diameter rotating anode tube can have a target area of approximately 3500 mm², which increases the heating capacity of the tube by a factor of nearly 1000.

Heat capacity can be further improved by increasing the speed of anode rotation. Most rotating anodes revolve at 3400 rpm (revolutions per minute). The anodes of high-capacity tubes rotate at 3400 rpm and 10,000 rpm.

The stem of the anode is the shaft between the anode and the rotor. The system is usually made of molybdenum because it is a poor heat conductor.

Occasionally, the rotor mechanism of a rotating anode tube fails. When this happens, the anode becomes overheated and pits or cracks, causing tube failure (Figure 9-14).

Induction Motor. How does the anode rotate inside an enclosure with no mechanical connection to the outside? Most things that revolve are powered by chains or axles or gears of some sort.

An electromagnetic induction motor is used to turn the anode. An induction motor consists of two principal parts separated from each other by the glass or metal enclosure (Figure 9-15). The part outside the enclosure, called the *stator*, consists of a series of electromagnets equally spaced around the neck of the tube. Inside the enclosure is a shaft made of bars of copper and soft iron fabricated into one mass. This mechanism is called the *rotor*.

 The rotating anode is powered by an electromagnetic *induction motor*.

The induction motor works through electromagnetic induction, similar to a transformer and based on Lenz's law of induced currents. Current in each stator winding induces a magnetic field that surrounds the rotor. The stator windings are energized sequentially so that the induced magnetic field rotates on the axis of the stator. This magnetic field interacts with the ferromagnetic rotor, causing it to rotate synchronously with the activated stator windings.

When the radiologic technologist pushes the exposure button of a radiographic imaging system, there is a short delay before an exposure is made. This allows the rotor to accelerate to its designed RPM while the filament is heated. Only then is the kVp applied to the x-ray tube.

During this time, filament current is increased to provide the correct x-ray tube current. When using a two-position exposure switch, the switch should be pushed to its final position in one motion. This minimizes the time that the filament is heated and prolongs tube life.

When the exposure is completed on imaging systems equipped with high-speed rotors, one can hear the rotor slow down and stop within approximately 1 minute. The high-speed rotor slows down as quickly as it does because the induction motor is put into reverse. The rotor is a precisely balanced, low-friction device that, if left alone, might take many minutes to coast to rest after use.

On registry

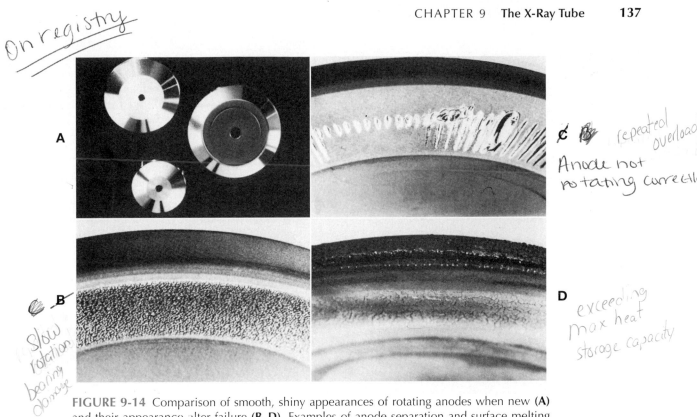

C — repeated overload
Anode not rotating correctly

B — slow rotation bearing damage

D — exceeding max heat storage capacity

FIGURE 9-14 Comparison of smooth, shiny appearances of rotating anodes when new **(A)** and their appearance after failure **(B–D)**. Examples of anode separation and surface melting shown were caused by slow rotation due to bearing damage **(B)**, repeated overload **(C)**, and exceeding of maximum heat storage capacity **(D)**. (Courtesy Philips Medical Systems.)

In a new x-ray tube, the **coast time** is approximately 60 s. With age, the coast time is reduced because of wear of the rotor bearings.

One design that allows the use of massive anodes uses a shaft fixed at each end (Figure 9-16). The principal advantage is improved heat dissipation and higher power capacity.

Line-Focus Principle. The focal spot is the area of the target from which x-rays are emitted. Radiology requires small focal spots because the smaller the focal spot, the better the spatial resolution of the image. Unfortunately, as the size of the focal spot decreases, the heating of the target is concentrated onto a smaller area. This is the limiting factor to focal spot size.

 The focal spot is the actual x-ray source.

Before the development of the rotating anode, another design was incorporated into x-ray tube targets to allow a large area for heating while maintaining a small focal spot. This design is known as the **line-focus principle**. By angling the target (Figure 9-17), one makes the effective area of the target much smaller than the actual area of electron interaction.

The effective target area, or **effective focal spot size**, is the area projected onto the patient and the image

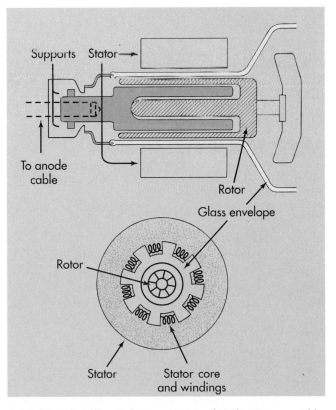

FIGURE 9-15 Target of a rotating anode tube is powered by an induction motor, the principal components of which are the stator and the rotor.

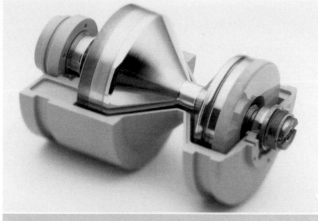

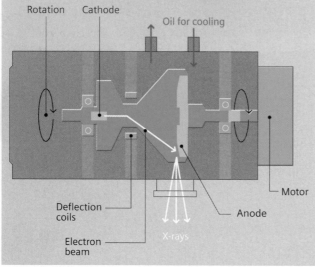

FIGURE 9-16 A, This very high capacity x-ray tube revolves in a bath of oil for complete heat dissipation. (Courtesy Philips Medical Systems.) **B,** The cooling capacity is greater than any heat load. (Courtesy Siemens Medical Systems.)

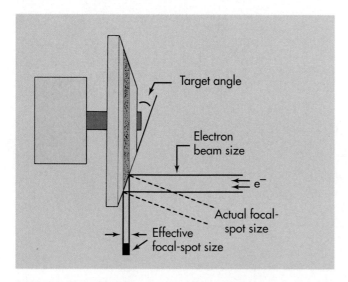

FIGURE 9-17 The line-focus principle allows high anode heating with small effective focal spots. As the target angle decreases, so does the effective focal spot size.

receptor. This is the value given when identifying large or small focal spots. When the target angle is made smaller, the effective focal spot size is also made smaller. Diagnostic x-ray tubes have target angles varying from approximately 5 to 15 degrees. The advantage of the line-focus principle is that it simultaneously improves spatial resolution and heat capacity.

 The line-focus principle results in an effective focal spot size much less than the actual focal spot size.

Biangular targets are available that produce two focal spot sizes because of two different target angles on the anode (Figure 9-18). Combining biangular targets with

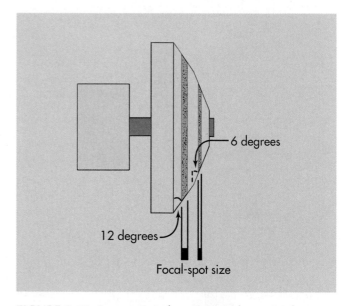

FIGURE 9-18 Some targets have two angles to produce two focal spots.

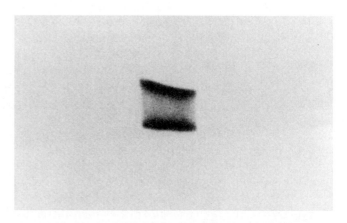

FIGURE 9-19 The usual shape of a focal spot is the double banana. (Courtesy Donald Jacobson.)

different-length filaments results in a very flexible combination.

A circular effective focal spot is preferred. Usually, however, it has a shape characterized as a double banana (Figure 9-19). These differences in x-ray intensity across the focal spot are controlled principally by the design of the filament and focusing cup and the voltage on the focusing cup. Round focal spots are particularly important for high-resolution magnification radiography and mammography.

The National Electrical Manufacturers Association (NEMA) has established standards and variances for focal spot sizes. When a manufacturer states a focal spot size, that is its nominal size. Table 9-2 shows the maximum measured size permitted that is still within the standard.

Heel Effect. One unfortunate consequence of the line-focus principle is that the radiation intensity on the cathode side of the x-ray field is higher than that on the anode side. Electrons interact with target atoms at various depths into the target.

The x-rays that constitute the useful beam emitted toward the anode side must traverse a greater thickness of target material than x-rays emitted toward the cathode direction (Figure 9-20). The intensity of x-rays that are emitted through the "heel" of the

TABLE 9-2	Nominal Focal Spot Size Compared With Maximum Acceptable Dimensions				
NOMINAL FOCAL SPOT SIZE (MM)			ACCEPTABLE MEASURED FOCAL SPOT SIZE (MM)		
Width	×	Length	Width	×	Length
0.1	×	0.1	0.15	×	0.15
0.3	×	0.3	0.45	×	0.65
0.4	×	0.4	0.6	×	0.85
0.5	×	0.5	0.75	×	1.1
1.0	×	1.0	1.4	×	2.0
2.0	×	2.0	2.6	×	3.7

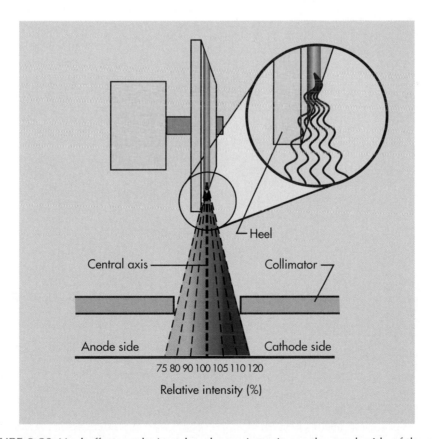

FIGURE 9-20 Heel effect results in reduced x-ray intensity on the anode side of the useful beam because of absorption in the "heel" of the target.

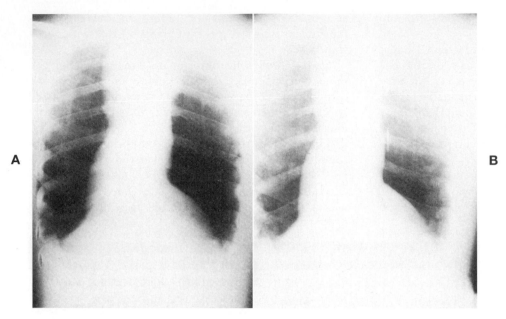

A

B

FIGURE 9-21 PA chest images demonstrating the heel effect. **A,** Images taken with the cathode up (superior). **B,** Image with cathode down (inferior). More uniform radiographic density is obtained with the cathode positioned to the thicker side of the anatomy, as in **B.** (Courtesy Pat Duffy.)

target is reduced because they have a longer path through the target, and therefore increased absorption. This is the **heel effect.**

 The smaller the anode angle, the larger is the heel effect.

The difference in radiation intensity across the useful beam of an x-ray field can vary by as much as 45%. The **central ray** of the useful beam is the imaginary line generated by the centermost x-ray in the beam. If the radiation intensity along the central ray is designated as 100%, then the intensity on the cathode side may be as high as 120% and that on the anode side may be as low as 75%.

The heel effect is important when imaging anatomic structures that differ greatly in thickness or mass density. In general, positioning the cathode side of the x-ray tube over the thicker part of the anatomy provides more uniform optical density on the film. The cathode and anode directions are usually indicated on the protective housing, sometimes near the cable connectors.

In chest radiography, for example, the cathode should be inferior. The lower thorax in the region of the diaphragm is considerably thicker than the upper thorax, and therefore requires higher radiation intensity if there is to be uniform exposure of the image receptor.

In abdominal imaging, on the other hand, the cathode should be superior. The upper abdomen is thicker than the lower abdomen and pelvis and requires higher x-ray intensity for uniform optical density.

Figure 9-21 shows two posteroanterior chest images, one taken with the cathode down, the other with the cathode up. Can you tell the difference? Which do you

think represents better radiographic quality? Resolve the difference before looking at the figure legend.

Another important consequence of the heel effect is changing focal spot size. The effective focal spot is smaller on the anode side of the x-ray field than on the cathode side (Figure 9-22). Some manufacturers of mammography equipment take advantage of this property by angling the x-ray tube to produce the smaller focal spot along the chest wall.

 The heel effect results in smaller effective focal spot and less radiation intensity on the anode side of the x-ray beam.

Extrafocal Radiation. X-ray tubes are designed so that projectile electrons from the cathode interact with the target only at the focal spot. However, some of the electrons bounce off the focal spot and then land on other areas of the target, causing x-rays to be produced from outside of the focal spot (Figure 9-23).

These x-rays are called *extrafocal radiation* or *offfocus radiation*. It is not unlike squirting a water pistol at a concrete pavement: Some of the water splashes off the pavement and lands in a larger area.

Extrafocal radiation is undesirable because it extends the size of the focal spot. The additional x-ray beam area increases skin dose modestly but unnecessarily. The extrafocal radiation can significantly reduce image contrast.

Finally, extrafocal radiation can image patient tissue that was intended to be excluded by the variable-aperture collimators. Examples of such undesirable images are the ears in a skull examination, soft tissue

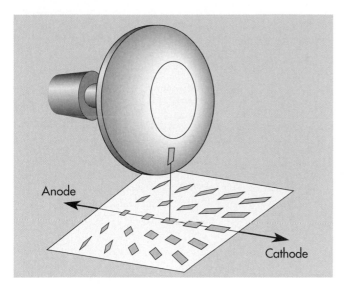

FIGURE 9-22 The effective focal spot changes size and shape across the projected x-ray field.

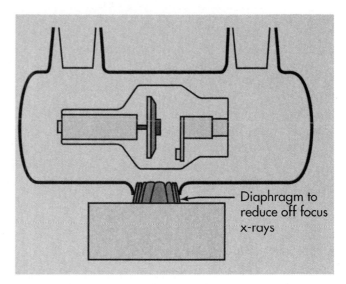

FIGURE 9-24 An additional diaphragm is positioned close to the focal spot to reduce extrafocal radiation.

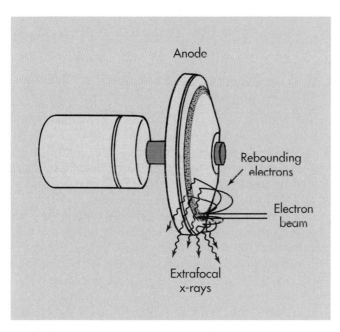

FIGURE 9-23 Extrafocal x-rays result from electrons interacting with the anode off of the focal spot.

beyond the cervical spine, and lung beyond the borders of the thoracic spine.

Extrafocal radiation is reduced by designing a fixed diaphragm in the tube housing near the window of the x-ray tube (Figure 9-24). This is a geometric solution.

Another effective solution is the metal enclosure x-ray tube. Electrons reflected from the focal spot are extracted by the metal enclosure and conducted away. Therefore, they are not available to be attracted to the target outside of the focal spot. The use of a grid does not reduce extrafocal radiation.

X-RAY TUBE FAILURE

With careful use, x-ray tubes can provide many years of service. With inconsiderate use, x-ray tube life may be shortened substantially.

The length of x-ray tube life is primarily under the control of the radiologic technologist. Basically, x-ray tube life is extended by using the minimum radiographic factors of mA, kVp, and exposure time that are appropriate for each examination. The use of faster image receptors has resulted in much longer tube life.

There are several causes of x-ray tube failure, most of which are related to the thermal characteristics of the x-ray tube. Enormous heat is generated in the anode of the x-ray tube during x-ray exposure. This heat must be dissipated for the x-ray tube to continue to function.

This heat can be dissipated in three ways: radiation, conduction, and convection (Figure 9-25). **Radiation** is the transfer of heat by the emission of infrared radiation. Heat lamps emit not only visible light but infrared energy. **Conduction** is the transfer of energy from one area of an object to another. The handle of a heated skillet becomes hot because of conduction. **Convection** is the transfer of heat by the movement of a heated substance from one place to another. Many homes and offices are heated by the convection of hot air.

 Excessive heat results in reduced x-ray tube life.

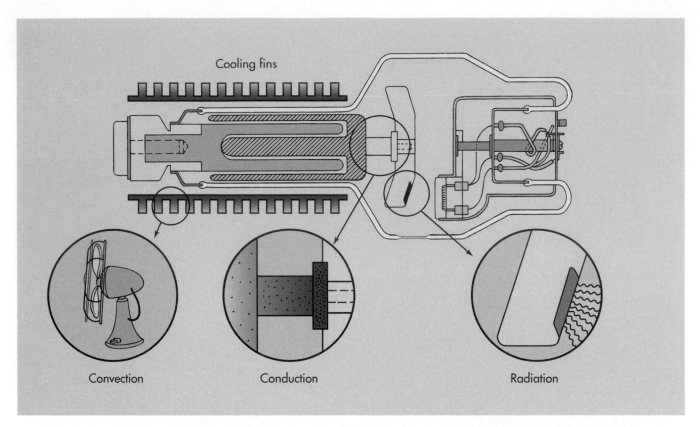

Cooling fins

Convection   Conduction   Radiation

FIGURE 9-25 Heat from an anode is dissipated by radiation, conduction, and convection.

All three modes of heat transfer occur in an x-ray tube. Most of the heat is dissipated by radiation during exposure. The anode may glow red hot. It always emits infrared energy. Some heat is conducted through the neck of the anode to the rotor and glass enclosure. The heated glass enclosure raises the temperature of the oil bath, which convects the heat to the tube housing and then to room air.

When the temperature of the anode is excessive during a single exposure, localized surface melting and pitting of the anode can occur. These surface irregularities result in variable and reduced radiation output. If the surface melting is sufficiently severe, the tungsten can be vaporized and can plate the inside of the glass enclosure. This can cause filtering of the x-ray beam and interference with electron flow from cathode to anode.

If the temperature of the anode increases too rapidly, the anode may crack, becoming unstable in rotation and rendering the tube useless. If maximum techniques are required for a particular examination, the anode should first be warmed by low-technique operation.

 Maximum radiographic techniques should never be applied to a cold anode.

A second type of x-ray tube failure results from maintaining the anode at elevated temperatures for prolonged periods. During exposures lasting 1 to 3 s, the temperature of the anode may be sufficient to cause it to glow like an incandescent light bulb. During exposure, heat is dissipated by radiation.

Between exposures, heat is dissipated, primarily through conduction, to the oil bath in which the tube is immersed. Some heat is conducted through the narrow molybdenum neck to the rotor assembly, and this can cause subsequent heating of the rotor bearings. Excessive heating of the bearings results in increased rotational friction and an imbalance of the rotor anode assembly. Bearing damage is another cause of tube failure.

If the thermal stress on the x-ray tube anode is maintained for prolonged periods, such as during fluoroscopy, the thermal capacity of the total anode system and of the x-ray tube housing is the limitation to operation. During fluoroscopy, the x-ray tube current is usually less than 5 mA, rather than hundreds of mA as in radiography.

Under such fluoroscopic conditions, the rate of heat dissipation from the rotating target attains equilibrium with the rate of heat input, and this rate rarely is sufficient to cause surface defects in the target. However, the x-ray tube can fail because of the continuous heat delivered to the rotor assembly, the oil bath, and the x-ray tube housing. Bearings can fail, the glass enclosure can crack, and the tube housing can fail.

A final cause of tube failure involves the filament. Because of the high temperature of the filament, tungsten atoms are slowly vaporized and plate the inside of the glass or metal enclosure, even with normal use. This tungsten, along with that vaporized from the anode, can disturb the electrical balance of the x-ray tube, causing abrupt, intermittent changes in tube current, which often leads to arcing and tube failure.

★ 6N Registry

The most frequent cause of abrupt tube failure is electron arcing from filament to enclosure due to vaporized tungsten.

With excessive heating of the filament caused by high mA operation for prolonged periods, more tungsten is vaporized. The filament wire becomes thinner and eventually breaks, causing an **open filament.** This same type of failure occurs when an incandescent light bulb burns out.

In the same way that the life of a light bulb is measured in hours—2000 hours is standard—that of an x-ray tube is measured in tens of thousands of exposures. Most computed tomography (CT) tubes are now guaranteed for 50,000 exposures.

Question: A 7-MHU spiral CT x-ray tube is guaranteed for 50,000 scans, each scan limited to 5 s. What is the x-ray tube life in hours?

Answer: Guaranteed tube life = (50,000 scans)

(.5 s/scan)

= 250,000 s

= 69 hr

RATING CHARTS

The radiologic technologist is guided in the use of x-ray tubes by x-ray **tube rating charts.** It is essential that the technologist be able to read and understand these charts. Three types of x-ray tube rating charts are particularly significant to the technologist: the radiographic rating chart, the anode cooling chart, and the housing cooling chart.

Radiographic Rating Chart

Of the three rating charts, the radiographic rating chart is the most important because it conveys which radiographic techniques are safe and which techniques are unsafe for x-ray tube operation. Each chart shown in Figure 9-26 contains a family of curves representing the various tube currents in mA. The x-axis and y-axis show scales of the two other radiographic parameters, time and kVp.

For a given mA, any combination of kVp and time that lies below the mA curve is safe. Any combination of kVp and time that lies above the curve representing the desired mA is unsafe. If an unsafe exposure was made, the tube might fail abruptly. Most x-ray imaging systems have a built-in safety feature that does not allow an exposure to be made when the technique selected would cause the tube to exceed the safe conditions of the radiographic rating chart.

A series of radiographic rating charts accompanies every x-ray tube. These charts cover the various modes of operation possible with that tube. There are different charts for filament in use (large or small focal spot), the speed of anode rotation (3400 rpm or 10,000 rpm), the target angle, and the voltage rectification (half-wave, full-wave, three-phase, high-frequency).

Be sure to use the proper radiographic rating chart with each tube. This is particularly important after the replacement of x-ray tubes. An appropriate radiographic rating chart is supplied with each replacement x-ray tube and can be different from that of the original tube.

The application of radiographic rating charts is not difficult.

Question: With reference to Figure 9-26, which of the following conditions of exposure are safe and which are unsafe?
   a. 95 kVp, 150 mA, 1 s; 3400 rpm; 0.6-mm focal spot
   b. 85 kVp, 400 mA, 0.5 s; 3400 rpm; 1-mm focal spot
   c. 125 kVp, 500 mA, 0.1 s; 10,000 rpm; 1-mm focal spot
   d. 75 kVp, 700 mA, 0.3 s; 10,000 rpm; 1-mm focal spot
   e. 88 kVp, 400 mA, 0.1 s; 10,000 rpm; 0.6-mm focal spot

Answer: a. Unsafe;   b. Unsafe;   c. Safe; d. Safe;   e. Unsafe

Question: Radiographic examination of the abdomen with a tube that has a 0.6-mm focal spot and anode rotation of 10,000 rpm requires technique factors of 95 kVp, 150 mAs. What is the shortest possible exposure time for this examination?

Answer: Locate the proper radiographic rating chart (upper right in Figure 9-26) and the 95-kVp line (horizontal line near middle of chart). Beginning from the left (shorter exposure times), determine the mAs for the intersection of each mA curve with the 95 kVp level.
   1. The first intersection is approximately 350 mA at 0.03 s = 10.5 mAs. Not enough.

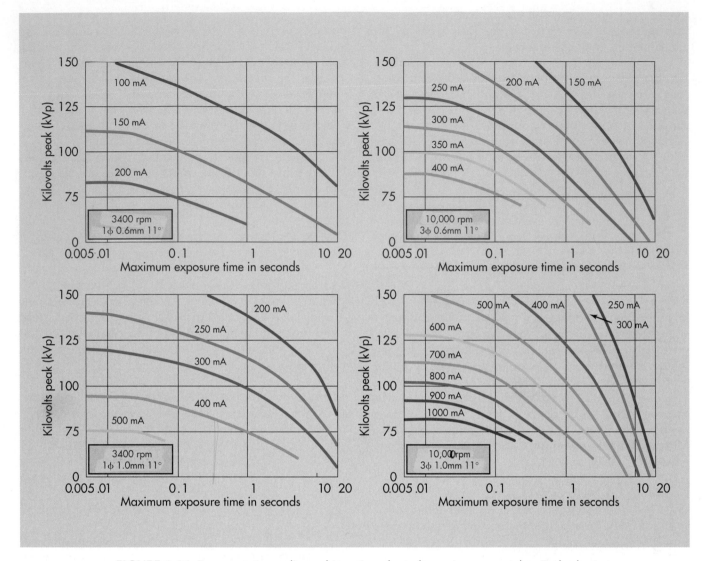

FIGURE 9-26 Representative radiographic rating charts for a given x-ray tube. Each chart specifies the conditions of operation to which it applies. (Courtesy General Electric Medical Systems.)

2. The next intersection is approximately 300 mA at 0.2 s = 60 mAs. Not enough.
3. The next intersection is approximately 250 mA at 0.6 s = 150 mAs. This is sufficient.

Consequently, 0.6 s is the minimum possible exposure time.

Anode Cooling Chart

The anode has a limited capacity for storing heat. Although heat is dissipated to the oil bath and x-ray tube housing, it is possible through prolonged use or multiple exposures to exceed the heat storage capacity of the anode.

Thermal energy is conventionally measured in units of calories, British thermal units (BTU), or joules. In x-ray applications, thermal energy is measured in **heat units (HU)**. The capacity of the anode and the housing to store heat is measured in heat units. One heat unit is equal to the product of 1 kVp, 1 mA, and 1 s.

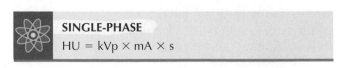

SINGLE-PHASE

$$HU = kVp \times mA \times s$$

Question: Radiographic examination of the lateral lumbar spine with a single-phase imaging system requires 98 kVp, 120 mAs. How many heat units are generated by this exposure?

Answer: Number of heat units = 98 kVp × 120 mAs

= 11,760 HU

Question: A fluoroscopic examination is performed with a single-phase imaging system at 76 kVp and 1.5 mA for 3.5 minutes. How many heat units are generated?

Answer: Number of heat units = 76 kVp × 1.5 mA × 3.5 min × 60 s/min = 23,940 HU

More heat is generated when three-phase and high-frequency equipment is used than when single-phase equipment is used. A modification factor is necessary for calculating three-phase or high-frequency heat units.

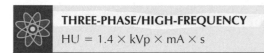

THREE-PHASE/HIGH-FREQUENCY
HU = 1.4 × kVp × mA × s

Question: Six sequential skull films are exposed with a three-phase generator operated at 82 kVp, 120 mAs. What is the total heat generated?

Answer: Number of heat units/film = 1.4 × 82 kVp × 120 mAs
= 13,776 HU
Total HU = 6 × 13,776 HU
= 82,656 HU

The thermal capacity of an anode and its heat dissipation characteristics are contained in a rating chart called an anode cooling chart (Figure 9-27). Unlike the radiographic rating chart, the anode cooling chart does not depend on the filament size or the speed of rotation.

The tube represented in Figure 9-27 has a maximum anode heat capacity of 350,000 HU. The chart shows that if the maximum heat load were attained, it would take 15 minutes for the anode to cool completely.

The rate of cooling is rapid at first and slows as the anode cools. In addition to determining the maximum heat capacity of the anode, the anode cooling chart is used to determine the length of time required for complete cooling after any level of heat input.

Question: A particular examination results in 50,000 HU being delivered to the anode in a matter of seconds. How long will it take the anode to cool completely?

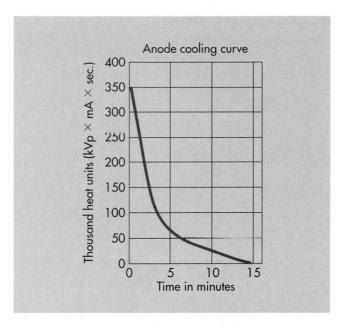

FIGURE 9-27 Anode cooling chart showing time required for heated anode to cool. (Courtesy General Electric Medical Systems.)

Answer: The 50,000-HU level intersects the anode cooling curve at approximately 6 min. From that point on the curve to complete cooling requires an additional 9 min (15 − 6 = 9). Therefore, 9 min is required for complete cooling.

Although the heat generated in producing x-rays is expressed in heat units, joules are the equivalent. By definition:

1 watt = 1 volt × 1 amp
= 1 J/C × 1 C/s
= 1 J/s
Therefore: 1 J/s = 1 kV × 1 mA
and 1 J = 1 kV × 1 mA × 1 s
and since 1 HU = 1 kVp × 1 mA × 1 s
1 HU = 1.4 J
1 J = 0.7 HU

Question: How much heat energy (in joules) is produced during a single high-frequency mammographic exposure of 25 kVp, 200 mAs?

Answer: 25 kVp × 200 mAs = 5000 HU
5000 HU × 1.4 J/HU = 7000 J
= 7 kJ

Housing Cooling Chart

The cooling chart for the housing of the x-ray tube has a shape similar to that of the anode cooling chart and is used in precisely the same way. Radiographic x-ray tube housings usually have maximum heat capacities in the range of several million heat units. Complete cooling after maximum heat capacity requires from 1 to 2 hours. Approximately twice that amount of time is required without auxiliary fan-powered air circulation.

SUMMARY

The primary support structure for the x-ray tube, which allows the greatest ease of movement and range of position, is the ceiling support system. The protective housing covers the x-ray tube and provides the following three functions: (1) it reduces leakage radiation to 100 mR/hr at 1 m, (2) it provides mechanical support protecting the tube from damage, and (3) it serves as a way to conduct heat away from the x-ray tube target.

The glass or metal enclosure surrounds the cathode (−) and anode (+), which are the electrodes of the vacuum tube. The cathode contains the tungsten filament, which is the source of electrons. The rotating anode is the tungsten-rhenium disk, which serves as a target for the electrons accelerated from the cathode. The line-focus principle results from angled targets. The heel effect is the variation in x-ray intensity across the x-ray beam because of absorption of x-rays in the heel of the target.

Safe operation of the x-ray tube is the responsibility of the radiographer. Tube failure can be prevented. The causes of tube failure are threefold:

1. A single excessive exposure causes pitting or cracking of the anode.
2. Long exposure times cause excessive heating of the anode, resulting in damage to the bearings in the rotor assembly. Bearing damage causes warping and rotational friction of the anode.
3. Even with normal use, vaporization of the filament causes tungsten to coat the glass or metal enclosure, which eventually causes arcing.

Tube rating charts printed by manufacturers of x-ray tubes aid the radiographer in using acceptable exposure levels to maximize x-ray tube life.

CHALLENGE QUESTIONS

1. Define or otherwise identify:
   a. Housing cooling chart
   b. Leakage radiation
   c. Heat unit (HU)
   d. Focusing cup
   e. Anode rotation speed
   f. Thoriated tungsten
   g. X-ray tube current
   h. Grid-controlled x-ray tube
   i. Convection
   j. Space charge
2. List the six main methods used to support the x-ray tube and briefly describe each.
3. Define SID.
4. What is the length and diameter of an x-ray tube?
5. Why are arcing and tube failure no longer a problem in modern x-ray tube design?
6. Explain the phenomenon of thermionic emission.
7. Describe the principal cause of x-ray failure. What addition to the filament material prolongs tube life?
8. What is the reason for the filament to be embedded in focusing cup?
9. Why are x-ray tubes manufactured with two focal spots?
10. Is the anode or the cathode the negative side of the x-ray tube?
11. List and describe the two types of anodes.
12. What are the three functions the anode serves in an x-ray tube?
13. How do atomic number, thermal conductivity, and melting point affect the anode target material?
14. Draw diagrams of a stationary and a rotating anode.
15. How does the anode rotate inside a glass enclosure with no mechanical connection to the outside?
16. Draw the difference between the actual focal spot and the effective focal spot.
17. Define the heel effect and describe how it can be used advantageously.
18. Explain the three causes of x-ray tube failure.
19. What happens when an x-ray tube is space-charge limited?
20. What is a detent position?

X-Ray Production

OBJECTIVES

At the completion of this chapter, the student should be able to do the following:

1. Discuss the interactions between projectile electrons and the x-ray tube target
2. Identify characteristic and bremsstrahlung x-rays
3. Describe the x-ray emission spectrum
4. Explain how mAs, kVp, added filtration, target material, and voltage ripple affect the x-ray emission spectrum

OUTLINE

Electron Target Interactions
    Anode Heat
    Characteristic Radiation
    Bremsstrahlung Radiation
X-Ray Emission Spectrum
    Characteristic X-Ray Spectrum
    Bremsstrahlung X-Ray Spectrum
    Minimum Wavelength
Factors Affecting the X-Ray Emission Spectrum
    Effect of mA and mAs
    Effect of kVp
    Effect of Added Filtration
    Effect of Target Material
    Effect of Voltage Waveform

CHAPTER 9 discussed the internal components of the x-ray tube, the cathode and anode, within the evacuated glass or metal enclosure. This chapter explains the interactions of the electrons accelerated from the cathode with the x-ray tube target. Those interactions produce two kinds of x-rays, characteristic and bremsstrahlung, which are described by the x-ray emission spectrum. Various conditions that affect the x-ray emission spectrum are discussed.

ELECTRON TARGET INTERACTIONS

The x-ray imaging system description in Chapter 9 emphasized that its primary function is to accelerate electrons from the cathode to the anode in the x-ray tube. The three principal parts of an x-ray imaging system—the operating console, the high-voltage generator, and the x-ray tube—are all designed to provide a large number of electrons with high kinetic energy focused to a small spot on the anode.

 Kinetic energy is the energy of motion.

Stationary objects have no kinetic energy; objects in motion have kinetic energy proportional to their mass and to the square of their velocity. The kinetic energy equation follows:

KINETIC ENERGY

$KE = \frac{1}{2} mv^2$

where m is the mass in kilograms,

V is the velocity in meters per second, and

KE is the kinetic energy in joules.

For example, a 1000-kg automobile has four times the kinetic energy of a 250-kg motorcycle traveling at the same speed (Figure 10-1). If the motorcycle were to double its velocity, however, it would have the same kinetic energy as the automobile.

In determining the magnitude of the kinetic energy of a projectile, velocity is more important than mass. In an x-ray tube, the projectile is the electron. All electrons have the same mass; therefore, electron kinetic energy is increased by raising the kVp. As electron kinetic energy is increased, both the intensity (quantity) and the energy (quality) of the x-ray beam are increased.

The modern x-ray imaging system is remarkable. It conveys to the x-ray tube target an enormous number of electrons at a precisely controlled kinetic energy. At 100 mA, for example, 6×10^{17} electrons travel from the cathode to the anode of the x-ray tube every second.

In an x-ray imaging system operating at 70 kVp, each electron arrives at the target with a maximum kinetic energy of 70 keV. Because there are 1.6×10^{-16} J per 1 keV, this energy is equivalent to the following:

$(70 \text{ keV})(1.6 \times 10^{-16} \text{ J/keV}) = 1.12 \times 10^{-14} \text{ J}$

Inserting this energy into the expression for kinetic energy and solving for the velocity of the electrons, the result is:

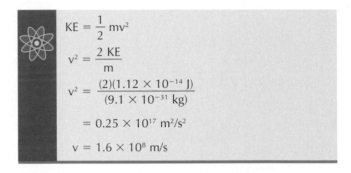

$$KE = \frac{1}{2} mv^2$$

$$v^2 = \frac{2 \text{ KE}}{m}$$

$$v^2 = \frac{(2)(1.12 \times 10^{-14} \text{ J})}{(9.1 \times 10^{-31} \text{ kg})}$$

$$= 0.25 \times 10^{17} \text{ m}^2/\text{s}^2$$

$$v = 1.6 \times 10^8 \text{ m/s}$$

Question: At what fraction of the velocity of light do 70-keV electrons travel?

Answer: $\dfrac{v}{c} = \dfrac{1.6 \times 10^8 \text{ m/s}}{3.0 \times 10^8 \text{ m/s}} = 0.53$

These calculations are not precisely correct; however, they do serve to illustrate the point and demonstrate the use of the preceding equation. According to the theory of relativity, an electron's mass increases as it approaches the speed of light, and thus the actual value of v/c is 0.47 at 70 keV.

The distance between the filament and the x-ray tube target is only approximately 1 cm. It is not difficult to imagine the intensity of the accelerating force required to raise the velocity of electrons from zero to half the speed of light in so short a distance.

The electrons traveling from cathode to anode constitute the x-ray tube current and are sometimes called **projectile electrons.** When these projectile electrons hit the heavy metal atoms of the x-ray tube target, they transfer their kinetic energy to the target atoms.

These interactions occur within a very small depth of penetration into the target. As they occur, the projectile electrons slow down and finally come nearly to rest, at which time they are conducted through the

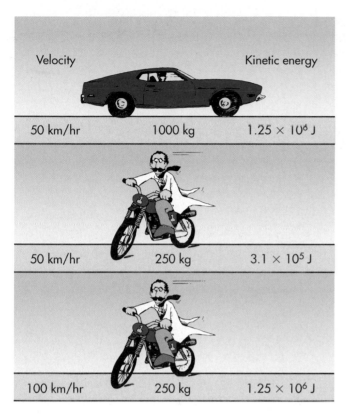

FIGURE 10-1 Kinetic energy is proportional to the product of mass and velocity squared.

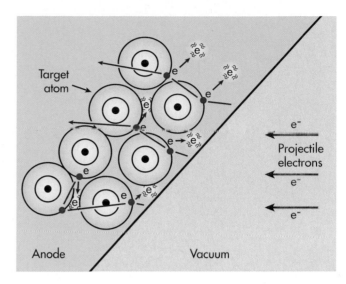

FIGURE 10-2 Most of the kinetic energy of projectile electrons is converted to heat by interactions with outer-shell electrons of target atoms. These interactions are primarily excitations rather than ionizations.

x-ray anode assembly and out into the associated electronic circuitry.

The projectile electron interacts with either the orbital electrons or the nuclear field of target atoms. These interactions result in the conversion of electron kinetic energy into thermal energy (heat) and electromagnetic energy in the form of infrared radiation (also heat) and x-rays.

Anode Heat

Most of the kinetic energy of projectile electrons is converted into heat (Figure 10-2). The projectile electrons interact with the outer-shell electrons of the target atoms but do not transfer sufficient energy to these outer-shell electrons to ionize them. Rather, the outer-shell electrons are simply raised to an excited, or higher, energy level.

The outer-shell electrons immediately drop back to their normal energy level with the emission of **infrared radiation.** The constant **excitation** and return of outer-shell electrons is responsible for most of the heat generated in the anodes of x-ray tubes.

Approximately 99% of the kinetic energy of projectile electrons is converted to heat.

Only approximately 1% of projectile electron kinetic energy is used for the production of x-radiation. Therefore, sophisticated as it is, the x-ray imaging system is very inefficient.

The production of heat in the anode increases directly with increasing x-ray tube current. Doubling the x-ray tube current doubles the heat produced. Heat production also increases directly with increasing kVp, at least in the diagnostic range. Although the relationship between varying kVp and varying heat production is approximate, it is sufficiently exact to allow the computation of heat units for use with anode cooling charts.

The efficiency of x-ray production is independent of the tube current. Consequently, regardless of what mA is selected, the efficiency of x-ray production remains constant.

The efficiency of x-ray production increases with increasing kVp. At 60 kVp, only 0.5% of the electron kinetic energy is converted to x-rays. At 100 kVp, approximately 1% is converted to x-rays, and at 20 MV, 70% is converted.

Characteristic Radiation

If the projectile electron interacts with an inner-shell electron of the target atom rather than with an outer-shell electron, **characteristic x-rays** can be produced. Characteristic x-rays result when the interaction is sufficiently violent to ionize the target atom by totally removing an inner-shell electron.

Characteristic x-rays are emitted when an outer-shell electron fills an inner-shell void.

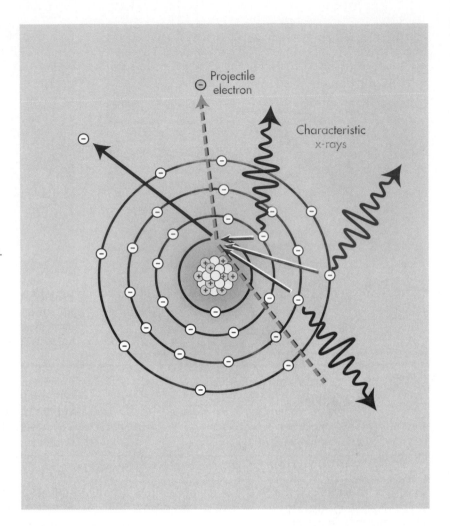

FIGURE 10-3 Characteristic x-rays are produced after the ionization of a K-shell electron.
When an outer-shell electron fills the vacancy
in the K shell, an x-ray is emitted.

Figure 10-3 illustrates how characteristic x-rays are produced. When the projectile electron ionizes a target
atom by removing a K-shell electron, a temporary electron void is produced in the K shell. This is a highly unnatural state for the target atom and is corrected by an
outer-shell electron falling into the void in the K shell.

The transition of an orbital electron from an outer
shell to an inner shell is accompanied by the emission of
an x-ray. The x-ray has energy equal to the difference in
the binding energies of the orbital electrons involved.

Question: A K-shell electron is removed from a tungsten atom and is replaced by an L-shell
electron. What is the energy of the characteristic x-ray that is emitted?

Answer: Reference to Figure 4-9 shows that for
tungsten, K-shell electrons have binding
energies of 70 keV, and L-shell electrons are
bound by 12 keV. Therefore, the characteristic x-ray emitted has energy of
70 − 12 = 58 keV

By the same procedure, the energy of x-rays resulting
from M-to-K, N-to-K, O-to-K, and P-to-K transitions
can be calculated. Tungsten, for example, has electrons
in shells out to the P shell, and when a K-shell electron
is ionized, its position can be filled with electrons from
any of the outer shells. All these x-rays are called
K x-rays because they result from electron transitions
into the K shell.

Similar characteristic x-rays are produced when the
target atom is ionized by removal of electrons from
shells other than the K shell. Note that Figure 10-3 does
not show the production of x-rays resulting from ionization of an L-shell electron.

Such a diagram would show the removal of an L-
shell electron by the projectile electron. The vacancy in
the L shell would be filled by an electron from any of
the outer shells. X-rays resulting from electron transitions to the L shell are called *L x-rays* and have much
less energy than K x-rays because the binding energy of
an L-shell electron is much lower than that of a K-shell
electron.

TABLE 10-1	Characteristic X-Rays of Tungsten and Their Effective Energies (keV)					
	ELECTRON TRANSITION FROM SHELL					
Characteristic	L-Shell	M-Shell	N-Shell	O-Shell	P-Shell	Effective Energy of X-ray
K	57.4	66.7	68.9	69.4	69.5	69
L		9.3	11.5	12.0	12.1	12
M			2.2	2.7	2.8	3
N				0.52	0.6	0.6
O					0.08	0.1

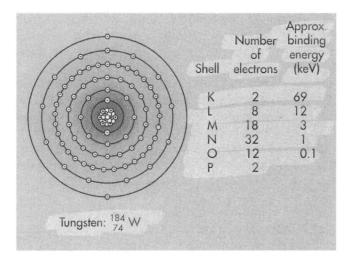

FIGURE 10-4 Atomic configuration and electron-binding energies for tungsten.

Only the K-characteristic x-rays of tungsten are useful for imaging.

Similarly, M-characteristic x-rays, N-characteristic x-rays, and even O-characteristic x-rays can be produced in a tungsten target. Figure 10-4 illustrates the electron configuration and Table 10-1 summarizes the production of characteristic x-rays in tungsten.

Although many characteristic x-rays can be produced, they can be produced only at specific energies, equal to the differences in the electron-binding energies for the various electron transitions.

Except for K x-rays, all the characteristic x-rays have very low energy. The L x-rays, with approximately 12 keV of energy, penetrate only a few centimeters into soft tissue. Consequently, they are useless as diagnostic x-rays, as are all the other low-energy characteristic x-rays. The last column in Table 10-1 shows the effective energy for each of the characteristic x-rays of tungsten.

This type of x-radiation is called *characteristic* because it is characteristic of the target element.

Because the electron-binding energy for every element is different, the energy of characteristic x-rays produced in the various elements is also different. The effective energy of characteristic x-rays increases with increasing atomic number of the target element.

Bremsstrahlung Radiation

The production of heat and characteristic x-rays involves interactions between the projectile electrons and the electrons of x-ray tube target atoms. A third type of interaction in which the projectile electron can lose its kinetic energy is an interaction with the nuclear field of a target atom. In this type of interaction, the kinetic energy of the projectile electron is also converted into electromagnetic energy.

A projectile electron that completely avoids the orbital electrons as it passes through a target atom may come sufficiently close to the nucleus of the atom to come under the influence of its electric field (Figure 10-4). Because the electron is negatively charged and the nucleus is positively charged, there is an electrostatic force of attraction between them.

The closer the projectile electron gets to the nucleus, the more it is influenced by the electric field of the nucleus. This field is very strong because the nucleus contains many protons and the distance between the nucleus and projectile electron is very small.

As the projectile electron passes by the nucleus, it is slowed down and changes its course, leaving with reduced kinetic energy in a different direction. This loss in kinetic energy reappears as an x-ray. This interaction is somewhat analogous to a comet in its course around the sun.

Bremsstrahlung x-rays are produced when a projectile electron is slowed by the electric field of a target atom nucleus.

These types of x-rays are called **bremsstrahlung x-rays.** *Bremsstrahlung* is a German word meaning "slowed-down radiation." Bremsstrahlung x-rays can be considered radiation resulting from the braking of projectile electrons by the nucleus.

A projectile electron can lose any amount of its kinetic energy in an interaction with the nucleus of a target atom and the bremsstrahlung x-ray associated with the loss can take on corresponding values. For example, when an x-ray imaging system is operated at 70 kVp, projectile electrons have kinetic energies up to 70 keV.

An electron with kinetic energy of 70 keV can lose all, none, or any intermediate level of that kinetic energy in a bremsstrahlung interaction. Therefore, the bremsstrahlung x-ray produced can have any energy up to 70 keV.

This is different from the production of characteristic x-rays, which have very specific energies. Figure 10-5 illustrates how one can consider the production of such a wide range of energies through the bremsstrahlung interaction.

A low-energy bremsstrahlung x-ray results when the projectile electron is barely influenced by the nucleus. A maximum-energy x-ray occurs when the projectile electron loses all its kinetic energy and simply drifts away from the nucleus. Bremsstrahlung x-rays with energies between these two extremes occur more frequently.

 In the diagnostic range, most x-rays are bremsstrahlung x-rays.

Bremsstrahlung x-rays can be produced at any projectile electron energy. K-characteristic x-rays require a tube potential of at least 70 kVp. At 65 kVp, for example, no useful characteristic x-rays are produced, and therefore the x-ray beam is all bremsstrahlung. At 100 kVp, approximately 15% of the x-ray beam is characteristic and the remaining is bremsstrahlung.

X-RAY EMISSION SPECTRUM

Most people have seen or heard of pitching machines (the devices used by baseball teams for batting practice so that the pitchers do not get worn out). There are similar machines for automatically ejecting bowling balls, tennis balls, and even ping-pong balls.

Suppose there was a device that could eject all these types of balls at random at a rate of one per second. The most straightforward way to determine how often each type of ball was ejected on average would be to catch each ball as it was ejected and then identify it and drop it into a basket; at the end of the observation period the total number of each type of ball could be counted.

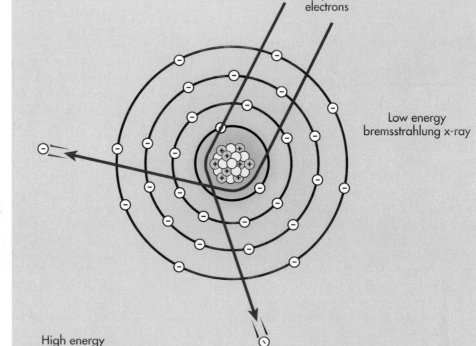

FIGURE 10-5 Bremsstrahlung x-rays result from an interaction between a projectile electron and a target nucleus. The electron is slowed and its direction is changed.

Let us suppose that the results obtained for a 10-minute period are those shown in Figure 10-6. A total of 600 balls were ejected. Perhaps the easiest way to represent these results graphically would be to plot the total number of each type of ball emitted during the 10-minute observation period and represent each total by a bar (Figure 10-7).

Such a bar graph can be described as a discrete ball-ejection spectrum representative of the automatic pitching machine. It is a plot of the number of balls ejected per unit of time as a function of the type of ball. It is called **discrete** because only five distinct types of balls are involved.

 A discrete spectrum contains only specific values.

Connecting the bars with a dashed curve as shown would indicate a large number of different types of balls. Such a curve is called a **continuous** ejection spectrum. The word **spectrum** refers to the range of types of balls or values of any quantity such as x-rays. The total number of balls ejected is represented by the sum of the areas under the bars in the case of the discrete spectrum and the area under the curve in the case of the continuous spectrum.

 A continuous spectrum contains all possible values.

Without regard to the absolute number of balls emitted, Figure 10-7 could also be identified as a relative ball-ejection spectrum because at a glance one can tell the relative frequency with which each type of ball was ejected. Relatively speaking, baseballs are ejected most frequently and basketballs least frequently.

This type of relationship is fundamental to describing the output of an x-ray tube. If one could stand in the middle of the useful x-ray beam, catch each individual x-ray and measure its energy, one could describe what is known as the **x-ray emission spectrum** (Figure 10-8).

Here, the relative number of x-rays emitted is plotted as a function of the energy of each individual x-ray. X-ray energy is the variable considered.

Although we cannot catch and identify each individual x-ray, there are instruments available that allow us to do essentially that. X-ray emission spectra have been measured for all types of x-ray imaging systems. Understanding x-ray emission spectra is a key to understanding how changes in voltage, kVp, mA, and added filtration affect the optical density (OD) and contrast of an image.

Characteristic X-Ray Spectrum

The discrete energies of characteristic x-rays are characteristic of the differences between electron-binding energies of a particular element. A characteristic x-ray from tungsten, for example, can have 1 of 15 different energies (Table 10-1) and no others. A plot of the frequency with which characteristic x-rays are emitted as a function of their energy would look like that shown for tungsten in Figure 10-9.

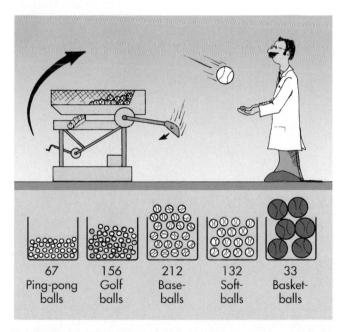

FIGURE 10-6 In a 10-minute period an automatic ball-throwing machine might eject 600 balls, distributed as shown.

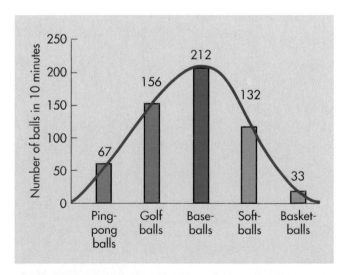

FIGURE 10-7 Bar graph representing the results of 10-minute observation of balls ejected by the automatic pitching machine in Figure 10-6. When the height of each bar is joined, a smooth emission spectrum is created.

Such a plot is called the **characteristic x-ray emission spectrum.** There are five vertical lines representing K x-rays and four vertical lines representing L x-rays. The other lower-energy lines represent characteristic emissions from the outer electron shells.

 Characteristic x-rays have precisely fixed (discrete) energies and form a discrete emission spectrum.

The relative intensity of the K x-rays is greater than that of the lower-energy characteristic x-rays because of the nature of the interaction process. K x-rays are the only characteristic x-rays of tungsten with sufficient energy to be of value in diagnostic radiology. Although there are five K x-rays, it is customary to represent them as one, as has been done with a single vertical line at 69 keV in Figure 10-10. Only this line will be shown in later graphs.

Bremsstrahlung X-Ray Spectrum

If it were possible to measure the energy contained in each bremsstrahlung x-ray emitted from an x-ray tube, one would find that these energies range from the peak electron energy all the way down to zero. In other words, when an x-ray tube is operated at 90 kVp, bremsstrahlung x-rays with energies up to 90 keV are emitted. A typical bremsstrahlung x-ray emission spectrum is shown in Figure 10-10.

 Bremsstrahlung x-rays have a range of energies and form a continuous emission spectrum.

Question: At what kVp was the x-ray imaging system presented in Figure 10-10 operated?

Answer: Because the bremsstrahlung spectrum intersects the energy axis at approximately 90 keV, the imaging system must have been operated at approximately 90 kVp.

The general shape of the bremsstrahlung x-ray spectrum is the same for all x-ray imaging systems. The maximum energy (in keV) of an x-ray is numerically equal to the kVp of operation.

The greatest number of x-rays is emitted with energy approximately one third of the maximum energy. The number of x-rays emitted decreases rapidly at very low energies.

Question: What would be the expected emission spectrum for an x-ray imaging system with a pure molybdenum target (effective energy of K x-ray = 19 keV) operated at 95 kVp?

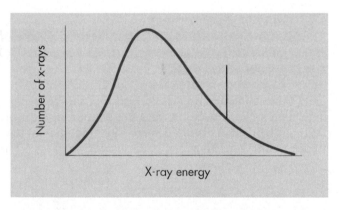

FIGURE 10-8 General form of an x-ray emission spectrum.

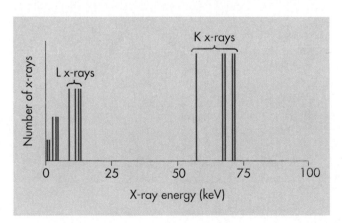

FIGURE 10-9 Characteristic x-ray emission spectrum for tungsten contains 15 different x-ray energies.

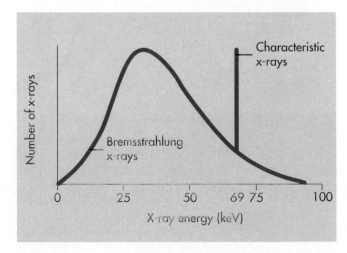

FIGURE 10-10 Bremsstrahlung x-ray emission spectrum extends from zero to maximum projectile electron energy, with the highest number of x-rays having approximately one-third the maximum energy. The characteristic x-ray emission spectrum is represented by a line at 69 keV.

Answer: The spectrum should look something like Figure 10-8. The curve intersects the energy axis at 0 and 95 keV and has the general shape shown in Figure 10-10. The bremsstrahlung spectrum is much lower because the atomic number of Mo is low, and x-ray production is much less efficient. A line extends above the curve at 19 keV to represent the K-characteristic x-rays.

Minimum Wavelength

As described in Chapter 5, the energy of an x-ray is equal to the product of its frequency *(f)* and Planck's constant *(h)*. X-ray energy is also inversely proportional to its wavelength. As x-ray wavelength increases, x-ray energy decreases.

> Maximum x-ray energy is associated with the minimum x-ray wavelength (λ_{min}).

The minimum wavelength of x-ray emission corresponds to the maximum x-ray energy and the maximum x-ray energy is numerically equal to the kVp.

FACTORS AFFECTING THE X-RAY EMISSION SPECTRUM

The total number of x-rays emitted from an x-ray tube could be determined by adding the number of x rays emitted at each energy over the entire spectrum, a process called **integration**. Graphically, the total number of x-rays emitted is equivalent to the area under the curve of the x-ray emission spectrum.

The general shape of an emission spectrum is always the same, but its relative position along the energy axis can change. The farther to the right a spectrum is, the higher the effective energy or **quality** of the x-ray beam.

The larger the area under the curve, the higher the x-ray intensity or **quantity**. A number of factors under the control of the radiologic technologist influence the size and shape of the x-ray emission spectrum, and therefore the quality and quantity of the x-ray beam. These factors are summarized in Table 10-2.

Effect of mA and mAs

If one changes the current from 200 to 400 mA, while all other conditions remain constant, twice as many electrons will flow from cathode to anode and the mAs will be doubled. This operating change will produce twice as many x-rays at every energy. In other words, the x-ray emission spectrum will be changed in amplitude but not in shape (Figure 10-11).

Each point on the curve labeled 400 mA is precisely two times higher than the associated point on the 200-mA curve. This relationship also is true for changes in mAs. Thus, the area under the x-ray emission spectrum varies in proportion to changes in mA or mAs, as does the x-ray quantity.

> A change in mA or mAs results in a proportional change in the amplitude of the x-ray emission spectrum at all energies.

Four Principal Factors Influencing the Shape of an X-Ray Emission Spectrum

1. The projectile electrons accelerated from cathode to anode do not all have the peak kinetic energy. Depending on the type of rectification and high-voltage generation, many of these electrons may have very low energies when they strike the target. Such electrons can produce only heat and low-energy x-rays.

2. The target of a diagnostic x-ray tube is relatively thick. Consequently, many of the bremsstrahlung x-rays emitted result from multiple interactions of the projectile electrons, and for each successive interaction, a projectile electron has less energy.

3. Low-energy x-rays are more likely to be absorbed in the target.

4. External filtration is always added to the x-ray tube assembly. This added filtration serves selectively to remove low-energy x-rays from the beam.

TABLE 10-2	Factors Affecting Size and Relative Position of X-Ray Emission Spectra	
	Factor	**Effect**
	Tube current	Amplitude of spectrum
	Tube voltage	Amplitude and position
	Added filtration	Amplitude, most effective at low energy
	Target material	Amplitude of spectrum and position of line spectrum
	Voltage waveform	Amplitude, most effective at high energy

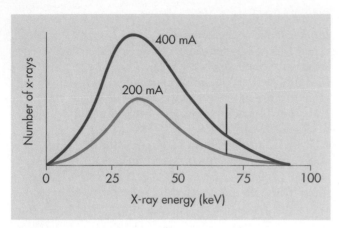

FIGURE 10-11 Change in mA results in a proportionate change in the amplitude of the x-ray emission spectrum at all energies.

increase quantity not quality

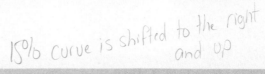

15% curve is shifted to the right and up

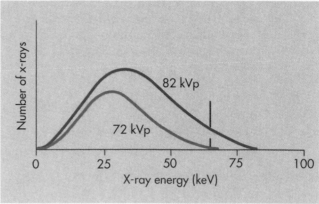

FIGURE 10-12 Change in kVp results in an increase in the amplitude of the emission spectrum at all energies, but a greater increase at high energies than at low energies. Therefore, the spectrum is shifted to the right or high-energy side.

increase quantity + quality

Question: Suppose the area under the 200-mA curve in Figure 10-11 totals 4.2 cm² and the x-ray quantity is 325 mR (3.25 mGy$_a$). What would the area under the curve and the x-ray quantity be if the tube current were increased to 400 mA, while other operating factors remain constant?

Answer: In going from 200 to 400 mA, the tube current has been increased by a factor of two. The area under the curve and the x-ray quantity are increased proportionately:

Area = 4.2 cm² × 2 = 8.4 cm²
Intensity = 325 mR × 2 = 650 mR

Effect of kVp

As the kVp is raised, the area under the curve increases to an area approximating the square of the factor by which kVp was increased. Accordingly, the x-ray quantity increases with the square of this factor.

When kVp is increased, the relative distribution of emitted x-ray energy shifts to the right, to a higher average x-ray energy. The maximum energy of x-ray emission always remains numerically equal to the kVp.

A change in voltage peak affects both the amplitude and the position of the x-ray emission spectrum.

Figure 10-12 demonstrates the effect of increasing the kVp while other factors remain constant. The lower spectrum represents x-ray operation at 72 kVp and the upper spectrum represents operation at 82 kVp, a 10 kVp (or 15%) increase.

The area under the curve has approximately doubled, while the relative position of the curve has shifted to the right, the high-energy side. More x-rays are emitted at all energies during operation at 82 kVp than during operation at 72 kVp. The increase, however, is relatively greater for high-energy x-rays than for low-energy x-rays.

A change in kVp has no effect on the position of the discrete x-ray emission spectrum.

Question: Suppose the curve labeled 72 kVp in Figure 10-12 covers a total area of 3.6 cm² and represents an x-ray quantity of 125 mR (1.25 mGy$_a$). What area under the curve and x-ray quantity would be expected for operations at 82 kVp?

Answer: The area under the curve and the output intensity are proportional to the *square* of the ratio of the kVp change. A ratio can be established.

$$\left(\frac{82}{72}\right)^2 (3.6 \text{ cm}^2) = (1.3)(3.6c \text{ cm}^2)$$

$$= 4.7 \text{ cm}^2$$
and
$$(1.3)(125 \text{ mR}) = 163 \text{ mR}$$

This example partially explains the rule of thumb used by radiologic technologists to relate the kVp and mAs changes necessary to produce a constant OD on a radiograph. The rule states that a 15% increase in kVp is equivalent to doubling the mAs. At low kVp, such as 50 to 60 kVp, approximately a 7-kVp increase is equivalent to doubling the milliampere-seconds. At tube potentials above about 100 kVp, a 15-kVp change may be necessary.

 In the diagnostic range, a 15% increase in kVp is equivalent to doubling the mAs.

A 15% increase in kVp does not double the x-ray intensity but is equivalent to doubling the mAs to obtain a given OD on the radiograph. To double the output intensity by increasing kVp, one would have to raise the kVp by as much as 40%.

Radiographically, only a 15% increase in kVp is necessary because with increased kVp, the penetrability of the x-ray beam is increased. Therefore, less radiation is absorbed by the patient, leaving proportionately more x-rays to expose the image receptor.

Effect of Added Filtration   *intensity = quantity*

Adding filtration to the useful x-ray beam reduces x-ray beam intensity while increasing average energy. This effect is shown in Figure 10-13, where an x-ray tube is operated at 95 kVp with 2-mm aluminum (Al) added filtration, compared with the same operation with 4-mm Al added filtration. Added filtration more effectively absorbs low-energy x-rays than high-energy x-rays, and therefore the bremsstrahlung x-ray emission spectrum is reduced more on the left than on the right.

 The overall result of added filtration is an increase in the average energy of the x-ray beam (higher quality, spectrum shift to the right) with an accompanying reduction in x-ray quantity (**reduced spectrum amplitude**).

Adding filtration is sometimes called **hardening** the x-ray beam because of the relative increase in average energy. The characteristic spectrum is not affected, nor is the maximum energy of x-ray emission. There is no simple method to calculate the changes in x-ray quality and quantity with a change in added filtration.

Effect of Target Material

The atomic number of the target affects both the number (quantity) and the effective energy (quality) of x-rays. As the atomic number of the target material increases, the efficiency of the production of bremsstrahlung radiation increases and high-energy x-rays increase in number more than low-energy x-rays.

The change in the bremsstrahlung x-ray spectrum is not nearly as pronounced as the change in the charac-

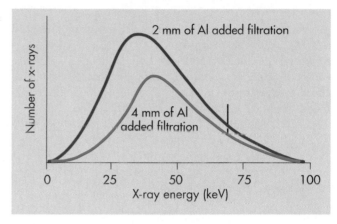

FIGURE 10-13 Adding filtration to an x-ray tube results in reduced x-ray intensity but increased effective energy. The emission spectra represented here resulted from operation at the same mA and kVp but with different filtration.

decrease quantity
increase quality

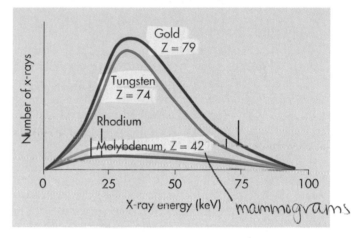

FIGURE 10-14 Discrete emission spectrum shifts to the right with an increase in the atomic number of the target material. The continuous spectrum increases slightly in amplitude, particularly to the high-energy side, with an increase in target atomic number.

mammograms

teristic spectrum. After an increase in the atomic number of the target material, the characteristic spectrum is shifted to the right, representing the higher-energy characteristic radiation. This phenomenon is a direct result of the higher electron-binding energies associated with increasing atomic numbers.

 Increasing target atomic number increases the efficiency of x-ray production and the energy of characteristic and bremsstrahlung x-rays.

These changes are shown schematically in Figure 10-14. Tungsten is the primary component of x-ray tube targets, but some specialty x-ray tubes use gold as target material. The atomic numbers for tungsten and gold are 74 and 79, respectively.

Molybdenum (Z = 42) and rhodium (Z = 45) are target elements used for mammography. Many dedicated mammography imaging systems have both elements separately incorporated into the target.

The x-ray quantity from such targets is low owing to the inefficiency of x-ray production. This occurs because of the low atomic number of these target elements. Elements of low atomic number also produce low-energy characteristic x-rays.

Effect of Voltage Waveform

There are five voltage waveforms: half-wave rectification, full-wave rectification, 3-phase/6-pulse, 3-phase/12-pulse, and high-frequency.

Half-wave–rectified and full-wave–rectified voltage waveforms are the same except for the frequency of x-ray pulse repetition. There are twice as many x-ray pulses per cycle with full-wave rectification as with half-wave rectification.

The difference between 3-phase/6-pulse and 3-phase/12-pulse power is simply the reduced ripple obtained with 12-pulse generation compared with 6-pulse generation. High-frequency generators are based on fundamentally different electrical engineering principles. They produce the lowest voltage ripple of all high-voltage generators.

Figure 10-15 shows an exploded view of a full-wave–rectified voltage waveform for an x-ray imaging system operated at 100 kVp. Recall that the amplitude of the waveform corresponds to the applied voltage and that the horizontal axis represents time.

At $t = 0$, the voltage across the x-ray tube is zero, indicating that at this instant no electrons are flowing and no x-rays are being produced. At $t = 1$ ms, the voltage across the x-ray tube has increased from 0 to approximately 10,000 V. The x-rays produced at this instant are of relatively low intensity and energy; none exceeds 10 keV. At $t = 2.1$ ms, the tube voltage has increased to approximately 25,000 V and is rapidly approaching its peak value.

At $t = 4.2$ ms, the maximum tube voltage is obtained, and the maximum energy and intensity of x-ray emission are produced. For the following one-quarter cycle between 4.2 and 8.3 ms, the x-ray quantity and quality decrease again to zero.

The number of x-rays emitted at each instant through a cycle is not proportional to the voltage. The number is low at lower voltages and increases at higher voltages. The quantity of x-rays is much higher at peak voltages than at lower voltages. Consequently, voltage waveforms of three-phase or high-frequency operation result in considerably more intense x-ray emission than those of single-phase operation.

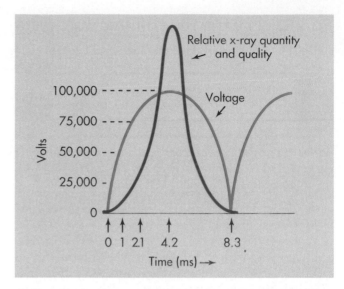

FIGURE 10-15 As the voltage across the x-ray tube increases from zero to its peak value, the x-ray intensity and energy increase slowly at first and then rapidly as peak voltage is obtained.

The relationship between x-ray quantity and type of high-voltage generator is the basis for another rule of thumb used by radiologic technologists. If a radiographic technique calls for 72 kVp on single-phase equipment, on three-phase equipment approximately 64 kVp, a 12% reduction, will produce similar results. High-frequency generators result in approximately the equivalent of a 16% increase in kVp or slightly more than a doubling of mAs over single-phase power.

Because of reduced ripple, operation with three-phase power or high frequency is equivalent to an approximate 12% increase in kVp or almost a doubling of mAs over single-phase power.

This discussion is summarized in Figure 10-16, where an x-ray emission spectrum from a full-wave–rectified unit is compared with that from a 3-phase, 12-pulse generator and a high-frequency generator, all operated at 92 kVp and the same mAs. The x-ray emission spectrum resulting from high-frequency operation is more efficient than that with either a single-phase or three-phase generator. The area under the curve is considerably greater and the x-ray emission spectrum is shifted to the high-energy side.

The characteristic x-ray emission spectrum remains fixed in its position on the energy axis but increases slightly in magnitude because of the increased number of projectile electrons available for K-shell electron interactions.

TABLE 10-3	Changes in X-Ray Beam Quality and Quantity by Factors That Influence the Emission Spectrum	
An Increase in	**Results in ...**
Current (mAs)	An increase in quantity. No change in quality.
Voltage (kVp)	An increase in quantity and quality.
Added filtration	A decrease in quantity. An increase in quality.
Increased target Z	An increase in quantity and quality.
Increased voltage ripple	A decrease in quantity and quality.

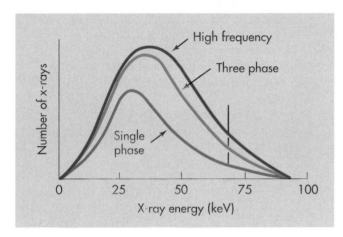

FIGURE 10-16 Three-phase and high-frequency operation are considerably more efficient than single-phase operation. Both the x-ray intensity (area under the curve) and the effective energy (relative shift to the right) are increased. Shown are representative spectra for 92-kVp operations.

Question: What would be the difference in the x-ray emission spectra between a full-wave–rectified operation compared with a half-wave–rectified operation if the kVp and mA are held constant?

Answer: Under constant conditions of kVp and mAs, there should be no difference in the x-ray emission spectra. The x-ray quantity and quality will remain constant for each x-ray pulse.

Table 10-3 presents a summary of the effect on x-ray quantity and quality from each of the factors that affect the x-ray emission spectrum. Although five factors are listed, only the first two, mAs and kVp, are routinely controlled by the radiologic technologist. Occasionally, the added filtration is changed if the imaging system design permits.

SUMMARY

When electrons are accelerated from the cathode to the target of the anode, three effects take place. There is the production of heat, the formation of characteristic x-rays, and the formation of bremsstrahlung x-rays.

Characteristic x-rays are produced when an electron ionizes an inner-shell electron of a target atom. As the inner-shell void is filled, an x-ray is emitted.

Bremsstrahlung x-rays are produced by the slowing down of an electron by the target atom's electrostatic nuclear field. Most x-rays in the diagnostic range (20 to 150 kVp) are bremsstrahlung x-rays.

X-ray emission spectra can be graphed as the number of x-rays for each increment of energy in keV volts. Characteristic x-rays of tungsten have a discrete energy of 69 keV. Bremsstrahlung x-rays have a range of energies up to X keV, where X is the kVp.

The following four factors influence the x-ray emission spectrum: (1) low-energy electrons interact to produce low-energy x-rays, (2) successive interactions of electrons result in the production of x-rays with lower energy, (3) low-energy x-rays are most likely to be absorbed by the target material, and (4) added filtration removes low-energy x-rays from the useful beam.

Factors that affect the size and relative position of x-ray emission spectra are summarized in Table 10-3.

CHALLENGE QUESTIONS

1. Define or otherwise identify the following:
   a. Projectile electron
   b. Binding energy
   c. Characteristic x-rays
   d. Bremsstrahlung x-rays
   e. X-ray quantity
   f. X-ray quality
   g. Effective energy
   h. Added filtration
   i. Emission spectrum
   j. Molybdenum
2. Calculate the energy and wavelength of the characteristic x-ray produced when a K-shell electron is replaced by M-shell electron.

3. At what fraction of the velocity of light do 90-keV electrons travel?

4. What does the discrete x-ray spectrum represent?

5. Draw the x-ray emission spectrum for an x-ray imaging system with a tungsten-targeted x-ray tube operated at 90 kVp.

6. When an x-ray imaging system is operated at 80 kVp, its emission spectrum represents an output intensity of 3.5 mR/mAs. What will be the output intensity if the voltage is increased to 90 kVp? How will the emission spectrum change?

7. Discuss the effect on the x-ray emission spectrum if a single-phase x-ray imaging system were changed to three-phase.

8. Explain the effect the addition of filtration to an x-ray tube has on the discrete and continuous x-ray emission spectra.

9. How is the kinetic energy of the projectile electrons streaming across the x-ray tube increased?

10. At 80 kVp, what is the energy in joules of the electrons arriving at the x-ray tube target?

11. Why is the x-ray tube considered an inefficient device?

12. Draw the diagram and write the description of the formation of characteristic radiation.

13. What is the importance of K-characteristic x-rays in forming a diagnostic radiograph?

14. What is the range of energies of bremsstrahlung x-rays?

15. What is the minimum wavelength associated with x-rays emitted from an x-ray tube operated at 90 kVp?

16. List three factors that affect the shape of the x-ray emission spectrum and briefly describe each.

17. Define and explain the 15% kVp rule.

18. What is the diagnostic range of x-rays?

19. What type of radiation is useful for mammography and not useful for general diagnostic exposures?

20. In your clinical setting, observe or ask what filtration is used on the x-ray tubes. Why is filtration important?

X-Ray Emission

OBJECTIVES

At the completion of this chapter, the student should be able to do the following:

1. Define radiation quantity and its relation to x-ray intensity
2. List and discuss the factors affecting the intensity of the x-ray beam
3. Explain x-ray quality and penetrability
4. List and discuss the factors affecting the quality of the x-ray beam

OUTLINE

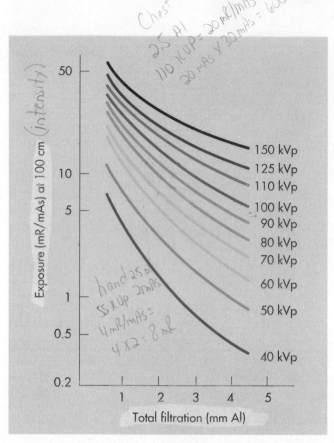

FIGURE 11-1 Nomogram for estimating intensity of x-ray beams. From the position on the x-axis corresponding to the filtration of the machine, draw a vertical line until it intersects with the appropriate voltage (kVp). A horizontal line from that point will intersect the y-axis at the approximate x-ray intensity for the imaging system. (Courtesy Edward McCullough.)

X-RAY QUANTITY
X-Ray Intensity

The intensity of the x-ray beam of an x-ray imaging system is measured in roentgens (R or mGy_a) or milliroentgens (mR) and is termed the x-ray **quantity**. Another term, **radiation exposure,** is often used instead of x-ray intensity or x-ray quantity. All have the same meaning and all are measured in roentgens.

The roentgen (mGy_a) is a measure of the number of ion pairs produced in air by a quantity of x-rays. Ionization of air increases as the number of x-rays in the beam increases. The relationship between the x-ray quantity as measured in roentgens and the number of x-rays in the beam is not always one-to-one. There are some small variations related to the effective x-ray energy.

Exposure rate expressed as mR/s, mR/min, or mR/mAs can also be used to express x-ray intensity.

 X-ray quantity is the number of x-rays in the useful beam.

These variations are unimportant over the x-ray energy range used in radiology, and we can therefore assume that the number of x-rays in the useful beam is the radiation quantity. Most general-purpose radiographic tubes, when operated at approximately 70 kVp, produce x-ray intensities of approximately 5 mR/mAs (50 μGy_a) at a 100-cm source-to-image receptor distance (SID).

Figure 11-1 is a nomogram for estimating x-ray intensity for a wide range of techniques. These curves apply only for single-phase, full-wave–rectified apparatus.

Factors Affecting X-Ray Quantity

A number of factors affect x-ray quantity. Most were discussed briefly in Chapter 10; consequently, this section may serve primarily as a review. The factors affecting x-ray quantity are nearly the same as those controlling optical density on a radiograph. These relationships are summarized in Table 11-1.

Milliampere-seconds (mAs). X-ray quantity is directly proportional to the mAs. When mAs is doubled, the number of electrons striking the tube target is doubled, and therefore the number of x-rays emitted is doubled.

X-RAY QUANTITY AND AMPERAGE

$$\frac{I_1}{I_2} = \frac{mAs_1}{mAs_2}$$

where I_1 and I_2 are the x-ray intensities at mAs_1 and mAs_2, respectively.

Question: A lateral chest technique calls for 110 kVp, 10 mAs, which results in an x-ray intensity of 32 mR (0.32 mGy_a) at the position of the patient. If the mAs is increased to 20 mAs, what will the x-ray intensity be?

TABLE 11-1	Factors Affecting X-Ray Quantity and Radiographic Optical Density	
The Effect of Increasing	**X-Ray Quantity Is:**	**Radiographic Optical Density Is:**
mAs	Increased proportionately	Increased
kVp	Increased by $\left(\dfrac{kVp_2}{kVp_1}\right)^2$	Increased
Distance	Reduced by $\left(\dfrac{d_1}{d_2}\right)^2$	Reduced
Filtration	Reduced	Reduced

Answer:
$$\frac{x}{32mR} = \frac{20\ mAs}{10\ mAs}$$

$$x = \frac{(32\ mAs)(20mR)}{10\ mAs}$$

$$= 64\ mR$$

X-ray quantity is proportional to mAs.

Question: The radiographic technique for a KUB (kidneys, ureters, and bladder) examination is 74 kVp/60 mAs. The result is a patient exposure of 250 mR (2.5 mGy$_a$). What will be the exposure if the mAs can be reduced to 45 mAs?

Answer:
$$\frac{x}{250\ mR} = \frac{45\ mAs}{60\ mAs}$$

$$x = \frac{(250\ mR)(45\ mAs)}{60\ mAs}$$

$$= 187.5\ mR$$

Remember that mAs is just a measure of the total number of electrons that travel from cathode to anode to produce x-rays.

mAs = mA × s
    = mC/s × s
    = mC

where C (coulomb) is a measure of electrostatic charges and 1 C = $6.25 × 10^{18}$ electrons.

Question: A radiograph is made at 74 kVp/100 mAs. How many electrons interact with the target?

Answer: 100 mAs = 100 mC
$$= 6.25 × 10^{17}\ \text{electrons}$$

Question: If the radiographic output intensity is 6.2 mR/mAs (62 µGy$_a$/mAs), how many electrons are required to produce 1.0 mR?

Answer: 6.2 mR/mAs = 6.2 mR/$6.25 × 10^{15}$ electrons
Stated inversely: $6.25 × 10^{15}$ electrons/ 6.2 mR = $1 × 10^{15}$ electrons/mR

Kilovolt Peak (kVp). X-ray quantity varies rapidly with changes in kVp. The change in x-ray quantity is proportional to the square of the ratio of the kVp; in other words, if kVp were doubled, the x-ray intensity would increase by a factor of four. Mathematically, this is expressed as follows:

X-RAY QUANTITY AND kVp

$$\frac{I_1}{I_2} = \left(\frac{kVp_1}{kVp_2}\right)^2$$

where I_1 and I_2 are the x-ray intensities at kVp_1 and kVp_2, respectively.

Question: A lateral chest technique calls for 110 kVp, 10 mAs and results in an x-ray intensity of 32 mR (0.32 mGya). What will be the intensity if the kVp is increased to 125 kVp and the mAs remains fixed?

Answer:
$$\frac{32mR}{I_2} = \left(\frac{110\ kVp}{125\ kVp}\right)^2$$

$$I_2 = (32\ mR)\left(\frac{125\ kVp}{110\ kVp}\right)^2$$

$$= (32\ mR)(1.14)^2$$
$$= (32\ mR)(1.29)$$
$$= 41.3\ mR$$

X-ray quantity is proportional to the kVp^2.

Question: An extremity is examined with a technique of 58 kVp/8 mAs, resulting in an entrance skin exposure (ESE) of 24 mR. If the technique is changed to 54 kVp/8 mAs to improve contrast, what will be the x-ray quantity?

Answer:
$$\frac{I}{24\ mR} = \left(\frac{54\ kVp}{58\ kVp}\right)^2$$

$$I = \left(\frac{54\ kVp}{58\ kVp}\right)^2$$
$$= (24\ mR)(0.93)^2$$
$$= (24\ mR)(0.867)$$
$$= 20.8\ mR$$

In practice, a slightly different situation prevails. Radiographic technique factors must be selected from a relatively narrow range of values, from approximately 40 to 150 kVp. Theoretically, doubling the x-ray intensity by kVp manipulation alone requires an increase of 40% in kVp.

This relationship is not adopted clinically because as kVp is increased, the penetrability of the x-ray beam is increased and relatively fewer x-rays are absorbed in the patient. More x-rays go through the patient and interact with the image receptor. Consequently, to maintain a constant exposure of the image receptor and constant average optical density (OD) would require that an increase of 15% in kVp should be accompanied by a reduction of one half in mAs.

Question: A radiographic technique calls for 80 kVp/30 mAs and results in 135 mR (1.4 mGy$_a$). What is the expected ESE if the kVp is increased to 92 kVp (+15%) and the mAs reduced by one half to 15 mAs?

Answer:
$$\frac{I}{135\ mR} = \left(\frac{15\ mAs}{30\ mAs}\right)\left(\frac{92kVp}{80\ kVp}\right)^2$$

$$I = 135\ mR\left(\frac{15\ mAs}{30\ mAs}\right)\left(\frac{92\ kVp}{80\ kVp}\right)^2$$
$$= 135\ mR(0.5)(1.32)$$
$$= 89\ mR$$

Note that by increasing kVp and reducing mAs so that optical density remains constant, patient dose is reduced significantly. The disadvantage to such a technique adjustment is reduced image contrast.

Distance. X-ray intensity varies inversely with the square of the distance from the x-ray tube target. This relationship is known as the **inverse square law** (see Chapter 5).

inverse square law

X-RAY QUANTITY AND DISTANCE
$$\frac{I_1}{I_2} = \left(\frac{d_2}{d_1}\right)^2$$
where I_1 and I_2 are the x-ray intensities at distances d_1 and d_2, respectively.

Question: A portable radiograph is normally conducted at 100 cm SID and results in an exposure of 12.5 mR (0.13 mGy$_a$) at the image receptor. If 91 cm is the maximum SID that can be obtained for a particular situation, what will be the image receptor exposure?

Answer:
$$\frac{1.25\ mR}{I_2} = \left(\frac{91\ cm}{100\ cm}\right)^2$$

$$I_2 = (12.5\ mR)\left(\frac{100\ cm}{91\ cm}\right)^2$$
$$= (12.5\ mR)(1.1)^2$$
$$= (12.5\ mR)(1.21)$$
$$= 15.1\ mR$$

ion pairs

X-ray quantity is inversely proportional to the square of the distance from the source.

Question: A PA chest examination (120 kVp/3 mAs) with a dedicated x-ray imaging system is taken at an SID of 300 cm. The exposure at the image receptor is 12 mR (0.12 mGya). If the same technique is used at a SID of 100 cm, what will be the x-ray exposure?

Answer:
$$\frac{I}{12\ mR} = \left(\frac{300\ cm}{100\ cm}\right)^2$$

$$I = 12\ mR\left(\frac{300\ cm}{100\ cm}\right)^2$$
$$= (12\ mR)(3)^2$$
$$= (12\ mR)(9)$$
$$= 108\ mR$$

When SID is increased, mAs must be increased by SID^2 to maintain constant OD.

Compensating for a change in SID by changing mAs by the factor SID² is known as the **square law,** a corollary to the **inverse square law.**

 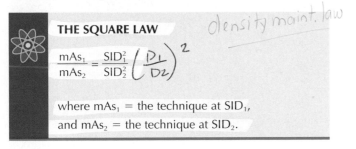

THE SQUARE LAW

density maint. law

$$\frac{mAs_1}{mAs_2} = \frac{SID_1^2}{SID_2^2}\left(\frac{D_1}{D_2}\right)^2$$

where mAs_1 = the technique at SID_1,
and mAs_2 = the technique at SID_2.

Question: What should be the new mAs in the previous question to reduce the x-ray quantity to 12 mR at 100 cm?

Answer: $\dfrac{x\ mAs}{3\ mAs} = \dfrac{12\ mR}{108\ mR}$

$$x\ mAs = (3\ mAs)\left(\frac{12\ mR}{108\ mR}\right)$$
$$= (3\ mAs)(0.111)$$
$$= 0.3\ mAs$$

Filtration. X-ray imaging systems have metal filters, usually 1 to 3 mm of aluminum (Al), positioned in the useful beam. The purpose of these filters is to reduce the number of low-energy x-rays that reach the patient.

Low-energy x-rays contribute nothing useful to the image. They only increase patient dose unnecessarily because they are absorbed in superficial tissues and do not penetrate to reach the image receptor.

 Adding filtration to the useful x-ray beam reduces patient dose.

When filtration is added to the x-ray beam, the patient dose is reduced because there are fewer low-energy x-rays in the useful beam. Calculation of the reduction in exposure requires a knowledge of half-value layer (HVL), which is discussed in the following section.

An estimate of exposure reduction can be made from the nomogram in Figure 11-1, where it is shown that the reduction is not proportional to the thickness of added filter but is related in a complex way. The disadvantage of x-ray beam filtration is reduced image contrast owing to beam hardening.

X-RAY QUALITY
Penetrability
As the energy of an x-ray beam is increased, the penetrability is also increased. **Penetrability** refers to the range of x-rays in tissue. High-energy x-rays are able to penetrate tissue farther than low-energy x-rays.

The penetrability of an x-ray beam is called the **x-ray quality.** X-rays with high penetrability are termed *high-quality x-rays.* Those with low penetrability are *low-quality x-rays.*

 Penetrability is one description of the ability of an x-ray beam to pass through tissue.

X-ray quality is identified numerically by HVL. The HVL is affected by the kVp and the added filtration in the useful beam. Therefore, x-ray quality is also influenced by kVp and filtration.

Factors that affect beam quality also influence radiographic contrast. Distance and mAs do not affect radiation quality; they do affect radiation quantity.

Half-Value Layer
Although x-rays are attenuated exponentially, high-energy x-rays are more penetrating than low-energy x-rays. Whereas 100-keV x-rays are attenuated at the rate of approximately 3%/cm of soft tissue, 10-keV x-rays are attenuated at approximately 15%/cm of soft tissue. X-rays of any given energy are more penetrating in material of low atomic number material than in material of high atomic number.

 Attenuation is the reduction in x-ray intensity resulting from absorption and scattering.

In radiography, the quality of x-rays is measured by the HVL. Therefore, HVL is a characteristic of the useful x-ray beam. A diagnostic x-ray beam usually has an HVL in the range of 3 to 5 mm Al or 3 to 6 cm of soft tissue.

 The HVL of an x-ray beam is the thickness of absorbing material necessary to reduce the x-ray intensity to half of its original value.

The HVL is determined experimentally, using a setup similar to that shown in Figure 11-2. There are three principal parts to this setup, the x-ray tube, a radiation detector, and graded thicknesses of filters, usually aluminum.

First, a radiation measurement is made with no filter between the x-ray tube and the detector. Then, measurements of radiation intensity are made for successively

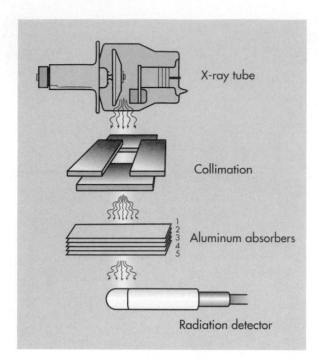

FIGURE 11-2 Typical experimental arrangement for determination of half-value layer.

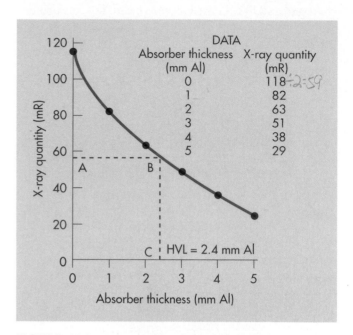

FIGURE 11-3 Data in table are typical for half-value layer (HVL) determination. The plot of these data shows an HVL of 2.4 mm Al.

DATA

Absorber thickness (mm Al)	X-ray quantity (mR)
0	118
1	82
2	63
3	51
4	38
5	29

thicker sections of filter. The thickness of filtration that reduces the x-ray intensity to half of its original value is the HVL.

A number of methods can be used to determine the HVL of an x-ray beam. Perhaps the most straightforward is to graph the results of x-ray intensity measurements made with an experimental setup like that in Figure 11-2. The graph in Figure 11-3 and the box in the right column show how this can be done when the following steps are completed.

Question: The following data were obtained with the radiographic tube operated at 70 kVp, while the detector is positioned 100 cm from the target with 0.5-mm Al filters inserted between the target and the detector. Estimate the HVL from a simple observation of this data. Then, plot the data to see how close you were.

mm Al	0	0.5	1.0	1.5	2.0	3.0	4.0	5.0
mR	94	81	69	62	55	42	38	34

Answer: One half of 94 is 47; therefore the HVL must be between 2 and 2.5 mm of AL. A plot of the data shows the HVL to be 2.4 mm Al.

HVL is the best method for specifying x-ray quality.

Steps to Determine the HVL

1. Determine the x-ray beam intensity with no absorbing material in the beam and then with different known thicknesses of absorber.

2. Plot the ordered pairs of data (thickness of absorber, x-ray quantity).

3. Determine the x-ray quantity equal to half the original quantity and locate this value on the y or vertical axis of the graph in Figure 11-3.

4. Draw a horizontal line parallel with the x-axis from the point A in step 3 until it intersects the curve (B).

5. From point B, drop a vertical line to the x-axis.

6. On the x-axis, read the thickness of absorber required to reduce the x-ray intensity to half of its original value point (C). This is the HVL.

Question: The following graph was plotted from measurements designed to estimate HVL. What does this graph suggest the HVL to be?

Answer: At zero filtration, x-ray quantity appears to be approximately 190 mR. One half of 190 mR is 95 mR. At the level of 95 mR, a horizontal line is drawn from the y-axis until it intersects the plotted curve. From that intersection, a vertical line is dropped to the x-axis, where it intersects at 2.8 mm Al, the HVL.

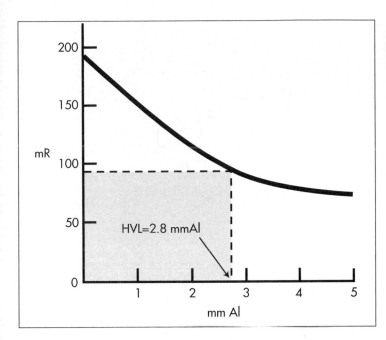

TABLE 11-2	Factors Affecting X-Ray Quality and Quantity	
		AFFECT ON
An Increase in	**X-Ray Quality**	**X-Ray Quantity**
mAs	None	Increase
kVp	Increase	Increase
Distance	None	Reduce
Filtration	Increase	Reduce

TABLE 11-3	Approximate Relationship Between kVp and HVL
kVp	**HVL (mm Al)**
50	1.9
75	2.8
100	3.7
125	4.6
150	5.4

X-ray beam penetrability changes in a complex way with variations in kVp and filtration. Different combinations of added filtration and kVp can result in the same x-ray beam HVL. For example, measurements may show that a single x-ray imaging system has the same HVL when operated at 90 kVp with 2-mm Al total filtration as when operated at 70 kVp with 4-mm Al total filtration. In this case, x-ray penetrability remains constant, as does the HVL. X-ray beam quality can be identified by either voltage or filtration, but HVL is most appropriate.

Factors Affecting X-Ray Quality

Some of the factors that affect x-ray quantity have no effect on x-ray quality. Other factors affect both x-ray quantity and x-ray quality. These relationships are summarized in Table 11-2.

Kilovolt Peak (kVp). As the kVp is increased, so is x-ray beam quality and therefore the HVL. An increase in kVp peak results in a shift of the x-ray emission spectrum toward the high-energy side, indicating an increase in the effective energy of the beam. The result is a more penetrating x-ray beam.

 Increasing the kVp peak increases the quality of an x-ray beam.

Table 11-3 shows the measured change in HVL as kVp is increased from 50 to 150 kVp for a representative x-ray imaging system. The total filtration of the beam is 2.5 mm of Al.

Filtration. The primary purpose of adding filtration to an x-ray beam is selectively to remove low-energy x-rays that have little chance of getting to the image receptor. Figure 11-4 shows the emission spectrum of an unfiltered x-ray beam and an x-ray beam with normal filtration.

The ideally filtered x-ray beam would be monoenergetic to reduce patient dose. It is desirable totally to remove all x-rays below a certain energy determined by the type of x-ray examination. To improve image contrast, it is also desirable to remove x-rays with energies above a certain level. Unfortunately, such removal of regions of an x-ray beam is not normally possible.

 Increasing filtration increases the quality of an x-ray beam.

Almost any material could serve as an x-ray filter. Aluminum (Z = 13) is chosen because it is efficient in removing low-energy x-rays through the photoelectric effect and because it is readily available, inexpensive, and easily shaped. Copper (Z = 29), tin (Z = 50), gadolinium (Z = 64), and holmium (Z = 67) have been used sparingly in special situations. As filtration is increased, so is beam quality, but quantity is decreased.

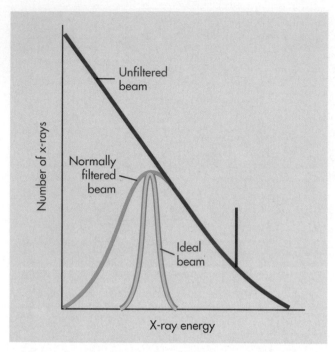

FIGURE 11-4 Filtration is used selectively to remove low-energy x-rays from the useful beam. Ideal filtration would remove all low-energy x-rays.

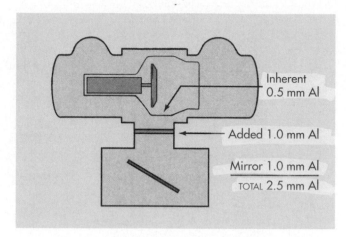

FIGURE 11-5 Total filtration consists of the inherent filtration of the x-ray tube, an added filter, and filtration by the mirror of the light-localizing collimator.

Types of Filtration

Filtration of diagnostic x-ray beams has two components—inherent filtration and added filtration.

Inherent Filtration. The glass or metal enclosure of an x-ray tube filters the emitted x-ray beam. This type of filtration is called **inherent filtration.** Inspection of an x-ray tube reveals that the part of the glass or metal enclosure through which x-rays are emitted—**the window**—is very thin. This provides for low inherent filtration.

The inherent filtration of a general purpose x-ray tube is approximately 0.5 mm Al equivalent. With age, inherent filtration tends to increase because some of the tungsten metal of both target and filament is vaporized and deposited on the inside of the window.

Special-purpose tubes, such as those used in mammography, have very thin x-ray tube windows. They are sometimes made of beryllium (Z = 4) rather than glass and have an inherent filtration of approximately 0.1 mm Al.

Added Filtration. A thin sheet of aluminum positioned between the protective x-ray tube housing and the x-ray beam collimator is the usual form of added filtration.

  Added filtration results in increased HVL.

The addition of a filter to an x-ray beam attenuates x-rays of all energies emitted, but it attenuates more low-energy x-rays than high-energy x-rays. This shifts the x-ray emission spectrum to the high-energy side, resulting in an x-ray beam with higher energy, greater penetrability, and higher quality. The HVL increases, but the extent of increase in the HVL cannot be predicted even when the thickness of added filtration is known.

Because added filtration attenuates the x-ray beam, it affects x-ray quantity. This value can be predicted if the HVL of the beam is known. The addition of filtration equal to the beam HVL reduces the beam quantity to half its prefiltered value and results in a **higher** x-ray beam quality.

Question: An x-ray imaging system has an HVL of 2.2 mm Al. The exposure is 2 mR/mAs (20 μGy$_a$/mAs) at 100 cm SID. If 2.2 mm Al is added to the beam, what will be the x-ray exposure?

Answer: This is an addition of one HVL; therefore, the x-ray exposure will be 1 mR/mAs (10 μGy$_a$/mAs).

Added filtration usually has two sources and totals 2 and 3 mm Al equivalent. First, 1- or 2-mm sheets of aluminum are permanently installed in the port of the x-ray tube housing, between the housing and the collimator.

With a conventional light-localizing variable-aperture collimator, the collimator contributes an additional 1 mm Al equivalent added filtration. This filtration results from the silver surface of the mirror in the collimator (Figure 11-5).

for chest

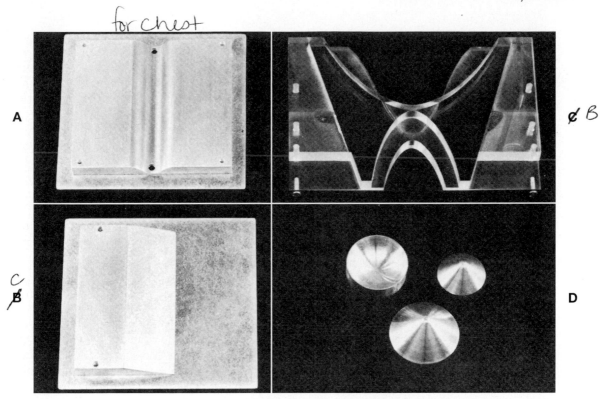

A   B   **∉ B**

C **B**   D

FIGURE 11-6 Compensating filters. **A,** Trough filter. **B,** "Bow-tie" filter for use in computed tomography. **C,** Wedge filter. **D,** Conic filters for use in digital fluoroscopy.

Compensating Filters. One of the most difficult tasks facing the radiologic technologist is producing an image with a uniform OD when examining a body part that varies greatly in thickness or tissue composition. When a filter is used in this fashion, it is called a **compensating filter** because it compensates for differences in subject radiopacity.

Compensating filters can be fabricated for many procedures, and therefore come in various sizes and shapes. They are nearly always constructed of aluminum, but plastic materials can also be used. Figure 11-6 shows some common compensating filters.

During PA chest radiography, for instance, if the left chest is relatively radiopaque because of fluid, consolidation, or mass, the image would appear with very low OD on the left side of the chest and very high OD on the right side of the chest. One could compensate for this OD variation by inserting a wedge filter so that the thin part of the wedge is positioned over the left side of the chest.

The wedge filter is principally used when radiographing a body part, such as the foot, that varies considerably in thickness (Figure 11-7). During an AP projection of the foot, the wedge would be positioned with its thick portion shadowing the toes and the thin portion toward the heel.

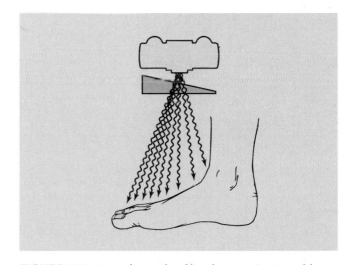

FIGURE 11-7 Use of a wedge filter for examination of foot.

A bilateral wedge filter, or a **trough filter,** is sometimes used in chest radiography (Figure 11-8). The thin central region of the wedge is positioned over the mediastinum, while the lateral thick portions shadow the lung fields. The result is a radiograph with more uniform OD. Specialty compensating wedges of this type are usually used with dedicated apparatus, such as an x-ray imaging system used exclusively for chest radiography.

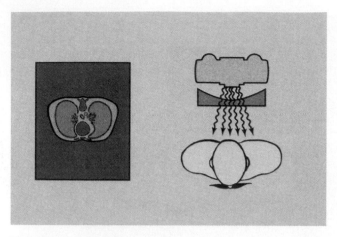

FIGURE 11-8 Use of a trough filter for examination of the chest.

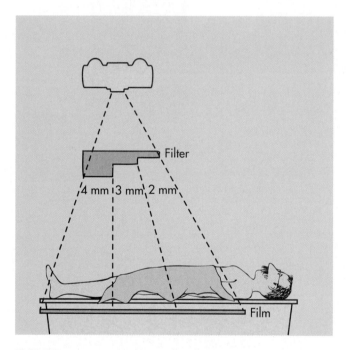

FIGURE 11-9 Arrangement of apparatus using an aluminum step-wedge for serial radiography of the abdomen and lower extremities.

Special "bow-tie"–shaped filters are used with some computed tomography imaging systems to compensate for the shape of the head or body. Conic filters, either concave or convex, find application in digital fluoroscopy, where the image receptor, the image intensifier tube, is round.

A step-wedge filter is an adaptation of the wedge filter (Figure 11-9). It is used in some special procedures, usually where long sections of the anatomy are imaged with two or three separate image receptors.

A common application of a step-wedge filter is a three-step aluminum wedge and three 14 × 17 in (30 × 36 cm) films in a rapid changer for translumbar and femoral arteriography and venography. These procedures call for careful selection of screens, grids, and radiographic technique.

Compensating filters are useful in maintaining image quality. They are not radiation protection devices.

SUMMARY

Radiation quantity is the number of x-rays in the useful beam. The factors affecting x-ray quantity are:

1. mAs: X-ray quantity is directly proportional to mAs.
2. kVp: X-ray quantity is proportional to the square of the kVp.
3. Distance: X-ray quantity varies inversely with distance from the source.
4. Filtration: X-ray quantity is reduced by filtration, which absorbs low-energy x-rays in the beam.

Radiation quality is the penetrating power of the x-ray beam. The penetrability is quantified by the HVL, which is the thickness of additional filtration that reduces x-ray intensity to half its original value. The factors affecting beam penetrability or radiation quality are:

1. kVp: X-ray penetrability is increased as kVp is increased.
2. Filtration: X-ray penetrability is increased when filtration is added to the beam.

The following are the three types of filtration: (1) inherent filtration of the glass or metal enclosure; (2) added filtration in the form of aluminum sheets; and (3) compensating filters, which provide variation in intensity across the x-ray beam.

CHALLENGE QUESTIONS

1. Define or otherwise identify:
   a. Inherent filtration
   b. The unit of x-ray quantity
   c. A filtered x-ray spectrum
   d. A kVp change equal to twice the mAs
   e. Three filter materials used with diagnostic x-ray beams
   f. Half-value layer
   g. Wedge filter
   h. The unit of x-ray quality
   i. The approximate HVL of your x-ray imaging system
   j. X-ray intensity
2. Graph the change in HVL with changing kVp (from 50 to 120 kVp) for an x-ray imaging system that has total filtration of 2.5 mm Al. Check your answer by plotting the data in Table 11-3.

3. An abdominal radiograph taken at 84 kVp, 150 mAs results in an exposure 650 mR. The image is too light and is repeated at 84 kVp, 250 mAs. What is the exposure?

4. An image of the lateral skull taken at 68 kVp, 200 mAs has sufficient optical density but too much contrast. If the kVp is increased to 78 kVp, what should be the new mAs?

5. A chest radiograph taken at 180 cm SID results in an exposure of 12 mR. What would the exposure be if the same radiographic factors were used at 100 cm SID?

6. The following data were obtained with a fluoroscopic x-ray tube operated at 80 kVp. The exposure levels were measured 50 cm above the table top with aluminum absorbers positioned on the surface. Estimate the HVL by visual inspection of the data; then, plot the data and determine the precise value of the HVL.

Added mm Al	mR
None	65
1	48
3	30
5	21
7	16
9	13.0

7. When operated at 74 kVp, 100 mAs with 2.2 mm Al added filtration and 0.6 mm Al inherent filtration, the HVL of an x-ray imaging system is 3.2 mm Al and its output intensity at 100 cm SID is 350 mR. How much additional filtration is necessary to reduce the x-ray intensity to 175 mR?

8. The following technique factors have been shown to produce good-quality radiographs of the cervical spine with an x-ray image having 3 mm Al total filtration. Refer to Figure 11-1 and estimate the x-ray intensity at 100 cm SID for each.
   a. 62 kVp, 70 mAs
   b. 70 kVp, 40 mAs
   c. 78 kVp, 27 mAs

9. A radiographic exposure is 80 kVp at 50 mAs. How many electrons will interact with the target?

10. An extremity is radiographed at 60 kVp, 10 mAs, resulting in an x-ray intensity of 28 mR. If the technique is changed to 55 kVp, 10 mAs, what is the resulting x-ray intensity?

11. What is the square law, and how is it used?.

12. What is the primary purpose of x-ray beam filtration?

13. The kVp is reduced from 78 to 68 kVp. What, if anything, should be done with mAs to maintain OD constant?

14. What is the relationship between x-ray quantity and mAs?

15. Define half-value layer.

16. List the two ways an x-ray beam can be shifted to a higher average energy.

17. Why is aluminum used for x-ray beam filtration?

18. Describe the use of a wedge filter when radiographing a foot.

19. Does adding filtration to the x-ray beam affect the quantity of x-rays reaching the image receptor?

20. Fill in the following chart:

Increasing	Effect on X-Ray Quality	Effect on Optical Density
mAs		
kVp		
Distance		
Filtration		

CHAPTER

12

X-Ray Interaction with Matter

OBJECTIVES

At the completion of this chapter, the student should be able to do the following:

1. Describe each of the five x-ray interactions with matter
2. Define differential absorption and its effect on image contrast
3. Explain the effect of atomic number and mass density of tissue on the differential absorption
4. Discuss why radiologic contrast agents are used to image some tissues and organs
5. Explain the difference between absorption and attenuation

OUTLINE

Five X-ray Interactions With Matter
    Coherent Scattering
    Compton Effect
    Photoelectric Effect
    Pair Production
    Photodisintegration
Differential Absorption
    Dependence on Atomic Number
    Dependence on Mass Density
Contrast Examination
Exponential Attenuation

-RAYS INTERACT with matter in the following five ways: (1) by coherent scattering, (2) through the Compton effect, (3) through the photoelectric effect, (4) by pair production, and (5) by photodisintegration. Only Compton effect and photoelectric effect are important to making an x-ray image. The conditions governing these two interactions control differential absorption, which results in the degree of contrast of an x-ray image.

FIVE X-RAY INTERACTIONS WITH MATTER

In Chapter 5, the interaction between electromagnetic radiation and matter was described briefly. The interaction was said to have wavelike and particle-like properties. Electromagnetic radiation interacts with structures similar in size to the wavelength of the radiation.

X-rays have very short wavelengths, no larger than approximately 10^{-8} to 10^{-9} m. The higher the energy of an x-ray, the shorter is its wavelength. Consequently, low-energy x-rays tend to interact with whole atoms, which have diameters of approximately 10^{-9} to 10^{-10} m; moderate-energy x-rays generally interact with electrons, and high-energy x-rays generally interact with nuclei.

There are five mechanisms by which x-rays interact at these various structural levels: coherent scattering, Compton effect, photoelectric effect, pair production, and photodisintegration. Two of these—Compton effect and photoelectric effect—are of particular importance to diagnostic radiology. They are discussed in some detail.

Coherent Scattering

X-rays with energies below approximately 10 keV interact with matter by coherent scattering, sometimes called classical scattering or Thompson scattering (Figure 12-1). J. J. Thompson described the coherent scattering of an x-ray with an electron.

In coherent scattering, the incident x-ray interacts with a target atom, causing it to become excited. The target atom immediately releases this excess energy as a scattered x-ray with wavelength equal to that of the incident x-ray ($\lambda = \lambda'$), and therefore of equal energy. However, the direction of the scattered x-ray is different from that of the incident x-ray.

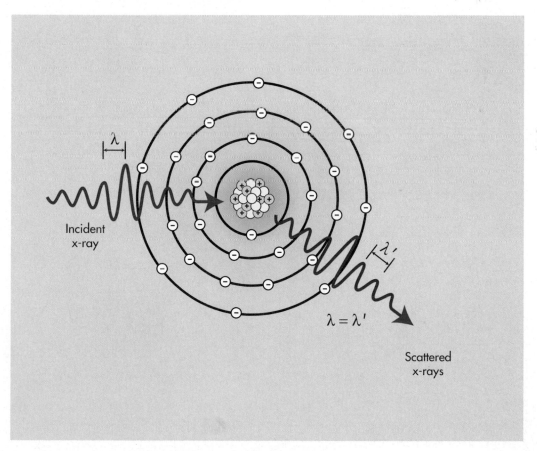

FIGURE 12-1 Classical scattering is an interaction between low-energy x-rays and atoms. The x-ray loses no energy but changes direction slightly. The wavelength of the incident x-ray is equal to the wavelength of the scattered x-ray.

The result of coherent scattering is a change in direction of the x-ray without a change in its energy. There is no energy transfer, and therefore no ionization. Most coherently scattered x-rays are scattered in the forward direction.

 Coherent scattering is of little importance to diagnostic radiology.

Coherent scattering primarily involves low-energy x-rays, which contribute little to the image. Some coherent scattering, however, occurs throughout the diagnostic range. At 70 kVp, a few percent of the x-rays undergo coherent scattering, which contributes slightly to **film fog**, the general graying of a radiograph that reduces image contrast.

Compton Effect

X-rays throughout the diagnostic range can undergo an interaction with outer-shell electrons that not only scatters the x-ray but reduces its energy and ionizes the atom as well. This interaction is called the **Compton effect** or **Compton scattering** (Figure 12-2).

In the Compton effect, the incident x-ray interacts with an outer-shell electron and ejects it from the atom, ionizing the atom. The ejected electron is called a *Compton electron* or a *secondary electron*. The x-ray continues in a different direction with less energy.

The energy of the Compton-scattered x-ray is equal to the difference between the energy of the incident x-ray and the energy of the ejected electron. The energy of the ejected electron is equal to its binding energy plus the kinetic energy with which it leaves the atom. Mathematically, this energy transfer is represented as follows:

 Compton Effect

$E_i = E_s + (E_b + E_{KE})$

where E_i = energy of the incident x-ray, E_s = energy of the scattered x-ray, E_b = electron binding energy, and E_{KE} = kinetic energy of the electron.

Question: A 30-keV x-ray ionizes an atom of barium by ejecting an O-shell electron with 12 keV

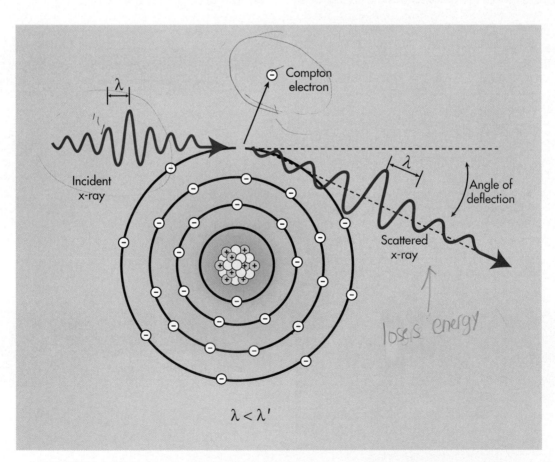

FIGURE 12-2 The Compton effect occurs between moderate-energy x-rays and outer-shell electrons. It results in ionization of the target atom, change in x-ray direction, and reduction of x-ray energy. The wavelength of the scattered x-ray is greater than that of the incident x-ray.

of kinetic energy. What is the energy of the scattered x-ray?

Answer: Figure 4-9 shows that the binding energy of an O-shell electron of barium is 0.04 keV; therefore,

$$30 \text{ keV} = E_s + (0.04 \text{ keV} + 12 \text{ keV})$$
$$E_s = 30 \text{ keV} - (0.04 \text{ keV} + 12 \text{ keV})$$
$$= 30 \text{ keV} - (12.04 \text{ keV})$$
$$= 17.96 \text{ keV}$$

During a Compton interaction, most of the energy is divided between the scattered x-ray and the Compton electron. Usually the scattered x-ray retains most of the energy. Both the scattered x-ray and the Compton electron may have sufficient energy to undergo more ionizing interactions before losing all their energy.

Ultimately, the scattered x-ray is absorbed photoelectrically. The Compton electron loses all of its kinetic energy by ionization and excitation and drops into a vacancy in an electron shell previously created by some other ionizing event.

Compton-scattered x-rays can be deflected in any direction, including 180 degrees from the incident x-ray. At a deflection of 0 degrees, no energy is transferred. As the angle of deflection increases to 180 degrees, more energy is transferred to the Compton electron, but even at 180 degrees of deflection, the scattered x-ray retains at least approximately two thirds of its original energy.

X-rays scattered back in the direction of the incident x-ray beam are called **backscatter radiation**. In diagnostic radiography, backscatter radiation is responsible for the cassette-hinge image sometimes seen on a radiograph even though the hinge was on the back side of the cassette. In such situations the x-radiation has backscattered from the wall or examination table, not the patient.

The probability that a given x-ray will undergo the Compton effect is a complex function of the energy of the incident x-ray. In general, the probability of the Compton effect decreases as x-ray energy increases.

The probability of the Compton effect is inversely proportional to energy (1/E) and independent of atomic number.

The probability of the Compton effect does not depend on the atomic number of the atom involved. Any given x-ray is just as likely to undergo the Compton effect with an atom of soft tissue as with an atom of bone (Figure 12-3). Table 12-1 summarizes Compton scattering.

Compton scattering reduces contrast in an x-ray image.

Compton scattering in tissue can occur with all x-rays and is therefore of considerable importance in x-ray imaging. However, its importance is in a negative sense. Scattered x-rays provide no useful information on the radiograph. Rather, they produce a uniform optical density on the radiograph that results in reduced image contrast. There are ways of reducing scattered radiation that are discussed later, but none is totally effective.

The scattered x-rays from Compton interactions can create a serious radiation exposure hazard in radiography and particularly in fluoroscopy. A large amount of radiation can be scattered from the patient during fluoroscopy. Such radiation is the source of most of the occupational radiation exposure that radiologic technologists receive.

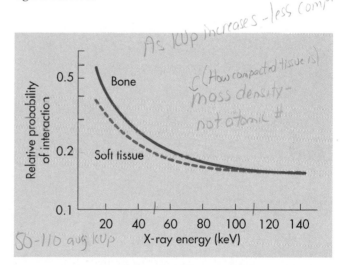

FIGURE 12-3 The probability that an x-ray will interact by the Compton effect is about the same for target atoms of soft tissue and bone. This probability decreases with increasing x-ray energy.

TABLE 12-1	Features of Compton Scattering
Most likely to occur	With outer-shell electrons
	With loosely bound electrons
As x-ray energy increases	Increased penetration through tissue without interaction
	Increased Compton scattering relative to photoelectric effect
	Reduced Compton scattering (~1/E)
As atomic number of absorber increases	No effect on Compton scattering
As mass density of absorber increases	Proportional increase in Compton scattering

During radiography, the hazard is less severe because no one but the patient is normally in the examining room. Nevertheless, scattered radiation levels are sufficient to necessitate protective shielding of the x-ray examining room.

Photoelectric Effect

X-rays in the diagnostic range also undergo ionizing interactions with inner-shell electrons. The x-ray is not scattered, but it is totally absorbed. This process is called the **photoelectric effect** (Figure 12-4).

The electron removed from the atom, called a **photoelectron,** escapes with kinetic energy equal to the difference between the energy of the incident x-ray and the binding energy of the electron. Mathematically, this is shown as follows:

Photoelectric Effect

$E_i = E_b + E_{KE}$

where E_i = the energy of the incident x-ray, E_b = electron-binding energy, and E_{KE} = kinetic energy of the electron.

The photoelectric effect is total x-ray absorption interaction.

For low atomic number atoms, such as those found in soft tissue, the binding energy of even K-shell electrons is low (e.g., 0.3 keV for carbon). Therefore, the photoelectron is released with kinetic energy nearly equal to the energy of the incident x-ray.

For higher atomic number target atoms, the electron-binding energies are higher (37 keV for barium K-shell electrons). Therefore, the kinetic energy of the photoelectron from barium is proportionately lower. Table 12-2 shows the approximate K-shell binding energy for elements of radiologic importance.

Characteristic x-rays are produced after a photoelectric interaction in a manner similar to that described in Chapter 10. The ejection of a K-shell photoelectron by the incident x-ray results in a vacancy in the K shell. This unnatural state is immediately corrected when an outer-shell electron, usually from the L shell, drops into the vacancy.

This electron transition is accompanied by the emission of an x-ray whose energy is equal to the difference in the binding energies of the shells involved. These characteristic x-rays are **secondary radiation** and behave in the same manner as scattered radiation. They con-

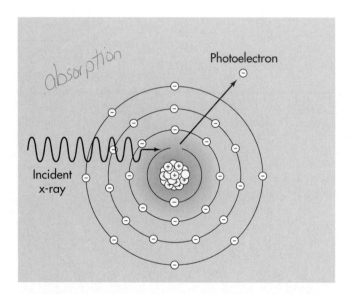

FIGURE 12-4 The photoelectric effect occurs when an incident x-ray is totally absorbed during the ionization of an inner-shell electron. The incident photon disappears and the K-shell electron, now called a *photoelectron,* is ejected from the atom.

TABLE 12-2	Atomic Number and K-shell Electron-Binding Energy of Radiologically Important Elements	
Element	**Atomic Number**	**K-shell Electron-Binding Energy**
Hydrogen	1	0.02 keV
Carbon	6	0.3 keV
Nitrogen	7	0.4 keV
Oxygen	8	0.5 keV
Aluminum	13	1.6 keV
Calcium	20	4.1 keV
Molybdenum	42	20 keV
Rhenium	45	24 keV
Iodine	53	33 keV
Barium	56	37 keV
Tungsten	74	69 keV
Lead	82	88 keV

tribute nothing of diagnostic value and fortunately do not occur often.

Question: A 50-keV x-ray interacts photoelectrically with (a) a carbon atom and (b) a barium atom. What is the kinetic energy of each photoelectron and the energy of each characteristic x-ray if an L-to-K transition occurs (see Figure 4-9)?

Answer: a. $E_{KE} = K_i - K_b$
                    $= 50 \text{ keV} - 0.3 \text{ keV}$
                    $= 49.7 \text{ keV}$
                $E_x = 0.3 \text{ keV} - 0.006 \text{ keV}$
                    $= 0.294 \text{ keV}$
            b. $E_{KE} = E_i - E_b$
                    $= 50 \text{ keV} - 37 \text{ keV}$
                    $= 13 \text{ keV}$
                $E_x = 37 \text{ keV} - 5.989 \text{ keV}$
                    $= 31.011 \text{ keV}$

The probability that a given x-ray will undergo a photoelectric interaction is a function of both the x-ray energy and the atomic number of the atom with which it interacts.

> The probability of the photoelectric effect is inversely proportional to the third power of the x-ray **energy $(1/E)^3$.** *a lot faster ↓*

A photoelectric interaction cannot occur unless the incident x-ray has energy equal to or greater than the electron-binding energy. A barium K-shell electron bound to the nucleus by 37 keV cannot be removed by a 36-keV x-ray.

If the incident x-ray has sufficient energy, the probability that it will undergo a photoelectric effect decreases with the third power of the photon energy $(1/E^3)$. This relationship is shown graphically in Figure 12-5 for soft tissue and bone.

> The probability of photoelectric effect is directly proportional to the third power of the atomic number of the absorbing material (Z^3).

As the relative vertical displacement between the graphs of soft tissue and bone demonstrates, a photoelectric interaction is much more likely to occur with high-Z atoms than with low-Z atoms (Figure 12-5). Table 12-3 presents the effective atomic numbers of materials of radiologic importance.

Question: If an 80-keV x-ray has a relative chance of one photoelectric effect with soft tissue,

what is its relative probability of interacting with
a. Fat?   (Z = 6.3)
b. Barium? (Z = 56)

Answer: a. $\left(\dfrac{6.3}{7.4}\right)^3 = 0.62$

            b. $\left(\dfrac{56}{7.4}\right)^3 = 433$

Semilogarithmic Graphs. Figure 12-5 is an example of a graph having a logarithmic (log, for short) scale along the vertical axis. A review of Table 2-1 shows that whole-log values represent orders of magnitude in power of 10 notation. Therefore, the difference between log 4 and log 2 is two orders of magnitude, or $10^4 - 10^2 = 10^2$.

A log scale is a power of 10 scale used to plot data that cover several orders of magnitude. In Figure 12-5,

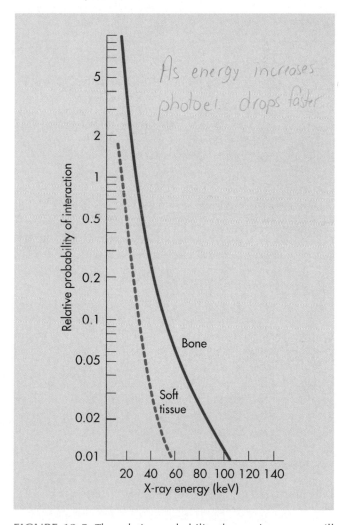

FIGURE 12-5 The relative probability that a given x-ray will undergo a photoelectric interaction is inversely proportional to the third power of the x-ray energy and directly proportional to the third power of the atomic number of the absorber.

TABLE 12-3	Effective Atomic Numbers of Materials Important to Diagnostic Radiology
Types of Substance	**Effective Atomic Number**
HUMAN TISSUE	
Fat	6.3
Soft tissue	7.4
Lung	7.4
Bone	13.8
CONTRAST MATERIAL	
Air	7.6
Iodine	53
Barium	56
OTHER	
Concrete	17
Molybdenum	42
Tungsten	74
Lead	82

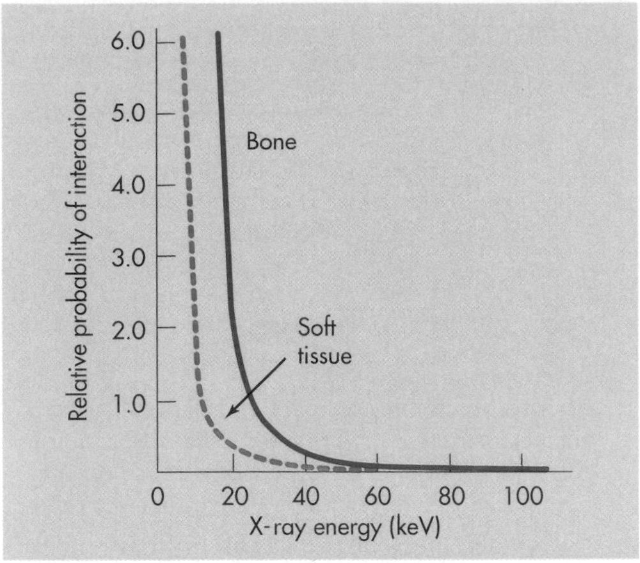

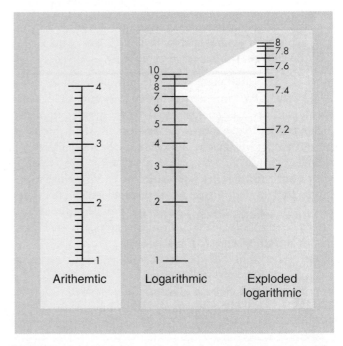

FIGURE 12-6 Relative probability for photoelectric interaction ranges over several orders of magnitude. If it is plotted in the conventional arithmetic fashion, as here, one cannot estimate its value above an energy of approximately 20 keV

for example, the relative probability of photoelectric interaction with soft tissue varies from approximately 2 to less than 0.01 over the energy range from 10 to 60 keV.

A plot of these data in conventional arithmetic form appears in Figure 12-6. Clearly, this type of graph is unacceptable because all probability values above 40 keV are so close to zero.

On an arithmetic scale, equal intervals have equal numerical value, but on a log scale, equal intervals represent equal ratios. This difference in scales is shown in Figure 12-7.

All major intervals on the arithmetic scale have a value of 1 and the subintervals a value of 0.1. On the other hand, the log scale contains major intervals that each equal one order of magnitude, and subintervals that are not equal in length. Figure 12-7 also shows an exploded view of one major log interval.

Cubic Relationships. A probability of interaction proportional to the third power changes rapidly. For the photoelectric effect, this means that a small variation in atomic number of the tissue atom or in x-ray energy results in a large change in the chance of photoelectric interaction. This is unlike the situation that exists for the Compton interaction.

FIGURE 12-7 Graphic scales can be arithmetic or logarithmic. The log scale is used to plot wide ranges of values.

Question: If the relative probability of photoelectric interaction with soft tissue for a 20-keV x-ray is 1, how much less likely will an interaction be for a 50-keV x-ray? How much more likely is interaction with iodine (Z = 53) than with soft tissue (Z = 7.4) for a 70-keV x-ray?

Answer:
$$\left(\frac{20\ keV}{50\ keV}\right)^3 = \left(\frac{2}{5}\right)^3 = 0.064$$

$$\left(\frac{53}{7.4}\right)^3 = 368$$

Table 12-4 summarizes the photoelectric effect.

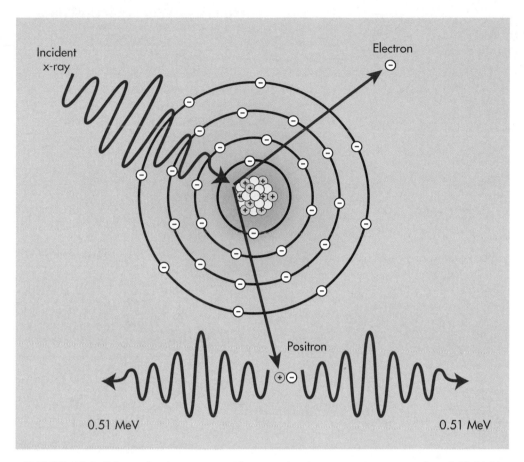

FIGURE 12-8 Pair production occurs with x-rays that have energies greater than 1.02 MeV. The x-ray interacts with the nuclear force field and two electrons that have opposite electrostatic charges are created.

TABLE 12-4	Features of Photoelectric Effect
Most likely to occur	With inner-shell electrons
	With tightly bound electrons
	When x-ray energy is just higher than electron-binding energy
As x-ray energy increases	Increased penetration through tissue without interaction
	Less photoelectric effect relative to Compton effect
	Reduced absolute photoelectric effect
As atomic number of absorber increases	Increases proportionately with the cube of the atomic number (Z^3)
As mass density of absorber increases	Proportional increase in photoelectric absorption

Pair Production

If an incident x-ray has sufficient energy, it may escape interaction with electrons and come close enough to the nucleus of the atom to be influenced by the strong electric field of the nucleus. The interaction between the x-ray and the nuclear electric field causes the x-ray to disappear, and in its place two electrons appear, one positively charged (**positron**) and one negatively charged. This process is called **pair production** (Figure 12-8).

 Pair production does not occur during x-ray imaging.

In Chapter 5, we calculated the energy equivalence of the mass of an electron to be 0.51 MeV. Because two electrons are formed in a pair production interaction, the incident photon must have at least 1.02 MeV of energy.

An x-ray with less than 1.02 MeV cannot undergo pair production. Any of the x-ray's energy in excess of 1.02 MeV is distributed equally between the two electrons as kinetic energy.

The electron resulting from pair production eventually fills a vacancy in an atomic orbital shell. The positron unites with a free electron and the mass of both particles is converted to energy in a process called **annihilation radiation.**

Because pair production involves only x-rays with energies greater than 1.02 MeV, it is unimportant in x-ray imaging but is very important for positron emission tomography (PET) imaging in nuclear medicine.

Photodisintegration

X-rays with energy above approximately 10 MeV can escape interaction with electrons and the nuclear electric field and be absorbed directly by the nucleus. When this happens, the nucleus is raised to an excited state and instantly emits a nucleon or other nuclear fragment. This process is called **photodisintegration** (Figure 12-9).

 Photodisintegration does not occur in diagnostic radiology.

DIFFERENTIAL ABSORPTION

Of the five ways an x-ray can interact with tissue, only two are important to radiology—the Compton effect and the photoelectric effect. Similarly, only two methods of x-ray production (see Chapter 10)—bremsstrahlung x-rays and characteristic x-rays—are important.

More important than the x-ray interacting by Compton or photoelectric effect, however, is the x-ray transmitted through the body without interacting. Figure 12-10 shows schematically how each of these types of x-ray contributes to an image.

 Differential absorption occurs because of Compton scattering, photoelectric effect, and x-rays transmitted through the patient.

The **Compton-scattered x-ray contributes no useful information** to the image. When a Compton-scattered x-ray interacts with the image receptor, the image receptor assumes that the x-ray came straight from the x-ray tube target (Figure 12-11). The image receptor does not recognize the scattered x-ray as representing an interaction off the straight line from the target.

These scattered x-rays result in **image fog,** a generalized dulling of the image by optical densities not repres-

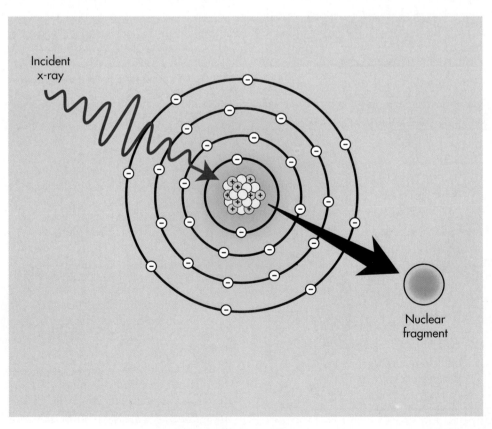

FIGURE 12-9 Photodisintegration is an interaction between high-energy x-rays and the nucleus. The x-ray is absorbed by the nucleus and a nuclear fragment is emitted.

enting diagnostic information. To reduce this type of fog, we use techniques and apparatus to reduce the number of scattered x-rays that reach the image receptor.

X-rays that undergo photoelectric interaction provide diagnostic information to the image receptor. Because they do not reach the image receptor, these x-rays are representative of anatomic structures with high x-ray absorption characteristics; such structures are **radiopaque.** The photoelectric absorption of x-rays results in the light areas of a radiograph (low optical density), such as those corresponding to bone.

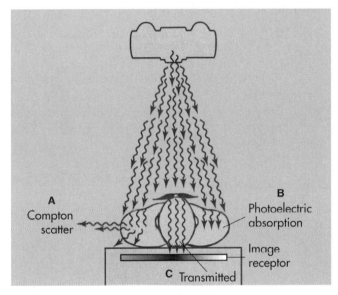

FIGURE 12-10 Three types of x-rays are important to the making of a radiograph: those scattered by Compton interaction (**A**); those absorbed photoelectrically (**B**); and those transmitted through the patient without interaction (**C**).

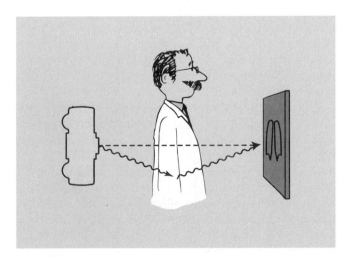

FIGURE 12-11 When an x-ray is Compton scattered, the image receptor thinks it came straight from the source.

Other x-rays penetrate the body and are transmitted to the image receptor with no interaction whatever. They result in the dark (high optical density) areas of a radiograph. The anatomic structures through which these x-rays pass are **radiolucent.**

Basically, an x-ray image results from the difference between those x-rays absorbed photoelectrically in the patient and those transmitted to the image receptor. This difference in x-ray interaction is called **differential absorption.**

Approximately 1% of the x-rays incident on a patient reach the image receptor. Less than half of those that reach the image receptor interact to form an image. Thus, the radiographic image results from approximately 0.5% of the x-rays emitted by the x-ray tube. Consequently, careful control and selection of the x-ray beam are necessary to produce high-quality radiographs.

> Differential absorption increases as the kVp is reduced.

Producing a high-quality radiograph requires the proper selection of kVp so that the effective x-ray energy results in maximum differential absorption. Unfortunately, reducing the kVp to increase differential absorption and therefore image contrast results in increased patient dose. A compromise is necessary for each examination.

Dependence on Atomic Number

Consider the image of an extremity (Figure 12-12). An image of the bone is produced because many more x-rays are absorbed photoelectrically in bone than in soft tissue. Recall that the probability of an x-ray undergoing photoelectric effect is proportional to the third power of the atomic number of the tissue.

According to Table 12-3, bone has an atomic number of 13.8, and soft tissue has an atomic number of 7.4. Consequently, the probability that an x-ray will undergo a photoelectric interaction is approximately seven times greater in bone than in soft tissue.

Question: How much more likely is an x-ray to interact with bone than muscle?

Answer: $\left(\dfrac{13.8}{7.4}\right)^3 = \dfrac{2628}{405} = 6.5$

These relative values of interaction are apparent in Figure 12-13 when one pays particular attention to the logarithmic scale of the vertical axis. Notice that the relative probability of interaction between bone and soft tissue (differential absorption) remains constant, whereas the absolute probability of each decreases with increasing energy. With higher x-ray energy, fewer interactions occur, so more x-rays are transmitted without interaction.

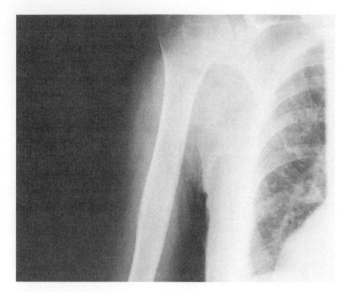

FIGURE 12-12 Radiograph of bony structures results from the differential absorption between bone and soft tissue.

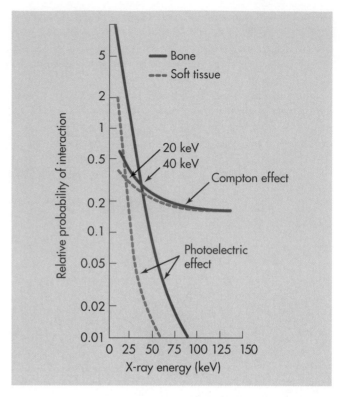

FIGURE 12-13 Graph showing probabilities of photoelectric and Compton interactions with soft tissue and bone. The interactions of these curves indicate those x-ray energies at which the change of photoelectric absorption equals the chance for Compton scattering.

Question: What is the relative probability that a 20-keV x-ray will undergo photoelectric interaction in bone compared with fat?

Answer: $Z_{bone} = 13.8$, $Z_{fat} = 6.8$

$$\left(\frac{13.8}{6.8}\right) = 8.36$$

The Compton effect is independent of the atomic number of tissue. The probability of Compton scattering for bone atoms and for soft tissue atoms is approximately equal and decreases with increasing x-ray energy.

This decrease in scattering, however, is not as rapid as the decrease in photoelectric effect with increasing x-ray energy. The probability of the Compton effect is inversely proportional to x-ray energy $(1/E)$. The probability of the photoelectric effect is inversely proportional to the third power of the x-ray energy $(1/E^3)$.

At low energies, most x-ray interactions with tissue are photoelectric. At high energies, Compton scattering predominates.

Of course, as x-ray energy is increased, the chance of any interaction at all decreases. As kVp is increased, more x-rays get to the image receptor, and therefore a lower x-ray quantity (lower mAs) is required.

Figure 12-13 combines all these factors into one graph. At 20 keV, the probability of photoelectric effect equals the probability of Compton effect in soft tissue. Below this energy, most x-rays interact with soft tissue photoelectrically. Above this energy, the predominant interaction with soft tissue is Compton effect. Low kVp resulting in increased differential absorption is the basis for mammography.

 To image small differences in soft tissue, one must use low kVp to get maximum differential absorption.

The relative frequency of Compton interaction compared with photoelectric interaction increases with increasing x-ray energy. The crossover point between photoelectric effect and Compton effect for bone is approximately 40 keV. Nevertheless, low-kVp technique is usually appropriate for bone radiography to maintain image contrast.

High-kVp technique is usually used for examination of barium studies and chest radiography where intrinsic contrast is high, resulting in much lower patient dose.

When high-kVp technique is used in this manner, the amount of scattered radiation from surrounding soft tissue contributes little to the image. When the amount of scattered radiation becomes too high, grids are used (see Chapter 17). Grids do not affect the magnitude of the differential absorption.

Differential absorption in bone and soft tissue results from photoelectric interactions, which greatly depend on the atomic number of tissue. The loss of contrast is due to fog caused by Compton scattering. Two other factors are also important in making an x-ray image: the x-ray emission spectrum and the mass density of patient tissue.

The crossover energies of 20 keV and 40 keV refer to a **monoenergetic** x-ray beam, that is, a beam containing x-rays that all have the same energy. In fact, as we saw in Chapter 10, clinical x-rays are **polyenergetic**. They are emitted over an entire spectrum of energies. The correct selection of voltage for optimum differential absorption depends on the other factors discussed in Chapter 11 that affect the x-ray emission spectrum. For instance, in AP radiography of the lumbar spine at 110 kVp, more x-rays are emitted with energy above the 40-keV crossover for bone than below it. Less filtration or a grid may then be necessary.

Dependence on Mass Density

Intuitively, we know that we could image bone even if differential absorption were not Z-related because bone has a higher mass density than soft tissue. **Mass density** is not to be confused with optical density. Mass density is the quantity of matter per unit volume, specified in units of kilograms per cubic meter (kg/m³). Sometimes mass density is reported in grams per cubic centimeter (g/cm³).

Question: How many g/cm³ are there in 1 kg/m³?

Answer: $$1 \text{ kg/m}^3 = \frac{1000\text{g}}{(100 \text{ cm})^3}$$

$$= \frac{10^3 \text{ g}}{10^6 \text{cm}^3}$$

$$= 10^{-3} \text{ g/cm}^3$$

Table 12-5 gives the mass densities of several radiologically important materials. Mass density is related to the mass of each atom and basically tells how tightly the atoms of a substance are packed.

Water and ice are composed of precisely the same atoms, but ice occupies more volume. The mass density of ice is 917 kg/m³ compared with 1000 kg/m³ for water. Ice floats in water because of this difference in mass density. Ice is lighter than water.

The interaction between x-rays and tissue is proportional to the mass density of the tissue regardless of the type of interaction.

When mass density is doubled, the chance for x-ray interaction is doubled because there are twice as many electrons available for interaction. Therefore, even without the Z-related photoelectric effect, nearly twice

TABLE 12-5	Mass Density of Materials Important to Diagnostic Radiology
Substance	**Mass Density (kg/m³)**
HUMAN TISSUE	
Lung	320
Fat	910
Soft tissue, muscle	1000
Bone	1850
CONTRAST MATERIAL	
Air	1.3
Barium	3500
Iodine	4930
OTHER	
Calcium	1550
Concrete	2350
Molybdenum	10,200
Lead	11,350
Rhenium	12,500
Tungstate	19,300

as many x-rays would be absorbed and scattered in bone as in soft tissue. The bone would be imaged.

Question: What is the relative probability that 60-keV x-rays will undergo Compton scattering in bone compared with soft tissue?

Answer:
Mass density of bone = 1850 kg/m³
Mass density of soft tissue = 1000 kg/m³
$$\frac{1850}{1000} = 1.85$$

Lungs are imaged in chest radiography primarily because of differences in mass density. According to Table 12-2, the mass density of soft tissue is 770 times that of air (1000/1.3) and 3 times that of lung (1000/320). Therefore for the same thickness, we can expect almost three times as many x-rays to interact with the soft tissue as with lung tissue.

The Z values of air and soft tissue are about the same, 7.4 for soft tissue and 7.6 for air; thus, differential absorption in air-filled soft tissue cavities is due primarily to differences in mass density. Figure 12-14 demonstrates differential absorption in air, soft tissue, and bone caused by mass density differences. Table 12-6 summarizes the various relationships of differential absorption.

Question: Assume that all x-ray interactions during mammography are photoelectric. What is the differential absorption of x-rays in microcalcifications (Z = 20, p = 1550 kg/m³)

TABLE 12-6	Characteristics of Differential Absorption
As x-ray energy increases	Fewer Compton interactions
	Many fewer photoelectric interactions
	More transmission through tissue
As tissue atomic number increases	No change in Compton interactions *loosely bound e's*
	Many more photoelectric interactions
	Less x-ray transmission
As tissue mass density increases	Proportional increase in Compton interactions
	Proportional increase in photoelectric interactions
	Proportional reduction in x-ray transmission

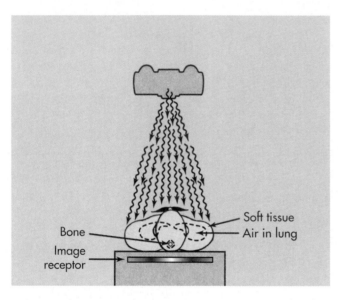

FIGURE 12-14 Even if x-ray interaction were not related to atomic number (Z), differential absorption would occur because of differences in mass density.

relative to fatty tissue (Z = 6.3, 910 kg/m³)?

Answer: Differential absorption due to atomic number

$$\left(\frac{20}{6.3}\right)^3 = \frac{8000}{250} = 32:1$$

Differential absorption due to mass density $= \dfrac{1550}{910} = 1.7:1$

Total differential absorption = 32 × 1.7 = 54.4:1

CONTRAST EXAMINATION

Barium and iodine compounds are used as an aid for imaging internal organs with x-rays. The atomic number of barium is 56; that of iodine is 53. Each has a much higher atomic number and mass density than soft

tissue. When used in this fashion, they are called **contrast agents,** and because of their high atomic numbers, they are positive contrast agents.

Question: What is the probability that an x-ray will interact with iodine rather than soft tissue?

Answer: Differential absorption as a result of atomic number $= \left(\dfrac{53}{7.4}\right)^3 = 367:1$

Differential absorption as a result of mass density $= \dfrac{4.93}{1.0} = 4.93:1$

Total differential absorption = 367 × 4.93 = 1809:1

When an iodinated compound fills the internal carotid artery or when barium fills the colon, these internal organs are readily visualized on a radiograph. Low-kVp technique (e.g., below 80 kVp) produces excellent, high-contrast radiographs of the organs of the gastrointestinal tract. Higher-kVp operation (e.g., above 90 kVp) can often be used in these examinations not only to outline the organ under investigation but to penetrate the contrast medium to visualize the lumen of the organ more clearly.

Air was used at one time as a contrast medium in procedures such as pneumoencephalography and ventriculography. In these procedures, the normal body fluids filling these internal cavities were replaced by air. Such procedures have disappeared, however, since the introduction of computed tomography and magnetic resonance imaging.

Air is still used for contrast in some examinations of the colon along with barium, called a **double-contrast examination.** When used in this fashion, air is a negative contrast agent.

EXPONENTIAL ATTENUATION

When x-rays are incident on any type of tissue, they can interact with the atoms of that tissue by any of the five mechanisms discussed previously. The relative frequency of interaction by each mechanism depends

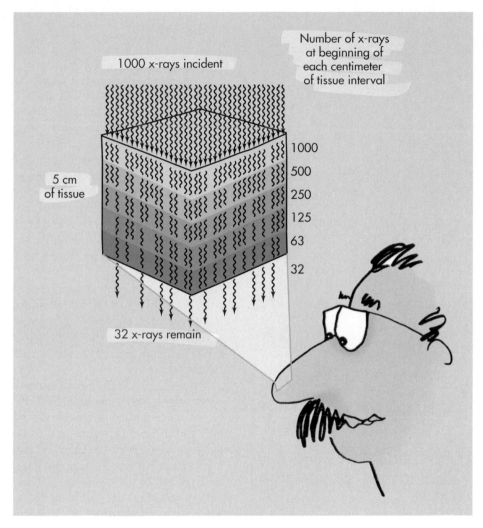

FIGURE 12-15 Interaction of x-rays by absorption and scatter is called *attenuation*. In this example, the x-ray beam has been attenuated 97%; 3% of the x-rays have been transmitted.

primarily on the atomic number of the tissue atoms and the x-ray energy.

An interaction such as the photoelectric effect is called an *absorption process* because the x-ray disappears. **Absorption** is an all-or-none condition for x-ray interaction.

Interactions in which the x-ray is only partially absorbed, such as the Compton effect, are scattering processes. Coherent scattering is also a scattering event because the x-ray emerging from the interaction travels in a direction different from that of the incident x-ray. Pair production and photodisintegration are absorption processes.

The total reduction in the number of x-rays remaining in an x-ray beam after penetration through a given thickness of tissue is called **attenuation**. When a broad beam of x-rays is incident on any tissue, some of the x-rays are absorbed and some are scattered. The result is a reduced number of x-rays, a condition referred to as *x-ray attenuation*.

 Attenuation is the product of absorption and scattering.

X-rays are attenuated exponentially, which means that they do not have a fixed range in tissue. They are reduced in number by a given percentage for each incremental thickness of tissue they go through.

Consider the situation diagrammed in Figure 12-15. One thousand x-rays are incident on a 25-cm-thick abdomen. The x-ray energy and the atomic number of the tissue are such that 50% of the x-rays are removed by the first 5 cm. Therefore, in the first 5 cm, 500 x-rays are removed, leaving 500 available to continue penetration.

By the end of the second 5 cm, 50% of the 500 or 250 additional x-rays have been removed, leaving 250 x-rays to continue. Similarly, entering the fourth 5-cm thickness are 125 x-rays, and entering the fifth and last 5 cm thickness are 63. Half of the 63 x-rays will be

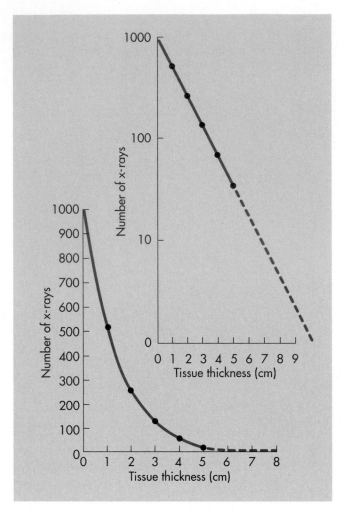

FIGURE 12-16 Linear and semilog plots of exponential x-ray attenuation data in Figure 12-15.

attenuated in the last 5 cm of tissue, and therefore, only 32 will be transmitted to interact with the image receptor. The total effect of these interactions is 97% attenuation and 3% transmission of the x-ray beam.

A plot of this hypothetical x-ray beam attenuation, which closely resembles the actual situation, appears in Figure 12-16. Is it obvious that the assumed HVL in soft tissue was 5 cm? It should be clear that, theoretically at least, the number of x-rays emerging from any thickness of absorber will never reach zero. Each succeeding thickness can attenuate the x-ray beam only by a fractional amount, and a fraction of any positive number is always greater than zero.

This is not the way that alpha particles and beta particles interact with matter. Regardless of the energy of the particle and the type of tissue, these particulate radiations can penetrate only so far before they are totally absorbed. For example, beta particles with 2 MeV of energy have a range of approximately 1 cm in soft tissue.

SUMMARY

The following are five fundamental interactions between x-rays and matter:

1. Coherent scattering is a change in the direction of an incident x-ray without a loss of energy.
2. The Compton effect occurs when incident x-rays ionize atoms and the x-ray then changes direction with a loss of energy.
3. The photoelectric effect occurs when the incident x-ray is absorbed in one of the inner electron shells and emits a photoelectron.
4. Pair production occurs when the incident x-ray interacts with the electric field of the nucleus. The x-ray disappears and two electrons appear, one positively charged (positron) and one negatively charged (electron).
5. Photodisintegration occurs when the incident x-ray is directly absorbed by the nucleus. The x-ray disappears and nuclear fragments are released.

The interactions that are important to diagnostic x-ray imaging are the Compton effect and the photoelectric effect.

Differential absorption controls the contrast of an x-ray image. The x-ray image results from the difference between those x-rays absorbed by photoelectric interaction and those x-rays that pass through the body as image-forming x-rays. Attenuation is the reduction of the x-ray beam intensity as it penetrates through tissue. Differential absorption and attenuation of the x-ray beam depend on the following factors:

1. The atomic number (Z) of the atoms in tissue
2. The mass density of the atoms in tissue
3. The x-ray energy

Radiologic contrast agents, such as iodine and barium, use the principles of differential absorption to image soft tissue organs. Iodine is used in vascular, renal, and biliary imaging. Barium is used for gastrointestinal imaging. Both elements have high atomic numbers (iodine is 53, barium is 56) and mass density much greater than soft tissue.

CHALLENGE QUESTIONS

1. Define or otherwise identify:
   a. Differential absorption
   b. Classical scattering
   c. Mass density
   d. 1.02 MeV
   e. Contrast agent
   f. Compton effect
   g. Attenuation
   h. Monoenergetic
   i. Secondary electron
   j. Photoelectric effect
2. What are the two factors of importance to differential absorption?

3. A 28-keV x-ray interacts photoelectrically with a K-shell electron of a calcium atom. What is the kinetic energy of the secondary electron (see Table 4-3)?

4. 1000 X-rays with energy of 140 keV are incident on bone and soft tissue of equal thickness. If 87 are scattered in soft tissue, approximately how many are scattered in bone?

5. Why are iodinated compounds such excellent agents for vascular contrast examinations?

6. Diagram the Compton interaction and identify the incident x-ray, positive ion, negative ion, secondary x-ray, and scattered x-ray.

7. Describe backscatter radiation. Can you think of examples in diagnostic radiology?

8. Tungsten is sometimes alloyed into the beam-defining collimators of an x-ray imaging system. If a 63-keV x-ray undergoes a Compton interaction with an L-shell electron and ejects that electron with 12 keV of energy, what is the energy of the scattered x-ray (see Figure 4-9)?

9. Of the five basic mechanisms of x-ray interaction with matter, three are not important to diagnostic radiology. Which are they and why are they not important?

10. On average, 33.7 eV is required for each ionization in air. How many ion pairs would a 22-keV x-ray probably produce in air, and approximately how many of these would be produced photoelectrically?

11. How is the energy of the Compton-scattered x-ray computed?

12. Does the probability of the Compton effect depend on the atomic number of the target atom?

13. When the kVp is increased, is there an increase or a reduction of Compton scattering?

14. Describe the photoelectric effect.

15. When the kVp is increased, what happens to the absolute probability of the photoelectric effect versus the Compton effect?

16. How much more likely is it that an x-ray will interact with bone than muscle?

17. What is the relationship between atomic number (Z) and differential absorption?

18. What is the relationship between mass density and differential absorption?

19. In a contrast radiographic examination using iodine, what is the relative probability that x-ray beam will interact with iodine rather than soft tissue?

20. What kVp is used to penetrate barium in a contrast examination?

PART III

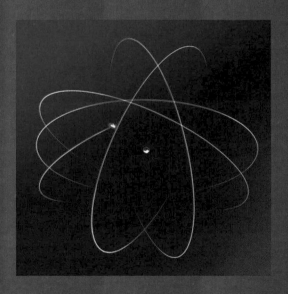

THE RADIOGRAPHIC IMAGE

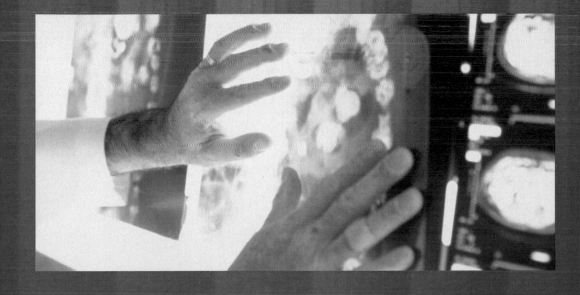

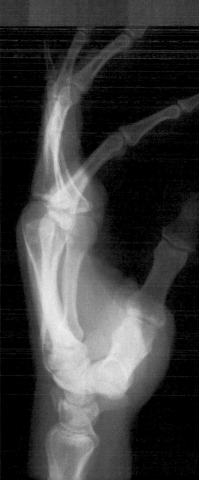

Radiographic Film

OBJECTIVES

At the completion of this chapter, the student should be able to do the following:

1. Discuss the construction of radiographic film
2. Describe the formation of the latent image
3. List and define the characteristics of x-ray film
4. Identify the types of film used in diagnostic imaging departments
5. Explain proper film handling and storage

OUTLINE

MAGE-FORMING x-rays exit the patient and expose the radiographic intensifying screen placed in the protective radiographic cassette. The radiographic intensifying screen emits light, which exposes the radiographic film placed between the two screens.

This chapter discusses the construction and various types of radiographic film, the use of x-rays to form a latent image, and tips for handling and storing film.

REMNANT RADIATION

The primary purpose of diagnostic radiologic apparatus and techniques is to transfer information from an x-ray beam to the eye-brain complex of the radiologist. The x-ray beam emerging from the x-ray tube is nearly uniformly distributed in space. After interaction with the patient, the beam of **image-forming x-rays** (see Chapter 12) is not uniformly distributed in space but varies in intensity according to the characteristics of the tissue through which it has passed.

 Image-forming x-rays are those that exit the patient and interact with the image receptor.

This beam of varied intensity is called the **exit beam** (formerly known as the *remnant beam*). The exit beam refers to the x-rays that remain as the useful beam exits the patient. It consists of x-rays scattered away from the image receptor and image-forming x-rays.

Image-forming x-rays are the x-rays that interact with the image receptor to form a radiographic image. The American Registry of Radiologic Technologists used the term *exit radiation* as a replacement for an earlier term.

The diagnostically useful information in this exit beam must be transferred to a form intelligible to the radiologist. X-ray film is one such medium. Other media include the fluoroscopic image intensifier, the television monitor, the laser imaging system, and solid-state detectors, all of which are discussed later. The medium that converts the x-ray beam into a visible image is called the **image receptor (IR)**. The most common IR is still photographic film, although other IRs are finding increased application.

Photography has its origins in the early nineteenth century. By the time of the American Civil War (1860 to 1865), photography was professionally used. Amateur photography surfaced early in the twentieth century.

The construction and characteristics of radiographic film are similar to those of regular photographic film. Radiographic film is manufactured with rigorous quality control and has a spectral response different from that of photographic film; however, its mechanism of operation is much the same. The following discussion concerns radiographic film, but with very few modifications it could be applied to photographic film.

FILM CONSTRUCTION

The manufacture of radiographic film is a precise procedure requiring tight quality control. Manufacturing facilities are extremely clean because the slightest bit of dirt or other contaminant in the film limits the film's ability to reproduce the information of the x-ray beam.

During the early 1960s, at the height of nuclear weapons testing, x-ray film manufacturers took extraordinary precautions to ensure that contamination from radioactive fallout did not invade their manufacturing environment. Such contamination could seriously **fog** the film.

Radiographic film basically has two parts: the **base** and the **emulsion** (Figure 13-1). Most x-ray film has the emulsion coated on both sides and therefore is called **double emulsion film**. Between the emulsion and the base is a thin coating of material called the **adhesive layer** to ensure uniform adhesion of the emulsion to the base. This adhesive layer allows the emulsion and base to maintain proper contact and integrity during use and processing.

The emulsion is enclosed by a protective covering of gelatin called the **overcoat**. This overcoat protects the emulsion from scratches, pressure, and contamination during handling, processing, and storage and allows for relatively rough manipulation of x-ray film before exposure. Processed film may be handled with even less regard for damage. The thickness of radiographic film is approximately 150 to 300 μm.

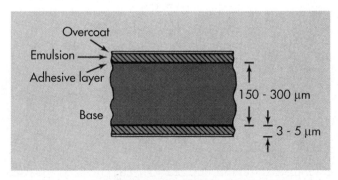

FIGURE 13-1 Cross-section of radiographic film. The bulk of the film is the base. The emulsion contains the diagnostic information.

Base

The base is the foundation of radiographic film. Its primary purpose is to provide a rigid structure onto which the emulsion can be coated. The base is flexible and fracture-resistant to allow easy handling but rigid enough to be snapped into a viewbox.

Conventional photographic film has a much thinner base than radiographic film and therefore is not as rigid. Can you imagine attempting to snap a 14 × 17 inch photographic negative into a viewbox?

 The base of radiographic film is 150 to 300 μm thick, semi-rigid, lucent, and made of polyester.

The base of radiographic film maintains its size and shape during use and processing so that it does not contribute to image distortion. This property of the base is known as **dimensional stability.** The base is of uniform **lucency** and nearly transparent to light, so there is no unwanted pattern or shading on the image.

During manufacturing, however, dye is added to the base of most radiographic film to slightly tint the film blue. Compared with untinted film, this coloring reduces eyestrain and fatigue, increasing the radiologist's diagnostic efficiency and accuracy.

The original radiographic film base was a glass plate. Radiologists used to refer to radiographs as **x-ray plates.** During World War I, high-quality glass became largely unavailable while medical applications of x-rays, particularly by the military, were increasing rapidly.

A substitute material, **cellulose nitrate,** soon became the standard base. Cellulose nitrate, however, had one serious deficiency: it was flammable. The improper storage and handling of some x-ray film files resulted in severe hospital fires during the 1920s and early 1930s.

By the mid-1920s, film with a "safety base," **cellulose triacetate,** was introduced. Cellulose triacetate has properties similar to those of cellulose nitrate but is not as inflammable.

In the early 1960s, a **polyester** base was introduced. Polyester has taken the place of cellulose triacetate as the film base of choice. Polyester is more resistant to warping from age and stronger than cellulose triacetate, permitting easier transport through automatic processors. Its dimensional stability is superior. Polyester bases are also thinner than triacetate bases (approximately 175 μm) but are just as strong.

Emulsion

The emulsion is the heart of the x-ray film. It is the material with which x-rays or light photons from screens interact and transfer information. The emulsion consists of a homogeneous mixture of **gelatin** and **silver halide crystals.** It is coated evenly in a layer that is 3 to 5 μm thick.

The gelatin is similar to that used in salads and desserts but is of much higher quality. It is clear, so that it transmits light, and is sufficiently porous for the processing chemicals to penetrate to the crystals of silver halide. Its principal function is to provide mechanical support for the silver halide crystals by holding them uniformly dispersed in place.

The silver halide crystal is the active ingredient of the radiographic emulsion. In the typical emulsion, 98% of the silver halide is **silver bromide;** the remainder is usually **silver iodide.** These atoms have relatively high atomic numbers ($Z_{Br} = 35$, $Z_{Ag} = 47$, $Z_I = 53$) compared with the gelatin and base (for both, $Z \approx 7$). The interaction of x-ray and light photons with these high-Z atoms ultimately results in the formation of a latent image on the radiograph.

Depending on the intended imaging application, silver halide crystals may have tabular, cubic, octahedral, polyhedral, or irregular shapes. Tabular grains are used in most radiographic films.

The tabular silver halide crystals are flat and typically 0.1 μm thick, with a triangular, hexagonal, or higher-order polygonal cross-section. The crystals are approximately 1 μm in diameter. The arrangement of atoms in a crystal is cubic, as shown in Figure 13-2.

The crystals are made by dissolving metallic silver (Ag) in nitric acid (HNO_3) to form silver nitrate ($AgNO_3$). The light-sensitive silver bromide (AgBr) crystals are formed by mixing the silver nitrate with potassium bromide (KBr) in the following reaction:

SILVER HALIDE CRYSTAL FORMATION
$$AgNO_3 + KBr \rightarrow AgBr \downarrow + KNO_3$$
The arrow ↓ indicates that the silver bromide is precipitated while the potassium nitrate, which is soluble, is washed away.

The entire process takes place in the presence of gelatin and with precise control of the temperature, the pressure, and the rate at which ingredients are mixed.

The shape and lattice structure of the silver halide crystals are not perfect, and some of the imperfections result in the imaging property of the crystals. The type of imperfection thought to be responsible is a chemical contaminant, usually silver sulfide, which is introduced by chemical sensitization into the crystal lattice, usually at or near the surface.

This contaminant has been given the name **sensitivity center.** During exposure, photoelectrons and silver ions are attracted to these sensitivity centers, where they combine to form a **latent image center** of metallic silver.

The differences in speed, contrast, and resolution among various radiographic films are determined by the process by which the silver halide crystals are manufactured and by the mixture of these crystals into the gelatin. The number of sensitivity centers per crystal, the concentration of crystals in the emulsion, and the size and distribution of the crystals also affect the performance characteristics of radiographic film.

Direct-exposure film contains a thicker emulsion with more silver halide crystals than screen-film. The size and concentration of silver halide crystals primarily affect film speed. The composition of the radiographic emulsion is a proprietary secret closely guarded by each manufacturer.

Radiographic film is manufactured in total darkness. From the moment the emulsion ingredients are brought together until final packaging, no light is present.

FORMATION OF THE LATENT IMAGE

The imaging-forming x-rays exiting the patient and incident on the radiographic film deposit energy in the emulsion primarily by photoelectric interaction with the atoms of the silver halide crystal. This energy is deposited in a pattern representative of the object or anatomic part being radiographed.

Immediately after exposure, no image can be observed on the film. An invisible image is present, however, and is called a **latent image.** With proper chemical processing, the latent image becomes a **manifest image.**

 The latent image is the invisible change induced in the silver halide crystal.

The interaction between photons and silver halide crystals is fairly well understood, as is the processing of the latent image into the manifest image. However, the formation of the latent image, sometimes called the **photographic effect,** is not well understood and continues to be the subject of considerable research. The following discussion is an extraction of the Gurney-Mott theory, the accepted, although incomplete, explanation of latent image formation.

Silver Halide Crystal

The silver, bromine, and iodine atoms are fixed in the **crystal lattice** in ion form (Figure 13-3). Silver is a positive ion, and bromide and iodide are negative ions. When a silver halide crystal is formed, each silver atom releases an outer-shell electron, which becomes attached to a halide atom (either bromine or iodine).

The silver atom is missing an electron and therefore is a positively charged ion, identified as Ag^+. The bromine and iodine atoms each have one extra electron and therefore are negatively charged ions, identified as bromide and iodide (Br^- and I^-), respectively.

 An ion is an atom that has either too many or too few electrons and therefore is electrically charged.

The silver halide crystal is not as rigid as some crystals such as diamonds. Under certain conditions, both atoms and electrons are free to migrate within the silver halide crystal.

The halide ions, bromide and iodide, are generally in greatest concentration along the surface of the crystal.

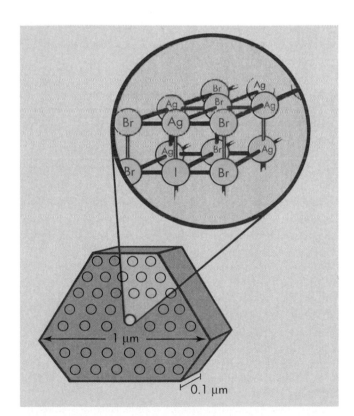

FIGURE 13-2 An example of a tabular silver halide crystal with triangular cross-section. The arrangement of atoms in the crystal is cubic.

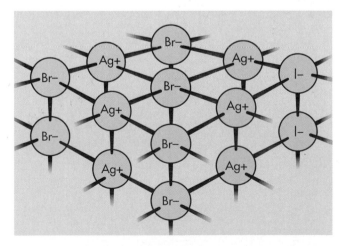

FIGURE 13-3 Silver halide crystal lattice contains ions. Electrons from Ag atoms have been loaned to Br and I atoms.

Therefore the crystal takes on a negative surface charge, which is matched by the positive charge of the **interstitial** silver ions, the silver ions inside the crystal. An inherent defect in the structure of silver halide crystals, the **Frankel defect,** consists of interstitial silver ions and silver ion vacancies. Figure 13-4 presents a model of the silver halide crystal.

Photon Interaction with Silver Halide Crystal

When radiation interacts with film, it is the interaction with the silver and halide atoms (Ag, Br, I) that forms the latent image. If the x-ray is totally absorbed, its interaction is photoelectric (Figure 13-5, *A*). If it is partially absorbed, its interaction is Compton.

In both cases a **secondary electron,** either a photoelectron or a Compton electron, is released with sufficient energy to travel a large distance in the crystal (Figure 13-5, *B*). While crossing the crystal, the secondary electron may have sufficient energy to dislodge additional electrons from the crystal lattice.

Consequently, as a result of one x-ray interaction, a number of electrons are released and travel through the crystal lattice. The release of these secondary electrons is represented as follows:

SECONDARY ELECTRONS FORMATION
$Br^- + photon \rightarrow Br + e^-$

Because light photons have lower energy, more are needed to produce a number of migrating secondary electrons equal to the number produced by a single x-ray.

The result is the same whether the interaction involves visible light from an intensifying screen or direct exposure by x-rays.

Secondary electrons liberated by the absorption event migrate to the sensitivity center and are trapped. Once a sensitivity center captures a photoelectron and becomes more negatively charged, the center is attractive to mobile interstitial silver ions (Figure 13-5, *C*). The interstitial silver ion combines with the electron trapped at the sensitivity center to form metallic silver atoms.

METALLIC SILVER FORMATION
$e^- + Ag^+ \rightarrow Ag$

Most of these electrons come from the bromide and iodide ions because these negative ions have one extra electron. These negative ions therefore are converted to neutral atoms, and the loss of ionic charge results in a disruption of the crystal lattice.

The bromine and iodine atoms are now free to migrate because they are no longer bound by ionic forces. They migrate out of the crystal into the gelatin portion of the emulsion. The deterioration of crystalline structure also makes it easier for remaining silver ions to migrate.

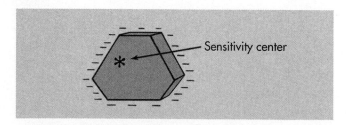

FIGURE 13-4 Model of a silver halide crystal emphasizing sensitivity center and concentration of negative ions on the surface.

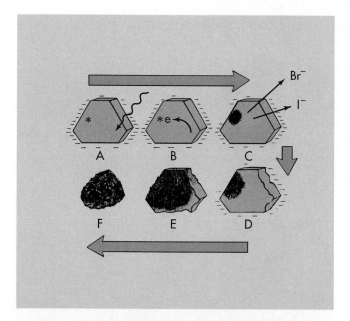

FIGURE 13-5 Production of the latent image and conversion of the latent image into a manifest image requires several simultaneous steps. **A,** Radiation interaction releases electrons. **B,** These electrons migrate to the sensitivity center. **C,** At the sensitivity center, atomic silver is formed by attracting an interstitial silver ion. **D,** This process is repeated many times, resulting in the buildup of silver atoms. **E,** The remaining silver halide is converted to silver during processing. **F,** The resulting silver grain.

Latent Image

The concentration of electrons at the sensitivity center produces a region of negative electrification. As the halide atoms are removed from the crystal, the positive silver ions are electrostatically attracted to the sensitivity center. After migrating to the sensitivity center, the silver ions are neutralized by electrons and converted to atomic silver.

In an optimally exposed film, most developable silver halide crystals have collected 4 to 10 silver atoms at a sensitivity center (Figure 13-5, *D*). Consequently, this silver deposition is not observable, even microscopically.

This group of silver atoms is called a **latent image center.** It is here that visible quantities of silver form during processing to create the radiographic image (Figure 13-5, *E*).

Crystals with silver deposited at the sensitivity center are developed into black grains (Figure 13-5, *F*). Crystals that have not been irradiated remain crystalline and inactive. The unobservable information contained in radiation-activated and inactivated silver halide crystals constitutes the latent image.

Processing is the term applied to the chemical reactions that transform the latent image into a manifest image. Because of its importance, processing is dealt with separately in the following chapter.

TYPES OF FILM

Medical imaging, especially radiologic imaging, is becoming extremely technical and sophisticated, and this is reflected in the number and variety of the films available. Each major film manufacturer produces over 25 different films for medical imaging. When combined with the various film formats offered, over 500 selections are possible.

Table 13-1 shows the standard film sizes in English and SI units. In most cases the sizes are not exactly equivalent but they are usually interchangeable. By far the most commonly used film is that customarily called **screen-film.** Screen-film is the type of film used with radiographic intensifying screens.

In addition to screen-film, there is **direct-exposure film,** sometimes called nonscreen film and special appli-cation film, such as those used in mammography, video recording, duplication, subtraction, cineradiography, and dental radiology. Each has particular characteristics that become more familiar to the technologist with use.

Screen-Film

Screen-film is the most widely used IR in radiology. Several characteristics need be considered when selecting screen-film: contrast, speed, spectral matching, anticrossover/antihalation dyes, and safe light required.

Contrast. Most manufacturers offer screen-film with multiple contrast levels. High-contrast film produces a very black-and-white image, whereas a low-contrast image is more gray. Contrast is discussed in more detail in Chapter 19.

The contrast of an IR is inversely proportional to its exposure **latitude,** that is, the range of exposure techniques that produce an acceptable image. Consequently, screen-film is available in multiple latitudes. Usually, the manufacturer identifies the contrast of these films as medium, high, or higher.

The difference depends on the **size and distribution of the silver halide crystals.** A high-contrast emulsion contains smaller silver halide grains with a relatively uniform grain size. Low-contrast films, on the other hand, contain larger grains having a wider range of sizes.

Speed. Screen-film IRs are also available with different speeds. Speed is the sensitivity of the screen-film combination to x-rays and light. Usually, a manufacturer offers several different IRs of different speeds that result from different film emulsions and different intensifying screen phosphors.

For direct-exposure film, speed is principally a function of the concentration and total amount of silver halide crystals. For screen-film, silver halide grain size and shape are the principal determinates of film speed.

Large-grain emulsions are more sensitive than small-grain emulsions.

To optimize speed, screen-films are almost always **double emulsion,** that is, an emulsion is layered on either side of the base. This double-layering is primarily due to the efficiency conferred by using two screens to expose the film from both sides. This provides for twice the speed that could be obtained with a single-emulsion film, even if the single emulsion were made twice as thick.

Film speed is limited, however, because the light from the radiographic intensifying screen is absorbed very rapidly in the superficial layers of the emulsion. If the emulsion is too thick, that portion next to the film base remains largely unexposed.

TABLE 13-1	Standard Film Sizes	
	English Units	**SI Units**
		18 × 43 cm
	8 × 10 in	20 × 25 cm
		24 × 30 cm
	10 × 12 in	28 × 35 cm
	14 × 14 in	35 × 35 cm
	14 × 17 in	35 × 43 cm

Compared to earlier technology, current emulsions contain less silver yet produce the same optical density per unit exposure. This more efficient use of silver in the emulsion is called the **covering power** of the emulsion.

The reported speed of a film is nearly always that for the IR: the film and two radiographic screens. When radiographic intensifying screens and film are properly matched, the reported speed is accurate. Mismatch can cause significant exposure error.

Crossover. Until recently, silver halide crystals were usually fat and three-dimensional (Figure 13-6, *A*). Most emulsions now (Figure 13-6, *B*) contain tabular grains, which are flat silver halide crystals so as to provide a large surface area/volume ratio. The result is not only improved covering power but significantly lower crossover.

When light is emitted by a radiographic intensifying screen, it not only exposes the adjacent emulsion but can also expose the emulsion on the other side of the base. When light **crosses over** the base it causes increased blur on the image (Figure 13-7).

 Crossover is the exposure of an emulsion by light from the opposite side of the radiographic intensifying screen.

Tabular grain emulsions reduce crossover because the covering power is increased, which relates not only to light absorption from the screen, which is increased, but also to light transmitted through the emulsion to cause crossover, which is reduced.

The addition of a light-absorbing dye in a crossover control layer reduces crossover to near zero (Figure 13-8). The crossover control layer has three critical characteristics: it absorbs most of the crossover light, it does not diffuse into the emulsion but remains as a separate layer, and it is completely removed during processing.

Crossover can also be reduced or eliminated by using radiographic intensifying screens, which emit short-wavelength light (blue or ultraviolet). Such light is more strongly absorbed by the silver halide crystals. Also, the polyester base is not transparent to ultraviolet light, so there is no crossover with ultraviolet-emitting screens.

Spectral Matching. Perhaps the most important consideration in selecting modern screen-film is its spectral absorption characteristics. Since the introduction of **rare earth screens** in the early 1970s, radiologic technologists must be particularly careful to use a film whose sensitivity to various colors of light—its **spectral response**—is properly matched to the spectrum of light emitted by the screen.

 Rare earth screens are made with rare earth elements, those with atomic numbers of 57 to 71.

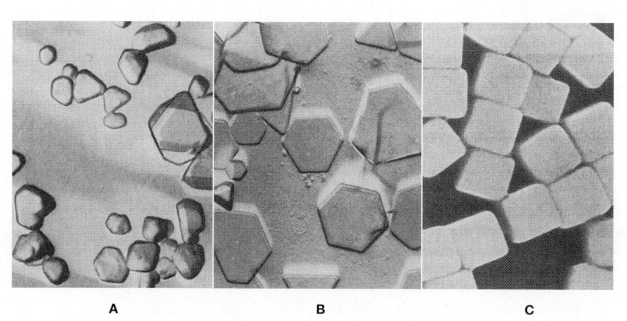

FIGURE 13-6 A, Conventional silver halide crystals are irregular in size. **B,** New technology produces flat, tablet-like grains. **C,** Cubic grains (Courtesy Eastman Kodak.)

Calcium tungstate screens emit blue and blue-violet light. Calcium tungstate screens have been largely replaced with rare earth screens, which are faster. There are now many rare earth phosphors that emit ultraviolet, blue, green, and red. All silver halide films respond to violet and blue light but not to green, yellow, or red unless they are spectrally sensitized with dyes.

If green-emitting screens are used, they should be matched with a film that is sensitive not only to blue light but also to green light. Such film is **orthochromatic** and is called green-sensitive film. This is distinct from **panchromatic film,** which is used in photography and is sensitive to the entire visible light spectrum.

Figure 13-9 shows the spectral response of blue-sensitive and green-sensitive films. Blue-sensitive film should be used only with blue- or ultraviolet-emitting screens. Green-sensitive film is usually exposed with green-emitting screens.

If films with sensitivity only in the ultraviolet and blue regions of the spectrum are used with green-emitting screens, then the IR speed is greatly reduced and patient dose increases. Proper **spectral matching** results in the correct screen-film combination.

Reciprocity Law. One would expect that the total exposure of a film would not depend on the time taken to expose it. That is the definition of the **reciprocity law,** which can also be stated:

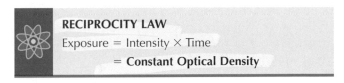

RECIPROCITY LAW
Exposure = Intensity × Time
= **Constant Optical Density**

The reciprocity law is true for film exposed to x-rays. Industrial radiographers do not have to compensate for this effect. The reciprocity law fails when film is exposed to light from radiographic intensifying screens. Radiographers must be aware of this.

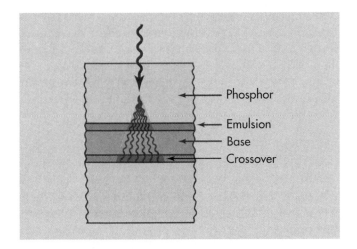

FIGURE 13-7 Crossover occurs when screen light crosses the base to expose the opposite emulsion.

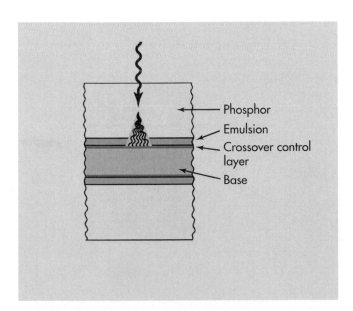

FIGURE 13-8 Crossover is reduced by adding a dye to the base, called a crossover control layer.

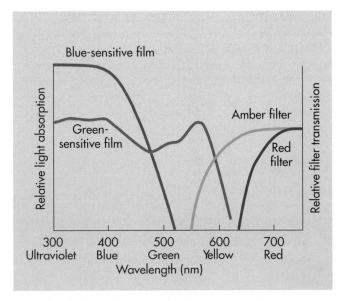

FIGURE 13-9 Radiographic films are either blue-sensitive or green-sensitive and they require amber-and red-filtered safelights, respectively.

Reciprocity law failure is important when exposure times are long (as in mammography) or short (as in angiography). The result for long or short exposures is reduced speed. An increase in radiographic technique may be required. Table 13-2 shows approximate speed lose as a function of exposure time.

Safelights. The use of radiographic film requires certain precautions in the darkroom. Most **safelights** are incandescent lamps with a color filter; safelights provide enough light to illuminate the darkroom while ensuring that the film remains unexposed.

Proper darkroom illumination depends not only on the color of the filter but also on the wattage of the bulb and the distance between the lamp and the work surface. A 15 W bulb should be no closer than 5 ft from the work surface.

With blue-sensitive film, an **amber filter** is used. The amber filter transmits light having wavelengths longer than approximately 550 nm, which is above the spectral response of blue-sensitive film.

The use of an amber filter would fog green-sensitive film; therefore, a **red filter**, which transmits only light above approximately 600 nm, must be used in this case. A red filter is suitable for both green- and blue-sensitive film. Figure 13-9 shows the approximate transmission characteristics for amber and red safelight filters.

Direct-Exposure Film

The use of radiographic intensifying screens with film allows reduced technique and therefore reduced patient dose. However, the image is more blurred than it would be following exposure without screens. In the past, certain films was manufactured for use without screens; they were used to image thin body parts, such as hands and feet, that have high subject contrast and present low radiation risk.

Most extremity examinations now use fine-grain, high-detail screens and double-emulsion film as the IR. Until the early 1970s, such film was also used for mammography, but patient dose was much too high. This film typically requires 10 to 100 times more radiation than screen-film and is rarely used today.

This type of film is identified as **direct-exposure film.** The emulsion of a direct-exposure film is thicker than that of screen-film and it contains higher concentration of silver halide crystals to improve direct x-ray interaction.

Direct-exposure film is less sensitive to light and therefore should not be used with screens. Direct-exposure film is usually used with a cardboard cassette, although some such films are available in individually packaged paper wrappings.

Following processing, double-emulsion film is flat because the expansion and contraction characteristics of the two emulsion layers compensate for one another. With single-emulsion film, however, special attention must be paid to the swelling of the emulsion during processing and its shrinking during drying. The backside of the base of single-emulsion film is coated with clear gelatin so that during processing, the emulsion swells and shrinkage is balanced, ensuring that the film will not curl.

Mammography Film

Mammography was originally performed with an industrial-grade, double-emulsion, direct-exposure film. The radiation doses associated with such a technique were much too high, and consequently specialty films were developed.

Most mammography film is single-emulsion film designed to be exposed with a single radiographic intensifying screen. All currently available mammography screen-film systems use green-emitting terbium-doped gadolinium oxysulfide screens with green-sensitive film.

TABLE 13-2	Approximate Reciprocity Law Failure
Exposure Time	**Relative Speed (%)**
1 ms	95
10 ms	100
100 ms	100
1 s	90
10 s	60

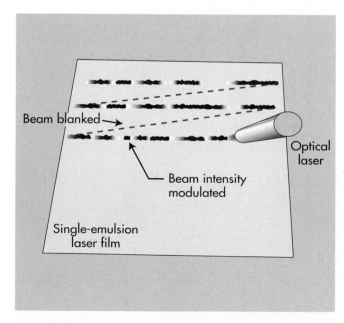

FIGURE 13-10 The laser beam writes in raster fashion.

The surface of the base opposite the screen is coated with a special light-absorbing dye to reduce reflection of screen light, which is transmitted through the emulsion and base. This effect is called **halation,** and the absorbing dye is an antihalation coating. Such antihalation coating is used on all single-emulsion screen-film, not just mammography film. The coating is removed during processing for better viewing.

Laser Film

A laser printer uses the digital electronic signal from an imaging device. The intensity of the laser beam is varied in direct proportion to the strength of the image signal. This process is called laser beam **modulation.** While being modulated, the laser beam writes in raster fashion over the entire film (Figure 13-10).

Laser printers provide exceptionally consistent image quality for multiple film sizes and multiple image formats per film. These printers can be electronically interfaced with multiple digital imaging modalities such as CT, MRI, and computed radiology. For even greater productivity, laser printers can be docked to an automatic film processor.

Laser film is silver halide film sensitized to the red light emitted by the laser in much the same way blue- and green-sensitive screen-film is sensitized. Different types of lasers are used in laser printers and laser film is light-sensitive; therefore, laser film must be handled in total darkness.

Figure 13-11 presents a cross-section of single-emulsion film, such as that used for mammography and laser imaging.

Specialty Film

Occasionally, a radiographer is requested to perform a different type of task that requires a different type of film. In order to duplicate an existing radiograph, **duplicating film** is used. Duplicating film is designed for same-size use—that is, the size of duplicating film is equal to the size of the film being duplicated.

Duplicating film is a single-emulsion film that is exposed to ultraviolet light or blue light through the existing radiograph to produce a copy. The way duplicating film responds to light is opposite that of radiographic film: exposure to light *reduces* optical density in duplicating film.

Cinefluorography is a special examination reserved almost exclusively for the cardiac catheterization laboratory. The radiologic technologist who becomes involved in such procedures uses **cine film.** Cine film is 35 mm and is supplied in rolls of 100 and 500 ft.

Spot films from 70 to 105 mm in width are used in a number of different types of spot film cameras. These films are similar in composition to cine film but are larger than cine film; therefore, spot film can be viewed directly on a conventional viewbox without resorting to a projector. Figure 13-12 shows the format of the more popular sizes of cine and roll-type spot films.

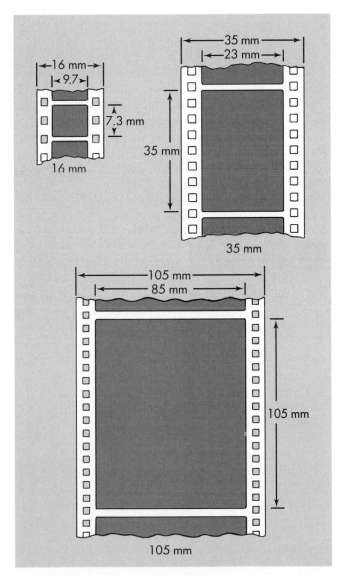

FIGURE 13-12 The format of 16 mm and 35 mm cine film and 105 mm spot film.

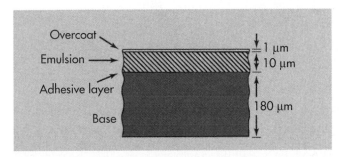

FIGURE 13-11 Cross-section of single-emulsion mammography film.

Processing of cine film and spot film is critical to providing a quality image. Roll-type spot film can usually be adequately processed in the automatic processor used for conventional radiographs. Cine film, on the other hand, should be processed with specially designed movie film processing equipment because artifacts are magnified along with the image during projection.

HANDLING AND STORAGE OF FILM

Radiographic film is a sensitive radiation detector and must be handled accordingly. Improper handling and storage results in poor radiographs with artifacts that interfere with diagnosis. For this reason it is essential that anyone handling radiographic film be careful not to bend, crease, or otherwise subject it to rough handling. Clean hands are a must, and hand lotion and cream should be avoided.

Improper handling or processing can cause **artifacts,** the marks or spurious images that sometimes appear on the processed radiograph. Artifacts can also be generated by the useful x-ray beam. Radiographic film is pressure-sensitive, so rough handling or the imprint of any sharp object, such as a fingernail, is reproduced as an artifact on the processed radiograph.

Creasing the film before processing produces a line artifact. Dirt on the hands or on radiographic intensifying screens results in specular artifacts. In a dry environment, static electricity can cause characteristic artifacts.

During automatic processing, a worn or dirty transport system can cause artifacts that are usually identifiable by their repetition. Identifying artifacts and their causes are covered in Chapter 32.

Heat and Humidity

Radiographic film is sensitive to the effects of elevated temperature and humidity, especially for long periods. Heat reduces contrast and increases the fog of a radiograph. Consequently, radiographic film should be stored at temperatures lower than approximately 20° C (68° F). With higher storage temperatures, the longer the time of storage, the more severe the loss of contrast because of the increase in fog.

Ideally, radiographic films should be in refrigerated storage. Storage for a year or longer is acceptable if the film is maintained at 10° C (50° F). Film should never be stored near steam pipes or other sources of heat.

Storage under conditions of elevated humidity (e.g., over 60%) also reduces contrast because of increased fog. Consequently, before use, radiographic film should be stored in a cool, dry place, ideally in a climate-controlled environment. Storage in an area that is too dry can be equally objectionable. Static artifacts are possible when the relative humidity dips below about 40%.

Light

Radiographic film must be stored and handled in the dark. No light can expose the emulsion before processing. If low-level, diffuse light exposes the film, fog is increased. If bright light exposes or partially exposes the film, a gross, obvious artifact is produced.

The control of light is ensured by a well-sealed darkroom and a light-proof storage bin for film that has been opened but not clinically exposed. The storage bin should have an electrical interlock that prevents it from being opened while the door to the darkroom is ajar or open.

Radiation

Ionizing radiation, other than the useful beam, creates an image artifact by reducing contrast and increasing fog. Film fog is the dull, uniform optical density that appears if the film has been inadvertently exposed to light, x-rays, heat, or humidity.

Darkrooms are usually located next to x-ray rooms and are lined with lead. However, this is not always necessary. It is usually acceptable to lead line only the storage shelf and film bin.

 The fog level for unprocessed film is approximately 0.2 mR (2μ Gy$_a$).

Radiographic film is far more sensitive to x-ray exposure than are people; therefore, more lead is required to protect film than people. The thickness of the lead barrier is designed to keep the total exposure of unprocessed film below this level. This, of course, requires some assumptions about the storage time of the film. Monthly turnover of film requires four times the lead shielding than weekly turnover.

Care should be taken to ensure that the receiving area for radiographic film is not the same as that for the radioactive material used in nuclear medicine. Even though the packaging of radioactive material ensures the safety of those who handle it, the low-level radiation emitted can fog radiographic film if the radioactive material and film are stored together for even a short time.

Shelf Life

Most radiographic film is supplied in boxes of 100 sheets. Some film is packaged in an interleaved fashion, with chemically treated protective paper between each sheet of film. Each box contains an expiration date, which indicates the maximum shelf life of the film.

Under no circumstances should film be stored for periods longer than the stated shelf life. Film must be used before its expiration date, usually a year or so after purchase. Aging results in a loss of speed and contrast and an increase in fog.

It is always wise to store boxes of film on edge rather than lying flat. When stored on edge, they are less likely to warp and, in the case of noninterleaved packaging, less likely to stick to one another.

The storage of film should be sequenced so that the oldest film is used first. A rotation of the film, much like the rotation of perishables in a supermarket, is appropriate.

Most hospitals receive film each month and purchase enough film for 5 weeks of use. The extra few days above monthly use are necessary to cover civil emergencies that require an unexpectedly large number of x-ray examinations. Given a 5-week supply schedule and the first-in, first-out rule, 45 days is **a reasonable maximum storage time for radiographic film.**

SUMMARY

Image-forming x-radiation is that part of the x-ray beam that exits a patient and exposes the IR. The conventional image radiographic IR is a cassette containing radiographic film sandwiched between two radiographic intensifying screens. Radiographic film is made up of a polyester base covered on both sides with a film emulsion.

The film emulsion contains light-sensitive silver-bromide crystals, which are made from the mixture of silver nitrate and potassium bromide. During manufacture, the emulsion is spread onto the base in darkness or under red lights because the AgBr molecule is sensitive to light.

The invisible latent image is formed in the film emulsion when light photons interact with the silver-halide crystals. Processing the radiographic film converts the latent image a visible image.

The following are some important characteristics of radiographic film:

- **Contrast.** High-contrast film produces black-and-white images. Low-contrast film produces images with shades of gray.
- **Latitude.** Latitude is the range of exposure techniques (kVp and mAs) that produces an acceptable image.
- **Speed.** Speed is the sensitivity of the screen-film combination to x-rays and light. Fast screen-film combinations need fewer x-rays to produce a diagnostic image.
- **Crossover.** When light is emitted from a radiographic intensifying screen, it exposes not only the adjacent film emulsion but also the emulsion on the other side of the base. The light crosses over the base and blurs the radiographic image.
- **Spectral Matching.** The x-ray beam does not directly expose the x-ray film. Radiographic intensifying screens emit light when exposed to x-rays and light, which then exposes the radiographic film. The color of light emitted must match the response of the film.
- **Reciprocity Law.** When exposed to the light of radiographic intensifying screens, radiographic film speed is less if the exposure time is very short or very long.

Film should be handled carefully and stored at specific temperatures and humidities to reduce artifacts. Artifacts on radiographic film can also be caused by rough handling.

CHALLENGE QUESTIONS

1. Define or otherwise identify the following:
   a. Polyester
   b. Sensitivity speck
   c. Latent image
   d. Emulsion covering power
   e. Orthochromatic film
   f. Silver halide
   g. Spectral matching
   h. Artifact
   i. Radiation fog
   j. Shelf life
2. Diagram the cross-sectional view of a radiographic film designed for use with a pair of radiographic intensifying screens.
3. What does the term **dimensional stability** mean when applied to radiographic film? Which part of the film is responsible for this characteristic?
4. List the principal ingredients in the radiographic emulsion and their respective atomic number (Z).
5. Silver bromide crystals are made from silver nitrate and potassium bromide. Following exposure, some of the silver bromide is reduced to metallic silver. What are the chemical equations representing these interactions?
6. Describe the process whereby a latent image is created in one crystal of the film emulsion.
7. What is the difference between panchromatic film and orthochromatic film?
8. What determines proper darkroom safelight selection?
9. What precautions are necessary when using films designed specifically for screen-film mammography?
10. What precautions are necessary when using and storing radiographic film?
11. Briefly discuss the historical development of x-ray film.

12. Write the silver-halide crystal reaction. What does the arrow pointing down represent?
13. What determines the speed of radiographic film?
14. What is the term for closely guarded information held by film manufacturers?
15. Explain the Gurney-Mott theory of latent-image formation.
16. What is the importance of spectral matching in choosing screen-film combinations?
17. Why do radiographers need to be aware of reciprocity law failure?
18. An amber filter on a safelight is used under what conditions? A red filter on a safelight is used under what conditions?
19. Discuss the difference between regular screen-film and mammography screen-film.
20. List the proper film storage conditions for (a) temperature, (b) humidity, and (c) shelf life.

CHAPTER 14

Processing the Latent Image

OBJECTIVES

At the completion of this chapter, the student should be able to do the following:

1. Discuss the historical development from hand processing to automatic processing
2. List the chemicals used in each processing step
3. Discuss the use of each chemical
4. Explain the systems of the automatic processor
5. Describe the alternative processing methods

OUTLINE

P ROCESSING THE invisible latent image creates the visible image. Processing causes the silver ions in the silver halide crystal that have been exposed to light to be converted into microscopic black grains of silver. The processing sequence has the following steps: (1) wetting, (2) developing, (3) stop bath, (4) fixing, (5) washing, and (6) drying.

These processing steps are completed in an automatic processor. This chapter discusses automatic processor design and use, as well as alternative processing methods.

FILM PROCESSING

The latent image is invisible because only a few silver ions have been changed to metallic silver and deposited at the sensitivity center. Processing the film magnifies this action many times until all the silver ions in an exposed crystal are converted to atomic silver; thus converting the latent image into a visible radiographic image.

The exposed crystal becomes a black grain that is visible microscopically. The silver contained in fine jewelry and tableware would also appear black except that it has been highly polished, which smoothes the surface and makes it reflective.

Processing is as important as technique and positioning in making a quality radiograph. A change in recommended processing conditions should never be a substitute for a poor radiographic exposure because the result is always a higher patient dose.

Manual Processing

Before the introduction of automatic film processing, x-ray films were processed manually. In manual processing, the exposed radiographic film was first immersed in a tank containing developer for approximately 5 min at 20° C (70° F). Films were then immersed in a stop bath, followed by immersion in a fixer solution.

The film was washed in running water and hung to drip dry. It took approximately 1 hr to obtain a completely dry and ready-to-read radiograph.

Automatic Processing

The first automatic x-ray film processor was introduced by Pako in 1942 (Figure 14-1). The first commercially available model could process 120 films/hr by using special film hangers. These film hangers were dunked from one tank to another. The total cycle time for processing one film was approximately 40 min.

Automatic x-ray film processing advanced significantly in 1956 when the Eastman Kodak Company introduced the first roller transport system for processing medical radiographs. The roller transport automatic processor shown in Figure 14-2 was about 10 ft long, weighed nearly three quarters of a ton, and sold for approximately $275,000 in today's dollars.

Automatic processing revolutionized busy departments. Finished radiographs became available in 6 min, and the variability in results caused by the human element was eliminated. Departmental efficiency, work flow, and radiographic quality all improved.

Another significant breakthrough was Eastman Kodak's introduction of 90 s rapid processing in 1965. Rapid processing was possible because of the development of new chemistry and emulsions as well as the faster drying permitted by a polyester film base. With this processor, the dry-to-drop time is 90 s. This type of automatic film processing system remains the standard.

In 1987, Konica introduced an automatic film processor that has a processing cycle of approximately 45 s. This processor requires special films and chemicals, however. In the future, 20 to 45 s processing may become the standard.

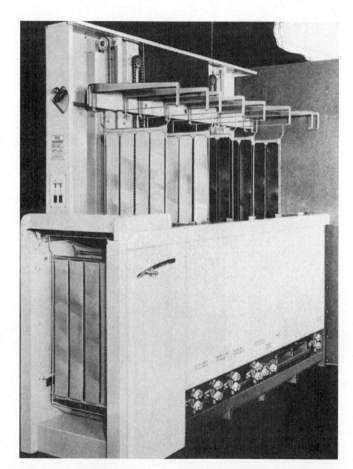

FIGURE 14-1 The first automatic processor, circa 1942. (Courtesy Art Haus.)

Processing Sequence

Radiographic film processing involves a number of steps, and these are summarized in Table 14-1.

All radiographic processing is automatic today; therefore, the following discussion does not cover manual processing. The chemicals involved in both are basically the same. In automatic processing the times for each step are shorter and the chemical concentrations and temperature are higher.

The first step in the processing sequence is wetting the film in order to swell the emulsion so that subsequent chemical baths can reach all parts of the emulsion uniformly. This step is often omitted, in which case the wetting agent is incorporated into the second step, developing.

 Developing is the stage of processing during which the latent image is converted to a visible image.

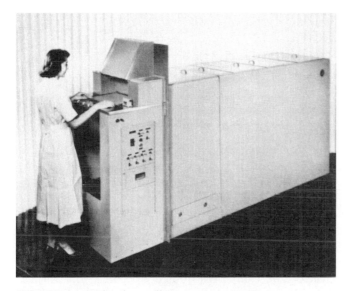

FIGURE 14-2 The first roller transport automatic processor, circa 1956. (Courtesy Eastman Kodak Company.)

The developing stage is very short and highly critical. After developing, the film is rinsed in an acid solution designed to stop the developing process and remove excess developer chemicals from the emulsion. Photographers call this step the **stop bath.** In radiographic processing, the stop bath is included in the next step, fixing.

 Fixing the silver halide that was not exposed to radiation is the process of clearing it from the emulsion and hardening the emulsion to preserve the image.

The gelatin portion of the emulsion is **hardened** at the same time to increase its structural soundness. Fixing is followed by a vigorous **washing** of the film to remove any remaining chemicals from the previous processing steps.

Finally, the film is **dried** to remove the water used to wash it and to make the film acceptable for handling and viewing.

Developing, fixing, and washing are important steps in the processing of radiographic film. The precise chemical reactions involved in these steps are not completely understood. However, a review of the general action is in order because of the importance of **processing** in a high-quality radiograph.

PROCESSING CHEMISTRY
Wetting

A **solvent** is a liquid into which various solids and powders can be dissolved. The **universal solvent** is water, which is the solvent for all the chemicals used in processing a radiograph.

For these chemicals to penetrate the emulsion, the radiograph must first be treated by a **wetting agent.** The wetting agent is water, and it penetrates the gelatin of the emulsion, causing it to swell. In automatic processing the wetting agent is in the developer.

TABLE 14-1	Sequence of Events in Processing a Radiograph			
			APPROXIMATE TIME	
Event	**Purpose**		**Manual**	**Automatic**
Wetting	Swells the emulsion to permit subsequent chemical penetration		15 s	—
Developing	Produces a visible image from the latent image		5 min	22 s
Stop bath	Terminates development and removes excess chemical from emulsion		30 s	—
Fixing	Removes remaining silver halide from emulsion and hardens gelatin		15 min	22 s
Washing	Removes excess chemicals		20 min	20 s
Drying	Removes water and prepares radiograph for viewing		30 min	26 s

Developing

The principal action of developing is to change the silver ions of the exposed crystals into metallic silver. The **developer** is the chemical that performs this task. The developer provides electrons to the sensitivity center of the crystal to change the silver ions to silver.

In addition to the solvent, the developer contains a number of other ingredients. The composition of the developer and the function of each ingredient are outlined in Table 14-2.

For the ionic silver to be changed to metallic silver, an electron must be supplied to the silver ion. Chemically, the reaction is described as follows:

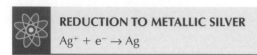

REDUCTION TO METALLIC SILVER

$$Ag^+ + e^- \rightarrow Ag$$

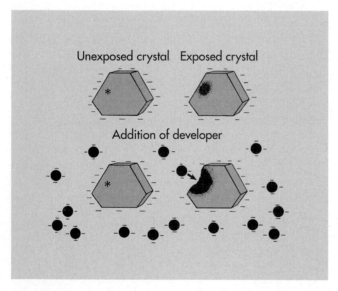

Unexposed crystal   Exposed crystal

Addition of developer

FIGURE 14-3 Development is the chemical process that amplifies the latent image. Only crystals that contain a latent image are reduced to metallic silver by the addition of developer.

When an electron is given up by a chemical, in this case the **developing agent**, to neutralize a positive ion, the process is called **reduction**. The silver ion is said to be **reduced** to metallic silver, and the chemical responsible for this is called a **reducing agent**.

The opposite of reduction is **oxidation**, a reaction that produces an electron. Oxidation and reduction occur simultaneously and are called **redox** reactions. To help recall the proper association, think of **EUR/OPE**: electrons are **u**sed in **r**eduction/**o**xidation **p**roduces **e**lectrons.

Film developers closely guard their precise chemical compositions as proprietary secrets. The principal component, however, is **hydroquinone**. Secondary constituents of the developing agent are **phenidone** and **metol**.

Usually, hydroquinone and phenidone are combined for rapid processing. As reducing agents, each of these molecules has an abundance of electrons that can be easily released to reduce silver ions. Chapter 19 discusses certain aspects of film sensitometry.

The optical density of a processed radiograph results from the development of crystals containing a latent image (Figure 14-3).

 Synergism occurs when the action of two agents working together is greater than the sum of the action of each agent working independently.

The characteristic curve of a radiograph is shaped by the synergistic action of developing agents. Hydroquinone acts rather slowly but is responsible for the very blackest shades. Phenidone acts rapidly and influences the lighter shades of gray. Phenidone controls the toe of the characteristic curve, and hydroquinone controls the shoulder (Figure 14-4).

An unexposed silver halide crystal has a negative electrostatic charge distributed over its entire surface. An exposed silver halide crystal, on the other hand, has a negative electrostatic charge distributed over its surface except at the sensitivity center. The similar electro-

TABLE 14-2	Components of the Developer and Their Function	
Component	**Chemical**	**Function**
Developing agent	Phenidone	Reducing agent; produces shades of gray rapidly
	Hydroquinone	Reducing agent; produces black tones slowly
Buffering agent	Sodium carbonate	Helps swell gelatin; produces alkalinity; controls pH
Restrainer	Potassium bromide	Antifog agent; protects unexposed crystals from chemical "attack"
Preservative	Sodium sulfite	Controls oxidation; maintains balance among developer components
Hardener	Glutaraldehyde	Controls emulsion swelling and increases archival quality
Sequestering agent	Chelates	Removes metallic impurities; stabilize developing agent
Solvent	Water	Dissolves chemicals for use

static charges on the developing agent and the silver halide crystal make it difficult for the developing agent to penetrate the crystal surface except in the region of the sensitivity center in an **exposed crystal.**

In such an exposed crystal, the developing agent penetrates the crystal through the sensitivity center and reduces the remaining silver ions to atomic silver. The sensitivity center can be considered a metallic conducting electrode through which electrons are transferred from the developing agent into the crystal. Development of exposed and unexposed crystals results in the kind of differences illustrated in Figure 14-5.

Development occurs over time and depends on factors such as crystal size, developer concentration, and temperature. Initially, metallic silver slowly builds up at the site of the sensitivity center. After complete development, exposed crystals are destroyed and a grain of black metallic silver is all that remains. Unexposed crystals remain unaffected.

The reduction of a silver ion is accompanied by the liberation of a bromide ion. The bromide ion migrates through the remnant of the crystal into the gelatin portion of the emulsion. From there the ion is dissolved into the developer and removed from the film.

The developer contains alkali compounds, such as **sodium carbonate** and **sodium hydroxide.** These **buffering agents** enhance the action of the developing agent by controlling the concentration of hydrogen ions: the pH.

These alkali compounds are caustic; that is, they are very corrosive and can cause a skin burn. Sodium hydroxide is the strongest alkali and is commonly called **lye.** Be very cautious if you mix a developer so

lution containing sodium hydroxide. You should wear rubber gloves and, of course, never let it get near your mouth or eyes.

Potassium bromide and **potassium iodide** are added to the developer as **restrainers.** Restrainers restrict the action of the developing agent to only those silver halide crystals that have been irradiated. Without the restrainer, even those crystals that had not been exposed would be reduced to metallic silver. This results in an increased fog that is called **development fog.**

A **preservative** is also included in the developer to control the oxidation of the developing agent by air. Air is introduced into the chemistry when it is mixed, handled, and stored; such oxidation is called **aerial oxidation.** By controlling aerial oxidation, the preservative helps maintain the proper development rate.

Mixed chemicals last only a couple of weeks; thus, replenishment tanks require close-fitting floating lids for the control of aerial oxidation. Hydroquinone is particularly sensitive to aerial oxidation. It is easy to tell when the developing agent has been oxidized because it turns brownish. The addition of a preservative causes the developer to remain clear. **Sodium sulfite** is the usual preservative.

Developers used in automatic processors contain a **hardener,** usually glutaraldehyde. If the emulsion swells too much or becomes too soft, the film will not be transported properly through the system because of the very close tolerances of the transport system.

The hardener controls the swelling and softening of the emulsion. When films that drop from the processor and are damp, the usual cause is depletion of the hardener.

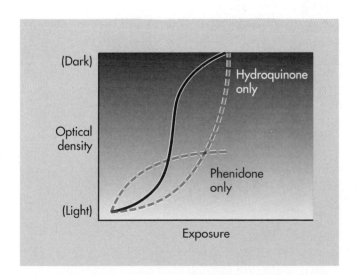

FIGURE 14-4 The shape of the characteristic curve is controlled by the developing agents. Phenidone controls the toe, and hydroquinone controls the shoulder.

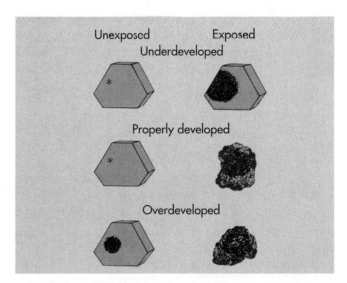

FIGURE 14-5 Underdevelopment results in a dull radiograph because the crystals that contain a latent image have not been completely reduced. Overdevelopment produces a similar radiograph because of the partial reduction of unexposed crystals. Proper development results in maximum contrast.

TABLE 14-3	Components of the Fixer and Their Function	
Component	**Chemical**	**Function**
Activator	Acetic acid	Neutralizes the developer and stops its action
Fixing agent	Ammonium thiosulfate	Removes undeveloped silver bromine from emulsion
Hardener	Potassium alum	Stiffens and shrinks emulsion
Preservative	Sodium sulfite	Maintains chemical balance
Buffer	Acetate	Maintains proper pH
Sequestering agent	Boric acids/salts	Removes aluminum ions
Solvent	Water	Dissolves other components

 Lack of sufficient glutaraldehyde may be the biggest cause of problems with automatic processing.

The developer may contain metal impurities and soluble salts. Such impurities can accelerate the oxidation of hydroquinone, rendering the developer unstable. **Chelates** are introduced as **sequestering agents** to form stable complexes with these metallic ions and salts.

With proper development, all exposed crystals containing a latent image are reduced to metallic silver and unexposed crystals are unaffected. The development process, however, is not perfect: some crystals containing a latent image remain undeveloped (unreduced), while other crystals that are unexposed may be developed. Both of these actions reduce the quality of the radiograph.

Film development is basically a chemical reaction. Like all chemical reactions, it is governed by three physical characteristics: time, temperature, and concentration (of the developer). Long development time increases reduction of the silver in each grain and increases development of the total number of grains. High developer temperature has the same effect.

Similarly, silver reduction is controlled by the concentration of the developing chemicals. With increased developer concentration, the reducing agent becomes more powerful and can more readily penetrate both exposed and unexposed silver halide crystals.

Manufacturers of x-ray film and developing chemicals have very carefully determined the optimal conditions of time, temperature, and concentration for proper development. Optimal conditions of contrast, speed, and fog (see Chapter 19, Figure 19-18) can be expected if the manufacturer's recommendations for development are followed.

Deviation from the manufacturer's recommendations can result in loss of image quality. Figure 14-5 illustrates three degrees of development for exposed and unexposed crystals. The importance of proper development is obvious.

The image on a fogged film is gray and lacks proper contrast. The causes of fog are many, but perhaps the most important are those just mentioned: time, temperature, and developer concentration. An increase in any of these factors above manufacturer recommendations results in increased development fog.

Fog can also be produced by chemical contamination of the developer, **chemical fog**, by unintentional exposure to radiation, **radiation fog**, and by improper storage at elevated temperature and humidity. Chemical antifoggants, such as indozoles and triazoles, are important ingredients in the developer.

Fixing

Once development is complete, the film must be treated so that the image will not fade but will remain permanently. This stage of processing is **fixing**. The image is said to be fixed on the film, and this produces film of **archival quality.**

 Archival quality refers to the permanence of the radiograph: the image thus does not deteriorate with age but remains in its original state.

When the film is removed from the developer, some developer is trapped in the emulsion and continues its reducing action. If developing is not stopped, development fog results. As discussed earlier, the step in manual processing that follows development is called **stop bath,** and its function is just that—to neutralize the residual developer in the emulsion and stop its action. The chemical used in the stop bath is **acetic acid.**

In automatic processing, a stop bath is not used because the rollers of the transport system squeeze the film clean. Furthermore, the fixer contains acetic acid that behaves as a stop bath. This acetic acid, however, is called an **activator.** An activator neutralizes the pH of the emulsion and stops developer action. Table 14-3 lists the chemical components of the fixer.

The terms **clearing agent, hypo,** and **thiosulfate** are often used interchangeably in reference to the fixing agent. Fixing agents remove unexposed and undeveloped silver halide crystals from the emulsion. Sodium thiosulfate is the agent classically known as *hypo,* but ammonium thiosulfate is the fixing agent used in most fixer chemistries.

Hypo retention is a term used to describe the undesirable retention of the fixer in the emulsion. Excess hypo slowly oxidizes and causes the image to discolor to brown over a long time. Fixing agents retained in the emulsion combine with silver to form silver sulfide, which appears yellow-brown.

 Silver sulfide stain is the most common cause of poor archival quality.

The fixer also contains a chemical called a **hardener.** As the developed and unreduced silver bromide is removed from the emulsion during fixation, the emulsion shrinks. The hardener accelerates this shrinking process and causes the emulsion to become more rigid or hardened.

The purpose of hardeners is to ensure that the film is transported properly through the wash-and-dry section and to ensure rapid and complete drying. The chemicals commonly used as hardeners are **potassium alum, aluminum chloride,** and **chromium alum.** Normally, only one is used in a given formulation.

The fixer also contains a **preservative** that is of the same composition and that serves the same purpose as the preservative in the developer. The preservative is **sodium sulfite,** and it is necessary to maintain the chemical balance because of the carryover of developer and fixer from one tank to another.

The alkalinity/acidity—the pH—of the fixer must remain constant. This is helped by adding a **buffer,** usually acetate, to the fixer.

In the same way that metallic ions are sequestered in the developer, so must they be sequestered in the fixer. Aluminum ions are the principal impurity at this stage. Boric acids and boric salts are used for sequestering.

Finally, the fixer contains water as the solvent. Other chemicals might be applicable as a solvent but they would be thicker and more likely to gum up the transport mechanism of the automatic processor.

Washing

The next stage in processing is to wash away any residual chemicals remaining in the emulsion, particularly hypo clinging to the surface of the film. Water is used as the wash agent. In automatic processing, **the temperature of the wash water should be maintained at approximately 3° C (5° F) below the developer temperature.**

In this way, the wash bath also serves to stabilize developer temperature. Inadequate washing leads to ex-

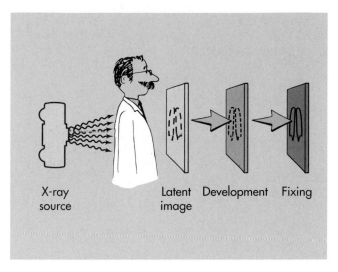

FIGURE 14-6 Converting the latent image to a visible image is a three-step process.

cess hypo retention and the production of an image that will fade, turn brown with time, and be of generally poor archival quality.

Drying

For the final step in processing, drying the radiograph, warm dry air is blown over both surfaces of the film as it is transported through the drying chamber.

The total sequence of events involved in manual processing requires over 1 hr. Most automatic processors are 90 s processors and require a total time from start to finish—the **dry-to-drop time**—of just that, 90 s.

The process of converting the latent image to a visible image can be summarized as a three-step process in the emulsion (Figure 14-6). First, the latent image is formed by exposure of silver halide grains. Next, the exposed grains and only the exposed grains are made visible by development. Finally, fixing removes the unexposed grains from the emulsion and makes the image permanent.

AUTOMATIC PROCESSING

With the introduction of roller transport automatic processing in 1956, the efficiency of radiology services increased considerably. Additionally, automatic processing has resulted in better image quality because each radiograph is processed exactly the same way. The opportunity for human variation and error is nearly absent.

The principal components of an automatic processor are the transport system, the temperature-control system, the circulation system, the replenishment system, the dryer system, and the electrical system (Table 14-4). Figure 14-7 is a cutaway view of an automatic processor.

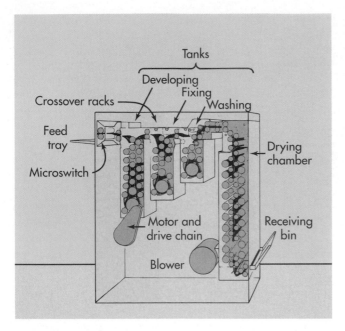

FIGURE 14-7 A cutaway view of an automatic processor. Major components are identified.

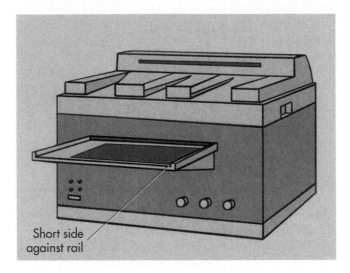

FIGURE 14-8 Place the short side of the film against the guide rail.

TABLE 14-4	Principal Components of an Automatic Processor	
System	**Subsystem**	**Purpose**
Transport		Transport film through various stages at precise intervals
	Roller	Support film movement
	Transport rack	Move and change direction of film via rollers and guide shoes
	Drive	Provide power to turn rollers at a precise rate
Temperature		Monitor and adjust temperature of each stage
Circulation		Agitate fluids
	Developer	Continuously mix, filter
	Fixer	Continuously mix
	Wash	Single pass water flowing at constant rate
Replenishment	Developer	Meter and replace
	Fixer	Meter and replace
Dryer		Remove moisture, vent exhaust
Electrical		Distribute fused power to above systems

Transport System

The transport system begins at the **feed tray,** where the film to be processed is inserted into the automatic processor in the darkroom. There, **entrance rollers** grip the film to begin its trip through the processor. A **microswitch** is engaged to control the replenishment rate of the processing chemicals.

Always feed the film evenly, using the side rails of the feed tray, and alternate sides from film to film (Figure 14-8). This ensures even wear of the transport system components. From the entrance rollers, the film is transported by rollers and racks through the wet chemistry tanks and drying chamber, finally being deposited in the receiving bin.

 The shorter dimension of the film should always be against the side rail in order to maintain the proper replenishment rate.

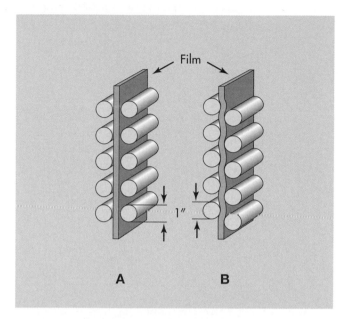

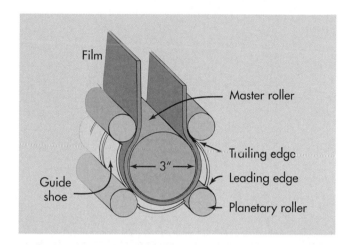

FIGURE 14-9 **A,** Transport rollers positioned opposite each other. **B,** Transport rollers positioned offset from one another.

FIGURE 14-10 A master roller with planetary rollers and guide shoes is used to reverse the direction of film in a processor.

The transport system not only transports the film but also controls processing by controlling the time the film is immersed in each wet chemical. Timing for each step in processing is governed by careful control of the rate of film movement through each stage. The transport system consists of the following three principal subsystems: **rollers, transport racks,** and **drive motor.**

Roller Subassembly. Three types of rollers are used in the transport system. **Transport rollers,** with a diameter of 1 in, convey the film along its path. They either are positioned opposite one another in pairs or are offset from one another (Figure 14-9).

A **master roller** (or solar roller), with a diameter of 3 in, is used when the film makes turns in the processor (Figure 14-10). A number of **planetary rollers** and metal or plastic guide shoes are usually positioned around the master roller.

Transport Rack Subassembly. Except for the entering rollers at the feed tray, most of the rollers in the transport system are positioned on a rack assembly (Figure 14-11). These racks are easily removable and provide for convenient maintenance and efficient cleaning of the processor.

When the film is transported in one direction along the rack assembly, only the 1 in rollers are required to guide and propel it. At each bend, however, a curved metal lip with smooth grooves guides the film around the bend. These are called **guide shoes.** For a 180-degree bend, the film is positioned for the turn by the leading guide shoe, is propelled around the curve by the master roller and its planetary rollers, and leaves the curve by

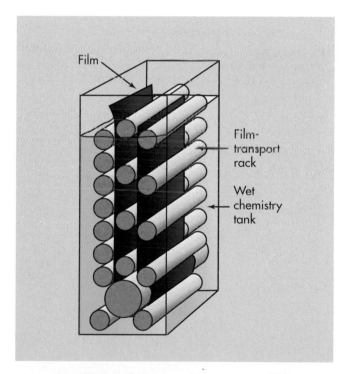

FIGURE 14-11 A transport rack subassembly.

entering the next straight run of rollers through the trailing guide shoe.

Such a system of a master roller, planetary rollers, and guide shoes is called a **turnaround assembly.** The turnaround assembly is located at the bottom of the transport rack assembly. For each chemistry cycle, a transport rack assembly is positioned in the tank.

When the film exits the top of the rack assembly, it is guided to the adjacent rack assembly through a **crossover rack.** The crossover rack is a smaller rack assembly composed of rollers and guide shoes.

Drive Subsystem. Power for the transport system is provided by a fractional horsepower drive motor. The shaft of the drive motor is usually reduced to 10 to 20 rpm through a gear reduction assembly. A chain, pulley, or gear assembly transfers power to the transport rack and drives the rollers. Figure 14-12 illustrates the three principal mechanical devices: a belt and pulley, a chain and sprocket, and gears. These devices connect the mechanical energy of the drive motor to the drive motor mechanism of the rack assembly.

 Film transport time should not vary by more than ± 2% of the time specified by the manufacturer.

The speed of the transport system is controlled by both the speed of the motor and the gear reduction system used. The tolerance on this mechanical assembly is rigid.

Temperature Control System

The developer, fixer, and wash require precise temperature control. The developer temperature is most critical and it is usually maintained at 35° C (95° F). Wash water is maintained at 3° C (5° F) lower. Temperature is monitored at each stage by a thermocouple or thermistor and controlled thermostatically by a controlled heating element in each tank.

Circulation System

Anyone who has manually processed a radiograph knows how important it is to agitate the film during processing. Agitation is necessary to continually mix the

processing chemicals, to maintain a constant temperature throughout the processing tank, and to aid exposure of the emulsion to the chemicals. In automatic processing, a circulation system continuously pumps the developer and fixer, maintaining constant agitation in each tank.

The developer circulation system requires a filter that traps particles as small as approximately 100 μm to trap flecks of gelatin that are dislodged from the emulsion. The particles thus have less chance of becoming attached to the rollers, where they can produce artifacts. These filters are not 100% efficient, and therefore sludge can build up on the rollers.

 Cleaning the tanks and the transport system should be a part of the routine maintenance of any processor.

Filtration in the fixer circulation system is normally unnecessary because the fixer hardens and shrinks the gelatin so that the rollers are not coated. Furthermore, the fixer neutralizes the developer, and therefore the products of this reaction do not affect the final radiograph.

Water must be circulated through the wash tank to remove all of the processing chemicals from the surface of the film before drying; this ensures archival quality. An open system, rather than a closed circulation system, is usually used. Fresh tap water is piped into the tank at the bottom and overflows out the top, where it is collected and discharged directly to the sewer system. The minimum flow rate for the wash tank in most processors is 12 l/min (3 gal/min).

Replenishment System

Each time a film makes its way through the processor, it uses some of the processing chemicals. Some developer is absorbed into the emulsion and then is neutralized during fixing. The fixer, likewise, is absorbed during that stage of processing and some is carried over into the wash tank.

If neither the developer nor the fixer is replenished, each quickly loses chemical balance and the level of solution in each tank drops, resulting in short contact times of the film with the chemicals.

The replenishment system meters the proper amount of chemicals into each tank to maintain volume and chemical activity. Although the replenishment of the developer is more important, the fixer also has to be replenished. Wash water is not recirculated and therefore is continuously and completely replenished.

When a film is inserted into the feed tray with its widest dimension gripped by the leading rollers and its narrow side against the guide fence, a microswitch

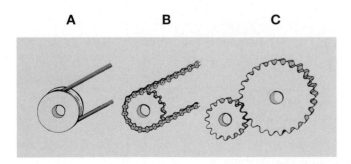

A   B   C

FIGURE 14-12 The three means of transferring power to the transport rack. **A,** Belt and pulley. **B,** Chain and sprocket. **C,** Gears.

is activated and turns on the replenishment for as long as film travels through the microswitch. Replenishment rates are approximately 60 to 70 ml of developer and 100 to 110 ml of fixer for every 14 in of film.

Exact film response to over- or underreplenishment depends on many emulsion variables, making it difficult to make accurate statements. Usually, if the replenishment rate is increased, radiographic contrast is slightly increased. If the rate is too low, contrast decreases significantly.

Dryer System

A wet or damp finished radiograph easily picks up dust particles that can result in artifacts. Furthermore, a wet or damp film is difficult to handle in a viewbox. When stored, it can become sticky and be destroyed.

The dryer system consists of a blower, ventilation ducts, drying tubes, and an exhaust system. The dryer system extracts all residual moisture from the processed radiograph so that it drops into the receiving bin dry.

The blower is a fan that sucks in room air and blows it across heating coils through ductwork to the drying tubes. Therefore, the room air should be low in humidity and free of dust. Sometimes as many as three heating coils of approximately 2500 W capacity are used. The temperature of the air entering the drying chamber is thermostatically regulated.

Most processing faults leading to damp film are due to a depletion of glutaraldehyde, the hardener in the developer.

The drying tubes are long hollow cylinders with slitlike openings extending the length of the cylinder and facing the film. They are positioned on both sides of the film as it is transported through the drying chamber.

The hot moist air is vented from the drying chamber to the outside, much like the air in a clothes dryer. Some fraction of the exhaust air may be recirculated in the dryer system.

A finished radiograph that is damp easily picks up dust particles that could result in artifacts.

When damp films drop into the receiving bin, the radiologic technologist should immediately suspect a malfunction of the dryer system, although developer and fixer replenishment should also be checked. Vendor replenishment reduces the concentration of the hardener and is a common cause of damp films.

Electrical System

The thermal and mechanical components of each of these systems require electrical power. This is done, of course, through proper wiring of the automatic processor. Normally, each major electrical component is fused. The fuse box is the only part of the electrical system of importance to the radiologic technologist.

ALTERNATIVE PROCESSING METHODS

We tend to think that most of the recent advances in medical x-ray imaging are associated with the imaging devices. This is certainly true. We forget, however, the excellent developments made by the radiographic film manufacturers that have improved image quality and the efficiency of radiology departments.

Rapid processing and extended processing are attractive alternatives in many imaging facilities. Daylight processing is fast becoming standard in medical imaging.

Rapid Processing

No matter what the task, today we want to do it faster. Medical imaging is no exception. The manufacturers of radiographic film have developed microprocessor-controlled equipment and specially formulated processing chemicals for this task. Processing can now be as rapid as 30 s.

These rapid processors are useful in angiography, special procedures, surgery, and emergency rooms, where time is most critical. Here, it is important to make radiographic images available for physicians as soon as possible. When used with proper chemistry, rapid processing produces images with sensitometric properties similar to those of 90 s processing.

For rapid processing, the chemicals are more concentrated and developer and fixer temperatures are higher. Consequently, it is not possible to switch from standard to rapid processing between films.

Extended Processing

Extended processing is particularly useful in mammography. Whereas the standard processing time is 90 s, extended processing may take as long as 3 min. Developer immersion time is nearly doubled, but it is not necessary to alter developer temperature. Furthermore, standard chemicals may be used. The only significant disadvantage is the longer dry-to-drop time.

There are two principal advantages with extended processing: greater image contrast and lower patient dose. Contrast is increased by approximately 15%. Image receptor sensitivity is increased by at least 30%. Thus, patient radiation dose is reduced by at least 30%.

Extended processing's improvements in contrast and patient dose occur only with single-emulsion film. Extended processing is not recommended for double-emulsion films because the improvement in contrast or dose is insignificant with such films.

Daylight Processing

Aside from the speed with which images are developed, another change is quietly taking place in radiology department darkrooms. They are disappearing! Consequently, the position of darkroom technologist is also disappearing.

Daylight systems are being adopted. In a daylight system (Figure 14-13), the radiologic technologist needs only position a cassette with an exposed film into the appropriate slot of the daylight system. The film is automatically extracted from the cassette and sent to the processor.

The processor may be an integral part of the daylight system or a separate unit docked to the daylight system. The cassette is reloaded with unexposed film of the proper size before it is released by the system for the next exposure.

Speed is the quality that makes the daylight system attractive. It takes only about 15 s for the radiologic technologist to insert the exposed cassette into the daylight loader and retrieve a fresh cassette. Total load, unload, and processing time is approximately 2 min. Multiple film sizes are automatically accommodated.

Microprocessor technology makes daylight systems possible. The microprocessor monitors and controls the unloading and reloading of the cassette automatically by sensing the cassette size and film consumption rate.

Most daylight systems can accommodate up to 1000 sheets of radiographic film of various sizes. Some units can also annotate the radiograph with data such as the date, time, and other examination characteristics. System status is continuously indicated with light-emitting diodes (LEDs) or liquid crystal displays (LCDs). Some models are on rollers for even greater flexibility.

Dry Processing

Dry processing refers to the development of images without the use of wet chemistry. It continues to rapidly replace the conventional chemical-based film processing. There are many advantages of dry processing driving its replacement of wet chemistry processing:

- Elimination of handling
- Maintenance and disposal of chemicals
- No darkroom required (space saved)
- No plumbing required
- Less environmental impact
- Reduced capital cost
- Reduced operating cost
- Higher throughput.

Although there are several approaches to dry processing, two technologies prevail at this time: photothermography (PTG) and thermography (TG).

The basic difference between the two is in the manner in which the latent image is recorded and the visible image processed onto the film media.

PTG utilizes a low power modulated laser beam to record the image signal on the film, thereby generating the latent image (Figure 14-14). The latent image so formed on the sensitized silver halide emulsion is subsequently developed by a thermal process at 125° C that takes approximately 15 s—the so called **dwell time**.

TG technology, on the other hand, utilizes a modulated heat source, referred to as a "print head" that heats the film and produces the image directly. The print head converts electrical energy into heat using resistive elements. No latent image is created in the TG technology as the organic silver salts are directly developed by the application of localized heat (Figure 14-15).

One of the advantages of PTG is that the laser beam can be modulated in a more accurate fashion in a very short interval (1 µs) compared to heat in the print head of a TG-based system (1 µs). This characteristic is shown in Figure 14-16 and can result in increased image blur in TG systems compared to PTG systems.

Due to the discrete size of the print head and its physical contact with the film media, the TG technique may result in a pixilated image. Furthermore, dust accumulated between the print head and the film media can result in loss of image.

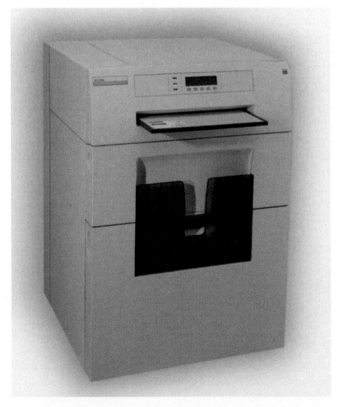

FIGURE 14-13 A daylight processing system. (Courtesy Eastman Kodak.)

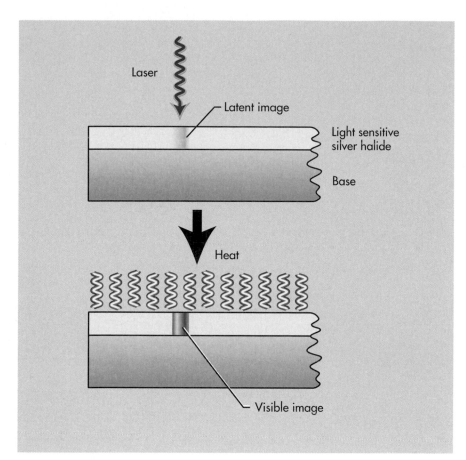

FIGURE 14-14 This photothermic method of dry processing uses a laser to form a latent image and heat to process the image.

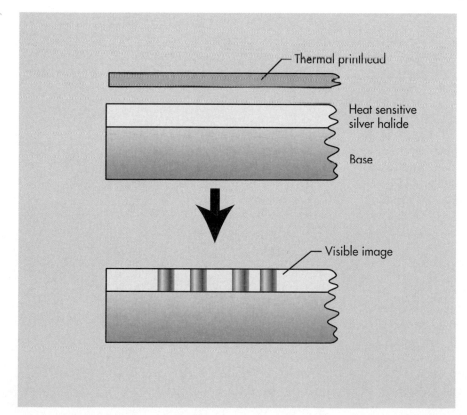

FIGURE 14-15 The thermographic process uses heat to directly produce a visible image.

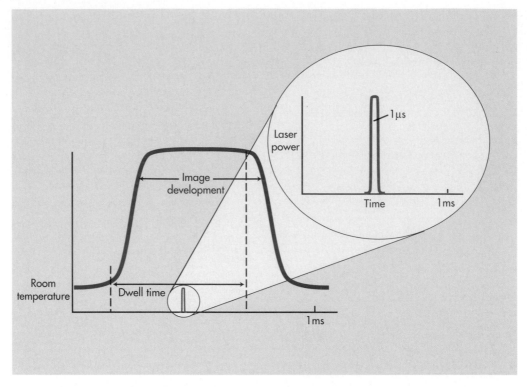

FIGURE 14-16 Photothermography has a much shorter dwell time than thermography.

SUMMARY

Converting the latent image to a visible image is a three-step process. First, the latent image is formed when silver-halide grains are exposed to light or x-rays. Next, only the grains so exposed are made visible by development. Finally, fixing removes the unexposed grains from the emulsion and makes the image permanent.

The 90 s radiographic film processor is the industry standard. The steps for manual and automatic processing are the same but because manual processing takes up to an hour, it is no longer used. The processing sequence consists of (1) wetting, (2) development, (3) stop bath, (4) fixing, (5) washing, and (6) drying. Tables 14-2 and 14-3 list the chemicals and their functions used in developing and fixing processes.

The components of the automatic processor are (1) the transport system, (2) the temperature control system, (3) the circulation system, (4) the replenishment system, (5) the dryer system, and (6) the electrical system. Diagnostic imaging departments may have alternative processing systems as well. Extended processing is used to develop specialty films such as single-emulsion mammography screen-film. Daylight processing allows radiographers to maintain uninterrupted patient care.

The daylight system commonly is used in critical care areas such as the emergency department.

CHALLENGE QUESTIONS

1. Define or otherwise identify:
   a. Solvent
   b. Glutaraldehyde
   c. Reducing agent
   d. Synergism
   e. Archival quality
   f. Planetary roller
   g. Guide shoe
   h. Extended processing
   i. LED
   j. Dry-to-drop
2. Identify the steps involved in the automatic processing of a radiograph and the time of each step for a 90 s processor.
3. Describe the action of phenidone and hydroquinone in producing optical density on a radiograph.
4. By what other name is fixer known?
5. What are characteristic features of daylight processing?

6. During the wash cycle, what restrictions are placed on temperature and flow rate?
7. What is a redox reaction?
8. When did automatic processing begin?
9. Which company invented the first roller transport processing system?
10. What type of processors are used in the clinical sites you visit?
11. What is the universal wetting agent?
12. What is the principal action of development?
13. Give an example of a redox reaction.
14. Name the principal component in developer solutions.
15. Why are gloves and goggles recommended for persons who mix or handle developer solutions?
16. What happens over time if the preservative is not added to the developer?
17. If a film is damp or wet when it drops into the receiving bin, what is the problem and probable cause?
18. Why does the film need to go through the fixer tank?
19. If a radiographic film turns brown once it has been stored in the file room, what may be the problem?
20. How should each x-ray film be fed onto the feed tray of the automatic processor? Why is this important?

Intensifying Screens

OBJECTIVES

At the completion of this chapter, the student should be able to do the following:

1. Describe the component layers of a radiographic intensifying screen
2. Discuss luminescence and its relationship to phosphorescence and fluorescence
3. Define and use the term *intensification factor*
4. Identify how detective quantum efficiency (DQE) and conversion efficiency (CE) affect screen speed
5. Describe image noise and image blur
6. Discuss the various screen-film combinations
7. Describe the handling and cleaning of radiographic intensifying screens

OUTLINE

RADIOGRAPHIC INTENSIFYING screens are part of the conventional image receptor. The image receptor (IR) includes the cassette (which is the protective holder), the radiographic intensifying screens, and the radiographic film.

Although some x-rays reach the film emulsion, it is actually visible light from the radiographic intensifying screens that exposes the radiographic film. Visible light is emitted from the phosphor of the radiographic intensifying screens, which is activated by the image-forming x-rays exiting the patient.

This chapter discusses the components of a radiographic intensifying screens, how these components contribute to a screen's performance characteristics, the properties of rare earth screens, and the importance of spectral matching.

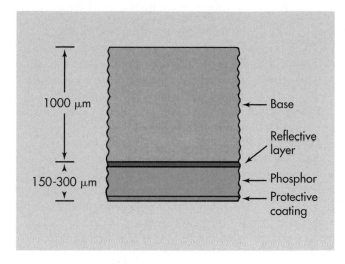

FIGURE 15-1 Cross-sectional view of an intensifying screen, showing its four principal layers.

SCREEN CONSTRUCTION

Using film to detect x-rays and image anatomic structures is inefficient. In fact, less than 1% of the x-rays incident on radiographic film interact with the film and contribute to the latent image.

Most radiographs are made with the film in contact with a radiographic intensifying screen because the use of film alone requires a high patient dose. A radiographic intensifying screen is a device that converts the energy of the x-ray beam into visible light. This visible light then interacts with the radiographic film, forming the latent image.

Approximately 30% of the x-rays striking a radiographic intensifying screen interact with the screen. For each such interaction, a large number of visible light photons are emitted.

 The radiographic intensifying screen amplifies the image-forming x-rays that reach the screen-film cassette.

On the one hand, using a radiographic intensifying screen lowers patient dose considerably; on the other hand, the image is slightly blurred. With modern screens, however, such image blur is not serious.

Radiographic intensifying screens resemble flexible sheets of plastic or cardboard. They come in sizes corresponding to film sizes.

Usually the radiographic film is sandwiched between two screens. The film used is called **double-emulsion film** because it has an emulsion coating on both sides of the base. Most screens have four distinct layers, shown in cross-section in Figure 15-1.

Protective Coating

The layer of the radiographic intensifying screen closest to the radiographic film is the **protective coating**. It is 10 to 20 μm thick and is applied to the face of the screen to make the screen resistant to the abrasion and damage caused by handling. This layer also helps eliminate the buildup of static electricity and provides a surface for routine cleaning without disturbing the active phosphor. The protective layer is transparent to light.

Phosphor

The active layer of the radiographic intensifying screen is the **phosphor**. The phosphor emits light during stimulation by x-rays. Phosphor layers vary in thickness from 50 to 300 μm, depending on the type of screen. The active substance of most phosphors before about 1980 was crystalline **calcium tungstate** embedded in a polymer matrix. The **rare earth** elements gadolinium, lanthanum, and yttrium are the phosphor material in newer, faster screens.

 The phosphor converts the x-ray beam into light.

The action of the phosphor can be demonstrated by viewing an opened cassette in a darkened room through the protective barrier of the control booth. The radiographic intensifying screen glows brightly when exposed to x-rays. Many materials react in this way, but radiography requires that materials possess the characteristics given in Box 15-1. Through the years, several materials have been used as phosphors because they exhibit these characteristics. These materials are **calcium tungstate, zinc sulfide, barium lead sulfate,** and the rare earths **gadolinium, lanthanum,** and **yttrium.**

Roentgen discovered x-rays quite by accident. He observed the luminescence of **barium platinocyanide,** a phosphor that was never successfully applied to diagnostic radiology. Within a year of Roentgen's discovery of x-rays, the American inventor Thomas A. Edison developed calcium tungstate. Although Edison demonstrated the use of radiographic intensifying screens before the beginning of the twentieth century, screen-film combinations did not come into general use until about the time of World War I. The phosphor used at that time was calcium tungstate.

For a time, barium lead sulfate screens were used, particularly with techniques involving high kVp. Zinc sulfide was once used for low kVp techniques but never gained wide acceptance. With improved manufacturing techniques and quality-control procedures, calcium tungstate proved superior for nearly all radiographic techniques and, until the 1970s, was used almost exclusively as the phosphor.

Since then, rare earth screens have been used in diagnostic radiology. These screens are faster than those made of calcium tungstate, rendering these screens more useful for most types of radiographic imaging. Use of rare earth screens results in lower patient dose, less thermal stress on the x-ray tube, and reduced shielding for x-ray rooms.

Differences in screen imaging characteristics are basically due to differences in phosphor composition. The thickness of the phosphor layer and the concentration and size of the phosphor crystals also influence the action of intensifying screens. The thickness of the phosphor layer is approximately 50 to 250 μm; individual phosphor crystals are 5 to 15 μm thick.

Reflective Layer

Between the phosphor and the base is a reflective layer, approximately 25 μm thick, made of a shiny substance such as magnesium oxide or titanium dioxide (Figure 15-2). When x-rays interact with the phosphor, light is emitted isotropically.

Less than half of this light is emitted in the direction of the film. The reflective layer intercepts light headed in other directions and redirects it to the film. The reflective layer increases the efficiency of the radiographic intensifying screen, nearly doubling the number of light photons reaching the film.

 Isotropic emission means radiation with equal intensity in all directions.

Some radiographic intensifying screens incorporate special dyes in the phosphor layer to selectively absorb those light photons emitted at a large angle to the film. These light photons increase image blur. Because they must travel a longer distance in the phosphor than those emitted perpendicular to the film, these photons are more easily absorbed by the dye. Unfortunately, this addition reduces screen speed somewhat.

BOX 15-1 **Favorable Properties of a Radiographic Intensifying Screen Phosphor**

The phosphor should have a **high atomic number** so that x-ray absorption is high. This is called **detective quantum efficiency (DQE).**

The phosphor should emit a large amount of light per x-ray absorption. This is called the x-ray **conversion efficiency (CE).**

The light emitted must be of proper wavelength (color) to match the sensitivity of the x-ray film. This is called **spectral matching.**

Phosphor **afterglow,** the continuing emission of light after exposure of the phosphor to x-rays should be minimal.

The phosphor should not be affected by heat, humidity, or other environmental conditions.

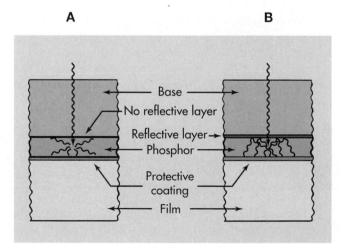

FIGURE 15-2 A, Screen without reflective layer. **B,** Screen with reflective layer. Screens without reflective layers are not as efficient as those with reflective layers because fewer light photons reach the film.

Base

The layer farthest from the film is the **base.** The base is approximately 1 mm thick and serves principally as a mechanical support for the active phosphor layer. Polyester is the popular base material in radiographic intensifying screens, just as it is for radiographic film. Box 15-2 presents the requirements for a base material of high quality.

LUMINESCENCE

Any material that emits light in response to some outside stimulation is called a **luminescent material,** or a **phosphor,** and the emitted visible light is called **luminescence.** A number of stimuli cause luminescence in materials; these stimuli include electric current (the fluorescent light), biochemical reactions (the lightning bug), visible light (a watch dial), and x-rays (a radiographic intensifying screen).

Luminescence is similar to characteristic x-ray emission. However, luminescence involves **outer-shell elec-**trons (Figure 15-3). In a radiographic intensifying screen, absorption of a single x-ray causes emission of thousands of light photons.

When a luminescent material is stimulated, the outer-shell electrons are raised to excited energy levels. This effectively creates a hole in the outer electron shell, which is an unstable condition for the atom. The hole is filled when the excited electron returns to its normal state. This transition is accompanied by electromagnetic energy emitted in the form of a visible light photon.

The range of excited energy states for an outer-shell electron is narrow, and these states depend on the structure of the luminescent material. The wavelength of the emitted light is determined by the level of excitation to which the electron was raised and is characteristic of a given luminescent material. In other words, luminescent materials emit light of a characteristic color.

There are two types of luminescence. If visible light is emitted only while the phosphor is stimulated, the process is called **fluorescence.** If, on the other hand, the phosphor continues to emit light after stimulation, then the process is called **phosphorescence.**

Some materials can phosphoresce for long periods following stimulation. For example, a light-stimulated watch dial will fade slowly in a dark closet. Radiographic intensifying screens fluoresce. Phosphorescence in an intensifying screen is called **screen lag** or **afterglow** and is undesirable.

If the electron returns to its normal state with the emission of light within one revolution following stimulation, then fluorescence has occurred. If more than one revolution is required, then phosphorescence has occurred. The time required for an electron to make one revolution about the nucleus is 10 ns.

BOX 15-2	**Favorable Properties of Radiographic Intensifying Screen Base**

Rugged and moisture-resistant
Resistant to radiation damage and discoloration with age
Chemically inert and not prone to interact with the phosphor layer
Flexible
Lacking impurities that would be imaged by x-rays

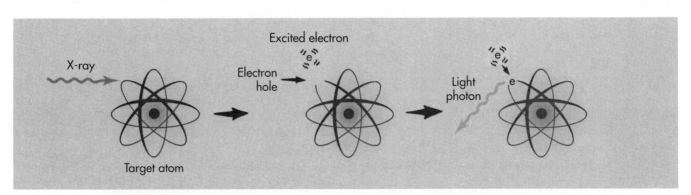

FIGURE 15-3 Luminescence occurs when an outer-shell electron is raised to an excited state and returns to its ground state with the emission of a light photon.

LUMINESCENCE

Fluorescence	Phosphorescence
No lag	Afterglow
$< 10^{-8}$ s	$> 10^{-8}$ s

SCREEN CHARACTERISTICS

The radiologic technologist is concerned with three primary characteristics of radiographic intensifying screens: screen speed, image noise, and spatial resolution.

Because screens are used to reduce patient dose, one characteristic is the magnitude of dose reduction. This property is called the **intensification factor** and is a measure of the **speed** of the screen.

With some exceptions, an increase in screen speed can result in increased **image noise**. Image noise is the speckled appearance on some images and has several sources (see Chapter 19).

Unfortunately, when image-forming x-rays are converted to visible light and the visible light in turn produces the latent image, the image is blurred somewhat. The **spatial resolution** of the screen is its ability to produce an accurate and clear image. Resolution is usually measured by the minimum line spacing that can be detected and imaged. See Chapter 29 for a discussion of spatial resolution measured in the line pair per millimeter (lp/mm).

Screen Speed

There are many types of radiographic intensifying screens, and each manufacturer uses different names to identify them. Collectively, however, screens are usually identified by their relative speed expressed numerically. Screen speeds range from 100 (slow, detail) to 1200 (very fast).

Screen speed is a relative number that describes how efficiently x-rays are converted into usable light. Par-speed calcium tungstate screens are assigned a value of 100 and are the basis for comparison of all other screens. Calcium tungstate screens are seldom used anymore. High-speed rare earth screens have speeds up to 1200; detail screens have speeds of approximately 50 to 80. These and other characteristics are summarized in Table 15-1.

The speed of a radiographic intensifying screen conveys no information concerning patient dose. This information is related by the **intensification factor** (IF). The IF is defined as the ratio of the exposure required to produce the same optical density *with* a screen to the exposure required to produce an optical density *without* a screen:

INTENSIFICATION FACTOR

$$IF = \frac{\text{Exposure required without screen}}{\text{Exposure required with screens}}$$

The optical density chosen for comparing one radiographic intensifying screen with another is usually 1.0. The value of the IF can be used to determine the dose reduction accompanying the use of a screen.

Question: A pelvic examination using a 100 speed radiographic intensifying screen is taken at 75 kVp, 50 mAs and results in an entrance skin exposure (ESE) of 200 mR (2 mGy$_a$). A similar examination taken without screens would result in an ESE of 6400 mR (64 mGy$_a$). What is the approximate IF of the screen-film combination?

Answer: $IF = \dfrac{6400}{200} = 32$

Several factors influence radiographic intensifying screen speed, some of which are controlled by the radiologic technologist. Ultimately, the screen speed is determined by the relative number of x-rays interacting with the phosphor and how efficiently x-ray energy is converted into the visible light that interacts with the film.

TABLE 15-1	Some Characteristics of Typical Radiographic Intensifying Screens	
CHARACTERISTIC	**TYPE OF SCREEN**	
Type of Phosphor	**Calcium Tungstate**	**Oxysulfides and Xybromides of Y, La, Gd**
Color of emission	Blue	Green or blue
Approximate speed	50–200	80–1200
Intensification factor	20–100	40–400
Resolution (lp/mm)	8–15	8–15

Box 15-3 gives the properties of radiographic intensifying screens that affect screen speed and **cannot be controlled by the radiologic technologist.** They are listed in their relative order of importance.

As said earlier, several conditions affect radiographic intensifying screen speed that **are controlled by the radiologic technologist.** They include radiation quality, image processing, and temperature.

Radiation Quality. As x-ray tube potential is increased, the IF increases also (Figure 15-4). Although this may seem contrary to the discussion of x-ray absorption in Chapter 12, it is not.

In Chapter 12, x-ray absorption was shown to decrease with increasing kVp. Remember, however, that the IF is the ratio of x-ray absorption in a radiographic intensifying screen to that in radiographic film alone.

Screens have higher effective atomic numbers than films; therefore, although true absorption in the screen decreases with increasing kVp, the relative absorption compared with that in film increases. At 70 kVp, the IF for a typical par-speed screen is 60, whereas that for a rare earth screen is 150.

Image Processing. Only the superficial layers of the emulsion are affected when radiographic film is exposed to light. However, the emulsion is affected uniformly throughout when the film is exposed to x-rays.

Therefore, excessive developing time for screen-film results in a lowering of the IF because the emulsion nearest the base contains no latent image, yet it can be reduced to silver if the developer is allowed sufficient time to penetrate the emulsion to the depth. This too is relatively unimportant because films manufactured for use with screens have thinner emulsion layers than those produced for direct exposure.

Temperature. Radiographic intensifying screens emit more light per x-ray interaction at low temperatures than at high temperatures. Consequently, the IF is lower at higher temperature. This characteristic, though relatively unimportant in a clinic with a controlled environment, can be significant in field work in hot or cold climates.

Image Noise

Image noise appears on a radiograph as a speckled background. It occurs most often when fast screens and high kVp techniques are used. Noise reduces image contrast. Chapter 19 discusses noise more completely.

Rare earth radiographic intensifying screens have increased speed because of two important characteristics, both of which are higher compared to other types of screens. The percentage of x-rays absorbed by the screen is higher. This is called **detective quantum efficiency (DQE).** The amount of light emitted for each x-ray absorbed is also higher. This is called **conversion efficiency (CE).**

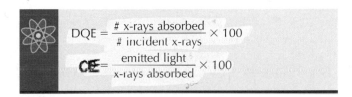

$$DQE = \frac{\text{\# x-rays absorbed}}{\text{\# incident x-rays}} \times 100$$

$$CE = \frac{\text{emitted light}}{\text{x-rays absorbed}} \times 100$$

Figure 15-5 illustrates why an increase in CE increases image noise, whereas an increase in DQE does not. In Figure 15-5, *A* a calcium tungstate screen has a DQE of 20% and a CE of 5%. A radiographic technique of 10 mAs results in 1000 x-rays incident on the screen, 200 of which are absorbed, resulting in light photons equivalent to 10 x-rays. We could say that this system has a speed of 100.

Higher conversion efficiency results in increased noise.

If the phosphor thickness is doubled as in Figure 15-5, *B,* the DQE increases to 40% so the mAs can be reduced to 5 mAs. The speed is now 200 but there is no increase in noise because the same number of x-rays are used.

However, if the phosphor is changed to one with a CE of 10%, the speed is doubled at the expense of increased noise (Figure 15-5, *C*). A 200 speed screen is attained because twice as much light is emitted per x-ray absorption. Only half as many x-rays are required, and this results in increased **quantum mottle,** a principal component of image noise.

BOX 15-3   Properties of Radiographic Intensifying Screens That Are Not Controlled by the Radiologic Technologist

Phosphor composition. Rare earth phosphors efficiently convert x-rays into usable light.

Phosphor thickness. The thicker the phosphor layer, the higher the DQE. High-speed screens have thick phosphor layers; fine-detailed screens have thin phosphor layers.

Reflective layer. The presence of a reflective layer increases screen speed but also increases image blur.

Dye. Light-absorbing dyes are added to some phosphors to control the spread of light. These dyes improve spatial resolution but reduce speed.

Crystal size. Larger individual phosphor crystals produce more light per x-ray interaction. The crystals of detail screens are approximately half the size of the crystals of high-speed screens.

Concentration of phosphor crystals. Higher crystal concentration results in higher screen speed.

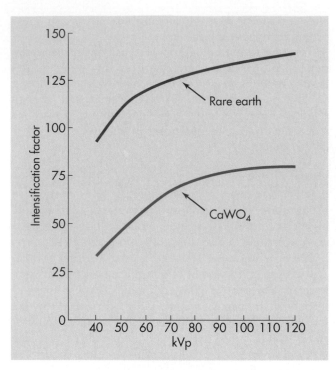

FIGURE 15-4 Graph showing approximate variation of the intensification factor (IF) with kVp.

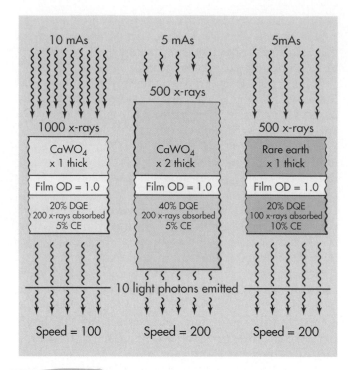

FIGURE 15-5 Image noise increases with higher CE but not with higher DQE.

Thicker emulsion w/ calcium tungstate

Noise is increased because of higher CE, not DQE

Quantum mottle is often a direct result of using very-fast-speed screen-film systems requiring very small amounts of exposure and resulting in a grainy, mottled, or splotchy image.

In practice, rare earth screens of the same spatial resolution are at least twice as fast as calcium tungstate with no significant increase in noise. Rare earth screens have higher DQE and CE, but the gain in speed is principally due to DQE.

Spatial Resolution

Radiographers often use the terms **image detail** or **visibility of detail** when describing image quality. These qualitative terms combine the quantitative measures of spatial resolution and contrast resolution. Spatial resolution refers to how small an object can be imaged. Contrast resolution refers to the ability to image similar tissues, such as liver and pancreas or gray matter and white matter.

Ability to image small objects with high subject contrast

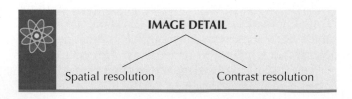

The use of radiographic intensifying screens adds one more step to the process of imaging with x-rays. Radiographic intensifying screens have the disadvantage of lower spatial resolution compared with direct-exposure radiographs.

Spatial resolution is measured in a number of ways and can be given a numerical value. Spatial resolution is limited principally by effective focal spot size. For our purposes, a general description should be sufficient.

A photograph in focus shows good spatial resolution; one out of focus shows poor spatial resolution and therefore much image blur. Figure 15-6 shows the differences in spatial resolution between a direct-exposure film and a par-speed screen-film combination obtained when imaging an x-ray test pattern.

Such a test pattern is called a **line-pair test pattern**. It has lead grid lines separated by interspaces of equal size. As discussed more completely in Chapter 29, spatial resolution may be expressed by the number of line pairs per millimeter (lp/mm) that are imaged. The higher this number, the smaller the object that can be imaged and the better the spatial resolution.

Very fast screens can resolve 7 lp/mm and fine-detail screens can resolve 15 lp/mm (see Table 15-1). Direct-exposure film can resolve 50 lp/mm. The unaided eye can resolve about 10 lp/mm.

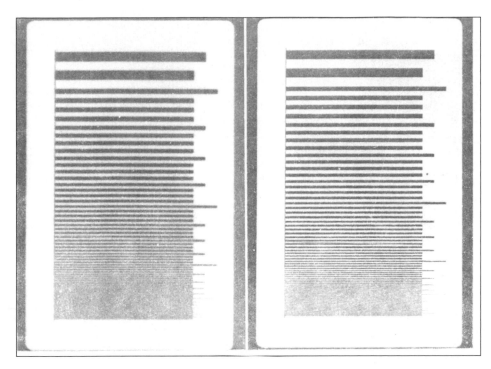

FIGURE 15-6 Radiographs of an x-ray test pattern made with direct-exposure film *(right)* and a par-speed screen-film combination *(left)*. The difference in image blur is obvious.

When x-rays interact with the screen's phosphor, the area of the film emulsion that is activated by the emitted light is larger than it would be with direct x-ray exposure. This results in reduced spatial resolution or more image blur.

 Generally, those conditions that increase the IF reduce spatial resolution.

High-speed screens have low spatial resolution and fine-detail screens have high spatial resolution. Spatial resolution improves with smaller phosphor crystals and thinner phosphor layers. Figure 15-7 shows how these factors affect image resolution. Unfortunately, these factors are not controlled by the radiologic technologist.

 In mammography, the screen is positioned in contact with the emulsion on the side of the film away from the x-ray source to reduce screen blur and improve spatial resolution.

In both parts of Figure 15-7 the x-ray is shown to interact with the phosphor soon after entering; this results in screen blur. Screen blur is reduced in thinner screens. Figure 15-8 illustrates how spatial resolution is improved in mammography by placing the single-emulsion film on the tube side of the cassette (see Chapter 22 for a more complete discussion).

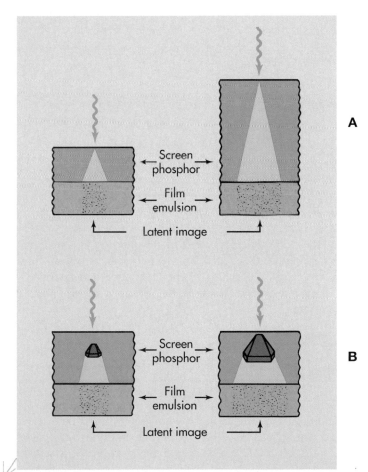

FIGURE 15-7 A, Reduction in spatial resolution is greater when phosphor layers are thick. **B,** Reduction is also greater when crystal size is large. These same conditions increase screen speed by producing more light photons per incident x-ray.

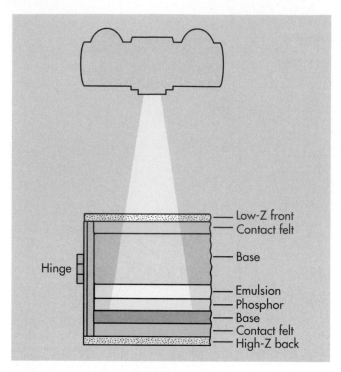

FIGURE 15-8 For mammography, the single screen is on the far side of the emulsion to reduce screen blur.

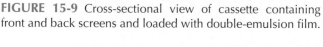

FIGURE 15-9 Cross-sectional view of cassette containing front and back screens and loaded with double-emulsion film.

SCREEN-FILM COMBINATIONS

Screens and films are manufactured for compatibility, which helps ensure good results.

Radiographic intensifying screens are nearly always used in pairs. Figure 15-9 is a cross-section of a properly loaded cassette containing front and back screens with a double-emulsion film. Production of the latent image is nearly evenly divided between front and back screens, with less than 1% being contributed directly by x-ray interaction. Each screen exposes the emulsion it contacts.

 Screen-film compatibility is essential; use only those films for which the screens are designed.

In addition to reduced patient dose, use of radiographic intensifying screens in an image receptor offer several advantages (Box 15-4). Attaining these advantages requires proper selection, handling, and use of a screen-film combination.

Cassette

The **cassette** is the rigid holder that contains the film and radiographic intensifying screens. The front cover,

BOX 15-4   Advantages of Proper Screen-Film Use

INCREASED
Flexibility of kVp selection
Adjustment of radiographic contrast
Spatial resolution when using smaller focal spots
Capacity for magnification radiography

DECREASED
Patient dose
Occupational exposure
X-ray tube heat production
X-ray exposure time
X-ray tube mA
Focal spot size

the side facing the x-ray source, should be made of material with a low atomic number such as plastic. It should be as thin as practicable, yet sturdy. The front cover of the cassette is designed for minimum attenuation of the x-ray beam.

Attached to the inside of the front cover is the front screen, and attached to the back cover is the back screen. The radiographic film is sandwiched between the two screens.

Between each screen and the cassette cover is some sort of **compression device**, such as felt or rubber, which maintains close screen-film contact when the cassette is closed and latched.

The back cover is usually made of heavy metal to minimize backscatter. The x-rays transmitted through the screen-film combination to the back cover more readily undergo photoelectric effect in a high-Z material than in a low-Z material.

X-rays can be transmitted through the entire cassette, and some might be scattered back to the film by the cassette holding device or a nearby wall. This is called **backscatter** radiation and results in image fog.

Sometimes the cassette hinges or hold-down clamps on the back cover are imaged. This is due to backscatter radiation and normally occurs only during high kVp radiography when the x-ray beam is sufficiently penetrating.

Carbon Fiber Material

One of the materials the United States developed early in its space exploration program was **carbon fiber.** This material was developed for nose cone applications because of its superior strength and heat resistance. It consists principally of graphite fibers ($Z_t = 6$) in a plastic matrix that can be formed to any shape or thickness.

In radiology, this material is now used widely in devices designed to reduce patient exposure. A cassette with a front consisting of carbon fiber material only absorbs approximately half the x-rays that an aluminum or plastic cassette does.

Carbon fiber is also being used as pallet material for fluoroscopic examination tables and computed tomography couches.

Carbon fiber not only reduces the patient exposure but may also result in longer x-ray tube life because of the lower-demand radiographic techniques required.

Direct Film Exposure versus Screen-Film Exposure

The principal advantage to the use of radiographic intensifying screens is that fewer x-rays are needed than in direct-exposure techniques. Table 15-2 shows the relative number of x-rays and light photons at various stages for radiographs taken directly and with a par-speed screen-film combination. This table assumes an IF of 50.

The major differences are due to the interaction of x-rays with the screen phosphor and to the large number of visible-light photons produced by each of these interactions. Unfortunately, the number of latent image

TABLE 15-2	Comparison of Relative Number of X-rays and Light Photons at Various Stages for Direct and Screen-Film Exposure*

	TYPE OF EXPOSURE	
Stage	Direct	Screen-Film
Incident x-rays	1000	20
X-rays absorbed by film	10	<1
X-rays absorbed by screens	—	5
Light photons produced	—	5000
Light photons incident on film	—	3000
Light photons absorbed by film	—	1000
Latent images formed	10	10

*Intensification factor = 1000/20 = 50.

centers formed is less than 1% of the number of light photons produced.

From its introduction in 1896 by Thomas Edison until the 1970s, calcium tungstate ($CaWO_4$) was used almost exclusively as the phosphor for radiographic intensifying screens. Such screens, however, exhibit only 5% CE.

One reason that calcium tungstate is a useful screen phosphor is that it emits light in the violet-to-blue region. The sensitivity of conventional radiographic film is highest in the violet-blue region of the spectrum. Consequently, the light emitted by calcium tungstate screens is readily absorbed in radiographic film (Figure 15-10).

If the screen phosphor emitted green or red light, its IF would be greatly reduced because it would require more light photons to produce a latent image. The light of the screen emission would be mismatched to the light sensitivity of the film.

Rare Earth Screens

Newer phosphor materials have become the material of choice for most radiographic applications. Table 15-3 lists these phosphors and the general identification of the screens into which they have been incorporated. Except for barium- and zinc-based phosphors, the other new phosphors are identified as rare earth, and therefore all these screens have come to be known as **rare earth screens.**

The term *rare earth* describes those elements of group IIIa in the periodic table (See Figure 3-3) having atomic numbers of 57 to 71. These elements are transitional metals that are scarce in nature. Those used in rare earth screens are principally **gadolinium, lanthanum,** and **yttrium.** The compositions of the

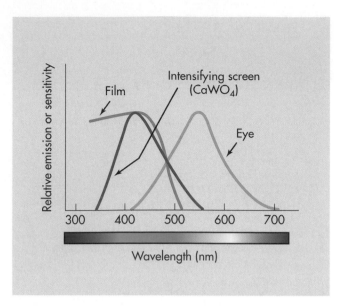

FIGURE 15-10 Importance of spectral matching is demonstrated by showing the relative emission spectrum for a radiographic intensifying screen and the relative sensitivity of radiograph film to the light from that screen.

TABLE 15-3	Composition and Emulsion of Radiographic Intensifying Screens	
Phosphor	**Activator**	**Emission**
Barium fluorochloride	Europium	Ultraviolet
Barium strontium sulfate	Europium	Ultraviolet
Barium sulfate	Lead	Ultraviolet
Zinc sulfide	Silver	Blue-ultraviolet
Calcium tungstate	Lead	Blue
Lanthanum oxybromide	Thulium	Blue
Yttrium oxysulfide	Terbium	Blue
Gadolinium oxysulfide	Terbium	Green
Lanthanum oxysulfide	Terbium	Green
Zinc cadmium sulfide	Silver	Yellow-green

four principal rare earth phosphors are terbium-activated gadolinium oxysulfide (Gd_2O_2S: Tb), terbium-activated lanthanum oxysulfide (La_2O_2S: Tb), terbium-activated yttrium oxysulfide (Y_2O_2S: Tb), and lanthanum oxybromide (LaOBr).

 Rare earth radiographic intensifying screens have the principal advantage of speed.

Rare earth radiographic intensifying screens are manufactured to perform at several speed levels, up to 1200. This increase in speed is obtained without loss of spatial or contrast resolution; however, with the fastest rare earth screens, the effects of **quantum mottle** (image noise) are noticeable and can become bothersome (see Chapter 19).

Because rare earth radiographic intensifying screens are faster, lower radiographic technique can be used and this results in lower patient dose. Rare earth screens provide a general reduction in the radiation environment and, when used exclusively, can influence the design of the radiographic facilities and reduce the need for protective lead shielding. The lower radiographic technique also results in increased x-ray tube life.

Rare earth radiographic intensifying screens obtain their increased sensitivity through higher x-ray absorption (DQE) and more efficient conversion of x-ray energy into light (CE). The light emitted by these screens,

however, differs from that of other screens; therefore, rare earth screens require specially matched film.

Higher X-ray Absorption. When diagnostic x-rays interact with a calcium tungstate screen, approximately 30% of the x-rays are absorbed. The mechanism of absorption is almost entirely the photoelectric effect. Recall that photoelectric absorption occurs readily with the inner electrons of atoms of high atomic number.

The tungstate atom determines the absorption properties of a calcium tungstate screen. Tungsten has an atomic number of 74 and a K-shell electron binding energy of 69 keV. In the diagnostic range, x-ray absorption in tungsten follows the relationship shown in Figure 15-11.

At very low energies photoelectric absorption is very high, but as the x-ray energy increases the probability of absorption decreases rapidly until the x-ray energy is equal to the binding energy of the K-shell electrons. At x-ray energies below the K-shell electron binding energy, the incident x-ray has too little energy to ionize K-shell electrons.

When the x-ray energy equals the K-shell electron binding energy, the two K-shell electrons become available for photoelectric interaction. Consequently, at this energy, the probability of photoelectric absorption increases abruptly.

This abrupt increase in absorption at this energy is called the **K-shell absorption edge,** and it is followed by another rapid reduction in photoelectric absorption with increasing x-ray energy.

The rare earth materials used for radiographic intensifying screens all have atomic numbers less than that for tungsten. Consequently, they each have a lower K-shell electron binding energy. Table 15-4 lists the important physical characteristics of the elements in radiographic intensifying screens.

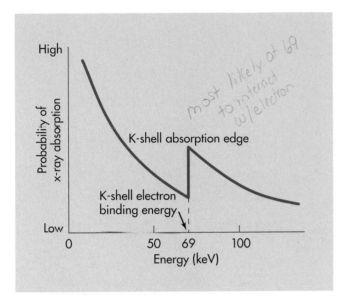

most likely at 69 to interact w/electron

FIGURE 15-11 Probability of x-ray absorption in a calcium tungstate screen as a function of the incident x-ray energy.

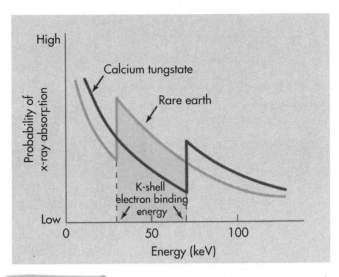

FIGURE 15-12 X-ray absorption probability in a rare earth screen compared with that for a calcium tungstate screen. In the energy interval between respective K-shell electron binding energies, absorption in a rare earth screen is higher.

TABLE 15-4	Atomic Number and K-Shell Electron Binding Energy of High-Z Elements in Radiographic Intensifying Screen Phosphors		
Element	**Chemical Symbol**	**Atomic Number (Z)**	**K-Shell Electron Binding Energy (keV)**
Yttrium	Y	39	17
Barium	Ba	56	37
Lanthanum	La	57	39
Gadolinium	Gd	64	50
Tungsten	W	74	70

Figure 15-12 shows that the probability of x-ray absorption in rare earth screens is lower than that for calcium tungstate screens at all x-ray energies except those between the respective K-shell electron binding energies. Below the K-shell absorption edge for the rare earth elements, x-ray absorption is higher in tungsten. At an x-ray energy equal to the K-shell electron binding energy of the rare earth elements, however, the probability of photoelectric absorption is considerably higher than that for tungsten.

As with tungsten, the absorption probability of the rare earth elements decreases with increasing x-ray energy. At x-ray energies above the K-shell absorption edge for tungsten, the rare earth elements again exhibit lower absorption than that for tungsten.

Each of the rare earth radiographic intensifying screens has an absorption curve characteristic of the phosphor that determines the speed of the screen and how it changes with kVp. Figure 15-13 shows the x-ray absorption in two phosphors relative to calcium tungstate. For instance, barium strontium sulfate has a higher DQE at a lower kVp than is the case with gadolinium oxysulfide.

The result of this complex interaction process is that in the x-ray energy range between the K-shell absorption edge for the rare earth elements and tungsten, a rare earth screen absorbs approximately five times more x-rays than a calcium tungstate screen. Furthermore, for each x-ray absorbed, more light is emitted by the rare earth screens.

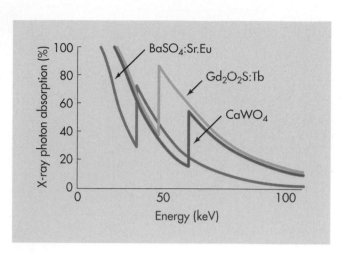

FIGURE 15-13 X-ray absorption for three intensifying screen phosphors.

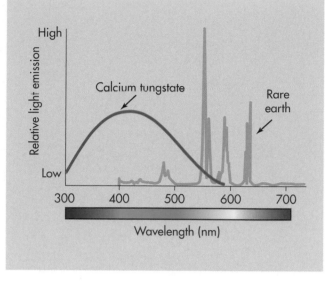

FIGURE 15-14 Calcium tungstate emits a broad spectrum of light centered in the blue region. Rare earth screens have discrete emissions centered near the green-yellow region.

Rare earth radiographic intensifying screens exhibit better absorption properties than calcium tungstate screens only in the energy range between the respective K-shell absorption edges. This energy range extends from approximately 35 to 70 keV and corresponds to most of the useful x-rays emitted during routine x-ray examinations. Outside this energy range, calcium tungstate radiographic intensifying screens absorb more x-rays than rare earth screens.

Higher Conversion Efficiency. An additional property of the rare earth phosphors, the **CE**, contributes to their extraordinary speed. The CE is defined as the ratio of visible light energy emitted to the x-ray energy absorbed.

When an x-ray interacts photoelectrically with a phosphor and is absorbed, its energy reappears as either heat or light through a rearrangement of electrons in the crystal lattice of the phosphor. If all the energy reappeared as heat, the phosphor would be worthless as an intensifying screen. In calcium tungstate, approximately 5% of the absorbed x-ray energy reappears as light. **The CE of rare earth phosphors is approximately 20%.**

 The combination of improved CE and higher DQE results in the increased speed of rare earth radiographic intensifying screens.

Faster Speed. Rare earth radiographic intensifying screens are available in many combinations with different films, resulting in varying relative speeds. Rare earth screen-film combinations have relative speeds from 200 to 1200.

When using rare earth screen-film systems with relative speeds as high as 1200, image quality may be degraded somewhat by increased quantum mottle, but this may be acceptable for some types of examinations in view of the significantly reduced patient dose.

Spectrum Matching. To be fully effective, rare earth radiographic intensifying screens must be used only in conjunction with film emulsions whose light absorption characteristics are matched to the light emission of the screen. This is called **spectrum matching.** Calcium tungstate screens emit light in a rather broad continuous spectrum centered in the violet-to-blue region, with a maximum intensity at approximately 430 nm (Figure 15-14).

The spectral emission of rare earth phosphors is more discrete, as indicated by the many peaks in the spectrum (see Figure 15-14). The spectral emission is centered in the green region of the visible spectrum at approximately 540 mm. Terbium activation is responsible for the shape and intensity of this emission spectrum.

The emission spectrum can be altered somewhat by varying the concentration of terbium atoms in the phosphor, by addition of activators, and by light-absorbing dyes. Phosphors are available that emit ultraviolet, blue, green, and red light.

Conventional x-ray film is sensitive to blue and blue-violet light and rather insensitive to light of longer

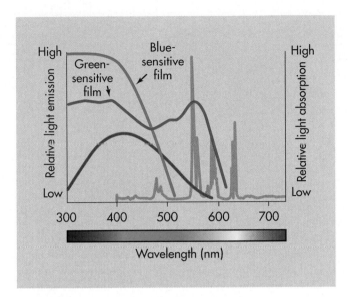

FIGURE 15-15 Blue-sensitive film must be used with blue-emitting screens and green-sensitive film with green-emitting screens.

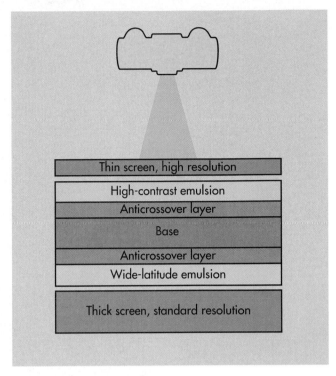

FIGURE 15-16 Asymmetric screens compensate for x-ray absorption in the front screen.

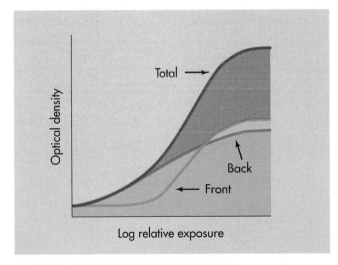

FIGURE 15-17 Characteristic curves from an asymmetric screen emulsion image receptor.

wavelengths. Such blue-sensitive films are used with calcium tungstate screens because their absorption spectrum matches the emission spectrum of calcium tungstate.

Specially designed green-sensitive film must be used with rare earth screens (Figure 15-15). If a green-emitting screen were used with blue-sensitive film, the strong emission in the green region would go undetected and system speed would be sharply reduced. To obtain maximum advantage and speed from rare earth screens, the film must be sensitized for the emission of the screen.

Safelights. Green-sensitive film creates problems in the darkroom. Safelight filters that are satisfactory for regular x-ray film fog film manufactured for use with rare earth screens. Rare earth screen-film requires the use of safelights that are colored even more toward the red portion of the spectrum.

Asymmetric Screen-Film. Consider the double-emulsion screen-film combination depicted in Figure 15-16 If each screen has a DQE of 50%, only 50% of the x-rays are transmitted to the back screen. Therefore, the back screen absorbs only 25% of the x-rays incident on the cassette, resulting in only one half of the exposure of the back emulsion as the front emulsion.

This difference in exposure can be remedied by thickening the back radiographic intensifying screen. Another remedy is to use a different screen, exposing a different emulsion. Such screens and/or emulsions are called **asymmetric** and are used to great advantage in some applications, such as chest, pediatric, and portable radiography.

In chest radiography, for example, the front screen/emulsion is slower and higher in contrast while the back screen/emulsion is faster and lower in contrast (Figure 15-17). The result is a more balanced image of wide latitude and high contrast over both the lung fields and the mediastinum (Figure 15-18).

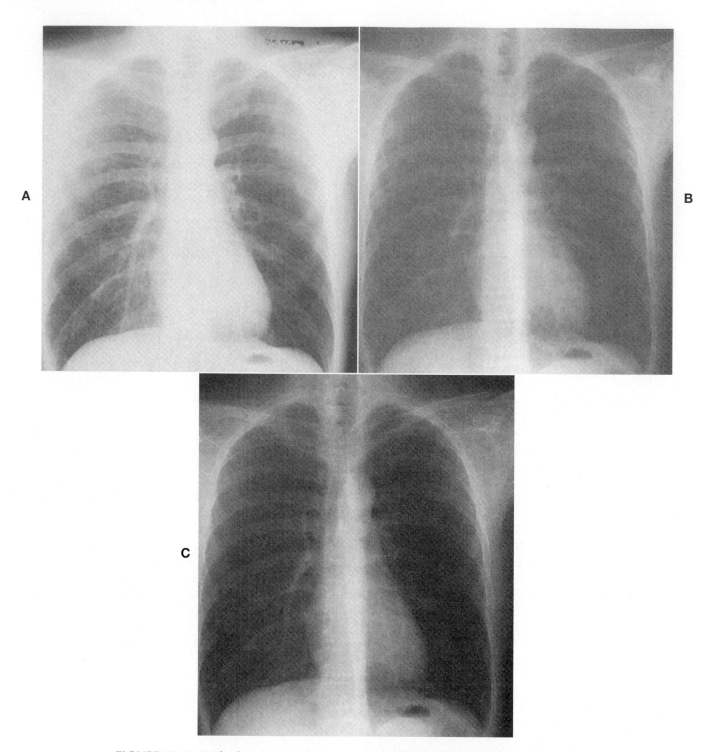

FIGURE 15-18 A, The front image of this asymmetric screen-emulsion image receptor shows high contrast. **B,** The back image shows wide latitude. **C,** The total image shows enhanced rendering of mediastinal and subdiaphragmatic tissue and pleural spaces. (Courtesy of Eastman Kodak.)

CARE OF SCREENS

High-quality radiographs require that radiographic intensifying screens receive proper care. Screen handling requires the utmost care because even a small fingernail scratch can produce artifacts and degrade the radiographic image. Screens should be handled only when they are new and being installed in cassettes and when they are being cleaned. When screens are mounted in a cassette, the manufacturer's instructions must be followed carefully.

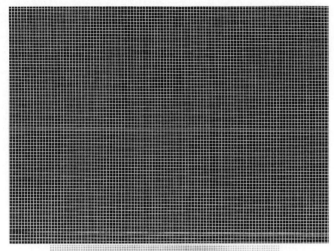

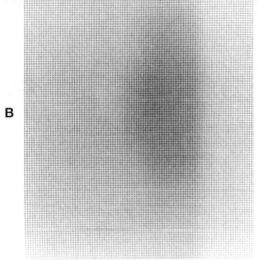

FIGURE 15-19 Radiographs of wire mesh are used to check for screen film contact. **A,** Good contact is evident. (Courtesy Nuclear Associates.) **B,** A warped cassette cover leads to a region of poor contact. (Courtesy Barbara Smith Pruner.)

When loading cassettes do not slide the film in. A sharp corner or the edge can scratch the screen. Place the film in the cassette. Remove the film by rocking the cassette on the hinged edge and letting it fall to your fingers. Do not dig the film out of the cassette with your fingernails. Do not leave cassettes open because the screens can be damaged by whatever might fall on them, be it dust or darkroom chemicals.

Radiographic intensifying screens must be cleaned periodically. This frequency of cleaning is determined primarily by two factors: the amount of use and the level of dust in the work environment. In a busy radiology department, it may be necessary to clean screens once each month or even more often. Under other circumstances, the cleaning frequency may safely be extended to 2 to 3 months.

Special screen cleaning materials exist. When they are used, the manufacturer's instructions should be followed carefully. One advantage to using these commercial preparations is that they often contain **antistatic** compounds, which can be helpful.

Radiographic intensifying screens can also be cleaned with mild soap and water. The screens should be carefully rinsed and thoroughly dried. If the screen is damp, the film emulsion layer may stick to it, possibly causing permanent damage.

An equally important requirement in caring for radiographic intensifying screens is maintaining good screen-film contact. Screen-film contact can be checked by radiographing a wire mesh (Figure 15-19, *A*). If there are any darker areas of blurring, as in Figure 15-19, *B*, then screen-film contact is poor and should be corrected or the cassette replaced.

To test for screen-film contact, expose the cassette through the wire mesh at 50 kVp at 5 mAs and an SID of 100 cm. To view the result optimally, back away 2 to 3 m from the viewbox. Areas of poor screen-film contact will appear blurred and cloudy, indicating that the cassette should be repaired or replaced.

This examination for screen-film contact is indicated when new radiographic intensifying screens are installed in a cassette, and the radiograph should be retained as a baseline evaluation. Additional wire mesh test radiographs for screen-film contact should be compared with the baseline film at least annually.

Box 15-5 summarizes the most common causes of poor screen-film contact. Nearly all of these causes can result from rough handling of cassettes, the principal cause of poor screen-film contact. Although the cassettes appear sturdy, they are precision pieces of equipment and should be treated accordingly.

Properly maintained radiographic intensifying screens will last indefinitely. X-ray interaction with the phosphor does not cause them to wear out. There is no such thing as **radiation fatigue.** The only way these screens become useless and need replacement is through improper handling and maintenance.

SUMMARY

Radiographic intensifying screens are permanently placed within the radiographic cassette. The x-ray film used for each exposure is placed between them. The radiographic intensify screens are so named because they change the energy of the image-forming x-ray beam exiting the patient into visible light, which exposes the radiographic film.

Radiographic intensifying screens are composed of the following four layers: (1) a protective coating, (2) the phosphor layer, (3) the reflective layer, and (4) the base. The phosphor layer has one purpose: to convert x-rays into visible light.

This process is called *luminescence*. Intensifying screens display a particular kind of luminescence called *fluorescence*, which means the phosphor is stimulated to emit light only when struck by x-ray or light energy. Once the x-ray exposure is terminated, no lag or afterglow of light is present.

Radiographic intensifying screens display an x-ray absorption efficiency and an x-ray-to-light CE. Intensification factor (IF) is a characteristic that compares nonscreen film exposure with screen-film exposure. The IF is defined as follows:

$$IF = \frac{\text{Exposure required without screens}}{\text{Exposure required with screens}}$$

Calcium-tungstate phosphors were used almost exclusively until 1972, when rare earth phosphors were developed for medical x-ray use. Radiographic intensifying screen speed is a number determined by the amount of radiation to which the patient is exposed. Par-speed screens ($CaWO_4$) are assigned a value of 100. Table 15-1 summarizes optical density, resolution in lp/mm, image noise, and applications of various intensifying screens.

Radiographic intensifying screens must be properly cared for. Avoid artifacts by handling the screens and film carefully. Spots will show up on the radiograph if dust or other deposits are on the screen. Because of dust accumulation, screens need to be cleared regularly.

CHALLENGE QUESTIONS

1. Define or otherwise identify:
   a. Afterglow
   b. Isotropic
   c. Spatial resolution
   d. Spectral matching
   e. Intensification factor
   f. Screen blur
   g. Image noise
   h. Phosphor
   i. Cassette compression
   j. Luminescence

2. Discuss the physical qualities required for a material to be used as a radiographic intensifying screen base.
3. Describe the composition of a typical radiographic intensifying screen.
4. Discuss the two types of luminescence and how they are associated with radiographic intensifying screens and fluoroscopic screens.
5. What can cause image fog?
6. The usual technique for an oblique radiograph of the foot uses direct-exposure film at 45 kVp, 180 mAs. If screens are used, the technique factors are changed to 45 kVp, 7.5 mAs to maintain the same average optical density. What is the approximate intensification factor for the screen-film combination?
7. Describe a technique designed to test for good screen-film contact.
8. What characteristics of phosphor materials make them especially suited for intensifying screens?
9. Describe the construction of a film cassette, listing each layer from tube side to back cover.
10. List the most common cassette malfunctions.
11. What percentage of the x-ray beam exposing the radiographic film contributes to the latent image?
12. Why are two intensifying screens placed in the radiographic cassette?
13. Why is afterglow objectionable as a characteristic of a radiographic intensifying screen?
14. Name five phosphors used in radiographic intensifying screens.
15. Name five properties of a radiographic intensifying screen base.
16. Discuss the difference between fluorescence and phosphorescence.
17. What is intensification factor? Write the formula for intensification factor.
18. Illustrate 20% x-ray absorption efficiency in the phosphor layer of a radiographic intensifying screen.
19. What is quantum mottle?
20. What is the importance of spectrally matching the radiographic film and the radiographic intensifying screen phosphor?

Beam-Restricting Devices

OBJECTIVES

At the completion of this chapter, the student should be able to do the following:

1. Identify the x-rays that constitute image-forming radiation
2. List three factors that contribute to scatter radiation
3. Discuss three devices developed to minimize scatter radiation
4. Describe beam-restricting and its effect on patient dose and image quality

OUTLINE

THREE FACTORS CONTRIBUTE to an increase in scatter radiation: increased kVp, increased x-ray field size, and increased patient thickness. Beam-restricting devices are designed to control and minimize scatter radiation by limiting the x-ray field size to only the anatomy of interest. The three principal types of beam-restricting devices are aperture diaphragm, cones, cylinders, and collimators.

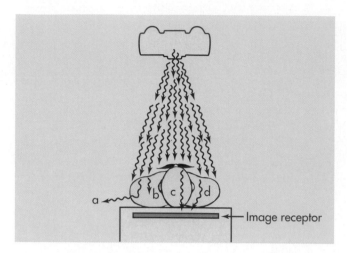

FIGURE 16-1 Some x-rays interact with the patient and are scattered away from the film *(a)*. Others interact with the patient and are absorbed *(b)*. X-rays that arrive at the image receptor are those transmitted through the patient without interacting *(c)* and those scattered in the patient *(d)*. X-rays of type *c* and *d* are called *image-forming x-rays*.

The two principal characteristics of any image are *spatial resolution* and *contrast resolution*. Some refer to these together as *image detail* or *visibility of detail*. In fact, these qualities are quite distinct and influenced by different links of the imaging chain.

Spatial resolution is determined by focal-spot size and other factors that contribute to blur. Contrast resolution is determined by scatter radiation and other sources of radiographic noise. There are two principal tools for controlling scatter radiation: beam-restricting devices and grids.

PRODUCTION OF SCATTER RADIATION

Two kinds of x-rays are responsible for the optical density and contrast on a radiograph: those that pass through the patient without interacting and those that are scattered in the patient through Compton interaction. X-rays that exit from the patient are remnant x-rays and those that interact with the image receptor are called **image-forming x-rays** (Figure 16-1).

Proper collimation of the x-ray beam has the primary effect of reducing patient dose by restricting the volume of irradiated tissue. Proper collimation also improves image contrast. Ideally, only those x-rays that do not interact with the patient should reach the image receptor.

 Collimation reduces patient dose and improves contrast resolution.

As scatter radiation increases, the radiograph loses contrast and appears gray and dull because of the fog caused by scatter. Three primary factors influence the relative intensity of scatter radiation reaching the image receptor: kVp, field size, and patient thickness.

Kilovolt Peak

As x-ray energy is increased, the absolute number of Compton interactions decreases with increasing x-ray energy but the number of photoelectric interactions de-

creases much more rapidly. Therefore, the relative number of x-rays that undergo Compton interaction increases (see Chapter 12).

Table 16-1 shows the percentage of x-rays incident on a 10 cm thickness of soft tissue that will undergo photoelectric interaction and Compton interaction at selected kVp levels of 50 to 120 kVp. Kilovoltage is one of the factors that affect the level of scatter radiation and can be controlled by the radiologic technologist.

It would be easy enough to say that all radiographs should be taken at the lowest reasonable kVp because this technique would result in minimum scatter and thus higher image contrast. Unfortunately, it is not that simple.

Figure 16-2 shows the relative contributions of photoelectric effect and Compton effect to the radiographic image. This increase results in a considerable increase in patient dose. Table 16-1 shows that the percentage of x-rays that interact photoelectrically increases greatly as kVp is lowered.

Also, fewer x-rays reach the image receptor at low kVp, a phenomenon that is usually compensated for by increasing the mAs. The result is still higher patient dose.

 Approximately 1% of incident x-rays reach the image receptor.

With large patients, kVp must be high to ensure adequate penetration of the portion of the body being radi-

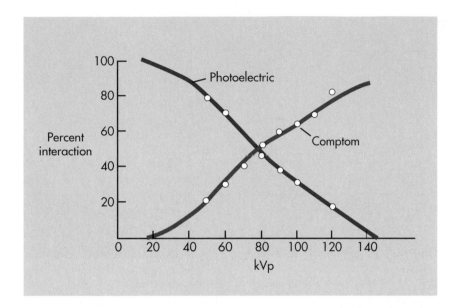

FIGURE 16-2 The relative contributions of photoelectric effect and Compton scattering to the radiographic image.

TABLE 16-1	Percent Interaction of X-rays by Photoelectric and Compton Processes and Percent Transmission Through 10 cm of Soft Tissue			
	PERCENT INTERACTION			
kVp	**Photoelectric**	**Compton**	**Total**	**Percent Transmission**
50	79	21	>99	<1
60	70	30	>99	<1
70	60	40	>99	<1
80	46	52	98	2
90	38	59	97	3
100	31	63	94	6
110	23	70	93	7
120	18	83	91	9

ographed. If, for example, the normal technique factors for an AP examination of the abdomen are inadequate, the technologist has a choice of increasing mA per second or kVp.

Increasing the mAs usually generates enough x-rays to provide a satisfactory image but may result in an unacceptably high patient dose. On the other hand, a much smaller increase in kVp is usually sufficient to provide enough x-rays, and this can be done at a much lower patient dose. Unfortunately, when kVp is increased, the level of scatter radiation also increases, leading to decreased image contrast.

Collimators and grids are used to reduce the level of scatter radiation. Figure 16-3 shows a series of radiographs of a skull phantom taken at 70, 80, and 90 kVp using appropriate collimation and grids, with the mAs adjusted to produce radiographs of nearly equal optical density (OD).

Most radiologists would accept any of these radiographs. Notice that the patient dose at 90 kVp is ap-

proximately one third that at 70 kVp. In general, because of this reduction in patient dose, a high kVp technique is preferred to a low kVp technique.

Field Size

Another factor affecting the level of scatter radiation and that is controlled by the radiologic technologist is x-ray beam field size. As field size is increased, scatter radiation also increases (Figure 16-4). The relative intensity of scatter radiation increases rapidly as x-ray field is increased (Figure 16-5).

 Scatter radiation increases as the field size of the x-ray beam increases.

Figure 16-6 shows two AP views of the lumbar spine. Figure 16-6, *A* was taken on a full-frame 14 × 17 in (35 × 43 cm) film; in Figure 16-6, *B*, field size is restricted to the spinal

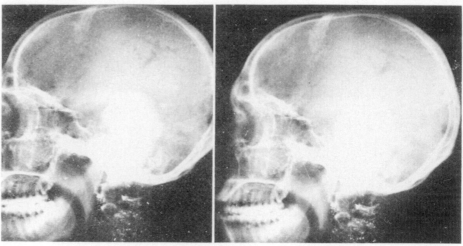

70 kVp / 120 mAs
665 mR

80 kVp / 60 mAs
545 mR

FIGURE 16-3 Each of these skull radiographs are of acceptable quality. The technique factors for each are shown, along with the resulting patient exposure. (Courtesy Donald Sommers.)

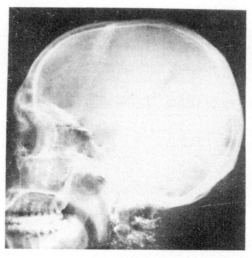

90 kVp / 30 mAs
230 mR

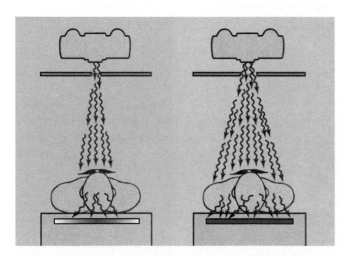

FIGURE 16-4 Collimation of the x-ray beam results in less scatter radiation, reduced dose, and improved contrast resolution.

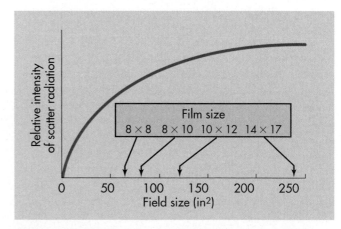

FIGURE 16-5 The relative intensity of scatter radiation increases with increasing field size.

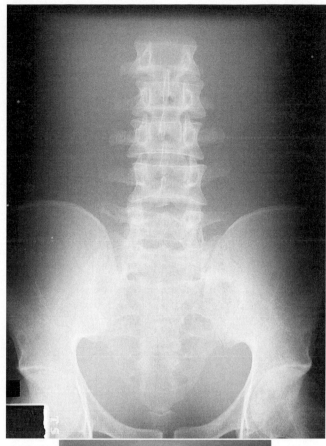

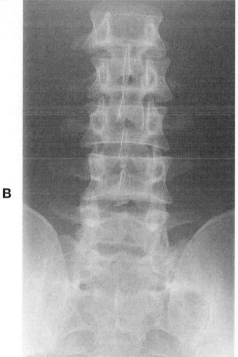

FIGURE 16-6 The recommended technique for lumbar spine radiography calls for collimation of the beam to the vertebral column. The full-field technique results in reduced image contrast. **A,** Full-field technique. **B,** Preferred collimated technique. (Courtesy Mike Enriquez.)

column. Contrast is noticeably lower in the full-frame radiograph because of the increased scatter radiation that accompanies larger field size.

The radiograph in Figure 16-6, *B* demonstrates proper collimation. Radiographic exposure factors may have to be increased during x-ray beam collimation. Reduced scatter radiation results in lower radiographic OD, which must be raised by increasing technique.

Restricting field size to improve image quality is perhaps even more important during fluoroscopy. Figure 16-7 shows a contrast/detail test object several centimeters thick. Such a test object is used to construct contrast/detail curves under various exposure conditions. Collimation results in better image contrast because of reduced scatter radiation.

Patient Thickness

Imaging thick parts of the body results in more scatter radiation than imaging thin parts does. Compare a radiograph of the bony structures in an extremity with a radiograph of the bony structures of the chest or pelvis. Even when the two are taken with the same screen-film combination, the extremity radiograph will be much sharper because of the reduced amount of scatter radiation (Figure 16-8).

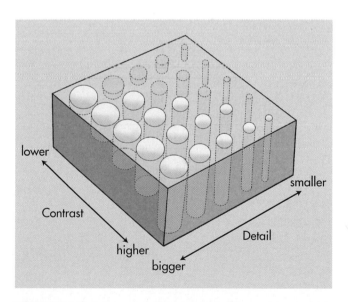

FIGURE 16-7 Schematic of a contrast/detail test object, which is used to construct contrast/detail curves for various imaging techniques.

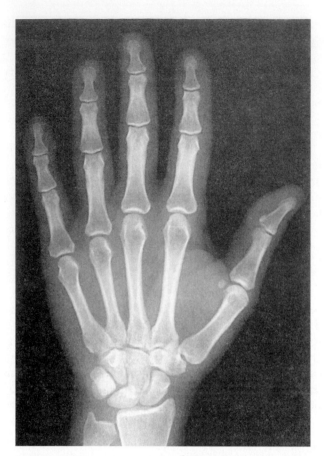

FIGURE 16-8 Extremity radiographs appear sharp because of less tissue and, hence, less scatter radiation. Posterior-anterior view of the hand. (Courtesy Rees Stuteville.)

Figure 16-9 shows the relative intensity of scattered x-rays as a function of the thickness of soft tissue for an 8 × 10 in (20 × 25 cm) field. Exposing a 3-cm thick extremity at 70 kVp results in about 45% scatter radiation. Exposing a 30-cm thick abdomen causes nearly 100% of the x-rays to exit the patient as scattered x-rays. With increasing patient thickness, more x-rays undergo multiple scattering so that the average angle of scatter in the remnant beam is greater.

Normally, patient thickness is not controlled by the radiologic technologist. If you recognize that more x-rays are scattered with increasing patient thickness, you can produce a high-quality radiograph by choosing the proper technique factors and by using devices that reduce scatter radiation to the image receptor, such as a compression paddle (Figure 16-10).

 Compression of anatomy improves spatial and contrast resolution and lowers patient dose.

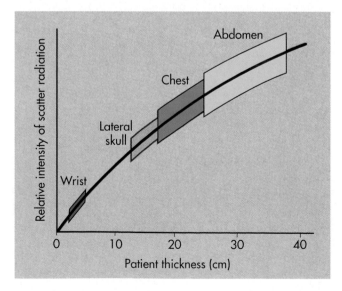

FIGURE 16-9 Relative intensity of scatter radiation increases with increasing thickness of anatomy.

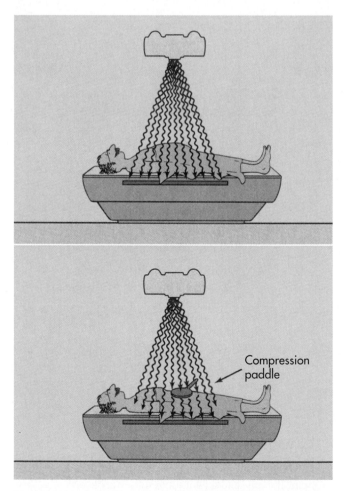

FIGURE 16-10 When tissue is compressed, scatter radiation is reduced, resulting in lower dose and improved contrast resolution.

Compression devices improve spatial resolution by reducing patient thickness and bringing the object closer to the image receptor. Compression also reduces patient dose and improves contrast resolution. Compression is particularly important during mammography.

CONTROL OF SCATTER RADIATION

Two types of devices reduce the amount of scatter radiation reaching the image receptor: **beam restrictors** and **grids**. Grids are discussed in Chapter 17. There are basically three types of beam-restricting devices: the aperture diaphragm, cones or cylinders, and the variable-aperture collimator (Figure 16-11).

There are two reasons to restrict any x-ray beam. (1) Only the tissue being examined should be exposed. Larger x-ray fields result in unnecessary patient exposure. (2) Large x-ray fields also result in more scatter radiation, which reduces image contrast.

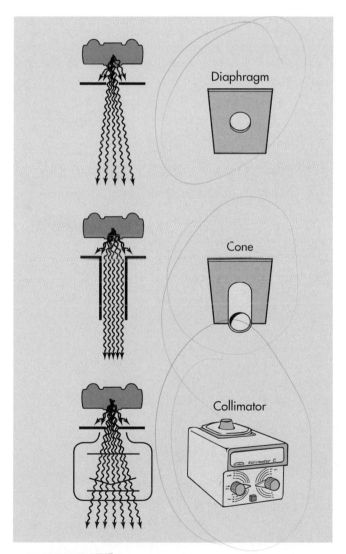

FIGURE 16-11 Three types of beam-restricting devices.

Aperture Diaphragm

An aperture is the simplest of all beam-restricting devices. It is basically a lead or lead-lined metal diaphragm attached to the x-ray tube head. The opening in the diaphragm is usually designed to cover just less than the size of the image receptor used. Figure 16-12 shows how the x-ray tube, aperture diaphragm, and image receptor are related.

With a properly designed aperture diaphragm, the image receptor receives an image that is 1 cm smaller on all sides than the image receptor itself. Therefore, an unexposed border should be visible on each edge of the radiograph. Aperture diaphragms are sometimes used with a cone or cylinder.

Question: If a 20 cm square film is to be imaged at 100 cm source-to-image receptor distance (SID) and the diaphragm is placed 10 cm from the target, what should be the dimension of one side of the diaphragm opening? *Note:* To leave an unexposed border of 1.0 cm on each side, we must reduce the beam size to 18 cm.

Answer:

$$\frac{X}{SSD} = \frac{18 \text{ cm}}{SID}$$

$$\frac{X}{10 \text{ cm}} = \frac{18 \text{ cm}}{100 \text{ cm}}$$

$$X = \frac{(10 \text{ cm})(18 \text{ cm})}{100}$$

$$= 1.8 \text{ cm}$$

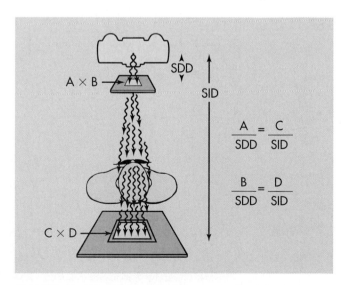

FIGURE 16-12 Aperture diaphragm is a fixed lead opening designed for a fixed image receptor size and constant SID. SDD, source-to-diaphragm distance.

The most familiar clinical example of aperture diaphragms may be radiographic imaging systems for trauma. The typical trauma system has a fixed SID and is equipped with diaphragms to accommodate film sizes of 5 × 7 in (13 × 18 cm), 8 × 10 in (20 × 25 cm), and 10 × 12 in (25 × 30 cm). Radiographic imaging systems for trauma can be positioned to image all parts of the body (Figure 16-13).

Radiographers should take care to insert aperture diaphragms into the x-ray tube head so that the long axis of the diaphragm is parallel to the long axis of the image receptor. Otherwise the diaphragm could be cut off, leaving large portions of the radiograph unexposed and possibly requiring repeat examinations and hence unnecessary patient exposure.

X-ray imaging systems dedicated specifically to chest radiography are supplied with fixed-aperture diaphragms. Usually, these diaphragms are securely fastened to the x-ray tube head and therefore are not easily removed. Aperture diaphragms for chest radiography are designed to expose all of a 14 × 17 in (35 × 45 cm) image receptor except for a 1 cm border.

Dental radiography is another application of aperture diaphragms. Dental radiographs are customarily obtained at 20 or 40 cm SID. The diaphragm used in these techniques must provide a circular x-ray beam not exceeding 7 cm in diameter at the entrance skin of the patient. Typically, the diameter of an aperture diaphragm for 20 cm SID is 18 mm and that for 40 cm SID is 9 mm.

Some dental apparatus are supplied with rectangular collimation, which requires that the dental radiologic technologist precisely align and position the x-ray tube head, the patient, and the image receptor.

Cones and Cylinders

Radiographic extension cones and cylinders are considered modifications of the aperture diaphragm. Figure 16-14 presents a diagram of a typical extension cone and cylinder. In both, an extended metal structure restricts the useful beam to the required size. The position and size of the distal end act as an aperture and determine field size.

Unlike the beam produced by an aperture diaphragm, the useful beam produced by an extension cone or cylinder is usually circular. Both of these beam restrictors are routinely called **cones,** even though the most commonly used type is actually a cylinder.

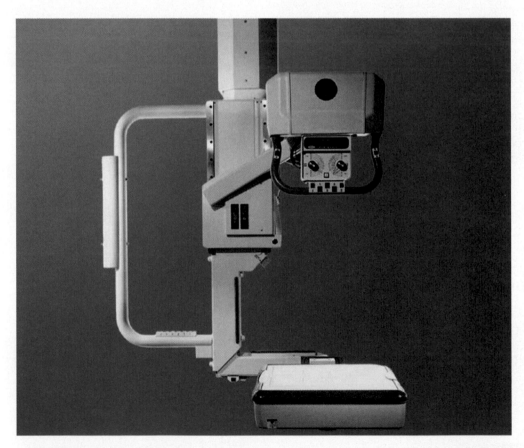

FIGURE 16-13 Typical trauma radiographic imaging system used for imaging the skull, spine, and extremities. Such units are flexible and adaptable for examination of many body parts. (Courtesy Fischer Imaging.)

One difficulty with using cones is alignment. If the x-ray source, cone, and image receptor are not aligned on the same axis, one side of the radiograph may not be exposed because the edge of the cone may interfere with the x-ray beam. Such interference is called **cone cutting.**

The same limitations that apply to aperture diaphragms apply to cones and cylinders. Their openings are fixed so that they are appropriate for only specific types of examinations.

At one time, cones were used extensively in diagnostic radiology. Today, they are reserved primarily for examinations of the head and spine. Figure 16-15 shows how a cone improves image contrast when used in the examination of the maxillary sinuses. In diagnostic radiography, the light-localizing variable-aperture collimator has largely replaced the cone.

Beam-defining cones, also known as position-indicating devices, are used extensively in dental radiography. Figure 16-16 is a photograph of six typical dental cones. Dental cones are usually fabricated of plastic and some are lined with lead. The long lead-lined dental cones result in slightly less exposure to the patient than the other types.

The 20 cm plastic pointer cones used on dental x-ray imaging systems result in unnecessarily high patient exposure due to scattering of the useful beam in the cone tip. Most dentists now use a long rectangular cone. Proper alignment is a little more difficult, but the resultant images have less distortion and the patient dose is reduced. The dental cone and circular diaphragm are often fabricated as one accessory; together they provide rather good beam restriction.

Variable Aperture Collimator

The light-localizing variable-aperture collimator is the most common beam-restricting device in diagnostic radiography. The photograph in Figure 16-17 is an example of a modern automatic variable-aperture collimator. Figure 16-18 identifies the principal parts of such a collimator.

 Collimation reduces patient dose and improves contrast resolution.

Not all x-rays are emitted precisely from the focal spot of the x-ray tube. Some x-rays are produced when projectile electrons stray and interact at positions on the anode other than the focal spot. Such radiation is called **off-focus radiation** and increases image blur.

To control off-focus radiation, a first-stage entrance-shuttering device that has multiple collimator blades protrudes from the top of the collimator into the x-ray tube housing.

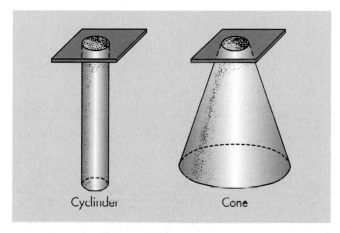

FIGURE 16-14 Radiographic cones and cylinders produce restricted useful x-ray beams of circular shape.

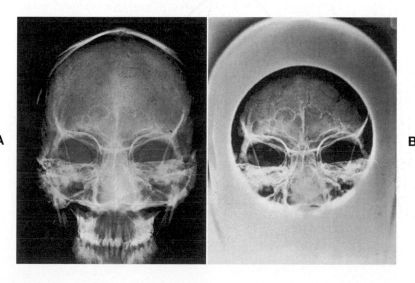

A   **B**

FIGURE 16-15 Radiographs of the frontal and maxillary sinuses without a cone (**A**) and using a cone (**B**). Cones reduce scatter radiation and improve contrast resolution. (Courtesy Lynn Davis.)

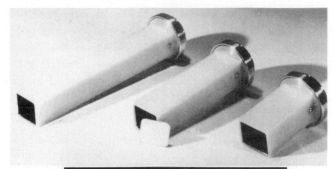

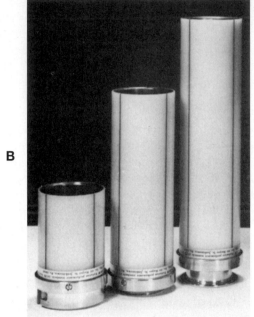

FIGURE 16-16 Six typical dental position-indicating devices: open-ended, lead-lined, 8 in, 12 in, 16 in, rectangles **(A),** and cylinders **(B).** (Courtesy Kenneth Abramovitch.)

The second-stage collimator shutters leaves are usually lead, at least 3 mm thick. They work in pairs and are independently controlled, thereby allowing for both rectangular and square fields.

Light localization in a typical variable-aperture collimator is accomplished with a small lamp and mirror. The mirror must be far enough on the x-ray tube side of the collimator leaves to project a sufficiently sharp light pattern through the collimator leaves when the lamp is on.

The collimator lamp and mirror must all be adjusted so that the projected light field coincides with the x-ray beam. If the light field and x-ray beam do not coincide, the lamp or mirror must be adjusted. Such coincidence checking is a necessary evaluation of any quality control program. Misalignment of the light field and x-ray beam can result in collimator cutoff of anatomic structures, as shown in Figure 16-19.

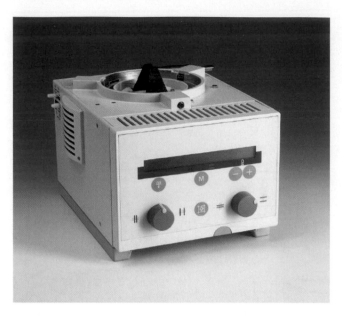

FIGURE 16-17 Automatic variable aperture collimator. (Courtesy Huestis Medical.)

Sometimes the light image indicates the location of the phototimer sensor. A scale is always marked on the collimator to indicate field size at fixed SIDs. The clear plastic exit surface of the collimator has two crossed lines that are used to project the center of the x-ray beam onto the center of the tissue being imaged. Often, a bright slit of light projects onto the table to assist the centering of the image receptor.

Today, nearly all light-localizing collimators manufactured in the United States for fixed radiographic equipment are automatic. They are called **positive-beam-limiting (PBL)** devices. Positive beam limitation was mandated by the United States Food and Drug Administration in 1974. That regulation was removed in 1994.

When a film-loaded cassette is inserted in the Bucky tray and clamped into place, sensing devices in the tray identify the size and alignment of the cassette. An electric signal is transmitted to the collimator housing and actuates the synchronous motors that drive the collimator leaves to a precalibrated position so that the x-ray beam is restricted to the image receptor size in use. Even with PBL devices, the radiologic technologist should manually collimate more tightly to reduce patient dose and improve image quality.

 Under no circumstances should the x-ray beam exceed the size of the image receptor.

Depending on the tube potential, additional **collimator filtration** may be necessary to produce high-quality ra-

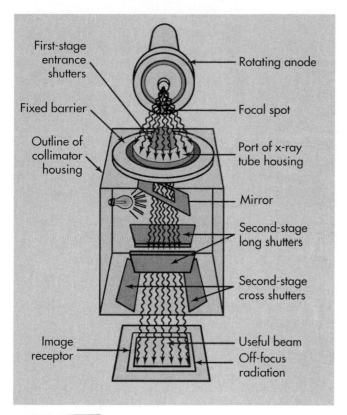

FIGURE 16-18 Simplified schematic of a variable-aperture light-localizing collimator.

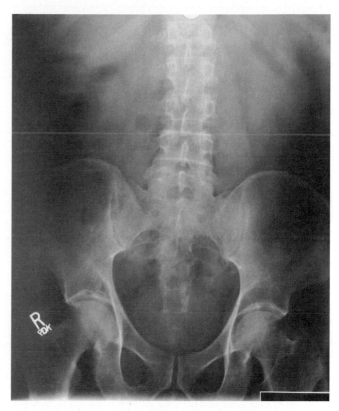

FIGURE 16-19 Anterior-posterior supine abdomen. In this radiograph, only the lower collimation is visible because the image receptor is not centered to the central ray, which cuts off the anatomic structure of the upper abdomen. (Courtesy Judy Williams.)

diographs with minimum patient exposure. Some collimator housings are designed to allow easy changing of the added filtration. Filtration stations of 0, 1, 2, and 3 mm Al are the most common.

TOTAL FILTRATION

Total Filtration = Inherent Filtration + Added Filtration

Even in the zero position, however, the added filtration to the x-ray tube is not zero because collimator structures intercept the beam. In addition to the inherent filtration of the tube, the exit port, usually plastic, and the reflecting mirror also provide filtration. The added filtration of the collimator assembly is usually equivalent to approximately 1 mm Al.

SUMMARY

Two types of image-forming x-rays exit the patient: (1) x-rays that pass through tissue without interacting and (2) x-rays that are scattered in tissue by the Compton interaction and therefore contribute only noise to the image. The three factors that contribute to increased scatter radiation and ultimately to image noise are increasing kVp, increasing x-ray field size, and increasing anatomic thickness.

Although increased kVp increases scatter radiation, the trade-off is reduced patient exposure. Beam-restricting devices can be used to control and minimize the increase in scatter; such devices include the aperture diaphragm, extension cones and cylinders, and the variable-aperture collimator. The variable-aperture collimator is the most commonly used beam-restricting device in diagnostic imaging.

CHALLENGE QUESTIONS

1. Define or otherwise identify:
   a. Three factors affecting scatter radiation
   b. Collimator filtration
   c. Aperture diaphragm
   d. Cone cutting
   e. Collimation
   f. Off-focus radiation
   g. PBL device
   h. Beam restrictors
   i. Image-forming x-rays
   j. Compression
2. Why should a radiograph of the lumbar vertebrae be well collimated?
3. A dedicated chest imaging system is designed for only 14 × 17 in (35 × 43 cm) radiographs. If the SID is 180 cm and the SDD is 10 cm, what diaphragm opening will allow an unexposed border of 1 cm around the film?
4. An acceptable IVP can be obtained with technique factors of (1) 74 kVp, 120 mAs or (2) 82 kVp, 80 mAs. Discuss possible reasons for selecting one technique over the other.
5. Does the radiograph of a long bone in a wet cast result in more or less scatter than a long bone in a dry cast?
6. One mode for skull radiography uses a 10 × 12 in (25 × 30 cm) film format. If the SID is 80 cm, what should be the size of the diaphragm located 12 cm from the source?
7. What happens to image contrast and patient dose as more filtration is added to the x-ray beam?
8. List and describe the two types of remnant radiation.
9. At the 80 kVp level, what percentage of the x-ray beam is scattered through Compton interaction?
10. Name the devices used to reduce the level of scatter radiation.
11. Compression of tissue is particularly important during what examination?
12. List the two reasons for restricting the x-ray beam.
13. Describe the design of the aperture diaphragm.
14. What is the reason to show an unexposed border on the edge of the radiograph?
15. Describe a possible difficulty with using extension cones.
16. What is viewed in the light field of a variable-aperture light-localizing collimator?
17. What is the origin of the two crossed lines that mark central ray location on the tissue to be radiographed?
18. Does a light-localizing collimator add filtration to the x-ray beam?
19. If the light field and the radiation field do not coincide, what needs to be adjusted?
20. When should the x-ray field exceed the size of the image receptor?

CHAPTER 17

The Grid

OBJECTIVES

At the completion of this chapter, the student should be able to do the following:

1. Recognize the relationship between scatter radiation and image contrast
2. Describe grid construction
3. Calculate grid ratio, grid frequency, contrast improvement factor, Bucky factor, and selectivity
4. Describe eight types of grids
5. Discuss the four common errors when using grids
6. Evaluate the circumstances for proper grid selection
7. Describe advantages and disadvantages to the use of grids in relation to patient dose

OUTLINE

ONTRAST AND CONTRAST RESOLUTION are important characteristics of image quality. Contrast arises from the areas of light, dark, and shades of gray on the x-ray image. These variations make up the radiographic image. Contrast resolution is the ability to image adjacent similar tissues.

Scatter radiation produced by the Compton effect produces noise, reducing image contrast and contrast resolution. It makes the manifest image less visible. The two types of devices that are used to reduce scatter radiation are beam-restricting devices (see Chapter 16) and radiographic grids. By removing scattered x-rays from the remnant beam, the grid removes a major source, thus improving image contrast.

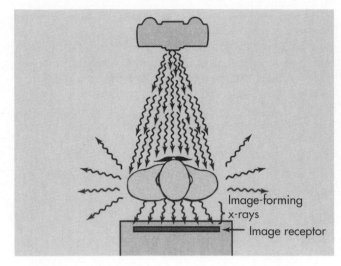

FIGURE 17-1 When primary x-rays interact with the patient, x-rays are scattered from the patient in all directions.

 Reduced image contrast results from scattered x-rays.

CONTROL OF SCATTER RADIATION

The relative intensity of scatter radiation was previously shown to be a complex function of many factors, primarily kVp, field size, and patient thickness. The amount of scatter radiation is reduced as kVp is lowered because of enhanced differential absorption. There are, however, a number of disadvantages to low-kVp radiography, principally increased patient dose.

The beam-restricting devices discussed in the previous chapter are very efficient in reducing scatter radiation. But their effect is not sufficient because they are positioned between the source and the patient. Even under the most favorable conditions, most of the **remnant x-rays** are scattered. Figure 17-1 illustrates that scattered x-rays are emitted in all directions from the patient.

Effect of Scatter Radiation on Image Contrast

Chapter 19 discusses in detail many characteristics that affect the quality of a radiograph. One of the most important characteristics of film quality is **contrast,** the visible difference between the light and dark areas of a radiograph. Contrast is the degree of difference in optical density (OD) between areas of an image. Contrast resolution is the ability to image and distinguish soft tissues.

If you could radiograph a long bone in cross section using only transmitted, unscattered x-rays, the image would be very sharp (Figure 17-2, *A*). The change in OD from dark to light, corresponding to the bone–soft tissue interface, would be very abrupt, and therefore the image contrast would be high.

On the other hand, if the radiograph were taken with only scatter radiation and no transmitted x-rays reached the image receptor, the image would be dull gray (Figure 17-2, *B*). The radiographic contrast would be very low.

In the normal situation, however, the x-rays arriving at the image receptor consist of both transmitted and scattered x-rays. If the radiograph were properly exposed, the image in cross-sectional view would appear as in Figure 17-2, *C*. The image would have moderate contrast. The loss of contrast results from the presence of scattered x-rays.

The scattered x-rays that reach the image receptor are part of the image-forming process; indeed, the x-rays that are scattered forward do contribute to the image. Most that are scattered at a large angle are removed by the grid and are part of the remnant x-rays, not the image-forming x-rays. Unlike beam-restricting devices, the grid is positioned between the patient and the image receptor.

Grid Characteristics

An extremely effective device for reducing the level of scatter radiation reaching the image receptor is the **grid,** a carefully fabricated series of sections of radiopaque material (**grid strips**) alternating with sections of radiolucent material (**interspace material**).

This technique for reducing the amount of scatter radiation reaching the image receptor was first demonstrated in 1913 by Gustave Bucky. Over the years,

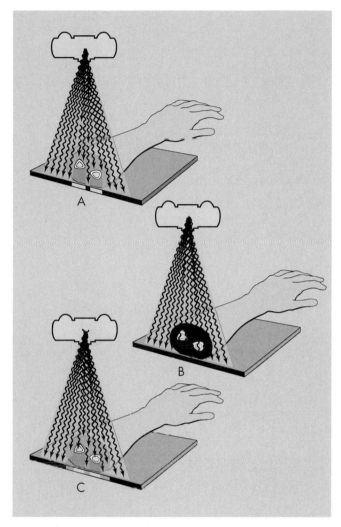

FIGURE 17-2 Radiographs of a cross-section of long bone. **A,** High contrast would result from using only transmitted, unattenuated x-rays. **B,** No contrast would result from using only scattered x-rays. **C,** Moderate contrast results from using both transmitted and scattered x-rays.

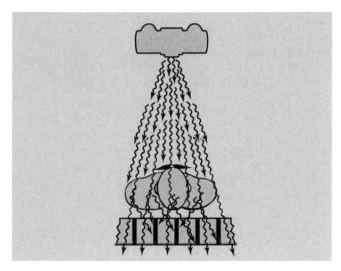

FIGURE 17-3 The only x-rays transmitted through a grid are those traveling in the direction of the interspace. X-rays scattered obliquely through the interspace are absorbed.

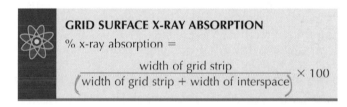

GRID SURFACE X-RAY ABSORPTION

% x-ray absorption =

$$\frac{\text{width of grid strip}}{\left(\text{width of grid strip} + \text{width of interspace}\right)} \times 100$$

Question: A grid is constructed with 50-μm strips and a 350-μm interspace. What percentage of x-rays incident on the grid will be absorbed by its entrance surface?

Answer: $\dfrac{50\ \mu m}{350\ \mu m + 50\ um} = 0.125$

$$= 12.5\%$$

Bucky's grid has been improved by more precise manufacturing, but the basic principle has not changed.

The grid is designed to transmit only those x-rays whose direction is on a straight line from the source to the image receptor. Scattered x-rays are absorbed in the grid material. Figure 17-3 is a schematic representation of how a grid "cleans up" scatter radiation.

X-rays exiting the patient that strike the radiopaque grid strips are absorbed and do not reach the image receptor. For instance, a typical grid may have grid strips approximately 50 μm wide separated by interspace material approximately 350 μm wide. Consequently, up to 12.5% of all x-rays striking the grid interact with the radiopaque grid strips and are absorbed.

Primary beam x-rays incident on the interspace material are transmitted to the image receptor. Scattered x-rays incident on interspace material may or may not be absorbed, depending on their angle of incidence and the physical characteristics of the grid.

If the angle of a scattered x-ray is great enough to cause it to intersect the lead grid strips, it will be absorbed. If the angle is slight, the scattered x-ray will be transmitted like a primary x-ray. Laboratory measurements show that high-quality grids can attenuate 80% to 90% of the scatter radiation. Such a grid is said to exhibit good "cleanup."

Question: When viewed from the top, a particular grid shows a series of lead strips 40 μm wide separated by interspaces 300 μm wide. How much of the radiation incident on this grid should be absorbed?

Answer: If 300 + 40 represents the total surface area and 40 the surface area of absorbing material, then the percentage absorption is

$$\frac{40\ \mu m}{340\ \mu m} = 0.118$$
$$= 11.8\%$$

Grid Ratio. There are three important dimensions on a grid: the thickness of the grid strip (T), the width of the interspace material (D), and the height of the grid (h). The **grid ratio** is the height of the grid divided by the interspace width:

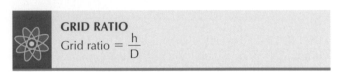

GRID RATIO

Grid ratio = $\dfrac{h}{D}$

The grid ratio can best be understood by reference to Figure 17-4.

High-ratio grids are more effective in cleaning up scatter radiation than low-ratio grids. This is because the angle of scatter allowed by high-ratio grids is less than that permitted by low-ratio grids (Figure 17-5).

Unfortunately, grids with high ratio are more difficult to manufacture than low-ratio grids. High-ratio grids are fabricated by reducing the width of the interspace or increasing the height of the grid strip. A combination of both is usually the case. The higher the grid ratio, the higher the radiation exposure necessary to get a sufficient number of x-rays through the grid to the image receptor.

High-ratio grids increase patient radiation dose.

In general, grid ratios range from 5:1 to 16:1, with the higher-ratio grids most often used in high-kVp radiography. An 8:1 to 10:1 grid is frequently used with general-purpose x-ray imaging systems. A 5:1 grid will clean up approximately 85% of the scatter radiation, whereas a 16:1 grid may clean up as much as 97%.

Question: A grid is fabricated of 30-μm lead grid strips sandwiched between interspace material 300 μm thick. The height of the grid is 2.4 mm. What is the grid ratio?

Answer: Grid ratio = $\dfrac{h}{D}$

$$= \frac{2400\ \mu m}{300\ \mu m}$$

$$= 8:1$$

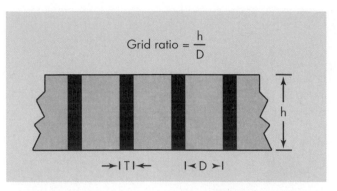

FIGURE 17-4 Grid ratio is defined as the height of the grid strip (h) divided by the thickness of the interspace material *(D)*. *T,* width of grid strip.

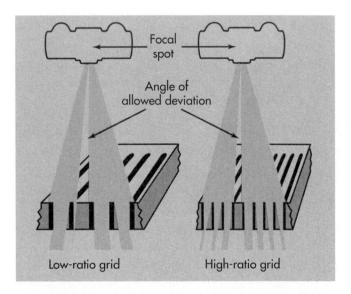

FIGURE 17-5 High-ratio grids are more effective than low-ratio grids because the angle of deviation is smaller.

Grid Frequency. The number of grid strips or grid lines per inch or centimeter is called the *grid frequency.* Grids with high frequency show less distinct grid lines on a radiograph than grids with low frequency.

If the grid strip width is held constant, the higher the frequency of a grid, the thinner its strips of interspace material must be and the higher the grid ratio.

The use of high-frequency grids requires high radiographic technique and results in higher patient radiation dose.

As grid frequency increases, there is relatively more grid strip to absorb x-rays, and therefore the patient dose is high because a higher radiographic technique is required. The disadvantage of the increased patient dose

TABLE 17-1	Construction Characteristics of Some of the More Popular Grids			
Type	**Interspace**	**Grid Frequency (Lines/in)**	**Grid Ratio**
Focused	Aluminum	145	14:1, 12:1, 10:1, 8:1
Focused	Aluminum	103	12:1, 10:1, 8:1, 6:1
Parallel	Aluminum	103	6:1
Focused	Aluminum	85	12:1, 10:1, 8:1, 6:1, 5:1
Parallel	Aluminum	85	6:1, 5:1
Parallel	Aluminum	196	3.5:1, 2:1
Crossed focused	Aluminum	85	6:1, 5:1
Focused	Fiber	80	12:1, 8:1, 5:1
Crossed focused	Fiber	80	8:1, 5:1
Focused	Fiber	60	6:1
Parallel	Fiber	60	6:1

associated with high-frequency grids can be overcome by reducing the width of the grid strips, but this effectively reduces the grid ratio and therefore the cleanup.

Most grids have frequencies in the range of 25 to 45 lines per centimeter (60 to 110 lines per inch). Grid frequency can be calculated if the widths of the grid strip and the interspace are known. Grid frequency is computed by dividing the thickness of one line pair (T + D), expressed in μm, into 1 cm:

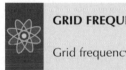

GRID FREQUENCY

$$\text{Grid frequency} = \frac{10,000 \ \mu m/cm}{(T + D) \ \mu m/\text{line pair}}$$

Question: What is the grid frequency of a grid having a grid strip width of 30 μm and an interspace width of 300 μm?

Answer: If one line pair = 300 μm + 30 μm = 330 μm, how many line pairs are in 10,000 μm (10,000 μm = 1 cm)?

$$\frac{10,000 \ \mu m/cm}{330 \ \mu m/\text{line pair}} = 30.3 \ \text{lines/cm}$$

30.3 lines/cm × 2.54 cm/in = 77 lines/in

Specially designed grids are used for mammography. Usually a 4:1 or a 5:1 ratio grid is used. These low-ratio grids have grid frequencies of approximately 80 lines/cm (200 lines/in).

Interspace Material. The purpose of the interspace material is to maintain a precise separation between the delicate lead strips of the grid. The interspace material of most grids is either **aluminum** or **plastic fiber;** there are conflicting reports as to which is better.

Aluminum has a higher atomic number than plastic, and therefore may provide some selective filtration of scattered x-rays not absorbed in the grid strip. Aluminum also has the advantage of producing less visible grid lines on the radiograph.

On the other hand, use of aluminum as interspace material increases the absorption of primary x-rays in the interspace, especially at low kVp. The result is higher mAs and higher patient dose. Above 100 kVp, this property is unimportant, but at low kVp, the patient dose may be increased by approximately 20%. For this reason, fiber interspace grids are usually preferred to aluminum interspace grids.

Still, aluminum has two additional advantages over fiber. It is **nonhygroscopic;** that is, it does not absorb moisture as plastic fiber does. Fiber interspace grids can become warped if they absorb moisture. Also, aluminum interspace grids are easier to manufacture with high quality because aluminum is easier to form and roll into sheets of precise thickness.

Grid Strip. Theoretically, the grid strip should be infinitely thin and have high absorption properties. There are several possible materials out of which to form these strips. Lead is the most widely used because it is easy to shape and is relatively inexpensive. Its high atomic number and high mass density make lead the material of choice in the manufacture of grids. Tungsten, platinum, gold, and uranium have all been tried, but none has the overall desirable characteristics of lead.

Grid Casing. Regardless of its composition, the grid is encased completely by a thin cover of aluminum. The aluminum casing provides rigidity for the grid and helps to seal out moisture. Table 17-1 is a summary of the characteristics of the most popular commercially available grids.

GRID PERFORMANCE

Perhaps the largest single factor responsible for poor radiographs is scatter radiation. By removing scattered x-rays from the remnant beam, the radiographic grid removes the source of poor contrast.

The principal function of a grid is to improve image contrast.

Contrast Improvement Factor

The characteristics of grid construction previously described, especially the grid ratio, are usually specified when identifying a grid. Grid ratio, however, does not relate the ability of the grid to improve radiographic contrast. This property of the grid is specified by the **contrast improvement factor** *(k)*.

The contrast improvement factor of a grid is the ratio of the contrast of a radiograph made with a grid to the contrast of a radiograph made without a grid. A contrast improvement factor of 1 indicates no improvement.

Most grids have contrast improvement factors of between 1.5 and 2.5. In other words, the radiographic contrast is approximately doubled when grids are used. Mathematically, the contrast improvement factor, *k,* is expressed as follows:

CONTRAST IMPROVEMENT FACTOR

$$k = \frac{\text{Radiographic contrast with grid}}{\text{Radiographic contrast without grid}}$$

Question: An aluminum step wedge is placed on a tissue phantom 20 cm thick and a radiograph is made. Without a grid, analysis of the radiograph shows an average gradient (a measure of contrast) of 1.1. With a 12:1 grid, radiographic contrast is 2.8. What is the contrast improvement factor of this grid?

Answer: $k = \dfrac{2.8}{1.1}$

          $= 2.55$

The contrast improvement factor is usually measured at 100 kVp, but it should be realized that *k* is a complex function of the x-ray emission spectrum, patient thickness, and the area irradiated. Other factors, such as lead content, also influence this measure of grid performance.

The contrast improvement factor is higher for high-ratio grids.

Bucky Factor

Although the use of a grid improves contrast, a penalty is paid in the form of patient dose. The amount of image-forming radiation transmitted through a grid is much less than the image-forming radiation incident on the grid. Therefore, when a grid is used, the radiographic technique must be increased to produce the same OD. The amount of this increase is given by the **Bucky factor (B):**

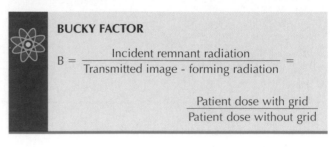

BUCKY FACTOR

$$B = \frac{\text{Incident remnant radiation}}{\text{Transmitted image - forming radiation}} =$$

$$\frac{\text{Patient dose with grid}}{\text{Patient dose without grid}}$$

The Bucky factor, sometimes called **grid factor,** is named for Gustave Bucky, the inventor of the grid. It is an attempt to measure the penetration of both primary and scatter radiation through the grid. Table 17-2 gives representative values of the Bucky factor for several popular grids.

Two generalizations can be made from the data presented in Table 17-2:

1. **The higher the grid ratio, the higher the Bucky factor.** The penetration of primary radiation through a grid is fairly independent of grid ratio. Penetration of scatter radiation through a grid becomes less likely with increasing grid ratio, and therefore, the Bucky factor increases.

2. **The Bucky factor increases with increasing kVp.** At high voltage, more scatter radiation is produced. This scatter radiation has a more difficult time penetrating the grid, and thus, the Bucky factor increases.

As the Bucky factor increases, radiographic technique and patient dose increase proportionately.

TABLE 17-2	Approximate Bucky Factor Values for Popular Grids			
	BUCKY FACTOR AT			
Grid Ratio	**70 kVp**	**90 kVp**	**120 kVp**	**Average**
No grid	1	1	1	1
5:1	2	2.5	3	2
8:1	3	3.5	4	4
12:1	3.5	4	5	5
16:1	4	5	6	6

Whereas the contrast improvement factor measures an improvement in image quality when using grids, the Bucky factor measures how much of an increase in technique will be required compared with nongrid exposure. The Bucky factor also indicates how large an increase in patient dose will accompany the use of a particular grid.

Selectivity

The ideal grid would be constructed so that all primary x-rays would be transmitted and all scattered x-rays would be absorbed. The ratio of transmitted primary radiation to transmitted scatter radiation is called the **selectivity** of the grid and is usually identified by a Greek sigma (Σ):

SELECTIVITY
$\Sigma = \dfrac{\text{Primary radiation transmitted through grid}}{\text{Scatter radiation transmitted through grid}}$

Selectivity is primarily a function of the construction characteristics of the grid rather than the characteristics of the x-ray beam. This is not the case for the contrast improvement factor.

Selectivity is related to grid ratio, but the total lead content in the grid has the primary influence on selectivity. Figure 17-6 shows how two grids can have the same grid ratio, yet greatly different lead content. This is usually accomplished with a small loss in grid frequency.

The heavier a grid is, the more lead it contains, the higher its selectivity, and the more efficient it is in cleaning up scatter radiation. Of course, the lead must be properly arranged. A flat sheet of lead with high mass would make a very poor grid.

The radiologic technologist normally selects a grid based on its ratio. The radiologic engineer or medical physicist takes into account grid ratio, grid frequency, contrast improvement factor, and selectivity in setting up apparatus for a particular radiologic suite or procedure. The relationships among these grid characteristics are complicated; however, a few general rules regarding them can be stated:

GRID CHARACTERISTICS

1. High-ratio grids have high contrast improvement factors.
2. High-frequency grids have low contrast improvement factors.
3. Heavy grids have high selectivity and high contrast improvement factors.

GRID TYPES
Parallel Grid

The simplest type of grid is the parallel grid diagrammed in cross-section in Figure 17-7. In the parallel grid, all lead grid strips are parallel. This type of grid is the easiest to manufacture but it has some properties that are clinically undesirable, namely **grid cutoff**, the undesirable absorption of primary x-rays by the grid.

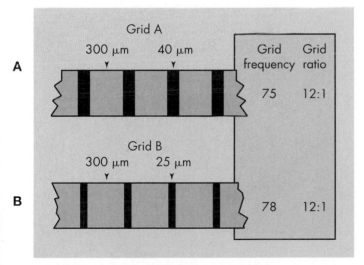

FIGURE 17-6 Because grids *A* and *B* have the same height and interspace thickness, they have the same grid ratio. Grid *A* has 60% more lead but a slightly lower frequency. Grid *A* has higher selectivity and, therefore, a higher contrast improvement factor.

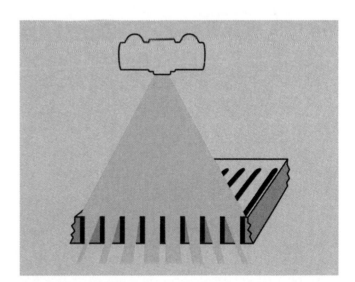

FIGURE 17-7 A linear grid is constructed with parallel grid strips. At a short source-to-image receptor distance (SID), some grid cutoff may occur.

Nearly all grids are large enough to cover a 35 × 43 cm (14 × 17 in) image receptor. As Figure 17-7 illustrates, the attenuation of primary x-rays becomes greater as the x-rays approach the edge of the image receptor. The lead strips in 35 × 43 cm grids are 43 cm long. Across the 35-cm dimension a variation in OD may be observed because of the primary x-ray attenuation. The OD reaches a maximum along the center line of the image receptor and decreases toward the sides.

Grid cutoff can be partial or complete and can result in reduced OD or total absence of film exposure, respectively. The term is derived from the fact that the primary x-rays are "cut off" from reaching the image receptor. Grid cutoff can occur with any type of grid if the grid is improperly positioned, but it is most common with parallel grids.

This characteristic of parallel grids is most pronounced when the grid is used at a short source-to-image receptor distance (SID) or with a large-area image receptor. Figure 17-8 demonstrates the geometric relationship for attenuation of primary x-rays by a parallel grid. The distance from the central ray at which complete cutoff will occur is given by the following:

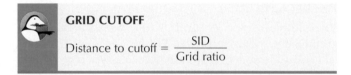

GRID CUTOFF

$$\text{Distance to cutoff} = \frac{\text{SID}}{\text{Grid ratio}}$$

For instance, in theory a 10:1 grid when used at 100 cm SID should completely absorb all primary x-rays farther than 10 cm from the central ray. When this grid is used with a 35 × 42 image receptor, OD should be apparent only over a 20 × 43 cm area of the image receptor.

The radiographs in Figure 17-9 were taken with a 6:1 parallel grid at 76 and 61 cm SID (A and B, respectively). They demonstrate increasing degrees of grid cutoff with decreasing SID.

Question: A 16:1 parallel grid is positioned for chest radiography at 180 cm SID. What is the distance from the central axis to complete

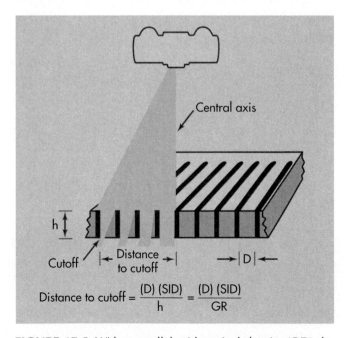

FIGURE 17-8 With a parallel grid, optical density (OD) decreases toward the edge of the image receptor. The distance to grid cutoff is the source-to-image receptor distance (SID) divided by the grid ratio.

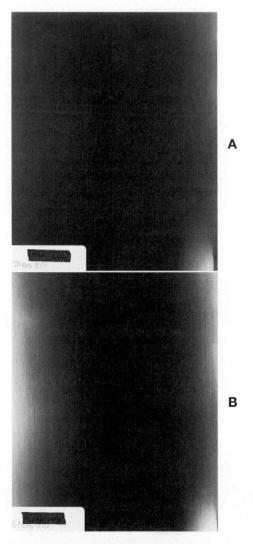

FIGURE 17-9 A, Radiograph taken with a 6:1 parallel grid at a source-to-image receptor distance (SID) of 76 cm. **B,** Radiograph taken with 6:1 parallel grid at an SID of 61 cm. Optical density decreases from the center to the edge of the image and to complete cutoff. (Courtesy Dawn Stark.)

grid cutoff? Will the image satisfactorily cover a 35 × 42 cm image receptor?

Answer: Distance to cutoff = $\dfrac{180}{16}$ = 11.3 cm

Distance to edge of
image receptor = 35 ÷ 2
= 17.5 cm

No! Grid cutoff will occur on the lateral 6.2 cm (17.5 − 11.3) of the image receptor.

Crossed Grid

Parallel grids clean up scatter radiation in only one direction, along the axis of the grid. Crossed grids are made to overcome this deficiency. Crossed grids have lead grid strips running parallel to both the long and short axes of the grid (Figure 17-10). They are usually fabricated by sandwiching two parallel grids together with their grid strips perpendicular to one another.

They are not too difficult to manufacture, and therefore are not excessively expensive. They have, however, found restricted application in clinical radiology. (Interestingly, Bucky's original grid was crossed.)

Crossed grids are much more efficient than linear grids in cleaning up scatter radiation. In fact, a crossed grid has a higher contrast improvement factor than a linear grid of twice the grid ratio. A 6:1 crossed grid will clean up more scatter radiation than a 12:1 linear grid.

This advantage of the crossed grid increases as the operating kVp is increased. A crossed grid identified as having a grid ratio of 6:1 is constructed with two 6:1 linear grids.

 The main disadvantage of parallel and crossed grid is grid cutoff.

There are two serious disadvantages to using crossed grids. First, positioning the grid is critical; the central ray of the x-ray beam must coincide with the center of the grid. Second, tilt-table techniques are possible only if the x-ray tube and table are properly aligned. If the table is horizontal and the tube is angled, grid cutoff will occur.

Focused Grid

The focused grid is designed to minimize grid cutoff. The lead grid strips of a focused grid lie on the imaginary radial lines of a circle centered at the focal spot so that they coincide with the divergence of the x-ray beam. The x-ray tube target should be placed at the center of this imaginary circle when a focused grid is used (Figure 17-11).

Focused grids are more difficult to manufacture than parallel grids. They are characterized by all the properties of parallel grids except that when properly positioned, they exhibit no grid cutoff. The radiologic technologist must take care when positioning focused grids because of their geometric limitations.

FIGURE 17-10 Crossed grids are fabricated by sandwiching two parallel grids together so that their grid strips are perpendicular.

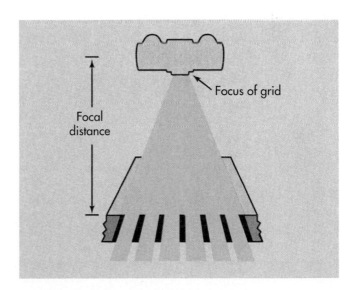

FIGURE 17-11 A focused grid is fabricated so that the grid strips are parallel to the primary x-ray path across the entire image receptor.

High-ratio grids have less positioning latitude than low-ratio grids.

Every focused grid is marked with its intended focal distance and the side of the grid that should face the tube. If radiographs are made at distances other than those intended, grid cutoff occurs.

A focused grid intended for use at 100 cm SID usually has sufficient latitude to produce acceptable radiographs when used at an SID between 90 and 110 cm. Use of a 100-cm SID 16:1 focused grid at 180 cm produces severe grid cutoff.

Moving Grid

An obvious and annoying shortcoming of the grids previously discussed is that they produce **grid lines** on the radiograph. Grid lines are the images made when primary x-rays are absorbed in the grid strips. Even though the grid strips are very small, their image is still observable.

The presence of grid lines can be demonstrated simply by radiographing a grid. Usually, high-frequency grids present less obvious grid lines than low-frequency grids. This is not always the case, however, because the visibility of grid lines is directly related to the width of the grid strips.

A major improvement in grid development occurred in 1920. Hollis E. Potter hit on a very simple idea: Move the grid while the x-ray exposure is being made. The grid lines disappear at little cost of increased radiographic technique. A device that does this is called a **moving grid** or Potter-Bucky diaphragm ("Bucky" for short).

Focused grids are usually used as moving grids. They are placed in a holding mechanism that begins moving just before the x-ray exposure and continues moving after the exposure ends. There are two basic types of moving grid mechanisms in use today: reciprocating and oscillating.

Reciprocating Grid. A reciprocating grid is a moving grid that is motor-driven back and forth several times during x-ray exposure. The total distance of drive is approximately 2 cm. The main advantage this type of moving grid mechanism has over the earlier single-stroke grid is that it does not require resetting after each exposure.

Oscillating Grid. An oscillating grid is positioned in a frame with a 2- to 3-cm tolerance on all sides between the frame and grid. Delicate, springlike devices located in the four corners hold the grid centered in the frame. A powerful electromagnet pulls the grid to one side and releases it at the beginning of the exposure. Thereafter, the grid oscillates in a circular fashion around the grid frame, coming to rest after 20 to 30 seconds.

The main difference between reciprocating and oscillating grids is their pattern of motion. The motion of a reciprocating grid is to and fro, whereas that of an oscillating grid is circular.

Disadvantages of Moving Grids. Moving grids require a bulky mechanism that is subject to failure. The distance between the patient and the image receptor is increased with moving grids because of this mechanism; that extra distance may create an unwanted increase in magnification and image blur. Moving grids can introduce motion into the cassette-holding device, which can result in additional image blur.

If not properly designed, moving grids can produce a stroboscopic effect when used with half- or full-wave–rectified x-ray generators because of synchronization between x-ray pulsation and grid movement. This effect results in the presence of pronounced grid lines. Also, the minimum exposure time is longer with moving grids than with stationary grids.

Fortunately, the advantages of moving grids far outweigh the disadvantages. The types of motion blur discussed are for descriptive purposes only. The motion blur generated by moving grids that are functioning properly is undetectable.

Only malfunctioning moving grid systems create problems, and those problems occur very infrequently. Moving grids are usually the technique of choice and therefore are widely used.

GRID PROBLEMS

Most grids in diagnostic imaging are of the moving type. They are permanently mounted in the moving mechanism just below the tabletop or just behind the vertical chest board.

To be effective, of course, the grid must move from side to side. If the grid is installed incorrectly and moves in the same direction as the grid strips, grid lines will appear on the radiograph (Figure 17-12).

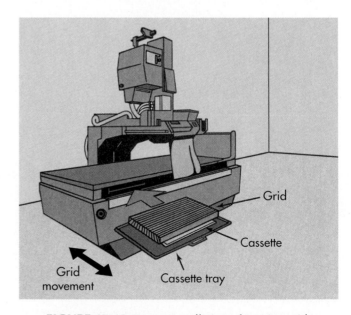

FIGURE 17-12 Proper installation of moving grid.

Stationary grids are either fastened to the front surface of a cassette or built into specially designed cassettes. Stationary grids are used for portable radiography and horizontal views of an upright patient.

The most frequent error in the use of grids is improper positioning. For the grid to function correctly, it must be precisely positioned relative to the x-ray tube target and to the central ray of the x-ray beam. Four situations characteristic of focused grids must be avoided (Table 17-3). Only an off-level grid is a problem with parallel and crossed grids.

Off-Level Grid

A properly functioning grid must lie in a plane perpendicular to the central ray of the x-ray beam (Figure 17-13). The **central ray** x-ray beam is the x-ray traveling along the center of the useful x-ray beam.

Despite its name, an **off-level grid** is in fact usually produced by having an improperly positioned radiographic tube and not an improperly positioned grid.

TABLE 17-3	Focused-Grid Misalignment
Type of Grid Misalignment	**Result**
Off-level	Grid cutoff across image; underexposed, light image
Off-center	Grid cutoff across image; underexposed, light image
Off focus	Grid cutoff toward edge of image
Upside-down	Severe grid cutoff toward edge of image

However, this can occur when the grid tilts during horizontal-beam radiography or during mobile radiography when the image receptor sinks into the patient's bed.

If the central ray is incident on the grid at an angle, then all incident x-rays will be angled and grid cutoff will occur across the entire radiograph, resulting in lower OD.

The condition can be prevented by paying careful attention to the installation of grids and the positioning of the x-ray tube. Grid cutoff caused by off-level grids can occur with all types of grids. It is the only positioning problem that occurs with parallel and crossed grids.

Off-Center Grid

A grid can be perpendicular to the central ray of the x-ray beam and still produce grid cutoff if it is shifted laterally. This is a problem with focused grids, as shown in Figure 17-14, where an off-center grid is shown with a properly positioned grid.

The center of a focused grid must be positioned directly under the x-ray tube target so that the central ray of the x-ray beam passes through the centermost interspace of the grid. Any lateral shift results in grid cutoff across the entire radiograph, resulting in lower OD. This error in positioning is called **lateral decentering**.

As with an off-level grid, an off-center grid is more a matter of positioning the x-ray tube than the grid. In practice, it means that the radiologic technologist must carefully line up the center of the light localized field with the center of the cassette. Marks on both the light field and the cassette, and sometimes on the table, are provided so that this can be done quickly and easily.

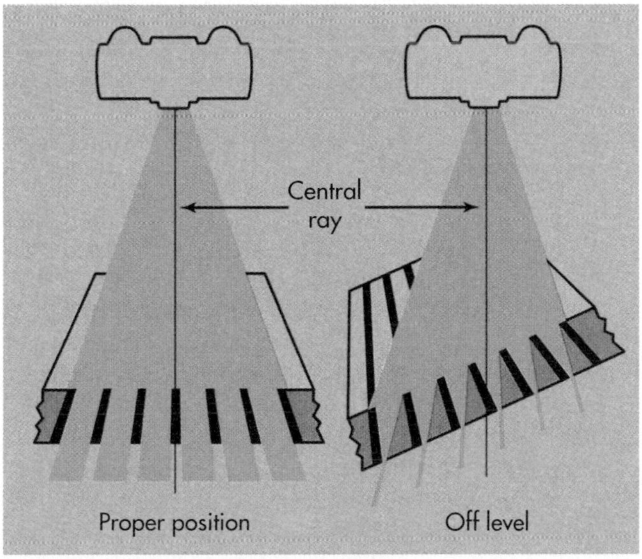

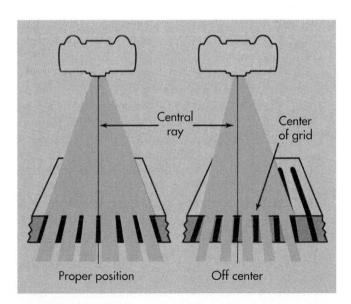

FIGURE 17-13 If a grid is off-level so that the central axis is not perpendicular to the grid, partial cutoff occurs over the entire image receptor.

FIGURE 17-14 When a focused grid is positioned off-center, partial grid cutoff occurs over the entire image receptor.

Off-Focus Grid

A major problem with using a focused grid arises when radiographs are taken at SIDs unspecified for that grid. Figure 17-15 illustrates what happens when a focused grid is not used at the proper focal distance. The farther the grid is from the specified focal distance, the more severe will be the grid cutoff. In Figure 17-15, the grid cutoff is not uniform across the image receptor, but instead is more severe to the periphery.

This condition is not normally a problem if all chest radiographs are taken at 180 cm SID and all table radiographs at 100 cm SID. Occasionally, table radiographs are taken at an SID other than 100 cm, with a grid having a 100-cm focal distance. Positioning the grid at the proper focal distance is more important with high-ratio grids; more positioning latitude is possible with low-ratio grids.

Upside-Down Grid

The explanation of an upside-down grid is obvious. It need occur only once and it will be noticed immediately. A radiographic image taken with an upside-down focused grid shows severe grid cutoff on either side of the central ray (Figure 17-16).

Every focused grid has a clear label on one side and sometimes on both. Labels indicate the tube side or image receptor side, or both, and the prescribed focal distance. With even moderate attention, upside-down grids will not occur.

Combined Off-Center, Off-Focus Grid. Perhaps the most common improper grid position occurs if the grid is both off-center and off-focus. Without proper attention, this can easily occur during mobile radiography. It is an easily recognized grid-positioning artifact because the result is uneven exposure. The resulting radiograph appears dark on one side and light on the other.

GRID SELECTION

Modern grids are sufficiently well manufactured that many radiologists do not find the grid lines of stationary grids objectionable, especially for portable radiography and horizontal views of an upright patient. Stationary grids are also cheaper than moving grids.

Moving grid mechanisms, however, rarely fail, and image degradation rarely occurs. Therefore, in most situations it is appropriate to design radiographic procedures around moving grids. When moving grids are used, parallel grids can be used, but focused grids are more common.

Focused grids are in general far superior to parallel grids, but they require care and attention in use. When focused grids are used, the indicators on the x-ray apparatus must be in good adjustment and properly calibrated. The SID indicator, the source-to-tabletop distance (STD) indicator, and the light-localizing collimator must all be properly adjusted.

Selection of a grid with the proper ratio depends on an understanding of three interrelated factors: kVp,

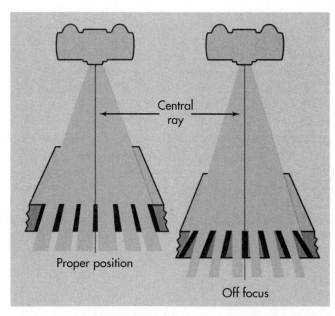

FIGURE 17-15 If a focused grid is not positioned at the specified focal distance, grid cutoff occurs and the optical density (OD) decreases with distance from the central ray.

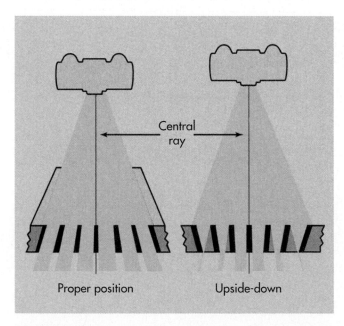

FIGURE 17-16 A focused grid positioned upside-down should be detected on the first radiograph. Complete grid cutoff occurs except in the region of the central ray.

degree of cleanup, and patient dose. When a high kVp is used, high ratio grids should be used as well. Of course, the choice of grid is also influenced by the size and shape of the anatomy being radiographed.

As grid ratio increases, the amount of cleanup also increases. Figure 17-17 shows the approximate percentage of scatter radiation and primary radiation transmitted as a function of grid ratio. Note that the difference between grid ratios of 12:1 and 16:1 is small.

The difference in patient dose is large, however, and therefore, 16:1 grids are not often used. Many general-purpose x-ray examination facilities find that an 8:1 grid is a good compromise between the desired levels of scatter radiation cleanup and patient dose.

> In general, grid ratios up to 8:1 are satisfactory at tube potentials below 90 kVp. Grid ratios above 8:1 are used when kVp exceeds 90 kVp.

The use of one grid also reduces the likelihood of grid cutoff because improper grid positioning can easily accompany frequent changes of grids. In those facilities where high-kVp technique for dedicated chest radiography is used, 16:1 grids can be installed.

Patient Dose

One major disadvantage that accompanies the use of x-ray grids is increased patient dose. For any examination, using a grid may result in several times more radiation to the patient than not using one. The use of a moving grid instead of a stationary grid with similar physical characteristics requires approximately 15% more radiation to the patient. Table 17-4 is a summary of approximate patient doses for various grid techniques with a 400-speed image receptor.

Low-ratio grids are used during mammography. All dedicated mammographic imaging systems are equipped with a 4:1 or a 5:1 ratio moving grid. Even at the low kVp used for mammography, considerable scatter radiation occurs.

The use of such grids greatly improves image contrast, with no loss of spatial resolution. The only disadvantage is the increased patient dose, which can be as much as twice that without a grid. However, with dedicated equipment and grid, patient dose still is very low.

The concern about exposure to the patient is important. Grid selection, however, should not be compromised so much that the loss of contrast enhancement interferes with diagnostic interpretation.

> **GRID SELECTION FACTORS**
> 1. Patient dose increases with increasing grid ratio.
> 2. High-ratio grids are usually used for high-kVp examinations.
> 3. Patient dose at high kVp is less than that at low kVp.

In general, compared with the use of low kVp and low-ratio grids, the use of high-kVp and high-ratio grids results in lower patient doses and radiographs of equal quality.

One additional disadvantage of using grids is the increased radiographic technique required. When a grid is used, the technique factors must be increased over what they were for nongrid examinations: either the mAs or the kVp must be increased. Table 17-5

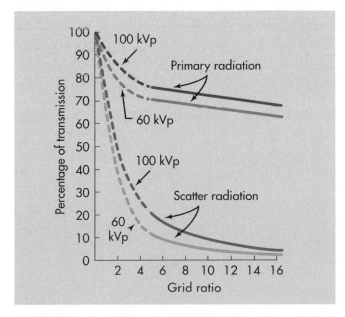

FIGURE 17-17 As grid ratio increases, transmission of scatter radiation decreases faster than transmission of primary radiation. Therefore, cleanup of scatter radiation increases.

TABLE 17-4	Approximate Entrance Skin Dose for Examination of the Adult Pelvis With a 200-Speed Image Receptor		
	ENTRANCE DOSE (mrad)		
Type of Grid	**70 kVp**	**90 kVp**	**110 kVp**
No grid	85	70	50
5:1	270	215	145
8:1	325	285	205
12:1	425	395	290
16:1	520	475	365
5:1 crossed	535	405	295
8:1 crossed	585	530	405

presents approximate changes in technique factors required by standards grids. Usually, the mAs are increased rather than the kVp. One exception to this is chest radiography; increased time can result in motion blur.

Table 17-6 summarizes the clinical factors that should be considered in the selection of various types of grids.

Air-Gap Technique

A clever technique as an alternative to the use of radiographic grids is the **air-gap technique.** The use of the air-gap technique is another method of reducing scatter radiation, thereby enhancing image contrast.

When the air-gap technique is used, the image receptor is moved 10 to 15 cm from the patient (Figure 17-18). A portion of the scattered x-rays generated in the patient would be scattered away from the image receptor and not be detected. Because fewer scattered x-rays interact with the image receptor, the contrast is enhanced.

Usually, when an air-gap technique is used, the mAs are increased approximately 10% for every centimeter of air gap. The technique factors usually are about the same as those for an 8:1 grid. Therefore, the patient dose is higher than that with the nongrid tech-

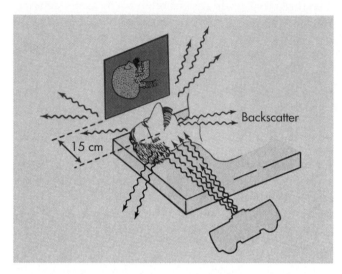

FIGURE 17-18 When the air-gap technique is used, the image receptor is positioned 10 to 15 cm from the patient. A large fraction of the scattered x-rays does not interact with the image receptor.

TABLE 17-5	Approximate Change in Radiographic Technique for Standard Grids	
Grid Ratio	**Milliampere-Second (mAs) Increase**	**Voltage (kVp) Increase**
No grid	1 ×	0
5:1	2 ×	+ 8 to 10
8:1	4 ×	+ 13 to 15
12:1	5 ×	+ 20 to 25
16:1	6 ×	+ 30 to 40

TABLE 17-6	Clinical Considerations in Grid Selection				
		POSITIONING LATITUDE			
Type of Grid	**Degree of Scatter Removal**	**Off Center**	**Off Focus**	**Recommended Technique**	**Remarks**
5:1, linear	+	Very wide	Very wide	Up to 80 kVp	It is the least expensive. It is the easiest to use.
6:1, linear	+	Very wide	Very wide	Up to 80 kVp	It is the least expensive. It is ideally suited for bedside radiography.
8:1, linear	++	Wide	Wide	Up to 100 kVp	It is used for general stationary grids.
10:1, linear	+++	Wide	Wide	Up to 100 kVp	Reasonable care is required for proper alignment.
5:1, crisscross	+++	Narrow	Very wide	Up to 100 kVp	Tube tile is limited to 5 degrees.
12:1, linear	++++	Narrow	Narrow	Over 110 kVp	Extra care is required for proper alignment. It is usually used in fixed mount.
6:1, crisscross	++++	Narrow	Very wide	Up to 110 kVp	It is not suited for tilted-tube techniques.
16:1, linear	+++++	Narrow	Narrow	Over 100 kVp	Extra care is required for proper alignment. It is usually used in fixed mount.
8:1, crisscross	+++++	Narrow	Wide	Up to 120 kVp	It is not suited for tilted-tube techniques.

Adapted from *Characteristics and applications of x-ray grids,* c. 1980, Liebel-Florsheim, Cincinnati.

nique and is approximately equivalent to that of an intermediate grid technique.

 One disadvantage of the air-gap technique is image magnification with associated focal spot blur.

The air-gap technique has found application particularly in areas of chest radiography and cerebral angiography. The magnification that accompanies these techniques is usually acceptable.

In chest radiography, however, some radiologic technologists increase the SID from 180 to 300 cm. This results in very little magnification and a sharper image. Of course, the technique factors must be increased, but the patient dose is not (Figure 17-19).

The air-gap technique is not normally as effective with high-kVp radiography, in which the direction of the scattered x-rays is more forward. At tube potentials below approximately 90 kVp, the scattered x-rays are directed more to the side, and therefore have a higher probability of being scattered away from the image receptor. Nevertheless, at some centers, 120 to 140 kVp air-gap chest radiography is used with good results.

The air-gap technique is sometimes called *air filtration*, but it should be obvious from Figure 17-18 that air filtration is an improper name for this procedure. In the air-gap technique the *air does not act as a filter* of low-energy scattered x-rays; rather, the distance between the patient and the image receptor permits the scattered x-rays to diverge from the image receptor without interaction. Because fewer x-rays reach the image receptor, technique factors must be increased relative to contact radiography.

SUMMARY

Contrast is one of the most important characteristics of the radiographic image. Scatter radiation, the result of Compton interaction, is the primary factor that reduces image contrast. Grids reduce the amount of scatter reaching the image receptor.

The two main components of grid construction are the interspace material (aluminum or plastic fiber) and grid material (lead strips). The principal characteristic of a grid is grid ratio, the height of the grid strip divided by the interspace width. Different grids are selected for use in particular situations. Under 90 kVp, grid ratios of 8:1 and lower are used. Above 90 kVp, grid ratios greater than 8:1 are used.

In all cases, the use of a grid increases patient dose. However, the use of grids combined with use of high-speed radiographic intensifying screens reduces patient radiation dose. Table 17-5 summarizes the changes in grid ratio and changes in mAs or kVp required. Problems can arise with the use of grids, including off-level, off-center, and upside-down grid errors.

An alternative to using a grid is the air-gap technique, in which the image receptor is moved 10 to 15 cm from the patient. Scatter is reduced with this technique because scatter exiting the patient escapes in the air space between the patient and the film.

CHALLENGE QUESTIONS

1. Define or otherwise identify:
   a. Contrast
   b. Remnant radiation
   c. Grid cutoff
   d. Lateral decentering
   e. Selectivity
   f. Air-gap technique
   g. Reciprocating grid
   h. Grid cleanup
   i. Grid focal distance
   j. Contrast improvement factor

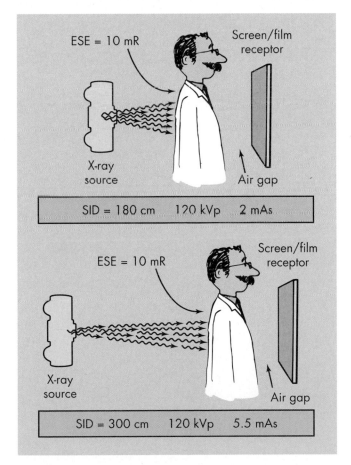

FIGURE 17-19 Increasing the source-to-image receptor distance (SID) to 300 cm from 180 cm improves spatial resolution with no increase in patient dose.

2. With particular reference to materials used and dimensions of various parts, discuss the construction of a grid.

3. A focused grid has the following characteristics: 100 cm focal distance, 27.2 lines/cm, 2.8 mm height, 40 μm grid strips, and 350 μm interspace. What is the grid ratio?

4. A focused grid has the following characteristics: 180 cm focal distance, 12:1 grid ratio, 20 μm grid strips, and 280 μm interspace. What is the grid frequency?

5. A parallel grid has the following characteristics: 14:1 grid ratio, 20 μm grid strips, and 250 μm interspace. What percentage of primary x-rays will this grid absorb?

6. A focused grid has the following characteristics: 100 cm focal distance, 3.2 mm height, 22 μm grid strips, and 26 lines/cm grid frequency. What is the interspace width?

7. What is the grid ratio of the grid described in question 6?

8. What percentage of primary x-rays will the grid described in question 6 absorb?

9. Why does tissue compression reduce image noise?

10. Compared with contact radiography, why does an air-gap technique increase patient dose?

11. What is the effect of scatter radiation on contrast?

12. Why does lowering the kVp increase patient dose?

13. What is the grid ratio for a grid made with 20 μm of lead between 200 μm of aluminum interspace material and a height of 2.5 mm?

14. Why is lead used as the grid strip material of choice?

15. A step-wedge is placed on a tissue phantom and two radiographs are made, one without a grid and one with a 10:1 grid. The contrast on the step-wedge image measures 1.25 without a grid and measures 2.8 with the grid. What is the contrast improvement factor of this 10:1 grid?

16. What is the approximate Bucky factor at 70 kVp for an 8:1 grid?

17. Explain why high-ratio grids have high contrast improvement factors.

18. Draw cross-sectional diagrams of a parallel grid and a focused grid.

19. Explain how grid cutoff can occur.

20. What is the advantage of a moving grid?

Radiographic Exposure

OBJECTIVES

At the completion of this chapter, the student should be able to do the following:

1. List the four prime exposure factors
2. Discuss mAs and kVp in relation to x-ray beam **quantity** and **quality**
3. Describe characteristics of the imaging system that affect x-ray beam quantity and quality

OUTLINE

EXPOSURE FACTORS are a few of the tools that radiographers use to create high-quality radiographs. Radiographic quality and its many components are discussed in Chapter 19. This chapter introduces the student radiographer to the factors that are under the radiographer's control. The prime exposure factors are kVp, mA, exposure time, and source-to-image receptor distance (SID).

Properties of the x-ray imaging system that influence the selection of exposure factors are reviewed, including focal-spot size, total x-ray beam filtration, and the source of high-voltage generation.

TABLE 18-1	Factors Influencing X-ray Quantity and Quality	
AN INCREASE IN THIS FACTOR	**WILL RESULT IN THE FOLLOWING CHANGE IN X-RAY:**	
	Quantity	Quality
Kilovolt peak	Increase	Increase
Milliampere	Increase	No change
Exposure time	Increase	No change
Milliampere-seconds	Increase	No change
Distance	Decrease	No change
Voltage ripple	Decrease	Decrease
Filtration	Decrease	Increase

EXPOSURE FACTORS

Proper exposure of a patient to x-radiation is necessary to produce a diagnostic radiograph. The factors that influence and determine the quantity and quality of x-radiation to which the patient is exposed are called **exposure factors** (Table 18-1). Recall from Chapter 12 that radiation quantity refers to radiation intensity measured in mR or mR/mAs, and radiation quality refers to x-ray beam penetrability, best measured by the half-value layer (HVL).

All of these factors are under the control of the radiologic technologist, except those fixed by the design of the x-ray imaging system. For example, focal-spot size is limited to two selections. Sometimes the added x-ray beam filtration is fixed. The high-voltage generator provides characteristic voltage ripple that cannot be changed.

The four prime exposure factors are kilovolt peak (kVp), current (given in milliamperes [mA]), exposure time, and source-to-image receptor distance (SID). Of these, the most important are kVp and mAs, the factors principally responsible for x-ray quality and quantity. Focal-spot size, distance, and filtration are secondary factors that may require manipulation for particular examinations.

kVp

The effects of kVp on the x-ray beam are described in previous chapters. To understand kVp as an exposure technique factor, assume that kVp is the primary control of beam quality, and therefore **beam penetrability**. A higher-quality x-ray beam is one with higher energy and thus is more likely to penetrate the anatomy of interest.

kVp controls radiographic contrast.

The kVp has more effect than any other factor on image receptor exposure because it affects beam quality and, to a lesser degree, influences beam quantity. With increasing kVp, more x-rays are emitted and they have higher energy and greater penetrability. Unfortunately, because they have higher energy, they also interact more by Compton effect and produce more scatter radiation, which results in increased image noise and reduced image contrast.

The kVp selected greatly determines the number of x-rays in the remnant-forming beam, and hence the resulting average optical density (OD). Finally, and perhaps most important, the kVp controls the scale of contrast on the finished radiograph because as kVp increases, there is less differential absorption and increased image noise. Therefore, high kVp results in reduced image contrast.

mA

The mA station selected for patient exposure determines the number of x-rays produced, and therefore the **radiation quantity.** Recall that the unit of electric current is the ampere (A). One ampere is equal to 1 coulomb (C) of electrostatic charge flowing each second in a conductor, as follows:

AMPERE
$1 A = 1 C/s = 6.3 \times 10^{18}$ electrons per second

Therefore, when the 100-mA station on the operating console is selected, 6.3×10^{17} electrons to flow through the x-ray tube each second.

Question: What is the electron flow from cathode to anode when the 500-mA station is selected?
Answer: 500 mA = 0.5 A
= (0.5 A) (6.3 × 10^{18} electrons/s/A)
= 3.15 × 10^{18} electrons/second

As more electrons flow through the x-ray tube, more x-rays are produced. Assuming a constant exposure time, this relationship is directly proportional. When one changes from 200 mA to 300 mA, the number of electrons flowing through the x-ray tube is increased by 50%. The number of x-rays produced is increased by 50%, and therefore so is patient dose. A change from 200 mA to 400 mA would be a 100% increase or a doubling of the x-ray tube current, a doubling of the x-rays produced, and a doubling of patient dose.

With a constant exposure time, mA controls x-ray quantity and therefore patient dose.

Question: At 200 mA the entrance skin exposure (ESE) is 752 mR (7.5 mGy$_a$). What will be the ESE at 500 mA?

Answer: $ESE = 752 \text{ mR} \left(\dfrac{500 \text{mA}}{200 \text{ mA}} \right)$
$= 1880 \text{ mR}$

A change in mA does not change the kinetic energy of electrons flowing from cathode to anode. It simply changes the number of electrons. Consequently, the energy of the x-rays produced is not changed, only the number is changed.

X-ray quality remains fixed with a change in mA.

Often, x-ray imaging systems are identified by the maximum x-ray tube current possible. Inexpensive radiographic imaging systems designed for private physicians' offices normally have a maximum capacity of 600 mA. The available mA stations may be 50 mA, 100 mA, 200 mA, 300 mA, 400 mA, and 600 mA.

High-power, special-procedure equipment may have a capacity of 1200 mA. The available mA stations are those previously listed plus 800 mA, 1000 mA, and 1200 mA.

Exposure Time

Radiographic exposure times are usually kept as short as possible. The purpose is not to minimize patient radiation dose, but rather to minimize motion blur that can occur because of patient motion.

Short exposure time reduces motion blur.

Producing a diagnostic radiograph requires a certain radiation exposure of the patient. Therefore, when expo-

TABLE 18-2	Relationships Among Different Units of Exposure Time	
Fractional (s)	**Seconds (s)**	**Milliseconds (ms)**
1.0	1.0	1000
4/5	0.8	800
3/4	0.75	750
2/3	0.67	667
3/5	0.6	600
1/2	0.5	500
2/5	0.4	400
1/3	0.33	333
1/4	0.25	250
1/5	0.2	200
1/10	0.1	100
1/20	0.05	50
1/60	0.017	17
1/120	0.008	8

sure time is reduced, the mA must be increased proportionately to provide the required x-ray intensity.

On older x-ray imaging systems, exposure time is expressed in fractional seconds, whereas current x-ray imaging systems identify exposure time in milliseconds (ms). Table 18-2 shows how the different units of time are related.

An easy way to identify an x-ray imaging system as either single phase, three phase, or high frequency is to note the shortest exposure time possible. Single-phase imaging systems cannot produce an exposure time less than ½ cycle or its equivalent 1/120 second or 8 ms. Three-phase and high-frequency generators can normally provide an exposure as short as 1 ms.

mAs and Exposure Time

mA and exposure time (in seconds) are usually combined and used as one mAs factor—in radiographic technique selection. Indeed, many x-ray consoles do not allow the separate selection of mA and exposure time, and permit only mAs selection.

mAs
Milliamperes (mA) × exposure time (s)

Although the radiologic technologist may be required to select an exposure time, it is always selected with consideration of the mA station. The important parameter is the product of the exposure time and tube current.

mAs controls OD.

The mAs value determines the number of x-rays in the primary beam, and therefore it principally controls radiation **quantity** in the same way that mA and exposure time, taken separately, do; it does not influence radiation quality. The mAs setting is the key factor in the control of OD on the radiograph.

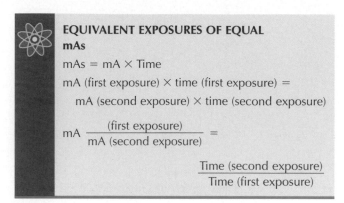

EQUIVALENT EXPOSURES OF EQUAL mAs

mAs = mA × Time

mA (first exposure) × time (first exposure) = mA (second exposure) × time (second exposure)

$$mA \frac{\text{(first exposure)}}{mA \text{ (second exposure)}} = \frac{\text{Time (second exposure)}}{\text{Time (first exposure)}}$$

Question: A radiographic technique calls for 600 mA at 200 ms. What is the mAs value?

Answer: 600 mA × 200 ms = 600 mA × 0.2 s
= 120 mAs

Time and mA can be used to compensate for each other in an indirect fashion. This is described by the following:

Question: A radiograph of the abdomen requires 300 mA and 500 ms. The patient is unable to breath-hold, which results in motion blur. A second exposure is made with an exposure time of 200 ms. Calculate the new mA that is required.

Answer: $\dfrac{x}{300 \text{ mA}} = \dfrac{500 \text{ ms}}{200 \text{ ms}}$

(200 ms)x = (500 ms) (300 mA)

(0.2 s)x = (0.5 s) (300 ms)

(0.2 s)x = 150 mAs

$x = \dfrac{150 \text{ mAs}}{0.2 \text{ s}}$

x = 750 mA

or

New mA = $\dfrac{\text{Original mAs}}{\text{New time}}$

New mA = $\dfrac{0.5 \text{ s} \times 300 \text{ mA}}{0.2 \text{ s}}$

New mA = 750 mA

If the high-voltage generator is properly calibrated, the same mAs value, and therefore the same OD, can be produced with various combinations of mA and exposure time (Table 18-3). This is according to the reciprocity law, which states that OD will be constant for any combination.

mAs are the product of x-ray tube current and exposure time. Because x-ray tube current is electron flow per unit time, the mAs value is therefore simply a measure of the total number of electrons conducted through the x-ray tube for a particular exposure.

TOTAL PROJECTILE ELECTRONS

mA = mC/s

therefore

mAs × = mC/s × s = mC

Question: How many electrons are involved in x-ray production at 100 mAs?

Answer: 100 mAs = 0.1 As = 0.1 C/s × s = 0.1 C
1 C = 6.3 × 10¹⁸ electrons
Therefore, 100 mAs = 6.3 × 10¹⁷ electrons

 mAs is one measure of electrostatic charge.

On an x-ray imaging system in which only mAs can be selected, exposure factors are automatically adjusted to the highest mA at the shortest exposure time allowed by the high-voltage generator. Such a design is called a **falling-load generator.**

Question: A radiologic technologist selects a technique of 200 mAs. The operating console is automatically adjusted to the maximum mA station, 1000 mA. What will be the exposure time?

TABLE 18-3	Products of Milliampere (mA) and Time (ms) for 10 mAs		
mA		**ms**	**mAs**
100	×	100	=	10
200	×	50	=	10
300	×	33	=	10
400	×	25	=	10
600	×	17	=	10
800	×	12	=	10
1000	×	10	=	10

Answer: $\dfrac{200 \text{ mAs}}{1000 \text{ mA}} = 0.2 \text{ s} = 200 \text{ ms}$

(The actual exposure time will be somewhat longer than 200 ms because the tube current falls as the anode heats up.)

Varying the mAs setting changes only the number of electrons conducted during an exposure, not the energy of those electrons. The relationship is directly proportional; a doubling of the mAs doubles the x-ray quantity.

 Only the x-ray quantity is affected by changes in mAs.

Question: A cervical spine examination calls for 68 kVp/30 mAs and results in an ESE of 114 mR (1.14 mGy$_a$). The next patient is examined at 68 kVp/25 mAs. What will be the ESE?

Answer: $\text{ESE} = 114 \text{ mR} \left(\dfrac{25 \text{ mAs}}{30 \text{ mAs}} \right) = 95 \text{ mR}$

Distance

Distance affects exposure of the image receptor according to the inverse square law, which was discussed in Chapter 5. The SID largely determines the intensity of the x-ray beam at the image receptor. *intensity + distance*

 Distance has no effect on radiation quality.

The following relationship, called the direct square law, is derived from the inverse square law. It allows a radiologic technologist to calculate the required change in mAs after a change in SID to maintain constant OD.

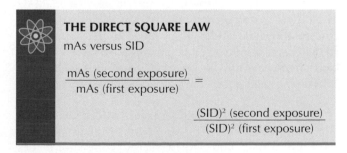

THE DIRECT SQUARE LAW
mAs versus SID

$$\frac{\text{mAs (second exposure)}}{\text{mAs (first exposure)}} = \frac{(\text{SID})^2 \text{ (second exposure)}}{(\text{SID})^2 \text{ (first exposure)}}$$

Note that both the original mAs value and the original SID are in the denominator rather than reversed, as in the inverse square law.

Question: An examination requires 100 mAs at 180 cm SID. If the distance is changed to 90 cm SID, what should be the new mAs setting?

Answer: $\dfrac{x}{100} = \dfrac{90^2}{180^2}$

$x = 100 \left(\dfrac{90}{180} \right)^2$

$= 100 \left(\dfrac{1}{2} \right)^2$

$= 100 \left(\dfrac{1}{4} \right)$

$= 25 \text{ mAs}$

 Distance (SID) affects OD.

When preparing to make a radiographic exposure, the radiologic technologist selects specific settings for each of the factors described: voltage, mAs, and SID. The control panel selections are based on an evaluation of the patient, the thickness of the anatomic part, and the type of accessories used.

Standard SIDs have been in use for many years. For tabletop radiography, 100 cm is common, whereas dedicated chest examination is usually conducted at 180 cm. With advances in generator design and image receptors, even larger SIDs are anticipated. Tabletop radiography at 120 cm and chest radiography at 300 cm are now in use.

The use of a longer SID results in less magnification, less focal spot blur, and improved spatial resolution. However, more mAs must be used because of the effects of the direct square law.

IMAGING SYSTEM CHARACTERISTICS
Focal-Spot Size

Most x-ray tubes are equipped with two focal-spot sizes. On the operating console, they are usually identified as small and large. Conventional tubes have two focal spots of normal size: 0.5 mm/1.0 mm, 0.6 mm/1.2 mm, or 1.0 mm/2.0 mm. X-ray tubes used in interventional procedures or magnification radiography have 0.3 mm/1.0 mm focal spots.

Most mammography tubes have 0.1 mm/0.3 mm focal spots. These are called **microfocus tubes** and are designed specifically for imaging very small microcalcifications at relatively short SIDs.

For normal imaging, the large focal spot is used. This ensures that a sufficient mAs time can be used to image thick or dense body parts. The large focal spot also provides for a shorter exposure time, which minimizes motion blur.

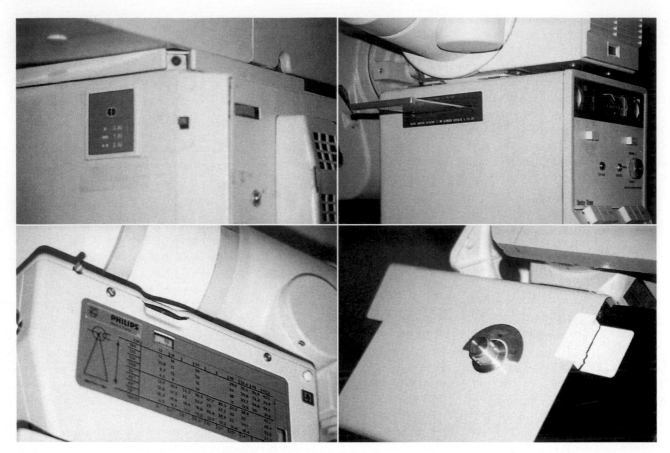

FIGURE 18-1 Examples of selectable added filtration.

One difference between the large and small focal spots is the capacity to produce x-rays. Many more x-rays can be produced with the large focal spot because anode heat capacity is higher. With the small focal spot, electron interaction occurs over a much smaller area of the anode and the resulting heat limits the capacity of x-ray production.

 Changing the focal spot for a given kVp/mAs setting does not change x-ray quantity or quality.

A small focal spot is reserved for fine-detail radiography, in which the quantity of x-rays is relatively low. Small focal spots are always used for magnification radiography. They are normally used during extremity radiography and in examination of other thin body parts in which higher x-ray quantity is not necessary.

Filtration

Inherent Filtration. All x-ray beams are affected by the inherent filtration properties of the glass or metal envelope of the x-ray tube. For general purpose tubes, the value of inherent filtration is approximately 0.5 mm Al equivalent.

The variable-aperture light localizing collimator usually provides an additional 1.0 mm Al equivalent. Most of this is due to the reflective surface of the mirror of the collimator. To meet the required total filtration of 2.5 mm Al, the manufacturer inserts an additional 1-mm Al filter between the x-ray tube housing and the collimator. The radiologic technologist has no control over these sources of filtration but may control stages of added filtration.

Added Filtration. Some x-ray imaging systems have selectable added filtration, as shown in Figure 18-1. Usually, the equipment is placed into service with the lowest allowable added filtration. Radiographic technique charts usually are formulated at the lowest filtration position. If any higher filter position is used, a radiographic technique chart must be developed at that position.

Figure 18-2 shows multiple layers of different filtration material designed for specialty examinations and patient dose reduction. The two sets of collimator blades are open, showing the filters and light field mirror.

Under normal conditions, it is unnecessary to change the filtration. Some facilities may be set for higher filtration during examinations of tissue with high subject contrast, such as extremities, joints, and chest. When

TABLE 18-4	Characteristics of the Various Types of High-Voltage Generators				
				EQUIVALENT TECHNIQUE (kVp/mAs)	
Generator Type	Percentage Ripple	Relative Quantity		Chest	Abdomen
Half-wave	100	100		120/20*	74/40*
Full-wave	100	200		120/20	74/40
3-Phase, 6-pulse	14	260		115/6	72/34
3-Phase, 12-pulse	4	280		115/4	72/30
High-frequency	<1	300		112/3	70/24

*The milliampere-second value equals that for full-wave generator; the exposure time is doubled.

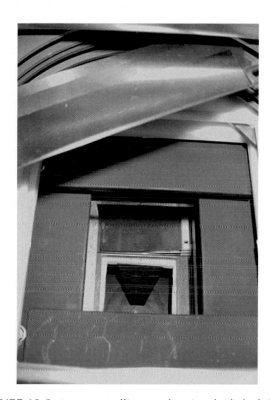

FIGURE 18-2 An open collimator showing the light field mirror and multiple layers of filtration. (Courtesy General Electric Medical Systems.)

properly used, higher filtration for these examinations results in lower patient dose. When filtration is changed, **be sure to return it to its normal position before the next examination.**

As added filtration is increased, the result is increased x-ray beam quality and penetrability. The result on the image is the same as that for increased kVp: more scatter radiation, increased image noise, and reduced image contrast.

High-Voltage Generation

The radiologic technologist **cannot** select the type of high-voltage generator to be used for a given examination. That is fixed by the type of x-ray imaging system. Still, it is important to understand how the various high-voltage generators affect radiographic technique and patient dose.

Three basic types of high-voltage generators are available: single phase, three phase, and high frequency. The radiation quantity and quality produced in the x-ray tube are influenced by the type of high-voltage generator.

Review Figure 8-25 for the shape of the voltage waveform associated with each type of high-voltage generator. Table 18-4 lists the percentage ripple of various types of high-voltage generators, the variation in their output, and the change in the radiographic technique for two common examinations associated with each generator.

Half-Wave Rectification. A half-wave–rectified generator has 100% voltage ripple. During exposure with a half-wave–rectified generator, x-rays are produced and emitted only half of the time. During each negative half-cycle, no x-rays are emitted.

 Half-wave rectification results in the same radiation quality as that for full-wave rectification, but the radiation quantity is halved.

Half-wave rectification is rarely used. Some mobile x-ray imaging systems and most dental x-ray imaging systems are half-wave rectified. No general-purpose x-ray imaging systems have this type of high-voltage generator.

Full-Wave Rectification. The voltage waveform for full-wave rectification is identical to half-wave rectification, except there is no dead time. During exposure, x-rays are continually emitted as pulses. Consequently, the required exposure time for full-wave rectification is only half that for half-wave rectification.

 The radiation quality does not change when going from half-wave to full-wave rectification; however, the radiation quantity doubles.

Three-Phase Power. Three-phase power comes in two principal forms: 6 pulse or 12 pulse. The difference is determined by the manner in which the high-voltage step-up transformer is engineered.

 Three-phase power results in higher x-ray quantity and quality.

The difference between the two forms is minor but does cause a detectable change in x-ray quantity and quality. Three-phase power is more efficient than single-phase power. More x-rays are produced for a given mAs setting, and the average energy of those x-rays is higher. The x-radiation emitted is nearly constant rather than pulsed.

High-Frequency Generation. High-frequency generators were developed in the early 1980s and are increasingly used. The voltage waveform is nearly constant, with less than 1% ripple.

 High-frequency generation results in even higher x-ray quantity and quality.

At present, high-frequency generators are being increasingly used with dedicated mammography systems, computed tomography systems, and mobile x-ray imaging systems. It is likely that most high-voltage generators of the future will be of the high-frequency type, regardless of the required power levels.

SUMMARY

Radiographic exposure factors (voltage, mAs, and distance) are manipulated by radiologic technologists to produce high-quality radiographs. The exposure factors influence quantity (number of x-rays) and quality (penetrability of the x-rays). Proper selection of these exposure factors optimizes both the spatial resolution and contrast resolution of the image.

CHALLENGE QUESTIONS

1. Define or otherwise identify:
   a. Kilovolt peak (kVp)
   b. Milliampere-second (mAs)
   c. Beam penetrability
   d. Radiation quality
   e. Source-to-image receptor distance (SID)
   f. Inherent filtration
   g. Falling-load generator
   h. High-voltage ripple
   i. Added filtration
   j. Radiation quantity
2. Discuss how an increase in kVp changes x-ray quantity, x-ray quality, and contrast scale.
3. What mAs stations are typically available on an operating console?
4. What is normally the shortest radiographic exposure time on single-phase, three-phase, and high-frequency imaging systems?
5. Describe how a change in SID from 100 cm to 180 cm should be accompanied by a change in mA and exposure time.
6. Why does an x-ray tube have two focal-spot sizes?
7. Discuss how an increase in mAs changes x-ray quantity, x-ray quality, and contrast scale.
8. Discuss the components of total x-ray beam filtration.
9. A radiographic technique calls for 800 mA at 50 ms. What is the mAs setting?
10. The normal lateral chest technique is 120 kVp, 100 mA, 15 ms. To reduce motion blur, the radiologic technologist shortens the exposure time to 5 ms. What is the new mA?
11. Explain the following statement: Changing the mA does not change the kinetic energy of electrons flowing across the x-ray tube.
12. Why is it important to keep exposure time as short as possible?
13. Write three mA and time exposure factors that equal 100 mAs. Explain the advantages of each exposure factor choice.
14. An examination requires 78 kVp/150 mAs at 100 cm SID. If the distance is changed to 180 cm, what should be the new mAs setting?
15. Describe the two focal spots available in x-ray tubes? Explain how each is typically used.
16. List the three types of high-voltage generators.
17. Explain how high-voltage generation influences x-ray beam quantity and quality.
18. What is the nature of variable x-ray beam filtration?
19. What is the principal advantage of exposure with a large focal spot compared with a small focal spot?
20. Identify each control and meter on an x-ray imaging system that you operate

CHAPTER

19

Image Quality

OBJECTIVES

At the completion of this chapter, the student should be able to do the following:

1. Define radiographic quality, resolution, noise, and speed
2. Interpret the shape of the characteristic curve
3. Identify the toe, shoulder, and straight-line portion of the characteristic curve
4. Distinguish the geometric factors affecting image quality
5. Analyze the subject factors affecting image quality
6. Examine the tools and techniques available to create high-quality images

OUTLINE

DEFINITIONS
Radiographic Quality

The term **radiographic quality** refers to the fidelity with which the anatomic structure being examined is imaged on the radiograph. A radiograph that faithfully reproduces structure and tissues is identified as a **high-quality radiograph.**

The radiologist needs high-quality radiographs to make accurate diagnoses. Poor-quality radiographs contain images that are difficult for the human eye to interpret. They can lead to reexamination or, sometimes, missed diagnoses.

The quality of a radiograph is not easy to define and it cannot be measured precisely. A number of factors affect radiographic quality, but there are no precise, universally accepted measures by which to judge it. The most important characteristics of radiographic quality are **spatial resolution, contrast resolution, noise,** and **artifacts.** Artifacts are discussed in Chapter 32.

Resolution

Resolution is the ability to image two separate objects and visually distinguish one from the other. **Spatial resolution** refers to the ability to image small objects that have high subject contrast, such as a bone–soft tissue interface, a breast microcalcification, or a calcified lung nodule. Conventional radiography has excellent spatial resolution. The measure of spatial resolution is discussed more completely in Chapter 29.

 Spatial resolution improves as screen blur decreases, motion blur decreases, and geometric blur decreases.

Contrast resolution is the ability to distinguish anatomic structures of similar subject contrast such as liver–spleen and gray matter–white matter. The actual size of objects that can be imaged will always be smaller under condi-

tions of high contrast than under conditions of low contrast. Computed tomography has excellent contrast resolution, and magnetic resonance imaging is even better.

Less precise terms, **detail** or **recorded detail,** are sometimes used instead of spatial and contrast resolution. These terms refer to the degree of sharpness of structural lines on a radiograph. **Visibility of detail** refers to the ability to visualize recorded detail when image contrast and optical density (OD) are optimized.

Noise

"Noise" is a term borrowed from electrical engineering. The flutter, hum, and whistle heard from a stereo system is **audio noise** that is inherent in the design of the system. The "snow" on television screens, especially in weak signal areas, is **video noise,** and it too is inherent in the system.

 Radiographic noise is the random fluctuation in the OD of the image.

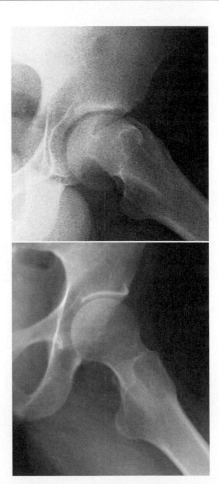

FIGURE 19-1 A, This hip radiograph demonstrates the mottled, grainy appearance associated with quantum mottle resulting from a low number of x-rays being used to produce the image. **B,** In comparison, an optimal hip image shows greater recorded detail. (Courtesy Tim Gienapp.)

Radiographic noise also is inherent in the imaging system (Figure 19-1). A number of factors contribute to radiographic noise, including some that are under the control of the radiologic technologist. Lower noise results in a better radiographic image because it improves contrast resolution.

Radiographic noise has four components: film graininess, structure mottle, quantum mottle, and scatter radiation. We discussed the principal source of radiographic noise–scatter radiation–in Chapters 17 and 18.

Film graininess refers to the distribution in size and space of the silver halide grains in the emulsion. **Structure mottle** is similar to film graininess but refers to the phosphor of the radiographic intensifying screen. Film graininess and structure mottle are inherent in the image receptor. They are not under the control of the radiologic technologist and they contribute very little to radiographic noise, with the exception of mammography.

Quantum mottle is somewhat under the control of the radiologic technologist and is a principal contributor to radiographic noise in many radiographic imaging procedures. Quantum mottle refers to the random nature in which x-rays interact with the image receptor.

If an image is produced with just a few x-rays, the quantum mottle will be higher than if the image is formed from a large number of x-rays. The use of very fast intensifying screens results in increased quantum mottle.

The use of high mAs, low kVp settings, and slower image receptors reduces quantum mottle.

Quantum mottle is like sowing grass seed. If very little seed is broadcast, the resulting grass will be thin, with only a few blades. Likewise, when fewer x-rays are "cast" at the image receptor, the resulting image appears mottled or blotchy. On the other hand, if a lot of seed is cast, the resulting grass will be thick and smooth. In the same way, when more x-rays interact with the image receptor, the image appears smooth, like a lush lawn.

Speed

Two of the characteristics of radiographic quality, resolution and noise, are intimately connected with a third characteristic—**speed.** Although the speed of the image receptor is not apparent on the radiographic image, it very much influences resolution and noise. In fact, a variation in any one of these characteristics alters the other two (Figure 19-2). As a general rule, the following apply:

RADIOGRAPHIC QUALITY RULES
1. Fast image receptors have high noise and low spatial resolution and contrast resolution.
2. High spatial resolution and contrast resolution require low noise and slow image receptors.
3. Low noise accompanies slow image receptors with high spatial resolution and contrast resolution.

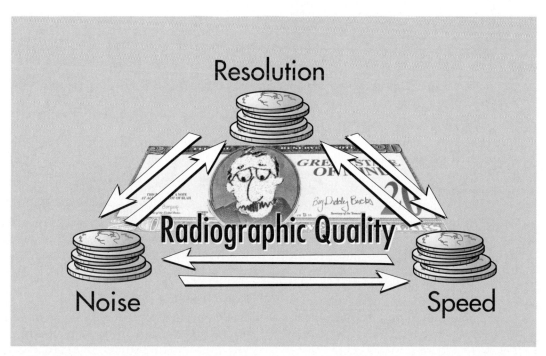

FIGURE 19-2 Resolution, noise, and speed are interrelated characteristics of radiographic quality.

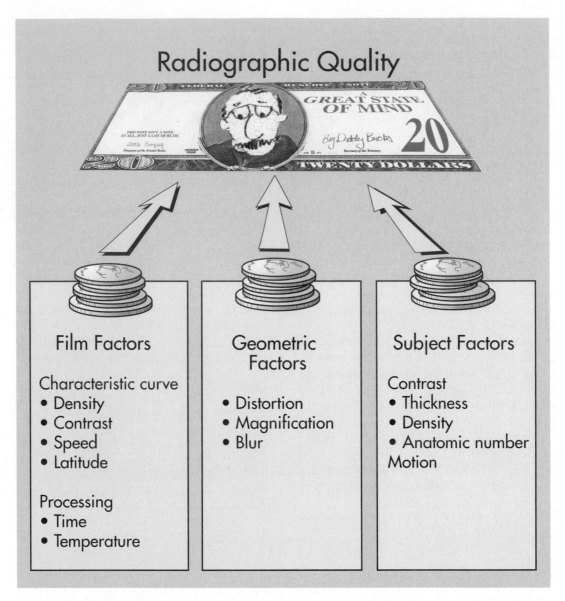

FIGURE 19-3 Organization chart of principal factors affecting radiographic quality.

The radiologic technologist is provided with all the physical tools required to produce high-quality radiographs. The skillful radiologic technologist properly manipulates these tools according to each specific clinical situation.

In general, the quality of a radiograph is directly related to an understanding of the basic principles of x-ray physics and the factors affecting radiographic quality. Figure 19-3 is an organizational chart of the principal factors affecting radiographic quality, most of which are under the control of the radiologic technologist. Each is considered in detail in this chapter.

FILM FACTORS

Unexposed x-ray film that has been processed appears quite lucent, like frosted window glass. It easily trans-

mits light but not images. On the other hand, exposed, processed x-ray film can be quite opaque. Properly exposed film appears with various shades of gray and heavily exposed film appears black.

The study of the relationship between the intensity of exposure of the film and the blackness after processing is called *sensitometry*. Knowledge of the sensitometric aspects of radiographic film is essential to maintain adequate quality control.

Characteristic Curve

The two principal measurements involved in sensitometry are the exposure to the film and the percentage of light transmitted through the processed film. Such measurements are used to describe the relationship between **OD** and radiation exposure. This relationship is

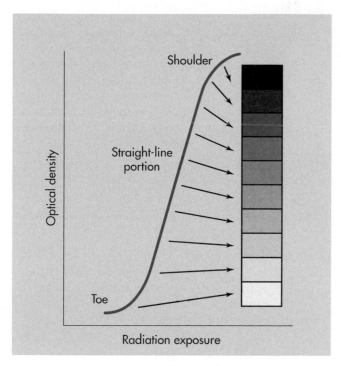

FIGURE 19-4 Characteristic curve of radiographic film is the graphic relationship between optical density (OD) and exposure.

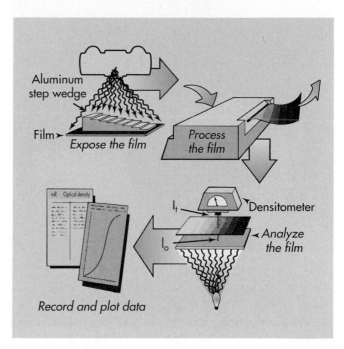

FIGURE 19-5 Steps involved in the construction of a characteristic curve.

called a **characteristic curve** or sometimes the H & D curve after Hurter and Driffield, who first described this relationship.

A typical characteristic curve is shown in Figure 19-4. At low and high exposure levels, large variations in exposure result in only a small change in OD. These portions of the characteristic curve are called the **toe** and **shoulder,** respectively.

At intermediate exposure levels, small changes in exposure result in large changes in OD. This intermediate region, called the **straight-line portion,** is the region in which a properly exposed radiograph appears.

Two pieces of apparatus are needed to construct a characteristic curve: an optical step wedge, sometimes called a **sensitometer,** and a **densitometer,** a device that measures OD. The steps involved are outlined in Figure 19-5, where an aluminum step wedge, or penetrameter, is shown as an alternative to the sensitometer. Figure 19-6 shows how these quality control devices appear.

First the film under investigation is exposed— flashed—through the sensitometer. When processed, the film will have areas of increasing OD corresponding to optical wedge steps. The sensitometer is fabricated so that the relative intensity of light exposure to the film under each step can be determined.

The processed film is analyzed in the densitometer, a device that has a light source focused through a pin-

hole. A light-sensing device is positioned on the opposite side of the film. The radiographic film is positioned between the pinhole and the light sensor and the amount of light transmitted through each step of the radiographic image is measured. These data are recorded and analyzed and, when plotted, result in a characteristic curve.

Radiographic film is sensitive over a wide range of exposures. Film-screen, for example, responds to radiation intensities from under 1 to over 1000 mR (0.01 to 10 mGy$_a$). Consequently, the exposure values for a characteristic curve are presented in logarithmic fashion.

Furthermore, it is not the absolute exposure that is of interest but rather the change in OD over each exposure interval. Therefore, **log relative exposure (LRE)** is used as the scale along the x-axis.

Figure 19-7 shows the exposure in mR, the LRE, and the relative mAs for a representative film-screen combination. The LRE scale is usually presented in increments of 0.3 because the log of 2, doubling the exposure, is 0.3. Doubling the exposure can be achieved by doubling the mAs, as the x-axis scale in Figure 19-7 shows.

An increase in LRE of 0.3 results from doubling the radiation exposure.

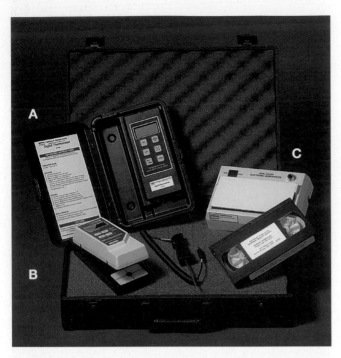

FIGURE 19-6 The digital thermometer **(A)**, densitometer **(B)**, and sensitometer **(C)** are tools necessary for fabricating a characteristic curve and for routine quality control. (Courtesy Cardinal Health.)

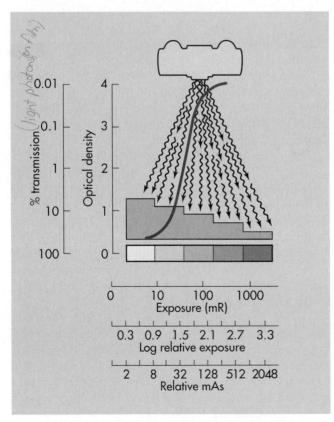

FIGURE 19-7 Relationship among log relative exposure (LRE) and relative milliampere-seconds for typical film-screen combination. Relationship between percentage transmission and optical density (OD) is shown along the y-axis.

Optical Density

It is not enough to say that OD is the degree of blackening of a radiograph or that a clear area of the radiograph represents low OD and a black area represents high OD. OD has a precise numeric value that can be calculated if the level of light incident on a processed film (I_o) and the level of light transmitted through that film (I_t) can be measured. The OD is defined as follows:

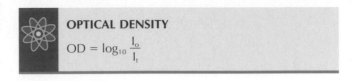

OPTICAL DENSITY

$$OD = \log_{10} \frac{I_o}{I_t}$$

Question: The lung field of a chest radiograph transmits only 0.15% of incident light as determined with a densitometer. What is the OD?

Answer: 0.15% = 0.0015

$$OD = \log_{10} \frac{1}{0.0015}$$
$$= 2.8$$

OD is a logarithmic function. Logarithms allow a wide range of values to be expressed by small numbers. Radiographic film contains ODs ranging from near 0 to 4. These ODs correspond to clear and black, respectively. An OD of 4 actually means that only 1 in 10,000 light photons (10^4) is capable of penetrating the x-ray film. Table 19-1 shows the range of light transmission corresponding to various levels of OD.

Question: The OD of a region of a lung field is 2.5. What percentage of visible light is transmitted through that region of the image?

Answer: Reference to Table 19-1 shows that an OD = 2.5 is equal to 2 of every 625 light photons being transmitted, or 0.32%.

High-quality glass has an OD of zero, which means that all light incident on such glass is transmitted. Unexposed radiographic film allows no more than approximately 80% of incident light photons to be transmitted. Most unexposed and processed radiographic film has an OD in the range of 0.1 to 0.3, corresponding to 79% and 50% transmission, respectively.

These ODs of unexposed film are due to **base density** and **fog density** (Figure 19-8). The base density is the OD inherent in the base of the film. It is due to the composition of the base and the tint added to the base to make the radiograph more pleasing to the eye. Base density has a value of approximately 0.1.

Fog density has been previously described as the development of silver grains that contain no useful informa-

TABLE 19-1	Relationship of Optical Density of Radiographic Film to Light Transmission Through the Film		
Percent of Light Transmitted	**Fraction of Light Transmitted**	**Optical Density**
($I_t/I_o \times 100$)	(I_t/I_o)	($\log I_o/I_t$)
100	1	0
50	1/2	0.3
32	8/25	0.5
25	1/4	0.6
12.5	1/8	0.9
10	1/10	1
5	1/20	1.3
3.2	4/25	1.5
2.5	1/30	1.6
1.25	1/80	1.9
1	1/100	2
0.5	1/200	2.3
0.32	2/625	2.5
0.125	1/800	2.9
0.1	1/1000	3
0.05	1/2000	3.3
0.032	1/3125	3.5
0.01	1/10,000	4

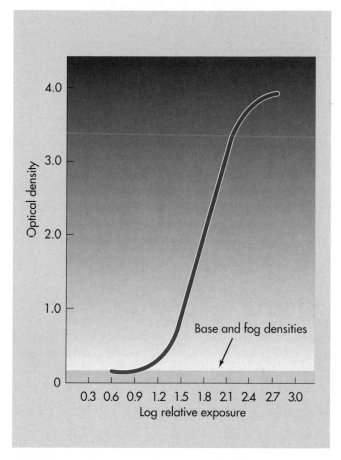

FIGURE 19-8 Base and fog densities reduce radiographic contrast and should be as low as possible.

tion. Fog density results from inadvertent exposure of film during storage, undesirable chemical contamination, improper processing, and a number of other influences. Fog density on a processed radiograph should not exceed 0.2.

 Higher fog density reduces the contrast of the radiographic image.

Question: The light incident on the radiograph of a long bone has a relative value of 1500. If the light transmitted through the radiopaque bony structures has an intensity of 480 (relatively white) and the light transmitted through the radiolucent soft tissue has an intensity of 2 (relatively black), what are the approximate respective ODs? Refer to Table 19-1 if necessary.

Answer: $OD = \log_{10} \dfrac{I_o}{I_t}$

a. For bone:

$$OD = \log_{10} \frac{1500}{480} = 0.5$$

b. For soft tissue:

$$OD = \log_{10} \frac{1500}{2} = 2.9$$

The useful range of OD is approximately 0.25 to 2.5. Most radiographs, however, show image patterns in the range of 0.5 to 1.25 OD. Attention to this part of the characteristic curve is essential. However, very low OD may be too light to contain an image pattern, whereas very high OD requires a hot light to view the image.

 Base plus fog OD has a range of approximately 0.1 to 0.3.

The most useful range of OD is highly dependent on viewbox illumination, viewing conditions, and the shape of the characteristic curve. For example, with high-contrast mammography image receptors, high-luminance viewboxes, and good viewing conditions, the most useful OD range is approximately 0.25 to 2.5 with gross features and as high as 3.5 with fine features such as skin lines.

Reciprocity Law. One would think that the OD on a radiograph would depend strictly on the total exposure (mAs), and be independent of the time of exposure. This, in fact, is the reciprocity law. Whether a radiograph is made with short exposure time or long exposure time, the reciprocity law states that the OD will be the same if the mAs value is constant.

 The reciprocity law states that the OD on a radiograph is proportional only to the total energy imparted to the radiographic film.

The reciprocity law holds for direct exposure with x-rays, but it does not hold for exposure of film by the visible light from radiographic intensifying screens. Consequently, **the reciprocity law fails for screen-film exposures** at exposure times less than approximately 10 ms or longer than approximately 5 s.

OD is somewhat less at such short or long exposure times than exposure times within that range, even though the radiation exposure is the same. The reciprocity law is important for some special procedures that require very short or very long exposure times, such as interventional radiography and mammography, respectively. For these few situations, increasing the mAs setting may be required if the automatic exposure control does not compensate for reciprocity law failure.

Contrast. When a high-quality radiograph is placed on an illuminator, the differences in OD are obvious in the image. Such OD variations are called **radiographic contrast.** A radiograph that has marked differences in OD is a high-contrast radiograph. On the other hand, if the OD differences are small and not distinct, the radiograph is of low contrast. Figure 19-9 illustrates the difference between high contrast and low contrast with a photograph.

Radiographic contrast is the product of two separate factors:

1. **Image receptor contrast** is inherent in the screen-film combination and influenced somewhat by processing of the film.
2. **Subject contrast** is determined by the size, shape, and x-ray–attenuating characteristics of the anatomy being examined and the energy (kVp) of the x-ray beam.

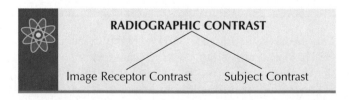

Radiographic contrast can be greatly affected by changes in either image receptor contrast or subject contrast. In the clinical setting, it is usually best to standardize the image receptor contrast and alter the subject contrast according to the needs of the examination. Subject contrast is dealt with in greater detail later.

Image receptor contrast is inherent in the type of film and radiographic intensifying screen being used. It can,

however, be influenced by two other factors: the range of ODs and the film processing technique.

Film selection is usually limited and determined somewhat by the intensifying screen used. Film-screen images always have higher contrast than direct exposure images.

The best control the radiologic technologist can exercise is exposing the image receptor properly so that the ODs lie within the diagnostically useful range, 0.25 to 2.5, and a bit higher in mammography. When the exposure of the image receptor results in an OD outside this range, contrast is lost because the image is in either the toe or the shoulder of the characteristic curve (Figure 19-10).

Standardized film processing techniques are absolutely necessary for consistent film contrast and good radiographic quality. Deviation from the manufacturer's recommendations results in reduced contrast.

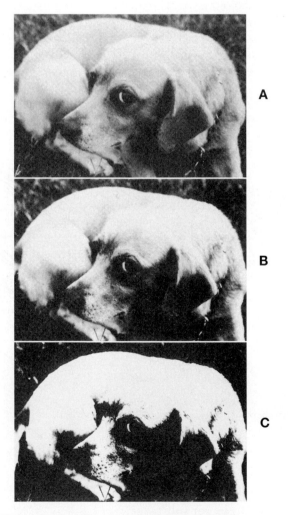

FIGURE 19-9 This vicious guard dog posed to demonstrate differences in contrast. **A,** Low contrast. **B,** Moderate contrast. **C,** High contrast. (Courtesy Butterscotch.)

Film contrast is related to the slope of the straight-line portion of the characteristic curve.

The characteristic curve of an image receptor allows one to judge at a glance the relative degree of contrast. If the slope or steepness of the straight-line portion of the characteristic curve had a value of 1, then it would be angled at 45 degrees. An increase of 1 unit along the LRE axis would result in an increase of 1 unit along the OD axis. The contrast would be 1.

An image receptor that has a contrast of 1 has very low contrast. Image receptors with a contrast higher than 1 amplify the subject contrast during x-ray examination. An image receptor with a contrast of 3, for instance, would show large OD differences over a small range of x-ray exposure.

In general, it is not necessary for the radiologic technologist to have a precise knowledge of image receptor contrast. However, from the appearance of the characteristic curve, the technologist should be able to distinguish high-contrast image receptors from low-contrast image receptors.

Figure 19-11 shows the characteristic curves for two different image receptors. Image receptor A has higher contrast than B, as shown by the fact that the slope of

the straight-line portion of the characteristic curve is steeper for A than for B.

Several methods are used to numerically specify image receptor contrast. The one most often used is **average gradient**. The average gradient is the slope of a straight line drawn between the two points on the characteristic curve at ODs 0.25 and 2.0 above base and fog densities. This is the approximate useful range of OD on most radiographs.

 IMAGE RECEPTOR CONTRAST

$$\text{Average gradient} = \frac{OD_2 - OD_1}{LRE_2 - LRE_1}$$

where OD_2 is the optical density of 2.0 plus base and fog densities, OD_1 is the optical density of 0.25 plus base and fog densities, and LRE_2 and LRE_1 are the LREs associated with OD_2 and OD_1, respectively.

This method is diagrammed in Figure 19-12 for a film having a combined base and fog density of 0.1.

Most radiographic image receptors have an average gradient in the range of 2.5 to 3.5. Because of this, the image receptor acts as an amplifier of subject contrast. The range of the number of x-rays producing the latent image is effectively expanded and the subject contrast is enhanced.

Question: A radiographic film has a base density of 0.06 and a fog density of 0.11. At what

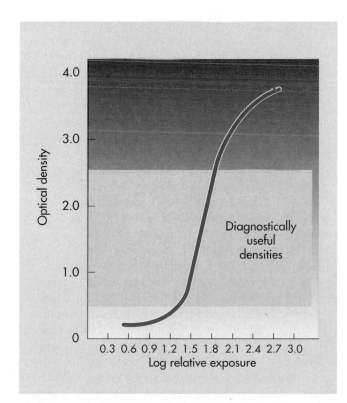

FIGURE 19-10 If the exposure of the film results in optical densities (OD) that lie in the toe or shoulder regions, where the slope of the curve is less, contrast is reduced.

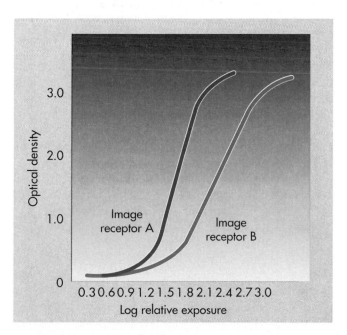

FIGURE 19-11 Slope of the straight-line portion of the characteristic curve is greater for image receptor A than for image receptor B. Image receptor A has higher contrast.

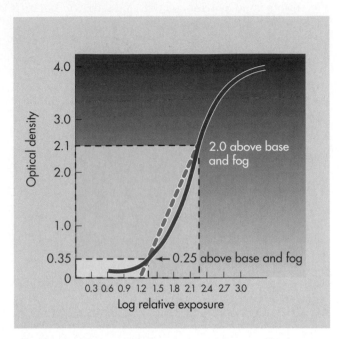

FIGURE 19-12 Average gradient is the slope of the line drawn between the points on the characteristic curve that correspond to the optical density (OD) levels 0.25 and 2.0 above base and fog densities.

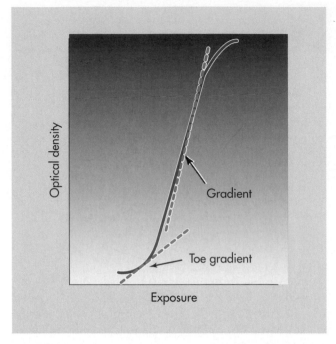

FIGURE 19-13 Gradient is the slope of the tangent at any point on the characteristic curve. Toe gradient is most important clinically.

ODs should one evaluate the characteristic curve to determine the film contrast?

Answer: The curve should be evaluated at OD 0.25 and 2.0 above base plus fog densities. Therefore, at ODs of:
$$OD_1 = 0.06 + 0.11 + 0.25 = 0.42$$
and
$$OD_2 = 0.06 + 0.11 + 2.0 = 2.17$$

Image receptor contrast may also be identified by **gradient**. The gradient is the slope of the tangent *at any point* on the characteristic curve (Figure 19-13). **Toe gradient** is probably more important than average gradient for general radiography because many clinical ODs appear in the toe region of the characteristic curve. **Midgradient** or **shoulder gradient** is more important for mammography.

Question: If the ODs of 0.42 and 2.17 on the characteristic curve in the preceding example correspond to LREs of 0.95 and 1.75, what is the average gradient?

Answer: Average gradient $= \dfrac{OD_2 - OD_1}{LRE_2 - LRE_1}$

$$= \frac{2.17 - 0.42}{1.75 - 0.95}$$

$$= \frac{1.75}{0.8}$$

$$= 2.19$$

Note that the numerator in the expression for average gradient always equals 1.75.

Another way to evaluate image receptor contrast is to replot the data of a characteristic curve (an H & D curve) into a H & H contrast curve, as done in Figure 19-14. "H & H" stands for Art Haus and Ed Hendrick, the medical physicists who first demonstrated this technique.

Speed. The ability of an image receptor to respond to a low x-ray exposure is a measure of its **sensitivity** or, more commonly, its **speed**. An exposure of less than 1 mR can be detected with a film-screen combination, whereas several mR are necessary to produce a measurable exposure with direct-exposure film.

The characteristic curve of an image receptor is also useful in identifying speed. Figure 19-15 shows the characteristic curves of two different image receptors. Because image receptor A requires less exposure than B to produce any OD, A is faster than B.

The characteristic curve of a fast image receptor is positioned to the left—closer to the y-axis—of that of a slow image receptor. Radiographic image receptors are identified as either fast or slow according to their sensitivity to x-ray exposure.

Usually the identification of a given image receptor as so many times faster than another is sufficient for the radiologic technologist. If A were twice as fast as B, image receptor A would require only half the mAs required by B to produce a given OD. Moreover, the image on image receptor A might be of poor quality because of increased radiographic noise.

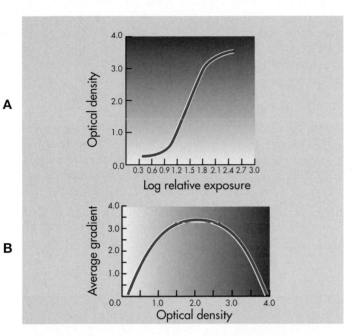

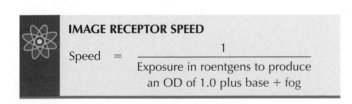

FIGURE 19-14 When the gradient of the characteristic curve (A) is plotted as a function of optical density, a contrast curve (B) results.

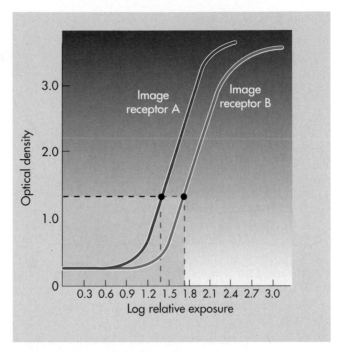

FIGURE 19-15 Speed of an image receptor is the reciprocal of the exposure, in roentgens, needed to produce an optical density (OD) of 1.0 above base plus fog. Image receptor A is faster than image receptor B (speed A = 1/1.3 = 0.78 R⁻¹; speed B = 1/1.6 = 0.63 R⁻¹).

When numbers are used to express speed, all are relative to 100, termed "par speed." Numbers higher than 100 refer to fast or high-speed image receptors. Numbers less than 100 refer to "detail" image receptors.

Do not be deceived that slower image receptors are better because they have less noise. Slower image receptors also require more patient radiation dose. A balance is required.

In sensitometry, the OD specified for determining image receptor speed is 1.0 above base plus fog density and the speed is measured in **reciprocal roentgens (1/R)** as follows:

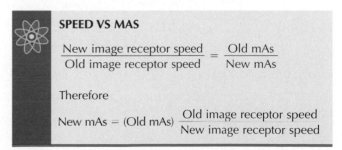

IMAGE RECEPTOR SPEED

$$\text{Speed} = \frac{1}{\text{Exposure in roentgens to produce an OD of 1.0 plus base + fog}}$$

Question: The characteristic curve of a given screen-film shows that 10 mR is needed to produce an OD of 1.0 above base plus fog density on that image receptor. What is the image receptor speed?

Answer: $\text{Speed} = \dfrac{1}{10\text{mR}} = \dfrac{1}{0.01\text{R}} = 100 \text{ R}^{-1}$

Question: How much exposure is required to produce an OD of 1.0 above base plus fog density on a 600 speed image receptor?

Answer: $\text{Speed} = \dfrac{1}{\text{exposure}}$

$\text{Exposure} = \dfrac{1}{\text{speed}}$

$= \dfrac{1}{600}$

$= 0.00167 \text{ R}$

$= 1.7 \text{ mR}$

When imaged receptors are replaced, a change in the mAs setting may be necessary to maintain the same OD. For example, if image receptor speed is doubled, the mAs must be halved. No change is required in kVp. This relationship is expressed as follows:

SPEED VS MAS

$$\frac{\text{New image receptor speed}}{\text{Old image receptor speed}} = \frac{\text{Old mAs}}{\text{New mAs}}$$

Therefore

$$\text{New mAs} = (\text{Old mAs})\frac{\text{Old image receptor speed}}{\text{New image receptor speed}}$$

Question: A posterior-anterior chest examination requires 120 kVp/8 mAs with a 250 speed image receptor. What radiographic technique should be used with a 400 speed image receptor?

Answer: New mAs = (8 mAs) $\dfrac{250}{400}$

$$= 5 \text{ mAs}$$

Therefore, the new technique is 120 kVp/5 mAs

Latitude. An additional image receptor feature easily obtained from the characteristic curve is the latitude. Latitude refers to the range of exposures over which the image receptor responds with ODs in the diagnostically useful range.

Latitude can also be thought of as the margin of error in technical factors. With wider latitude, the mAs can vary more and still result in a diagnostic image. Figure 19-16 shows two image receptors with different latitudes. Image receptor *B* responds to a much wider range of exposures than *A* and is said to have a wider latitude than *A*.

 Latitude and contrast are inversely proportional.

Image receptors with wide latitude are said to have **long gray scale** and those with narrow latitude have **short gray scale.** When slopes of the curves in Figure 19-16 are compared, it should be clear that a high-contrast image receptor has narrow latitude and a low-contrast image receptor has wide latitude.

Film Processing

Proper film processing is required for optimal image receptor contrast because the degree of development has a pronounced effect on the level of fog density and on the ODs resulting from a given exposure at a given image receptor speed. The important factors affecting the degree of development are listed in Box 19-1.

Development Time. As development time is varied, the characteristic curve for any film changes in shape and position along the LRE axis (Figure 19-17). If the

> **BOX 19-1   Factors Affecting the Finished Radiograph**
>
> The concentration of processing chemicals
> The degree of chemistry agitation during development
> The development time
> The development temperature

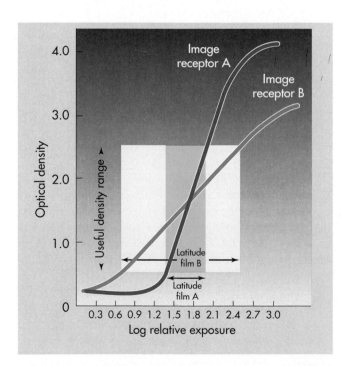

FIGURE 19-16 The latitude of an image receptor is the exposure range over which it responds with diagnostically useful optical density (OD).

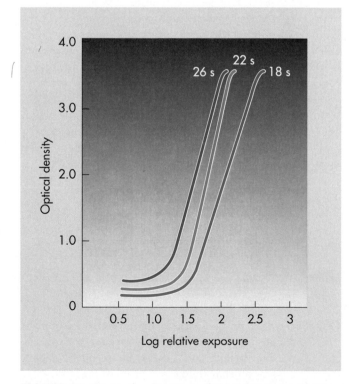

FIGURE 19-17 As development of time increases, changes occur in the shape and relative position of the characteristic curve.

characteristic curves were analyzed for contrast, speed, and fog level, each would be shown to vary as in Figure 19-18. Speed and fog increase with longer development time.

The development time recommended by the manufacturer is the time that will result in maximum contrast, at relatively high speed and with low levels of fog. When development time extends far beyond the recommended period, the image receptor contrast decreases, the relative speed increases, and the fog level increases.

Development Temperature. The relationships just described for variations in development time apply equally well to variations in development temperature. When the average gradient, speed, and fog level for any film are plotted as a function of development temperature, the results appears as in Figure 19-18.

As with time of development, the maximum contrast is obtained at the recommended development temperature. The fog level increases with increasing temperature, as does the image receptor speed.

Within a small range, a change in either time or temperature can be compensated for by a change in the other. However, a small change in either time or temperature alone can result in a large change in the sensitometric characteristics of the image receptor.

GEOMETRIC FACTORS

Making a radiograph is similar in many ways to taking a photograph. Proper exposure time and intensity are required for both processes. Images are recorded in both because the x-rays and the visible light photons travel in straight lines.

In that regard, an x-ray image may be considered analogous to a shadowgraph. Figure 19-19 shows the familiar shadowgraph that can be made to appear on a wall if light is shone on a properly contorted hand.

The sharpness of the shadow image on the wall is a function of a number of geometric factors. For example, the closer to the wall the hand is placed, the sharper the shadow image. Similarly, as the light source is moved farther from the hand, the shadow becomes sharper.

These geometric conditions also apply to the production of high-quality radiographs. Three principal geometric factors affect radiographic quality: magnification, distortion, and focal-spot blur.

GEOMETRIC FACTORS

Magnification
Distortion
Focal-spot blur

Magnification

All images on the radiograph are larger than the object they represent, a condition called **magnification.** For most clinical examinations, the smallest magnification possible should be maintained.

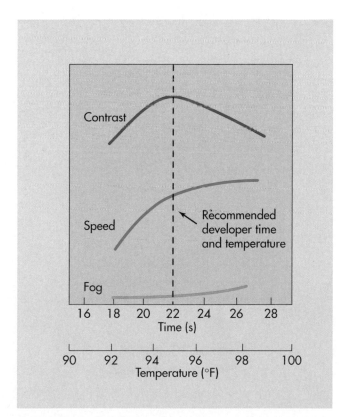

FIGURE 19-18 Analysis of characteristic curves at various development times and temperatures yields these relationships for contrast, speed, and fog for 90-second automatically processed film.

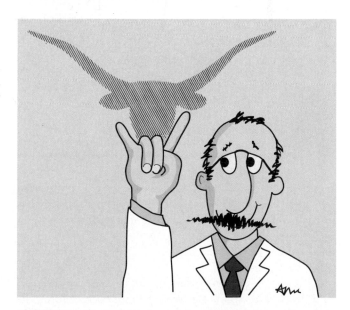

FIGURE 19-19 A shadowgraph is analogous to a radiograph. (Dedicated to Xie Nan Zhu, Guangzhou, People's Republic of China.)

During some examinations, however, magnification is desirable and is carefully planned into the radiographic examination. This type of examination is called **magnification radiography,** and is discussed in Chapter 21.

Quantitatively, magnification is expressed by the magnification factor (MF), which is defined as follows:

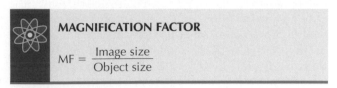

MAGNIFICATION FACTOR

$$MF = \frac{Image\ size}{Object\ size}$$

The MF depends on the geometric conditions of the examination. For most radiographs taken at a source-to-image receptor (SID) of 100 cm, the MF is approximately 1.1. For radiographs taken at 180 cm SID, the MF is approximately 1.05.

Question: If a heart measures 12.5 cm at its maximum width and its image on a chest radiograph measures 14.7 cm, what is the MF?

Answer: $MF = \dfrac{14.7\ cm}{12.5\ cm} = 1.176$

Many imaging departments are changing from the traditional 100 cm SID to 120 cm SID. Such a change results in reduced magnification, improved spatial resolution, and reduced patient dose.

In the usual radiographic examination, it is not possible to determine the object size. The image size may be measured directly from the radiograph. In such situations, the MF can be determined from the ratio of the SID to the source-to-object distance (SOD):

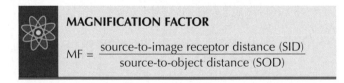

MAGNIFICATION FACTOR

$$MF = \frac{source\text{-}to\text{-}image\ receptor\ distance\ (SID)}{source\text{-}to\text{-}object\ distance\ (SOD)}$$

Figure 19-20 shows that this method of calculating the MF results from the basic geometric relationship between similar triangles. If two right triangles have a common hypotenuse, the ratio of the height of one to its base will be the same as the ratio of the height of the other to its base.

This is the situation that usually is encountered in radiology. The SID is known and can be measured directly. The SOD can be estimated relatively accurately by a radiologic technologist who has a good foundation in human anatomy. The image size can be measured accurately; therefore, the object size can be calculated as follows:

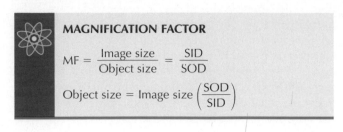

MAGNIFICATION FACTOR

$$MF = \frac{Image\ size}{Object\ size} = \frac{SID}{SOD}$$

$$Object\ size = Image\ size\left(\frac{SOD}{SID}\right)$$

Question: A renal calculus measures 1.2 cm on the radiograph. The SID is 100 cm and the SOD is estimated at 92 cm. What is the size of the calculus?

Answer: Object size = $1.2\left(\dfrac{92}{100}\right)$

= 1.1 cm

Question: A lateral film of the lumbar spine taken at 100 cm SID results in the image of a vertebral body with maximum and minimum dimensions of 6.4 cm and 4.2 cm. What is the object size if the vertebral body is 25 cm from the image receptor?

Answer: $MF = \dfrac{100}{100 - 25} = \dfrac{100}{75} = 1.33$

Therefore, the object size is

$$\frac{6.4}{1.33} \times \frac{4.2}{1.33} = 4.81\ cm \times 3.16\ cm$$

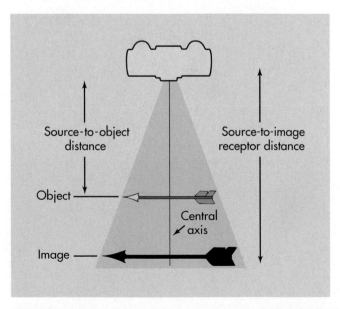

FIGURE 19-20 Magnification is the ratio of image size to object size or source-to-image receptor distance (SID) to source-to-object distance (SOD).

You might ask if these relationships hold for objects off the central axis (Figure 19-21). The MF will be the same for objects positioned off the central axis as for those lying on the central axis if the object-to-image receptor distance (OID) is the same and if the object is essentially flat.

In summary, there are two factors that affect image magnification: SID and OID.

> **MINIMIZING MAGNIFICATION**
>
> Large SID: use as large a source-to-image receptor
>   distance as possible.
> Small OID: place the object as close to the image
>   receptor as possible.

The SID is standard in most radiology departments at 180 cm for chest imaging, 100 cm for routine examinations, and 90 cm for some special studies, such as mobile radiography and trauma radiography.

There are three familiar clinical situations in which magnification is routinely minimized. Most chest radiographs are taken at 180 cm SID from the posterior-anterior projection. Compared with an examination at 100 cm SID, this projection results in a larger SID/SOD ratio and the OID is constant. Magnification is reduced because of the large SID.

Dedicated mammography imagers are designed for 50 to 70 cm SID. This is a relatively short SID, but it is necessary, considering the low kVp and low radiation intensity of mammography imaging systems. Such systems have a device for vigorous compression of the breast to reduce magnification by reducing OID.

Distortion

The previous discussion assumed a very simple object, an arrow, positioned parallel to the image receptor at a fixed OID. If any one of these conditions is changed, as they all are in most clinical examinations, the magnification will not be the same over the entire object.

> Unequal magnification of different portions of the same object is called shape distortion.

Distortion can interfere with diagnosis. Three conditions contribute to image distortion: object thickness, object position, and object shape.

> **DISTORTION DEPENDS ON:**
> 1. Object thickness
> 2. Object position
> 3. Object shape

Object Thickness. With a thick object, the OID changes measurably across the object. Consider, for instance, two rectangular structures of different thicknesses (Figure 19-22). Because of the change in OID across the thicker structure, the image of that structure is more distorted than the image of the thinner structure.

> Thick objects are more distorted than thin objects.

Consider the images produced by a disc and a sphere of the same diameter (Figure 19-23). When positioned on the central axis, the images of both objects appear as circles. The image of the sphere appears less distinct because of its varying thickness, but it does appear circular.

When these objects are positioned laterally to the central axis, the disc still appears circular. The sphere appears not only less distinct but elliptical because of its thickness. This distortion resulting from object thickness is shown more dramatically in Figure 19-24 by the image of an irregular object.

These statements about discs and spheres are clinically insignificant because lateral distances off the central axis are too small. Only irregular objects, such as those shown in Figure 19-24 or the human body, show significant distortion.

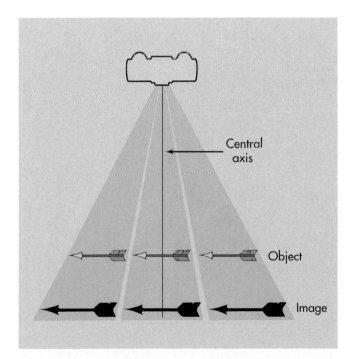

FIGURE 19-21 Magnification of an object positioned off the central x-ray axis is the same as that for an object on the central axis if the objects are in the same plane.

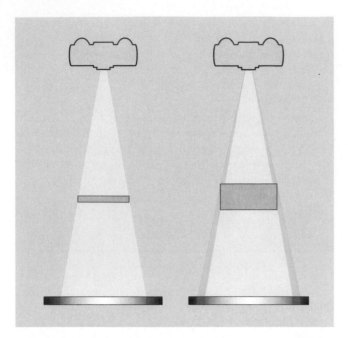

FIGURE 19-22 Thick objects result in unequal magnification and thus more distortion than thin objects.

Object Position. If the object plane and the image plane are parallel, the image is not distorted. However, distortion is possible in every radiographic examination if proper patient positioning is not maintained.

 If the object plane and image plane are not parallel, distortion occurs.

Figure 19-25 is an example of gross distortion and shows that the image of an inclined object can be smaller than the object itself. In such a condition, the image is said to be **foreshortened.** The amount of foreshortening, the amount of reduction in image size, increases as the angle of inclination increases.

If an inclined object is not located on the central x-ray beam, the degree of distortion is affected by the object's angle of inclination and its lateral position from the central axis. Figure 19-26 illustrates this situation and shows that the image of an inclined object can be severely foreshortened, or **elongated.**

With multiple objects positioned at various OIDs, **spatial distortion** can occur. Spatial distortion is the misrepresentation in the image of the actual spatial relationships among objects. Figure 19-27 demonstrates this condition for two arrows of the same size, one of which lies on top of the other. Because of the position of the arrows, only one image should be seen, representing the superposition of the arrows.

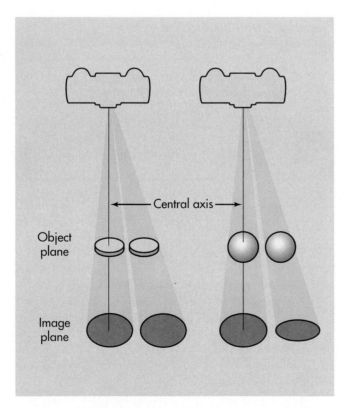

FIGURE 19-23 Object thickness influences distortion. Radiographs of a disc or sphere appear as circles if the object is on the central axis. When lateral to the central axis, the disc appears as a circle and the sphere as an ellipse.

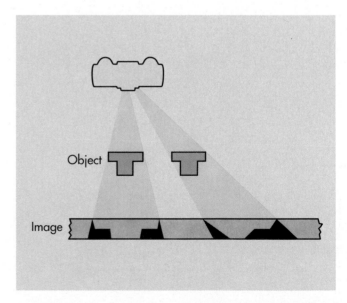

FIGURE 19-24 Irregular anatomy or objects such as these can cause considerable distortion when radiographed off the central axis.

Unequal magnification, however, of the two objects causes arrow *A* to appear larger than arrow *B* and to be positioned more laterally. This distortion is minimal for objects lying along the central x-ray beam. As object position is shifted laterally from the central axis, spatial distortion can become more significant.

This illustrates the projection nature of x-ray images; a single image is not enough to define the three-dimensional configuration of a complex object. Therefore, most x-ray examinations are made with two or more projections.

Focal-Spot Blur

Thus far, our discussion of the geometric factors affecting radiographic quality has assumed that x-rays are emitted from a point source. In actual practice there is no point source of x-radiation but, rather, a roughly rectangular source varying in size from approximately 0.1 to 1.5 mm on a side, depending on the type of x-ray tube in use.

Figure 19-28 illustrates the result of using x-ray tubes with measurable effective focal spots as imaging devices. The point of the object arrow in Figure 19-28 does not appear as a point in the image plane because the x-rays used to image that point originate throughout the rectangular source.

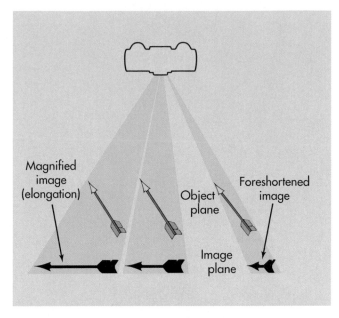

FIGURE 19-26 An inclined object positioned lateral to the central ray may be severely distorted by elongation or foreshortening.

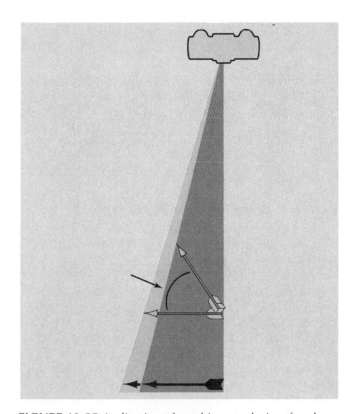

FIGURE 19-25 Inclination of an object results in a foreshortened image.

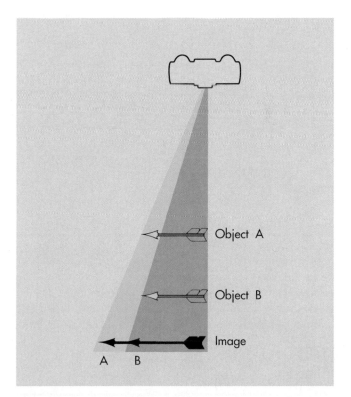

FIGURE 19-27 When objects of the same size are positioned at different distances from the image receptor, spatial distortion occurs.

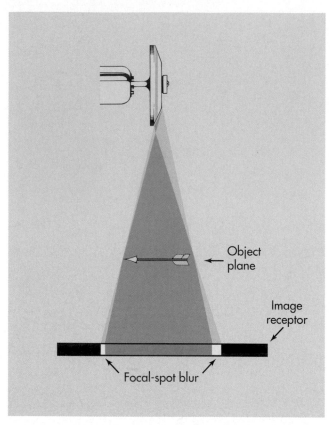

FIGURE 19-28 Focal-spot blur is caused by the effective size of the focal spot, which is larger to the cathode side of the image.

area projected on to pt & IR

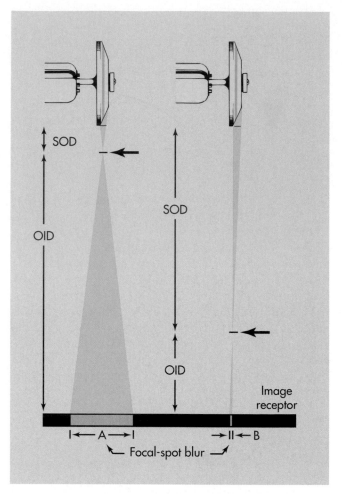

FIGURE 19-29 Focal-spot blur is small when the object-to-image receptor distance (OID) is small.

 Focal-spot blur occurs because the focal spot is not a point.

A blurred region on the radiograph over which the radiologic technologist has little control results because the effective focal spot has size. This phenomenon is called **focal-spot blur** and, as illustrated, it is greater on the cathode side of the image. Focal-spot blur is undesirable.

 Focal-spot blur is the most important factor in determining spatial resolution.

The geometric relationships governing magnification also influence focal-spot blur. As the geometry of the source, object, and image are altered to produce greater magnification, they also produce increased focal-spot blur. Consequently, these conditions should be avoided when possible.

The region of focal-spot blur can be calculated using similar triangles. If an arrowhead were positioned near the x-ray tube target, the size of the focal-spot blur would be larger than that of the effective focal spot (Figure 19-29, *A*). In general, the object is much closer to the image receptor, and therefore the focal-spot blur is much smaller than the effective focal spot (Figure 19-29, *B*).

From these drawings, you can see that two similar triangles are described. Therefore, the ratio of SOD to OID is the same as the ratio of the sizes of the effective focal spot and the focal-spot blur.

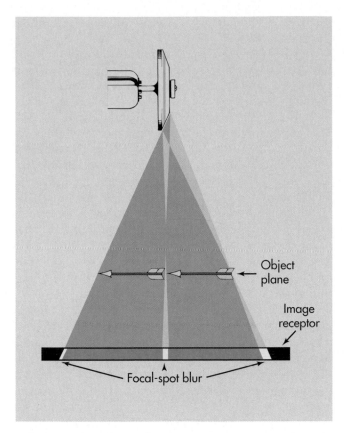

TABLE 19-2	Patient Positioning for Examinations That Can Take Advantage of the Heel Effect	
Examination	**Position Toward the Cathode**	**Position Toward the Anode**
Posterior-anterior chest	Abdomen	Neck
Abdomen	Abdomen	Pelvis
Femur	Hip	Knee
Humerus	Shoulder	Elbow
AP thoracic spine	Abdomen	Neck
AP lumbar spine	Abdomen	Pelvis

AP, Anterior-posterior.

FIGURE 19-30 Effective focal spot size is largest on the cathode side, and therefore focal-spot blur is greatest on the cathode side.

To minimize focal-spot blur, you should use small focal spots and position the patient so that the anatomic part under examination is close to the image receptor. The SID is usually fixed but should be as large as possible. High-contrast objects that are smaller than the focal-spot blur cannot normally be imaged.

Heel Effect

The heel effect, introduced in Chapter 10, is described as a varying intensity across the x-ray field in the anode–cathode direction caused by attenuation of x-rays in the heel of the anode. Another characteristic of the heel effect is unrelated to x-ray intensity but affects focal-spot blur.

The size of the effective focal spot is not constant across the radiograph. An x-ray tube said to have a 1-mm focal spot has a smaller effective focal spot on the anode side and a larger effective focal spot on the cathode side (Figure 19-30).

 The focal-spot blur is small on the anode side and large on the cathode side.

This variation in focal-spot size results in a variation in focal-spot blur. Consequently, images toward the cathode side of a radiograph have higher blur and poorer spatial resolution than those to the anode side. This is clinically significant when x-ray tubes with small target angles are used at short SIDs. Table 19-2 lists radiographic examinations that should be performed with regard for the heel effect.

SUBJECT FACTORS

The third general group of factors affecting radiographic quality concerns the patient (Box 19-2).

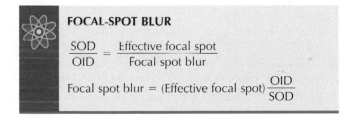

FOCAL-SPOT BLUR

$$\frac{SOD}{OID} = \frac{Effective\ focal\ spot}{Focal\ spot\ blur}$$

$$Focal\ spot\ blur = (Effective\ focal\ spot)\frac{OID}{SOD}$$

Question: An x-ray tube target having a 0.6-mm effective focal spot is used to image a calcified nodule estimated to be 8 cm from the anterior chest wall. If the radiograph is taken in a posterior-anterior projection at 180 cm SID, with a tabletop to image receptor separation of 5 cm, what will be the size of the focal-spot blur?

Answer: Focal spot blur $= (0.6\ mm)\dfrac{8 + 5}{180 - (8 + 5)}$

$$= (0.6\ mm)\frac{13}{167}$$

$$= (0.6\ mm)(0.078)$$
$$= 0.047\ mm$$

The smaller the angle the greater the heel effect

These factors are those associated not so much with the positioning of the patient as with the selection of a radiographic technique that properly compensates for the patient's size, shape, and tissue composition. Patient positioning is basically a requirement associated with the geometric factors affecting radiographic quality.

Subject Contrast

The contrast of a radiograph viewed on an illuminator is called **radiographic contrast**. As indicated previously, radiographic contrast is a function of film contrast and subject contrast. In fact, the radiographic contrast is simply the product of film contrast and subject contrast.

RADIOGRAPHIC CONTRAST

Radiographic contrast = Film contrast × Subject contrast

Question: Screen-film with an average gradient of 3.1 is used to radiograph a long bone having subject contrast of 4.5. What is the radiographic contrast?
Answer: Radiographic contrast = (3.1)(4.5)
= 13.95

Several of these subject factors were discussed in Chapter 12 in their relation to the attenuation of an x-ray beam. The effect of each on subject contrast is a direct result of differences in attenuation in body tissues.

Patient Thickness. Given a standard composition, a thick body section attenuates more x-rays than a thin body section (Figure 19-31). The same number of x-rays is incident on each section, and therefore the contrast of the incident x-ray beam is zero; there is no contrast.

If the same number of x-rays left each section, the subject contrast would be 1.0. Because more x-rays are transmitted through thin body sections than through thick ones, however, subject contrast is greater than 1. The degree of subject contrast is directly proportional to the relative number of x-rays leaving those sections of the body.

Tissue Mass Density. Different sections of the body may have equal thicknesses, yet different mass densities. Tissue mass density is an important factor affecting subject contrast. Consider, for example, the radiograph of different salad ingredients (Figure 19-32). The materials have the same thickness and chemical composition. However, they have slightly different mass density from water and therefore will be imaged. The effect of mass density on subject contrast is demonstrated in Figure 19-33.

Effective Atomic Number. Another important factor affecting subject contrast is the effective atomic number of the tissue being examined. In Chapter 12, it is shown that Compton interactions are independent of atomic number but photoelectric interactions vary in proportion to the cube of the atomic number.

The effective atomic numbers of tissues of interest are reported in Table 12-1. In the diagnostic range of x-ray energies, the photoelectric effect is of considerable importance; therefore, the subject contrast is greatly influenced by the effective atomic number of the tissue being radiographed. When the effective atomic number of adjacent tissues is very much different, subject contrast is very high.

Subject contrast can be greatly enhanced by the use of contrast media. The high atomic numbers of iodine (Z = 53) and barium (Z = 56) result in extremely high subject contrast. Contrast media are effective because they accentuate subject contrast through increased photoelectric absorption.

Object Shape. The shape of the anatomic structure under investigation influences the radiographic quality not only through its geometry but also through its contribution to subject contrast. Obviously, a structure having a form that coincides with the x-ray beam has maximum subject contrast (Figure 19-34, *A*).

All other anatomic shapes have reduced subject contrast because of the change in thickness that they present across the x-ray beam. Figure 19-34, *B* and *C* show examples of two shapes that result in reduced subject contrast.

This characteristic of the subject affecting subject contrast is sometimes termed **absorption blur**. It reduces both spatial resolution and contrast resolution of any anatomic structure, but it is most troublesome during interventional procedures where vessels with small diameters are being examined.

kVp. The radiologic technologist has no control over the four previous factors influencing subject contrast. The absolute magnitude of subject contrast, however, is greatly controlled by the kVp of operation. Kilovolt peak also influences film contrast but not to the extent it controls subject contrast.

BOX 19-2 Subject Factors

Subject contrast
Patient thickness
Tissue mass density
Effective atomic number
Object shape
Kilovolt peak

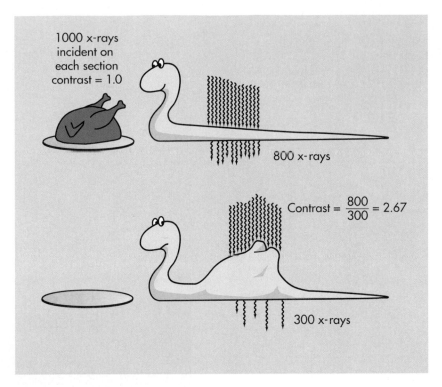

FIGURE 19-31 Different anatomic thicknesses contribute to subject contrast.

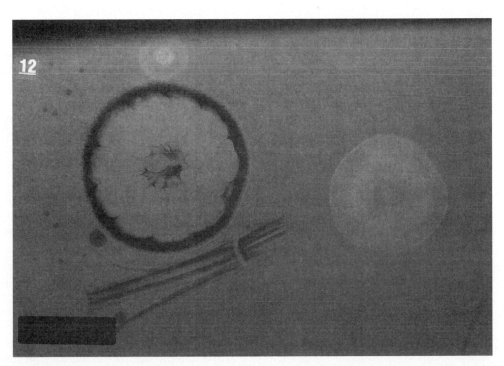

FIGURE 19-32 Radiograph of an orange, kiwi, piece of celery, and chunk of carrot shows the effect of subtle differences in mass density. (Courtesy Marcy Barnes.)

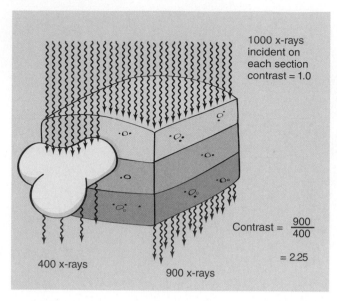

FIGURE 19-33 The variation in tissue mass density contributes to subject contrast.

FIGURE 19-35 Radiographs of an aluminum step wedge (penetrometer) demonstrating change in contrast with varying voltage. (Courtesy Eastman Kodak Co.)

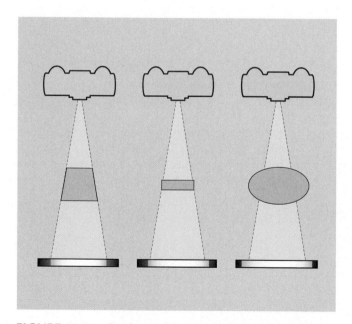

FIGURE 19-34 The shape of the structure under investigation contributes to absorption blur.

 kVp is the most important influence on subject contrast.

Figure 19-35 shows a composite of a series of radiographs of an aluminum step wedge taken at kVp peaks ranging from 40 to 100. A low kVp results in high sub-

ject contrast, sometimes called **short gray-scale contrast,** because the radiographic image appears either black or white with few shades of gray. On the other hand, high kVp results in low subject contrast or **long gray-scale contrast.**

It would be easy to jump to the conclusion that low-kVp techniques are always more desirable than high-kVp techniques. However, low-kVp radiography has two major disadvantages.

As the kVp is lowered for any radiographic examination, the x-ray beam becomes less penetrating, requiring a higher mAs setting to produce an acceptable range of ODs. The result is higher patient dose. A method to estimate this increased patient dose is given in Chapter 40.

A radiographic technique that produces low subject contrast allows for wide latitude in exposure factors. Optimization of radiographic technique by mAs selection is not so critical when using high kVp.

TABLE 19-3	Procedures for Reducing Motion Blur

Use the shortest possible exposure time.
Restrict patient motion by instruction or restraining device.
Use a large source-to-image receptor distance (SID).
Use a small object-to-image receptor distance (OID).

Motion Blur

Movement of either the patient or the x-ray tube during exposure results in a blurring of the radiographic image. This loss of radiographic quality, called **motion blur**, may result in repeated radiographs and therefore should be avoided.

Normally, motion of the x-ray tube is not a problem. In tomography, the x-ray tube is deliberately moved during exposure to blur the images of structures on either side of the plane of interest (see Chapter 21). Sometimes the table or a restraining device is caused to move by auxiliary equipment, such as moving grid mechanism.

 Patient motion is usually the cause of motion blur.

The radiographer can reduce motion blur by carefully instructing the patient, "Take a deep breath and hold it. Don't move."

There are two types of patient motion. Voluntary motion of limbs and muscles is controlled by immobilization. Involuntary motion of heart and lungs is controlled by short exposure time.

Motion blur is primarily affected by four factors. By observing the guidelines listed in Table 19-3, the radiologic technologist can reduce motion blur. Note that the last two items in this list have the same relation to motion blur as to focal-spot blur. With the use of low ripple power and high-speed image receptors, motion has been virtually eliminated as a common clinical problem.

TOOLS FOR IMPROVED RADIOGRAPHIC QUALITY

The radiologic technologist normally has the tools available to produce high-quality radiographs. Proper patient preparation, the selection of proper imaging devices, and proper radiographic technique are complex, related concepts.

For any given radiographic examination, a proper interpretation and application of each of these factors must be made. A small change in one may require a compensating change in another.

Patient Positioning

The importance of patient positioning should now be clear. Proper patient positioning requires that the anatomic structure under investigation be placed as close to the image receptor as is practical and that the axis of this structure lie in a plane parallel to the plane of the image receptor. The central-axis x-ray beam should be incident on the center of the structure. Finally, the patient must be effectively immobilized to minimize motion blur.

To be able to position patients properly, the radiologic technologist must have a good knowledge of human anatomy. If multiple structures are being radiographed and are to be imaged with uniform magnification, they must be the same distance from the image receptor. The various techniques applied to radiographic positioning are designed to produce radiographs with minimal image distortion and maximum image resolution.

Image Receptors

Usually, a standard type of screen-film combination is used throughout a radiology department for a given examination. In general, extremity and soft tissue radiographs are taken with the fine-detail screen-film combinations.

Most other radiographs use double-emulsion film with screens. The new, structured-grain x-ray films used with high-resolution intensifying screens produce exquisite images with limited patient dose.

 Principles to be considered when planning a particular examination:
1. Use of intensifying screens decreases patient dose by a factor of at least 20.
2. As the speed of the image receptor increases, radiographic noise increases and spatial resolution is decreased.
3. Low-contrast imaging procedures have a wider latitude, margin of error, in producing an acceptable radiograph.

Selection of Technique Factors

Before each examination, the radiologic technologist must select the optimum radiographic technique factors: kVp, mAs, and exposure time. Many considerations determine the value of each of these factors, and they are complexly interrelated. Few generalizations are possible.

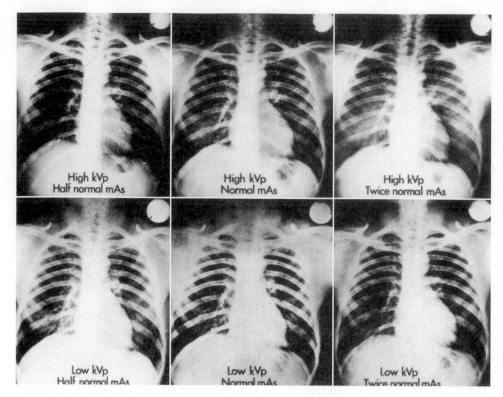

FIGURE 19-36 Chest radiographs demonstrating two advantages of high-voltage technique: greater latitude and margin for error. (Courtesy Eastman Kodak Co.)

One generalization that can be made for all radiographic exposures is that the time of exposure should be as short as possible. Image quality is improved with short exposure times as a result of reduced motion blur. One of the reasons three-phase and high-frequency generators are better than single-phase generators is that shorter exposure times are possible with the former.

 Keep exposure time as short as possible.

Similar simple statements cannot be made about the selection of kVp or mA. Because time is to be kept at a minimum, the selection of kVp, mA, and the resulting mAs value should be considered. The radiographer should strive for optimum radiographic contrast and ODs by exposing the patient to the proper quantity and quality of x-radiation.

 The primary control of radiographic contrast is kVp.

As kVp is increased, both the quantity and quality of x-radiation increases; more x-rays are transmitted through the patient so that a higher portion of the primary beam reaches the image receptor. Thus, kVp also affects OD. Of the x-rays that interact with the patient, the relative number of Compton interactions increases with increasing kVp, resulting in less differential absorption and reduced subject contrast.

Furthermore, with increased kVp the scatter radiation reaching the image receptor is higher, and therefore radiographic noise is higher. The result of increased kVp is loss of contrast. When radiographic contrast is low, latitude is high, and there is greater margin for error.

The principal advantages to the use of high kVp are the reduction in patient dose and the wide latitude of exposures allowed in the production of a diagnostic radiograph. Figure 19-36 shows a series of chest radiographs that demonstrates the increased latitude resulting from high-kVp technique. The relative technique factors are indicated on each radiograph. To some extent, the use of grids can compensate for the loss of contrast accompanying high-kVp technique.

TABLE 19-4	Principal Factors Affecting the Making of a Radiograph*						
	Patient Dose	**Magnification**	**Focal-Spot Blur**	**Motion Blur**	**Absorption Blur**	**Optical Density**	**Radiographic Contrast**
Film speed	−	0	0	−	0	+	0
Screen speed	−	0	0	−	0	+	0
Grid ratio	+	0	0	0	0	−	+
Processing time/temperature	0	0	0	0	0	+	−
Patient thickness	+	+	+	+	+	−	−
Field size	+	0	0	0	0	+	−
Use of contrast media	0	0	0	0	0	+	−
Focal-spot size	0	0	+	0	0	0	0
SID	−	−	−	−	0	−	0
OID	0	+	+	+	0	0	+
Screen-film contact	0	0	0	0	0	0	−
Milliampere-seconds	+	0	0	0	0	I	+ or −
Time	+	0	0	+	0	+	+ or −
Voltage	+	0	0	0	0	+	−
Voltage ripple	+	0	0	−	0	−	−
Total filtration	−	0	0	0	0	−	−

SID, Source-to-image receptor distance; *OID,* object-to-image receptor distance.

*As the factors in the left-hand column are increased, **while all other factors remain fixed,** cross-referenced conditions are affected as shown: +, increase; − , decrease; 0, no change.

The primary control of OD is mAs.

As the mAs value is increased, the radiation quantity increases, and therefore the number of x-rays arriving at the image receptor increases, resulting in higher OD and lower radiographic noise.

In a secondary way, the mAs value also influences contrast. Recall that maximum contrast is obtained only when the film is exposed over a range that results in OD along the straight-line portion of the characteristic curve. Too low a mAs setting results in low OD and reduced radiographic contrast because the H & D curve has flattened. Too high a mAs value results in high OD and a loss of radiographic contrast for the same reason.

A number of other factors influence OD and radiographic contrast, and hence radiographic quality. Adding filtration to the x-ray tube reduces the x-ray beam intensity but increases the quality. A change in SID results in a change in OD because x-ray intensity varies with distance. Table 19-4 summarizes the principal factors that influence the making of a radiograph.

The continuing trend in radiographic technique is to use high kVp with a compensating reduction in mAs to produce a radiograph of satisfactory quality while reducing patient exposure and the likelihood of reexamination because of an error in technique. Such considerations are taken up in detail in Chapter 20.

SUMMARY

Radiographic quality is the exactness of representation of the anatomic structure on the radiograph. Characteristics that make up radiographic quality are as follows:

1. Spatial resolution or the ability to detect separate structures on the radiograph
2. Low noise or elimination of ODs that do not reflect anatomic structures
3. Proper speed of the screen-film combination, which limits patient dose but produces a high-quality, low-noise radiograph

These characteristics and three others—film factors, geometric factors, and subject factors—combine to determine radiographic quality. Film factors involve quality control in film processing and characteristics of film.

The graph on semilogarithmic paper resulting from sensitometry and densitometry data of film optical density is the characteristic curve. The characteristic curve shows film contrast, speed, and latitude.

Geometric factors affecting radiographic quality include preventing magnification and distortion, as well as using object thickness, position, focal-spot blur, and the heel effect advantageously.

Subject factors that involve radiographic quality depend on the patient. A radiographer must prevent motion blur by encouraging patient cooperation. Also, by measuring patient thickness, recognizing tissue mass density, examining anatomic shape, and evaluating optimal kVp levels, a radiographer can create a high-quality radiograph.

CHALLENGE QUESTIONS

1. Define or otherwise identify the following:
   a. Average gradient
   b. Optical density
   c. Foreshortening
   d. Focal-spot blur
   e. Opaque, radiopaque
   f. Densitometer
   g. Motion blur
   h. Spatial distortion
   i. Quantum mottle
   j. Latitude
2. What principally determines radiographic spatial resolution?
3. Describe the equipment used in sensitometry.
4. What is the importance of processor quality control in an imaging department?
5. Have the manufacturer's representative help construct a characteristic curve from the data obtained from sensitometry and densitometry of a screen-film combination used in your department.
6. The intensity of light emitted by a viewbox is 1000. The intensity of the light transmitted through the film is 1. What is the optical density of the film? Will it be light, gray, or black?
7. Base and fog densities on a given radiograph are 0.35. At densities 0.25 and 2 above base and fog densities, the characteristic curve shows log relative exposure values of 1.3 and 2. What is the average gradient?
8. List the factors affecting the finished radiograph in relation to film processing.
9. X-ray image receptors A and B require 15 mR and 45 mR to produce an optical density of 1.0. Which is faster and what is the speed of each?
10. What are the three principal geometric factors that affect radiographic quality?
11. What are standard SIDs?
12. List and explain the five factors that affect subject contrast.
13. What is the difference between foreshortening and elongation?
14. Describe the H & H contrast curve.
15. Discuss the factors that influence radiographic optical density and contrast.
16. Construct a characteristic curve for a typical screen-film combination and carefully label the axes.
17. An x-ray examination of the heart taken at 100 cm SID shows a cardiac silhouette measuring 13 cm in width. If the OID distance is estimated at 15 cm, what is the actual width of the heart?
18. The subject contrast of a thorax is 5.3. Image receptor contrast is 3.2. What is the radiographic contrast?
19. State the reciprocity law and its influence on radiography.
20. Does the use of a radiographic intensifying screen increase contrast compared with direct exposure?

CHAPTER

20

Radiographic Technique

OBJECTIVES

At the completion of this chapter, the student should be able to do the following:

1. List the four patient factors and explain their affect on radiographic technique
2. Identify four image-quality factors and how they influence the characteristics of a radiograph
3. Discuss the three types of technique charts
4. Explain the three types of automatic exposure controls

OUTLINE

RADIOGRAPHIC TECHNIQUE is usually described as the combination of settings selected on the control panel of the x-ray imager to produce a high-quality image on the radiograph. The geometry and position of the x-ray tube, the patient, and the image receptor are included in this description.

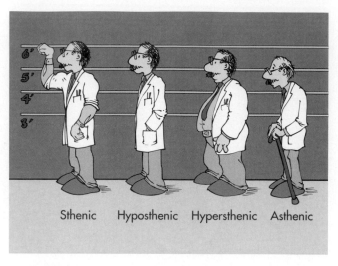

FIGURE 20-1 The four general states of body habitus.

Radiographic techniques may be described by identifying three groups of factors. The first group includes **patient factors,** such as anatomic thickness and body composition. The second group consists of the **image-quality factors,** such as optical density (OD), contrast, detail, and distortion. Also of importance is how these image-quality factors are influenced by the patient.

The final group includes the **exposure-technique factors,** such as kilovolt peak, milliamperage, exposure time, and source-to-image receptor distance (SID), as well as grids, screens, focal-spot size, and filtration. These factors determine the basic characteristics of radiation exposure of the image receptor and patient dose. They have been covered in previous chapters.

These factors provide the radiologic technologist with a specific and orderly means to produce, evaluate, and compare radiographs. Understanding each of these factors is essential for the production of high-quality images.

PATIENT FACTORS

Perhaps the most difficult task for the radiologic technologist is evaluation of the patient. The patient's size, shape, and physical condition greatly influence the required radiographic technique.

The general size and shape of a patient is called the **body habitus,** and there are four such states (Figure 20-1). The **sthenic**—meaning "strong, active"—patient is the average patient. The **hyposthenic** patient is thin but healthy appearing. Such a patient requires less radiographic technique. The **hypersthenic** patient is big in frame and usually overweight. The **asthenic** patient is small, frail, sometimes emaciated, and often elderly.

 Radiographic technique charts are based on the sthenic patient.

Recognition of body habitus is essential to radiographic technique selection. Once this is established, the thickness and composition of the anatomy being examined must be determined.

Thickness of Part

The thicker the patient, the more x-radiation is required to penetrate through the patient to the image receptor. For this reason, the radiologic technologist must use **calipers** to measure the thickness of the anatomy being irradiated.

 Patient thickness should not be guessed.

Depending on the type of radiographic technique being practiced, either the mAs setting or the kVp will be altered as a function of the thickness of the part. Table 20-1 shows an example of how the mAs setting changes when imaging the abdomen if a fixed-kVp technique is used. Table 20-2 reports the change in radiographic technique factors as a function of thickness of part when a variable-kVp technique is used.

Body Composition

Measurement of the thickness of the anatomic part does not release the radiologic technologist from exercising some additional judgment when selecting a proper radiographic technique. The thorax and the abdomen may have the same thickness, but the radiographic technique used for each will be considerably different. The radiologic technologist must estimate the mass density of the anatomic part and the range of mass densities involved.

In general, when only soft tissue is being imaged, low kVp and high mAs are used. With an extremity, however, which has both soft tissue and bone, low kVp is used because the body part is thin.

When imaging the chest, the radiologic technologist takes advantage of the high subject contrast. Lung tis-

TABLE 20-1	Fixed-kVp Technique for an Anterior-Posterior Abdominal Examination							
kVp	80	80	80	80	80	80	80	80
Patient thickness (cm)	16	18	20	22	24	26	28	30
mAs	12	15	22	30	45	60	90	120

TABLE 20-2	Variable-kVp Technique for an Anterior-Posterior Pelvic Examination							
mAs	100	100	100	100	100	100	100	100
Patient thickness (cm)	15	16	17	18	19	20	21	22
kVp	56	58	60	62	64	66	68	70

sue has very low mass density, the bony structures have high mass density, and the mediastinal structures have intermediate mass density. Consequently, high kVp and low mAs can be used to good advantage. This results in an image with satisfactory contrast and low patient radiation exposure.

 The chest has high subject contrast; the abdomen has low subject contrast.

These various tissues are often described by their degree of **radiolucency** or **radiopacity** (Figure 20-2). Radiolucent tissue attenuates few x-rays and appears black on the radiograph. Radiopaque tissue absorbs x-rays and appears white on the radiograph. Table 20-3 shows the relative degree of radiolucency for various body habitus and tissues.

Pathology

The type of pathlogy, its size, and its composition influence radiographic technique. In this case, the patient examination request form and previous images may be of some help. The radiologic technologist should not hesitate to seek more information from the referring physician, the radiologist, or the patient regarding the suspected pathology.

 Pathology can appear with increased radiolucency or radiopacity.

Some pathology is **destructive,** causing the tissue to be more radiolucent. Other pathology can **constructively** increase mass density or composition, causing the tissue to be more radiopaque. Such pathology is often called *additive.* Practice and experience will guide the radiologic technologist's clinical judgment, but Box 20-1 presents a beginning classification scheme.

TABLE 20-3	Relative Degrees of Radiolucency		
		Body Habitus	Tissue Type
Radiolucent	Black		
		Asthenic	Lung
		Hyposthenic	Fat
		Sthenic	Muscle
		Hypersthenic	Bone
Radiopaque	White		

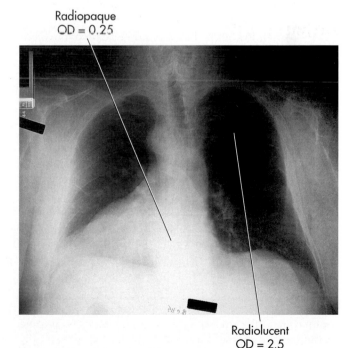

Radiopaque OD = 0.25

Radiolucent OD = 2.5

FIGURE 20-2 Relative radiolucency and optical density (OD) are shown on this radiograph. (Courtesy Bette Shans.)

BOX 20-1 Classifying Pathology

RADIOLUCENT (DESTRUCTIVE)	RADIOPAQUE (CONSTRUCTIVE)
Active tuberculosis	Aortic aneurysm
Atrophy	Ascites
Bowel obstruction	Atelectasis
Cancer	Cirrhosis
Degenerative arthritis	Hypertrophy
Emphysema	Metastases
Osteoporosis	Pleural effusion
Pneumothorax	Pneumonia
	Sclerosis

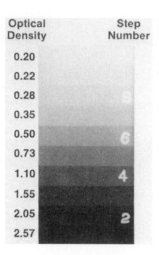

Optical Density	Step Number
0.20	
0.22	
0.28	9
0.35	
0.50	6
0.73	
1.10	4
1.55	
2.05	2
2.57	

FIGURE 20-3 Amount of light transmitted through a radiograph is determined by the optical density (OD) of a film. The step-wedge radiograph shows a representative range of OD.

IMAGE-QUALITY FACTORS

The phrase **image-quality factors** refers to the characteristics of the radiographic image; these include OD, contrast, image detail, and distortion. These factors provide a means for the radiologic technologist to produce, review, and evaluate radiographs. Image-quality factors are considered the "language" of radiography, and often it is difficult to separate one factor from another.

Optical Density

Optical density (OD), sometimes called **radiographic density,** is the degree of blackening of the finished radiograph. OD has a numeric value (see Chapter 19) and can be present in varying degrees, from completely black, where no light is transmitted through the radiograph, to almost clear. Black is numerically equivalent to an OD of 4 or greater, whereas clear is less than 0.2 (Figure 20-3).

In medical radiography, many problems involve an image being "too dark" or "too light." A radiograph that is too dark has a high OD resulting from **overexposure.** This situation is caused by too much x-radiation reaching the image receptor. A radiograph that is too light has been exposed to too little x-radiation, resulting in **underexposure** and a low OD.

Both overexposure and underexposure can result in unacceptable image quality, which may require that the examination be repeated. Figure 20-4 shows clinical examples of these two extremes of exposure.

OD can be controlled in radiography by two major factors: **mAs** and **SID.** A significant number of problems would arise if the SID were continually changed. Therefore, SID is usually fixed at 90 cm for mobile examinations, 100 cm for table studies, and 180 cm for upright chest examinations. Figure 20-5 illustrates the change in OD at these SIDs when other exposure-technique factors remain constant.

When distance is fixed, however, as is usually the case, the mAs value becomes the primary variable technique factor used to control OD. OD increases directly with mAs, which means that if the OD is to be increased on a radiograph, the mAs setting needs to be increased accordingly.

 When the OD of the radiograph is the only characteristic that is to be changed, the appropriate factor to adjust would be the mAs.

OD can be affected by other factors, but the mAs value becomes the factor of choice for its control (Figure 20-6). A change in mAs of approximately 30% is required to produce a visible change in OD. As a general rule, when only the mAs setting is changed, it should be halved or doubled (Figure 20-7). If a change is not required, the repeat examination is probably not required.

 The mAs value must be changed by approximately 30% to produce a perceptible change in OD.
The kVp setting must be changed by approximately 4% to produce a perceptible change in OD.

Because an increase in OD on the finished radiograph is accomplished with a proportionate increase in mAs, is the same true with kilovoltage? Yes, but the increase is not proportionate. As kVp is increased, the quality of the beam is increased and more x-rays penetrate the anatomic part. This results in more

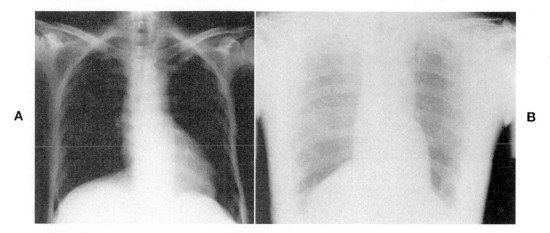

FIGURE 20-4 **A,** Overexposed radiograph of the chest is too black to be diagnostic. **B,** Likewise, underexposed chest radiograph is unacceptable because there is no detail to the lung fields. (Courtesy Richard Bayless.)

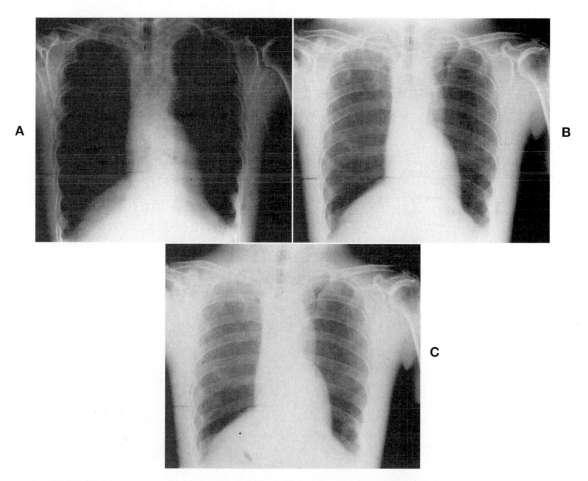

FIGURE 20-5 Normal chest radiograph taken at 100 cm source-to-image receptor distance (SID). **B,** If the exposure technique factors are not changed, a similar radiograph at 90 cm SID **(A)** will be overexposed and at 180 cm SID **(C)** underexposed. (Courtesy Kurt Loveland.)

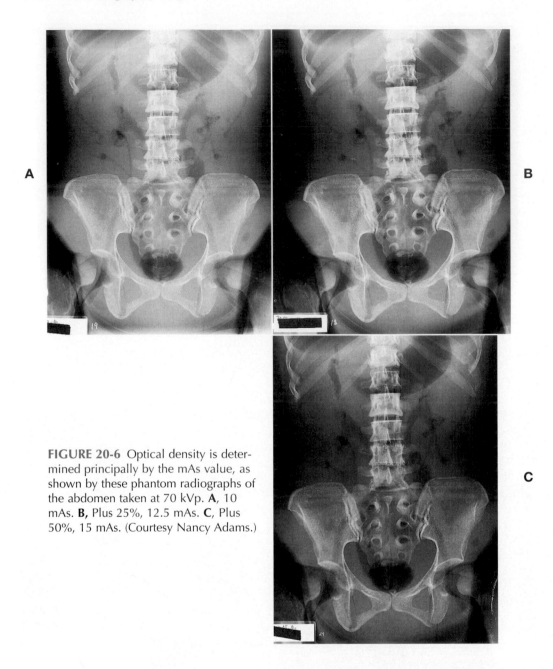

FIGURE 20-6 Optical density is determined principally by the mAs value, as shown by these phantom radiographs of the abdomen taken at 70 kVp. **A**, 10 mAs. **B**, Plus 25%, 12.5 mAs. **C**, Plus 50%, 15 mAs. (Courtesy Nancy Adams.)

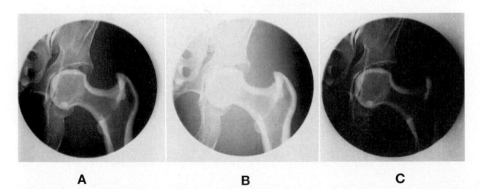

FIGURE 20-7 Changes in the mAs value have a direct effect on OD. **A**, The original image. **B**, The decrease in OD when the mAs value is decreased by half. **C**, The increase in OD when the mAs value is doubled. (Courtesy Euclid Seeram.)

image-forming x-rays. As discussed in Chapter 12, x-ray intensity at the patient is proportional to kVp^2 and at the image receptor to kVp^5.

Image contrast is affected when kVp is changed to adjust OD. This makes it much more difficult to optimize OD with kVp. It takes the eye of an experienced radiologic technologist to determine if OD is the only factor to be changed or if contrast should also be changed to optimize the radiographic image.

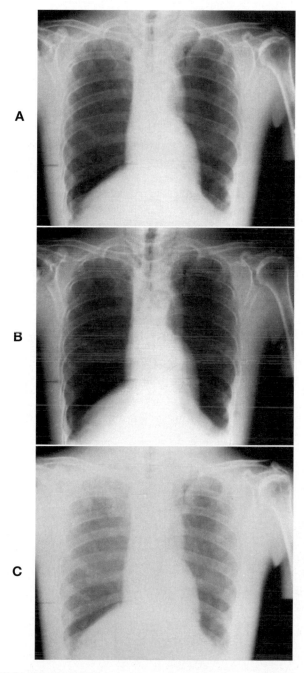

A

B

C

FIGURE 20-8 Normal chest radiograph taken at 70 kVp **(B)**. If the kilovoltage is increased 15% to 80 kVp **(A),** overexposure occurs. Similarly, at 15% less, 60 kVp **(C),** the radiograph is underexposed. (Courtesy Euclid Seeram.)

Technique changes involving kVp become complicated. A change in kVp affects penetration, scatter radiation, patient dose, and especially contrast. It is generally accepted that if the OD on the radiograph is to be increased using kVp, an increase in kVp by 15% is equivalent to doubling the mAs. This is known as the **fifteen percent rule.**

Figure 20-8 illustrates the OD change when the fifteen percent rule is applied. If OD only is to be changed, the fifteen percent rule should not be used because such a large change in kVp will change image contrast.

 A 15% increase in kVp accompanied by a half reduction in mAs results in the same OD.

The simplest method to increase or decrease OD on a radiograph is to increase or decrease the mAs. This reduces other possible factors that could affect the finished image. The various factors that affect OD are listed in Table 20-4.

Contrast

The function of contrast in the image is to make anatomy more visible. Contrast is the difference in OD between adjacent anatomic structures or the variation in OD on a radiograph. Contrast, therefore, is one of the most important factors in radiographic quality.

Contrast on a radiograph is necessary for the outline or border of a structure to be visible. Contrast is the result of differences in attenuation of the x-ray beam as it passes through various tissues of the body. The relative penetrability of the x-ray beam through different tissues determines the image contrast.

Figure 20-9 shows an image of the abdomen, illustrating the difference in OD between adjacent structures. High contrast is visible at the bone–soft tissue interface along the spinal column. The soft tissues of the psoas

TABLE 20-4	Technique Factors Affecting Optical Density
Factor Increased	**Effect on Optical Density**
Milliampere-seconds (mAs)	Increase
Kilovoltage (kVp)	Increase
Source-to-image receptor distance (SID)	Decrease
Thickness of part	Decrease
Mass density	Decrease
Development time	Increase
Image receptor speed	Increase
Collimation	Decrease
Grid ratio	Decrease

muscle and kidneys exhibit much less contrast, although details of these structures are readily visible. The contrast resolution of the soft tissues can be enhanced with reduced kVp, but at the expense of higher patient dose.

 kVp is the major factor for controlling radiographic contrast.

The penetrability of the x-ray beam is controlled by kVp. Obtaining adequate contrast requires that the anatomic part be adequately penetrated; therefore, penetration becomes the key to understanding radiographic contrast. Compare the radiographs shown in Figure 20-10: Figure 20-10, *A*, shows high contrast or

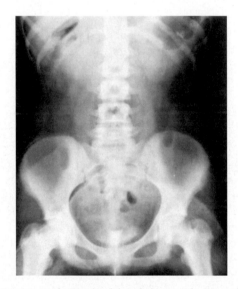

FIGURE 20-9 Radiograph of the abdomen showing the vertebral column with its inherent high contrast. The kidneys, pelvis, and psoas muscle are low-contrast tissues that are better visualized with low kVp. (Courtesy Euclid Seeram.)

"short gray scale," whereas Figure 20-10, *B*, shows low contrast or "long gray scale."

Gray scale of contrast means the range of ODs from the whitest to the blackest part of the radiograph. For example, think of using scissors to cut a small patch representing each OD on the radiograph, then arranging the patches in order from the lightest to darkest. The resulting OD range would be the gray scale of contrast.

High-contrast radiographs produce short gray scale. They exhibit black to white in just a few apparent steps. Low-contrast radiographs produce long gray scale and have the appearance of many shades of gray.

Figure 20-11 presents two radiographs of an aluminum step wedge—a penetrameter—that demonstrate scales of contrast. The one taken at 50 kVp shows that only five steps are visible. At 90 kVp, all 13 steps are visible because of the long scale of contrast.

Often the radiologic technologist is required to increase or decrease contrast because of an unacceptable image. To increase contrast, the range of ODs must be made more black and white with a greater difference in the OD of adjacent structures. In other words, a radiograph with a shorter contrast scale must be produced. Accomplishing this requires a reduction in kVp.

To reduce contrast, the radiographer must produce a radiograph with longer gray scale contrast, and therefore with more grays. This is done by increasing the kVp. Normally, a change of approximately 4% in kVp is required visually to affect the scale of contrast in the 50- to 90-kVp range. At lower kVp, a 2-kVp change may be sufficient, whereas at higher kVp a 10-kVp change may be required (Figure 20-12).

The phrases **high contrast, high degree of contrast,** and "a lot of contrast" all define short scale of contrast and are obtained by using low-kVp exposure techniques. **Low contrast** and **low degree of contrast** are the same as "long scale of contrast" and result from high-kVp exposure techniques. These relation-

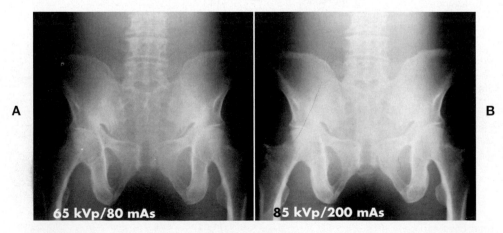

65 kVp/80 mAs   85 kVp/200 mAs

FIGURE 20-10 Radiographs of a pelvis phantom demonstrate short scale of contrast **(A)** and long scale of contrast **(B).** (Courtesy Kyle Thornton.)

ships in radiographic contrast are summarized in Table 20-5.

In addition to kilovoltage, many other factors influence radiographic contrast. Although the mAs setting affects only x-ray quantity, not quality, it still influences contrast. If the mAs value is too high or too low, the predominant OD will fall on the shoulder or toe of the characteristic curve, respectively.

Radiographic contrast is low on the shoulder and toe regions because the gradient of the characteristic curve is low in these regions. The images of different structures will have similar ODs despite differences in subject contrast.

The use of radiographic intensifying screens results in shorter contrast scale compared with nonscreen exposures. Collimation removes some scatter radiation, producing a radiograph of shorter contrast scale. Grids also reduce the amount of scatter that reaches the film,

thus also producing radiographs of shorter contrast scale. Grids with a high ratio increase the contrast. The exposure-technique factors that affect contrast are summarized in Table 20-6.

A typical clinical problem faced by the radiologic technologist is the adjustment of radiographic contrast. An image is made but the contrast scale is either too long (too many grays) or too short (too much black and white). Usually, it is the latter, so a longer scale of contrast is required. To solve such a problem, apply the

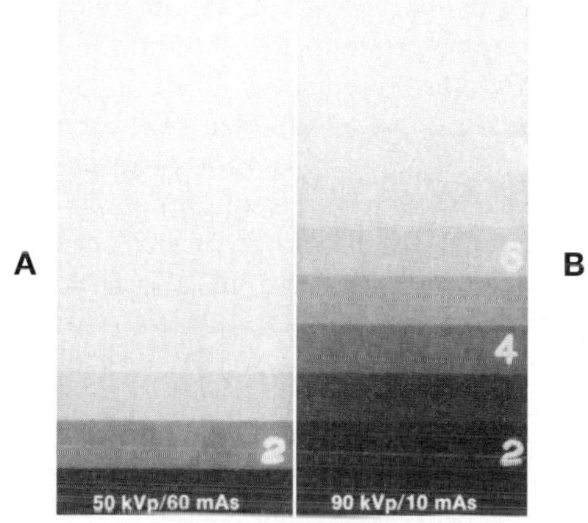

TABLE 20-5	The Relationship Between kVp and Scale of Contrast
High kVp Produces	**Low kVp Produces**
Long scale	Short scale
Low contrast	High contrast
Less contrast	More contrast

TABLE 20-6	Exposure Technique Factors That Affect Radiographic Contrast (in Approximate Order)
An Increase in This Factor	**Results in the Following Change in Contrast**
Kilovoltage	Decrease
Grid ratio	Increase
Beam restriction	Increase
Image receptor used	Variable
Development time	Decrease
Milliampere-seconds	Decrease (toe, shoulder)

FIGURE 20-11 Images of a step wedge exposed at low kVp (**A**) and high kVp (**B**) illustrate the meaning of short scale and long scale of contrast, respectively. (Courtesy Kyle Thornton.)

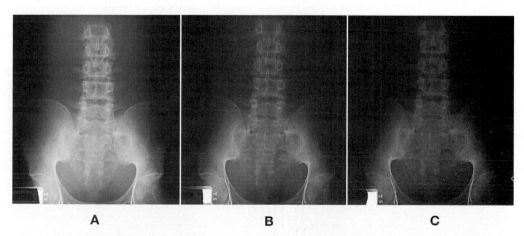

FIGURE 20-12 These radiographs of the pelvis and abdomen show that a 4-kVp increase results in a perceptible change in contrast. **A**, 75 kVp and 28 mAs. **B**, 79 kVp and 28 mAs. **C**, 81 kVp and 28 mAs. (Courtesy Mike Enriquez.)

fifteen percent rule. Increase the kVp by 15%, while reducing the mAs by one half.

Question: A patient's knee measures 14 cm and an exposure is made at 62 kVp/12 mAs. The resulting contrast scale is too short. What should the repeat technique be?

Answer: Increase kVp by 15%
$$62 \text{ kVp} \times 0.15 = 9.3 \text{ kVp}$$
Therefore, new kVp = 62 + 9 = 71 kVp
Reduce mAs to $\frac{1}{2}$
$$12 \text{ mAs} \times 0.5 = 6 \text{ mAs}$$
Repeat technique = 71 kVp/6 mAs

A smaller technique compensation for a change in contrast scale may be required. An increase of 5% in kVp may be accompanied by a 30% reduction in mAs to produce the same OD at a slightly reduced contrast scale. This is known as the **five percent rule.**

The proper technique compensation by the radiologic technologist is a judgment call. The anatomic part, body habitus, suspected pathology, and x-ray image receptor characteristics must all be considered by the skillful radiologic technologist. With practice and experience, this will become routine.

Question: A modest reduction in image contrast is required for a knee exposed at 62 kVp/12 mAs. What technique should be tried?

Answer: Apply the five percent rule:
$$62 \text{ kVp} \times 0.05 = 3.1 \text{ kVp}$$
$$62 + 3 = 65 \text{ kVp}$$
$$12 \text{ mAs} \times 0.30 = 3.6 \text{ mAs}$$
$$12 - 4 = 8 \text{ mAs}$$
Repeat technique = 65 kVp/8 mAs

Image Detail

Image detail describes the sharpness of appearance of small structures on the radiograph. With adequate detail, even the smallest parts of anatomy are visible and the radiologist can more readily detect tissue abnormalities. Image detail must be evaluated by two means—**recorded detail** and **visibility of image detail.**

Sharpness of image detail refers to the structural lines or borders of tissues in the image and the amount of blur of the image. The factors that generally control the sharpness of image detail are the geometric factors discussed in Chapter 19—focal spot size, SID, and object-to-image receptor distance (OID). Sharpness of image detail is also influenced by the type of intensifying screens used and the presence of motion.

 Sharpness of image detail is best measured by spatial resolution.

To produce the sharpest image detail, one should use the smallest appropriate focal spot and the longest SID and place the anatomic part as close to the image receptor as possible (i.e., minimize OID). Figure 20-13 shows two radiographs of a foot phantom. One was taken under optimum conditions and the other with poor technique. The difference in sharpness of image detail is obvious.

Visibility of image detail describes the ability to see the detail on the radiograph and is best measured by contrast resolution. Loss of visibility refers to any factor that causes the deterioration or obscuring of the image detail. For example, fog reduces the ability to see structural lines on the image.

An attempt to produce the best-defined image can be made by using all the correct factors, but if the film is

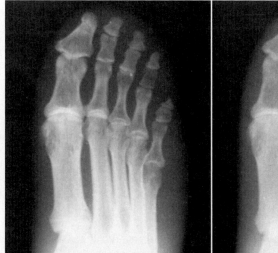
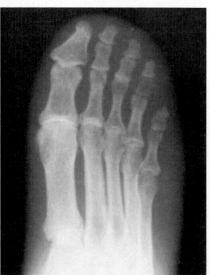

FIGURE 20-13 A radiograph taken with a 1-mm focal spot x-ray tube **(A)** exhibits far greater detail than one that taken with a 2-mm focal spot x-ray tube **(B).** (Courtesy Mike Enriquez.)

fogged by light or radiation, the detail present will not be fully visible (Figure 20-14). You might conclude that good detail is still present but that its visibility is poor. Because kVp and the mAs value influence image contrast, these factors must be chosen with care for each examination.

 The visibility of image detail is best measured by contrast resolution.

The assumption is that any factor that affects OD and contrast affects the visibility of image detail. Key factors that provide the best visibility of image detail are

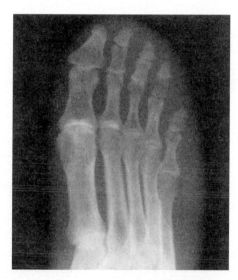

FIGURE 20-14 Same radiograph as shown in 20-13, *A* except the visibility of image detail is reduced because of safelight fog. (Courtesy Mike Enriquez.)

collimation, use of grids, and other methods that prevent scatter radiation from reaching the image receptor.

Distortion

The fourth image-quality factor is distortion, the misrepresentation of object size and shape on the radiograph. Because of the position of the x-ray tube, the anatomic part, and the image receptor, the final image may misrepresent the object.

Poor alignment of the image receptor or the x-ray tube can result in **elongation** of the image. Elongation means the object or part of interest appears longer than normal.

Poor alignment of the anatomic part may also result in **foreshortening** of the image. Foreshortening means that the anatomic part appears shorter than normal. Figure 20-15 provides examples of elongation and foreshortening. Many body parts are naturally foreshortened as a result of shape (e.g., ribs and facial bones).

Distortion can be minimized by proper alignment of the tube, the anatomic part, and the image receptor. This alignment is fundamentally important for **patient positioning.**

 Distortion is reduced by positioning the anatomic part of interest in a plane parallel to that of the image receptor.

Table 20-7 summarizes the principal radiographic image-quality factors. The primary controlling technique factor for each image-quality factor is given, as well as secondary technique factors that influence each image-quality factor.

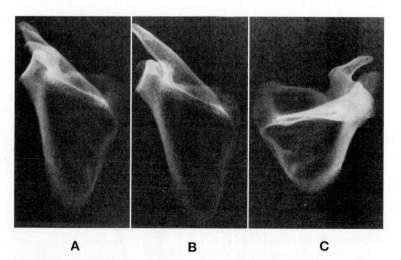

FIGURE 20-15 A, Normal projection of the scapula. **B,** Elongation of the scapula. **C,** Foreshortening of the scapula. (Courtesy Lynne Davis.)

TABLE 20-7	Principal Radiographic Image-Quality Factors	
Factor	**Controlled by**	**Influenced by**
Optical density	mAs	kVp Distance Thickness of part Mass density Development time/temperature Image receptor speed Collimation Grid ratio
Contrast	kVp	mAs (toe, shoulder) Development time/temperature Image receptor used Collimation Grid ratio
Detail	Focal-spot size	SID OID Motion All factors related to density and contrast
Distortion	Patient positioning	Alignment of tube, anatomic part, and image receptor

EXPOSURE-TECHNIQUE FACTORS

kVp, mA, exposure time, and SID are the principal exposure-technique factors. It is important for the radiologic technologist to know how to manipulate these exposure-technique factors to produce the desired OD, radiographic contrast, image detail, and distortion on the finished radiograph.

It is not necessary, however, to become creative with each new patient. For each radiographic imaging system, a guide or chart should be available that describes standard methods for consistently producing high-quality images. Such an aid is called a **radiographic technique chart.** Radiographic technique charts are tables that provide a means for determining the specific technical factors to be used for a given radiographic examination.

For a radiographic technique chart to meet with success, the radiologic technologist must understand its purpose, how it was constructed, and how it is to be used. Most important, the technologist must know how to make adjustments for body habitus and pathologic processes.

When used properly, the radiographic technique chart allows for consistently good diagnostic images. The scale of contrast and OD are more predictable than if no chart is used.

Radiographic technique charts can be prepared to accommodate all types of facilities. The four principal types of charts are based on **variable kilovoltage, fixed kilovoltage, high kilovoltage,** and **automatic exposure.** Each chart provides the radiologic technologist with a guide in the selection of exposure factors for all patients and all examinations.

Most facilities select a particular type of chart for use and then prepare similar charts for each radiographic examination room. The type of chart selected usually depends on the technical director of radiology, the type of imaging systems available, the screen-film combination, and the accessories available.

Radiographic technique charts and their use become an important issue in patient protection. Radiologic technologists are required to use their skills in producing the best possible image with a single exposure.

Repeat examinations serve only to increase the radiation dose to the patient. The preparation of these charts becomes an important and challenging task, and once in use, the charts must constantly be evaluated and changed when necessary.

A principal advantage to using technique charts is consistency in exposure from one technologist to another and comparison of examinations on the same patient on different dates and with different technologists.

The preparation of a technique chart does not require that it be created completely from scratch. Many authors have guides that can be used in preparation of specific charts. Each radiographic imaging system is unique in its radiation characteristics. Therefore, a specific chart should be prepared and tested for each examination room.

 Radiographic technique charts from books, pamphlets, and manufacturers should not be used as printed.

Before the preparation of the radiographic technique chart begins, the x-ray equipment must be calibrated by a medical physicist and the processing system must be thoroughly evaluated. The total filtration should also be determined. Although 2.5 mm Al is the prescribed standard, 3 mm Al total filtration or more may be available on the collimator housing. This significantly alters contrast and makes a considerable difference in any technique chart.

The type of grid to be used should be known and the collimator or beam restrictor checked for accurate light field and x-ray beam coincidence. This is most important so that all variables are reduced to a minimum. When a radiographic technique chart is found to be inadequate, these factors should be checked first.

Variable-kVp Technique Chart

The variable-kVp radiographic technique chart uses a fixed mAs value and a kVp that varies according to the thickness of the anatomic part. The basic characteristic of the variable-kVp chart is an inherently short scale of contrast. In general, exposures made with this method provide radiographs of shorter contrast scale because of the use of lower kVp.

 kVp varies with the thickness of the anatomic part by 2 kVp/cm.

Exposure directed by the variable-kVp chart usually results in higher patient dose and less exposure latitude. For success, the radiologic technologist must be accurate in measuring the anatomic part before selecting the exposure factors from the chart. Without such care and attention, the anatomic part may not be fully penetrated as a result of the lower kVp.

There are approximate procedures for establishing a kVp to begin formulating a variable-kVp technique chart. The beginning kVp depends on the voltage ripple as follows:

VARIABLE kVp
Beginning kVp (high frequency) = 2 × thickness of anatomy (cm) + 23

To begin preparation of a variable-kVp radiographic technique chart, select the body part for examination. For example, if the knee is chosen, use a knee phantom for all test exposures.

First, measure the thickness of the knee phantom, using a caliper designed for that purpose. Multiply the part thickness by 2 and add 23; this indicates a kVp with which to begin if the high-voltage generator is high frequency. If

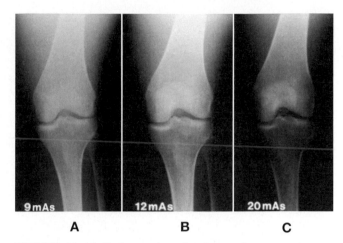

| **A** | **B** | **C** |

FIGURE 20-16 Radiographs of a knee phantom taken at 58 kVp. That obtained at 12 mAs (**B**) was selected to begin the variable-kilovoltage chart. (Courtesy Lynne Davis.)

the high-voltage generator is single phase or three phase, 30 or 25, respectively, are the additive factors.

Question: A phantom knee measures 14 cm thick. What single-phase kVp should be used to begin construction of a variable-kVp technique chart?

Answer: 14 cm × 2 = 28 + 30
= 58 kVp

The kilovoltage setting for examination of the knee is 58 kVp. The next task is to select the optimal mAs setting at this kVp. This depends on the image receptor characteristics and effectiveness of scatter radiation control. For example, when using a 200 speed image receptor with an 8:1 grid, make test exposures at 58 kVp with 9 mAs, 12 mAs, and 20 mAs (Figure 20-16). Select the radiograph that produces the best OD or make additional exposures at other mAs settings values if necessary.

The result of this exercise is the first line of the variable-kVp technique chart. The kVp and mAs setting to be used when radiographing a knee measuring 14 cm have been established at 58 kVp and 12 mAs, as shown in Table 20-8.

At this point, the chart can be expanded to include knees with other thicknesses. The same procedure is used. To prepare a variable-kVp radiographic technique chart for other anatomic parts, the same procedure is used. Because radiologists prefer similar contrast scales for examination of the same anatomy, the variable-kVp technique chart has been replaced largely by the fixed-kVp technique chart.

TABLE 20-8	Variable-kVp Chart for Examination of the Knee	
Knee—AP/Lat	**Part Thickness (cm)**	**kVp**
mAs: 12	8	50
SID: 100 cm	9	52
Grid: 12:1	10	54
Collimation: to part	11	56
Image receptor speed: 200	**12**	**58**
	13	60
	14	62
	15	64
	16	66

AP, Anterior-posterior; *Lat,* Lateral; *SID,* Source-to-image receptor distance.

Fixed-kVp Technique Chart

The fixed-kVp radiographic technique chart is the one used most often. Developed by Arthur Fuchs, it is a method for selecting exposures that produce radiographs with a longer scale of contrast. The kVp is selected as the optimum required for penetration of the anatomic part. This usually results in somewhat higher kVp values for most examinations than with the variable-kVp technique.

 For each anatomic part there is an optimum kVp.

Once selected, the kVp is fixed at that level for each type of examination and not varied according to different thicknesses of the anatomic part. The mAs value, however, is changed according to the thickness of the anatomic part to provide the proper OD. For example, all examinations of the knee might require 60 kVp with mAs adjusted to accommodate for differences in thickness.

Because the fixed-kVp technique usually requires higher kVp, one benefit is lower patient dose. There is greater latitude and more consistency with exposures of the same anatomic part.

Measurement of the part is not as critical because part size is grouped as small, medium, or large. For most x-ray examinations of the spine and trunk of the body, the optimal kVp is approximately 80 kVp. Approximately 70 kVp is appropriate for the soft tissue

of the abdomen. For most extremities, the optimum would be approximately 60 kVp.

To prepare a fixed-kVp radiographic technique chart, the first step is to separate the anatomic part thickness into three groups—small, medium, and large—by identifying the range of thickness that is to be included in each group. Using the abdomen as an example, small might be 14 to 20 cm; medium, 21 to 25 cm; and large, 26 to 32 cm.

For test exposures, use a medium-size phantom and begin with 80 kVp. Produce radiographs at mAs increments of 40, 60, 80, and so on until the proper OD is obtained (Figure 20-17). Again, the OD selected depends on the type of image receptor and available scatter radiation control devices.

Once the proper OD has been established, the chart can then be expanded to include small and large anatomic parts. For small anatomic parts, reduce the mAs by 30%. For large anatomic parts, increase the mAs by 30%. For a part that is swollen as a result of trauma, a 50% increase may be required. Table 20-9 presents the results of a representative procedure.

Fixed-kVp charts can also be calculated with specific mAs values for every 2-cm thickness. This approach is more accurate than the subjective small, medium, and large labels.

High-kVp Technique Chart

The kVp selected for high-kVp technique charts is usually greater than 100. For example, overhead radiographs for procedures using barium contrast medium would use 120 kVp for each exposure. High-kVp exposure techniques are ideal for barium work to ensure adequate penetration of the barium.

This type of exposure technique could also be used for routine chest radiography to provide improved visualization of the various tissue mass densities present in the lung fields and mediastinum. Lower or more conventional kVp settings provide increased subject contrast between bone and soft tissue. When 120 kVp is selected for chest radiography, however, all skeletal tissue is penetrated and there is increased visualization of the different soft tissue mass densities present.

To prepare a high-kVp technique chart, the procedure is basically the same as for preparing the fixed-kVp technique chart. All exposures for a particular anatomic part would use the same kVp. Obviously, the mAs value would be much less.

Test exposures are made using a phantom to determine the appropriate mAs setting for adequate OD. Figure 20-18 shows a chest radiograph made at 120 kVp. Note the improved visualization of the tissue markings of the bronchial tree and the mediastinal structures, compared with the low-kVp radiographs of Figure 20-8. An additional advantage to the high-kVp exposure technique is reduced patient dose.

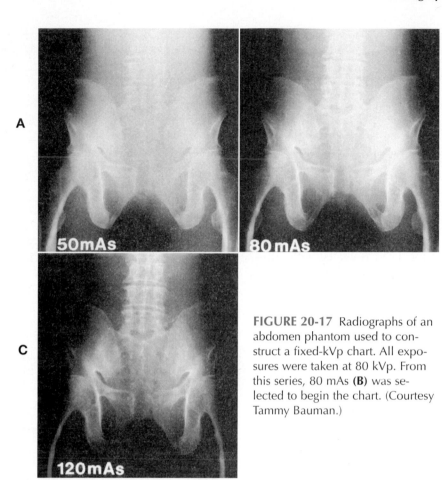

FIGURE 20-17 Radiographs of an abdomen phantom used to construct a fixed-kVp chart. All exposures were taken at 80 kVp. From this series, 80 mAs **(B)** was selected to begin the chart. (Courtesy Tammy Bauman.)

TABLE 20-9	Fixed-kVp Chart for Examination of the Abdomen		
Abdomen— AP	Part Thickness (cm)		Required mAs
kVp: 80	Small:	14–20	56
SID: 100 cm	Medium:	21–25	80
Grid: 12:1	Large:	26–31	104
Collimation: to part			
Image receptor speed: 200			

AP, Anterior-posterior; *SID,* Source-to-image receptor distance.

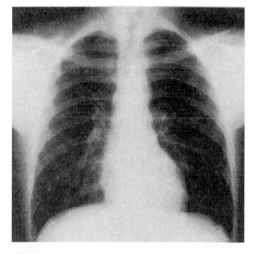

FIGURE 20-18 High-voltage chest radiograph illustrates the improved visualization of mediastinal structures. (Courtesy Andrew Woodward.)

AUTOMATIC EXPOSURE TECHNIQUES

The appearance of the operating console of x-ray imaging systems is changing in response to the ability to incorporate computer-assisted technology. Several automated exposure techniques are now available, but none relieves the radiologic technologist of the responsibility of identifying certain characteristics of the patient and the anatomic part to be imaged.

Computer-assisted automatic exposure systems use an electronic exposure timer, such as those described in Chapter 8. The radiation intensity is measured by either a photocell or an ionization chamber and terminates the

TABLE 20-10	Factors to Consider When Constructing an Exposure Chart for Automatic Systems	
Factor for Selection	**Rationale for Selection**	
Kilovolt peak	To select for each anatomic part	
Density control	To adjust according to the thickness of part	
Collimation	To reduce patient dose and ensure proper response of automatic exposure control	
Accessory selection	To optimize the radiation dose–image quality ratio	

exposure when the proper OD on the image receptor has been reached. The principles associated with automatic exposure systems have already been described, but the importance of using radiographic exposure charts with these systems has not.

Automatic control x-ray systems are not completely automatic. It is incorrect to assume that because the radiologic technologist does not have to select kVp and mAs settings and time for each examination, a less qualified or less skilled operator can use the system.

Usually, the radiologic technologist must use a guide for the selection of kVp similar to that of the fixed-kVp method. OD selections are numerically scaled to allow for "tweaking" the calibration of the sensors for changes in field size or anatomy requiring OD adjustment.

Patient positioning *must be absolutely accurate* because the specific body part must be placed over the phototiming device to ensure proper exposure.

The factors shown in Table 20-10 must be considered when preparing the radiographic exposure chart for an automatic x-ray system. The kVp is selected according to the specific anatomic part being examined.

The specific accessories to be used, such as film, screens, and grids, determine to a great extent the previous selections. It is critical to ensure that collimation confines the x-ray beam only to the anatomic part under investigation or to the image receptor, whichever is smaller. Excessive scatter radiation causes the automatic exposure control (AEC) to reduce exposure time and reduce image contrast.

Automatic Exposure Control

Radiation exposure during radiography in most x-ray imagers is determined by AEC. AEC incorporates a device to sense the amount of radiation falling on the image receptor. Through an electronic feedback circuit, the radiation exposure is terminated when a sufficient number of x-rays has reached the image receptor to produce an acceptable OD.

To image with the use of an AEC, the radiologic technologist selects the appropriate kVp, and the AEC does the rest. Exposure is terminated when the image recep-

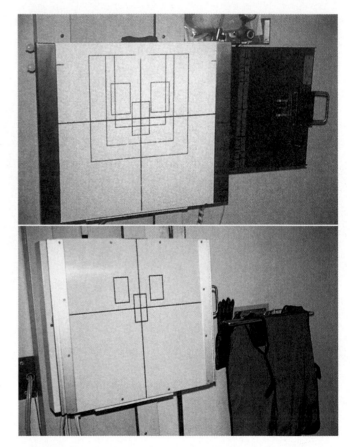

FIGURE 20-19 Vertical chest Bucky shows the position of three phototimers, two circles, and a rectangle and the dimensions of four standard image receptor sizes.

tor has received the appropriate radiation exposure to correspond with the acceptable OD.

AEC devices usually have two or more exposure sensors available for control (Figure 20-19). For instance, three radiation-sensing cells may be available, and the technologist is responsible for selecting which of the sensors to use for the examination. During a chest examination, if the mediastinum is the region of interest, only the central sensing cell is used. If the lung fields are of principal importance, the two lateral cells are activated.

Regulations require that AECs have a 600-mAs safety override. If the AEC fails to terminate the exposure, the secondary safety circuit terminates it at 600 mAs, which is equivalent to a few seconds depending on the mA.

In addition to the selection of the exposure cells, the radiologic technologist usually has a three- to seven-position dial labeled "OD" with numeric steps. Each step on the dial is calibrated to increase or decrease the preset average OD of the image receptor by 0.1. This control can be used to accommodate any unusual patient characteristics or to overcome the slowly changing calibration or sensitivity of the AEC.

A technique chart for AEC may be helpful. Such a chart would include mA, kVp, back-up time, sensor selection, and OD setting.

Programmed Exposure

Microprocessors are being incorporated ever more frequently into operating consoles. A microprocessor allows the operator digitally to select any kVp or mAs setting and the microprocessor automatically activates the appropriate mA station and exposure time.

With falling-load generators, the microprocessor begins the exposure at a maximum mA setting and then causes the tube current to be reduced during exposure. The overall objective is to minimize exposure time to reduce motion blur.

Anatomically Programmed Radiography

The ultimate in patient exposure control is termed **anatomically programmed radiography (APR)**. APR also uses microprocessor technology. Rather than have the radiologic technologist select a desired kVp and mAs, graphics on the console or on a video touch screen guide the technologist (Figure 20-20).

To produce an image, the radiologic technologist simply touches a picture or a written description of the anatomic part to be imaged and the body habitus. The microprocessor selects the appropriate kVp and mAs settings automatically. The whole process uses AECs, resulting in near-flawless radiographs. Thus, fewer repeats are necessary. However, precise patient positioning relative to the phototiming sensor is still critical in producing high-quality radiographs.

The principle of APR is similar to AEC, with the radiographic technique chart stored in the microprocessor of the control unit. The service engineer loads the controlling programs during installation and calibrates the exposure control circuit for the general conditions of the facility.

The radiologic technologist needs only to select the part and its relative size before each exposure. The programmed instructions, however, must be continuously adjusted by the radiologic technologist until the entire panel of examinations is optimized for best image quality.

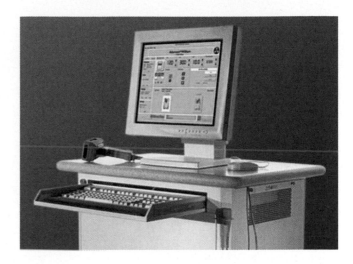

FIGURE 20-20 Anatomically programmed radiography (APR) operating console with lower ribs and automatic exposure control selected.

SUMMARY

Radiographic technique is the combination of factors used to expose an anatomic part to produce a high-quality radiograph. Radiographic technique is characterized by the following: (1) patient factors, (2) image-quality factors, and (3) exposure-technique factors.

Patient factors are anatomic thickness, body composition, and any pathology that is present. Body thickness is measured by calipers. Radiographers recognize sthenic, asthenic, hyposthenic, and hypersthenic body habitus types as a way to determine body composition and, thus, proper radiographic technique. Pathology in the body may be either destructive and therefore radiolucent, which requires a reduction in technique, or constructive and therefore radiopaque, which requires an increase.

Image-quality factors that define the quality of the image are OD, contrast, image detail, and distortion. OD is the blackening of the radiograph and is defined as the log of the incident light over the transmitted light. Contrast is the difference in optical density between adjacent anatomic structures.

High kVp produces low-contrast images, whereas low kVp produces high-contrast images. Image detail is the sharpness of the image on the radiograph. To produce the sharpest image detail, use the smallest focal spot, the longest SID, and the least OID. Distortion refers to the misrepresentation of object size or shape on the radiograph.

The principal radiographic exposure factors are kVp, mAs, and SID. The two most common technique charts for use by radiographers to produce consistently high-quality radiographs are the fixed-kVp chart and the high-kVp chart. The high-kVp chart is used for barium studies and chest radiographs with kVp from 120 to 135 kVp. The fixed-kVp chart uses approximately 60 kVp for extremity radiography and approximately 80 kVp for examinations of the trunk of the body.

Even with AEC, radiographic exposure charts are required. APR uses microprocessor technology to program the technique chart into the control unit. The radiographer selects an anatomic display of the part and the microprocessor selects the appropriate kVp and mAs settings automatically.

CHALLENGE QUESTIONS

1. Define or otherwise identify:
   a. Fifteen percent rule
   b. Image detail
   c. Body habitus
   d. Image-quality factors
   e. Scale of contrast
   f. APR
   g. Optical density
   h. Elongation
   i. Variable-kVp chart
   j. Distortion
2. List and discuss the four exposure-technique factors. How does each affect OD?
3. Explain how kVp influences the scale of contrast.
4. A radiographic technique calls for 82 kVp at 400 mA, 200 ms, and an SID of 90 cm. What is the mAs value?
5. A radiographic technique of 150 mA, 200 ms is used but there is motion blur. If the exposure time is reduced to 25 ms, what should be the mA?
6. An acceptable chest radiograph was taken at 180 cm SID with 10 mAs. If the 400-mA station is used, what will be the new exposure time at 90 cm SID?
7. Identify the range of optical densities that are too light, too dark, and within the useful range.
8. When a change in OD is required, what exposure technique factor should be changed and why?
9. When a change in radiographic contrast is required, what exposure technique factor should be changed and why?
10. List and discuss the nature of the four types of radiographic exposure charts.
11. What are the three groups of variables or factors that determine the quality of the finished radiograph?
12. How does body habitus affect the selection of technical factors?
13. Describe the two classifications of pathology and how technical factors may be affected by each classification.
14. Name the tool used to measure the thickness of an anatomic part when a radiographer is determining technical factor selection.
15. How does the radiographer determine the type of pathology a patient may have before a radiographic examination?
16. Write the formula for optical density (OD).
17. Identify the numeric equivalent range of ODs from black to clear.
18. What is the relationship between OD and mAs?
19. Define contrast. Give an example of tissues with high contrast and an example of tissues with low contrast.
20. List the three ways to produce the sharpest image detail.

Special Imaging Methods

OBJECTIVES

At the completion of this chapter, the student should be able to do the following:

1. List the directional movements of a conventional tomographic imaging system
2. Explain tomographic motion blur
3. Discuss the relationship between tomographic angle and section thickness
4. Identify the sequence of steps in producing and viewing a stereoradiograph
5. Describe magnification radiography and its use

OUTLINE

Tomography
  Linear Tomography
  Zonography
  Panoramic Tomography
  Practical Considerations
Magnification Radiography

ANY AREAS of x-ray diagnosis require special equipment and specialized techniques to obtain the required information. Such procedures are designed to visualize more clearly a given anatomic structure, usually at the expense of nonvisualization of other structures.

The equipment and procedures discussed in this chapter include tomography, stereoradiography, and magnification radiography. These x-ray examinations are not routine, and therefore, require the radiologic technologist to be specially trained.

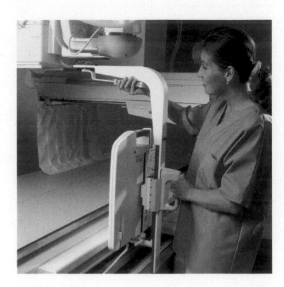

FIGURE 21-1 This tomography system is designed for linear movement with a general purpose R&F imaging system. (Courtesy General Electric Medical Systems.)

TOMOGRAPHY

A conventional radiograph of the chest or abdomen images all structures contained in these parts of the body with approximately equal fidelity. The structures, however, are superimposed on one another, and often this superimposition results in a masking of the structure of interest. When this occurs, a procedure called **tomography** may be necessary.

The tomographic examination is designed to bring into focus only that anatomy lying in a plane of interest while blurring structures on either side of that plane. Actually, the object is **not focused** in the normal sense but rather its radiographic contrast is enhanced by the blurring of the anatomic structure above and below.

A tomographic x-ray imaging system appears similar to a conventional radiographic imaging system in most features (Figure 21-1). Note the vertical rod that attacks the x-ray tube above the table with the image receptor below the patient to enable both to move in reciprocal fashion about the fulcrum. That is the feature unique to tomography.

 The principal advantage of tomography is improved contrast resolution.

Since the introduction of computed tomography (CT) and magnetic resonance imaging (MRI) with their excellent contrast resolution, tomography is used less frequently. Tomography is now applied principally to high contrast procedures, such as imaging calcified kidney stones. Table 21-1 lists the more common tomographic examinations and their representative techniques.

During the tomographic examination, the radiographic tube is caused to move in a precise fashion, while the image receptor moves synchronously. There are five types of tomographic movement: linear, circular, elliptical, hypocycloidal, and trispiral. Only the linear motion is now used with any regularity because of the dedicated equipment requirements of the others and the common availability of CT and MRI.

Linear Tomography

The simplest tomographic examination is linear tomography. During linear tomography (Figure 21-2), the x-ray tube is mechanically attached to the image receptor and moves in one direction, while the image receptor moves in the opposite direction.

The ability to perform tomography can be obtained inexpensively by altering a conventional radiographic imaging system to accommodate x-ray tube and image receptor motion. With this type of linear tomography, the x-ray tube and the image receptor remain in the same plane during motion (Figure 21-2, *A*).

Some equipment specially designed for linear tomography is constructed so that the x-ray tube and the image receptor move in similar arcs during the examination (Figure 21-2, *B*). This latter method of linear tomography results in higher quality tomography but it is more expensive and has limited use.

Other aspects of the linear tomographic examination are shown in Figure 21-3. The **fulcrum** is the imaginary pivot point about which the x-ray tube and the image receptor move. The position of the fulcrum determines the **object plane** and only those anatomic structures lying in this plane are clearly imaged. The plane of the section is determined by adjusting the height of the fulcrum from the table or by repositioning the table height between exposures.

TABLE 21-1	Representative Linear Tomography Techniques			
Examination	**Projection**	**kVp**	**mAs***	**Section thickness**
Cervical spine	Anterior-Posterior	75	60	3 - 5 mm
	Lateral	77	60	2 mm
Thoracic spine	Anterior-Posterior	77	80	5 mm
Lumbar spine	Anterior-Posterior	77	140	5 mm
Chest	Anterior-Posterior	96	80	2 - 5 cm
Intravenous pyelogram	Anterior-Posterior	70	140	1 cm
Wrist	Anterior-Posterior	48	20	2 mm

* Usually automatic exposure control.

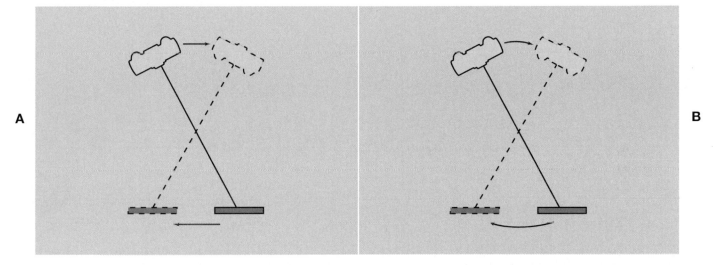

A   B

FIGURE 21-2 A, Image receptor and tube head of a general-purpose x-ray imaging system designed to move tomographically in a plane. **B,** An imaging system designed for tomography to move in an arc.

The angle of movement is known as the **tomographic angle.** The tomographic angle determines the **section thickness,** or that thickness of tissue that will not be blurred. The determination of the section thickness is made by selecting the proper tomographic angle.

Figure 21-4 illustrates how anatomic structures in the object plane are imaged but structures above and below this plane are not. The examination begins with the x-ray tube and the image receptor positioned on opposite sides of the fulcrum. The exposure begins as the x-ray tube and image receptor move simultaneously in opposite directions. The image of an anatomic structure lying in the object plane, such as the arrow, will have a fixed position on the radiograph throughout the tube travel.

On the other hand, the images of structures lying above or below the object plane, such as the ball and box, will have varying positions on the image receptor during the tomographic movement (Figure 21-4). Consequently the ball and box will be blurred. The larger

the tomographic angle, the more blurred the images of structures above and below the object plane appear.

 The farther from the object plane an anatomic structure is, the more blurred its image will be.

The blurring of anatomic structures lying outside the object plane is simply an example of **motion blur** caused by the moving x-ray source. In theory, only objects lying precisely in the object plane, which is the plane of the fulcrum, will be properly imaged.

Objects lying outside this plane will exhibit increasing motion blur with increasing distance from the object plane. Objects within a section of tissue between two parallel planes are in focus. This thickness of tissue that will be imaged is called the **tomographic section** and its width is described numerically by the section thickness (Figure 21-5).

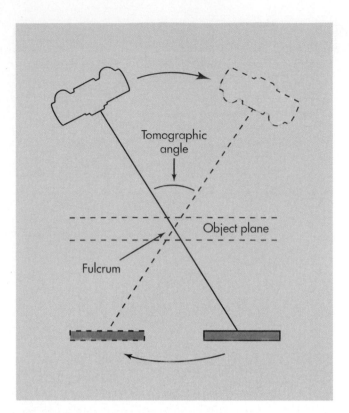

FIGURE 21-3 Relationship of fulcrum, object plane, and tomographic angle.

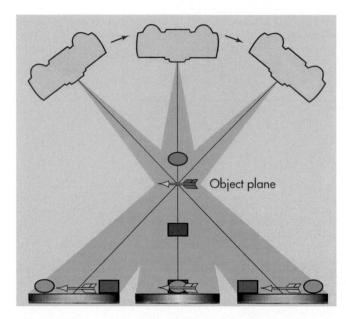

FIGURE 21-4 Only objects lying in the object plane are properly imaged. Objects above and below this plane are blurred because they are imaged across the film.

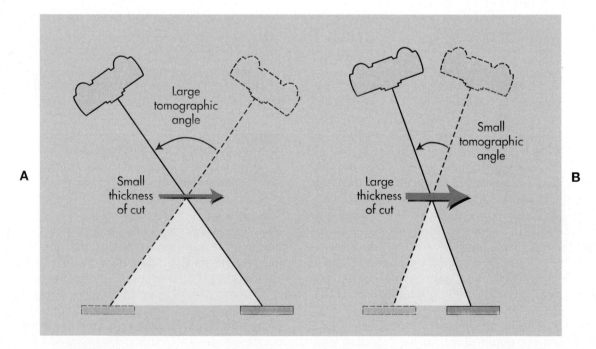

FIGURE 21-5 Section thickness is determined by the tomographic angle. **A**, A large tomographic angle, results in a thin section. **B**, A small tomographic angle, results in a thick section.

The larger the tomographic angle, the thinner the tomographic section.

The tomographic section thickness is controlled by the tomographic angle. Table 21-2 shows the approximate relationship between tomographic angle and tomographic section thickness. This relationship is shown graphically in Figure 21-6.

When the tomographic angle is very small (for example, 0 degrees), the section thickness is the entire anatomic structure resulting in a conventional radiograph. When the tomographic angle is 10 degrees, the section thickness is approximately 6 mm; structures lying farther than approximately 3 mm from the object plane will appear blurred.

A linear anatomic structure can be imaged with less blur if the length of the structure is positioned parallel to the x-ray tube motion. This is illustrated with a

TABLE 21-2	Approximate Values for Section Thickness During Linear Tomography as a Function of Tomographic Angle
Tomographic angle (degrees)	**Section thickness (mm)**
0	Infinity
2	31
4	16
6	11
10	6
20	3
35	2
50	1

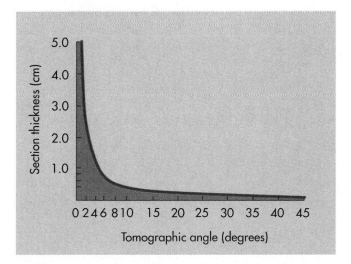

FIGURE 21-6 Image section becomes thinner as the tomographic angle is increased.

tomographic test object (Figure 21-7). Conversely, Figure 21-8 shows how linear structures that lie perpendicular to the x-ray tube motion are more easily blurred. These foot tomographs were taken parallel to the long axis of the patient (Figure 21-8, *A*) and perpendicular to the long axis of the patient (Figure 21-8, *B*).

Zonography

If the tomographic angle is less than about 10 degrees, the section thickness will be quite large (Table 21-2). This type of tomography is called **zonography** because a relatively large zone of tissue is imaged.

Zonography is used when the subject contrast is so low that thin-section tomography would result in a poor image. Zonography finds most application in chest and renal examination where tomographic angles of 5 to 10 degrees are usually used.

Panoramic Tomography

Panoramic tomography was first developed for a fast dental survey but finds increasing diagnostic application of the curved bony structures of the head, such as the mandible. For this procedure the x-ray tube and image receptor move around the head as shown in Figure 21-9. The x-ray beam is collimated to a slit as shown. The image receptor is likewise slit-collimated. During the

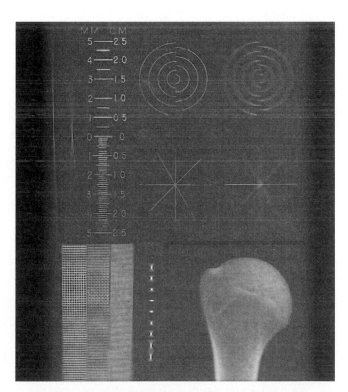

FIGURE 21-7 This test object image shows properly calibrated elevation and increased blur of objects perpendicular to the motion of the x-ray tube. (Courtesy Sharon Glaze.)

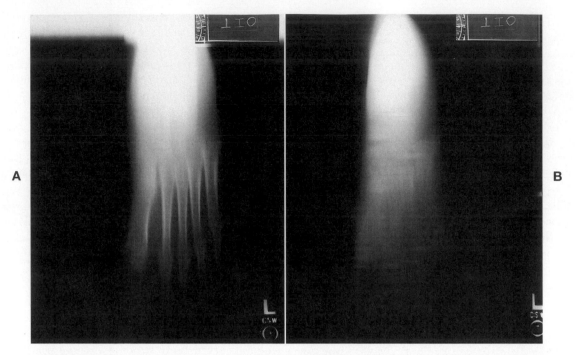

FIGURE 21-8 Foot tomographs obtained with x-ray tube motion. **A**, Parallel with the body axis. **B**, Perpendicular to the body axis. (Courtesy Rees Stuteville.)

examination, the image receptor translates behind the slit collimator so that it is exposed for several seconds along its length. Figure 21-10 is a clinical example.

Practical Considerations

The principal advantage to tomography is improved radiographic contrast. By blurring overlying and underlying tissues, the subject contrast of tissue of the tomographic section is enhanced. The more irregular the movement of the x-ray tube and image receptor, the greater will be the contrast enhancement. Multidirectional movement of the x-ray tube and image receptor does not affect section thickness of the tomographic layer. Only the tomographic angle does.

The principal disadvantage of tomography is increased patient dose. The x-ray tube is on during the entire period of tube travel, which can be several seconds. A single nephrotomographic exposure (examination of the kidneys), for example, can result in a patient dose of 1000 mrad (10 mGy_t).

Furthermore, most tomographic examinations require several exposures to make certain that the tomographic section of interest is imaged. A sixteen film tomographic examination can result in a patient dose of several rad (mGy_t).

 During tomography, parallel grids must be used and the grid lines must be oriented in the same direction as the tube movement.

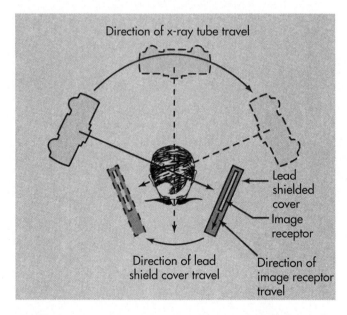

FIGURE 21-9 The x-ray source-image receptor motion for panoramic tomography.

Grids are used during a tomography for the same reason that they are used during radiography. For linear tomography, this usually means that the grid will be positioned with its grid lines parallel with the length of the table.

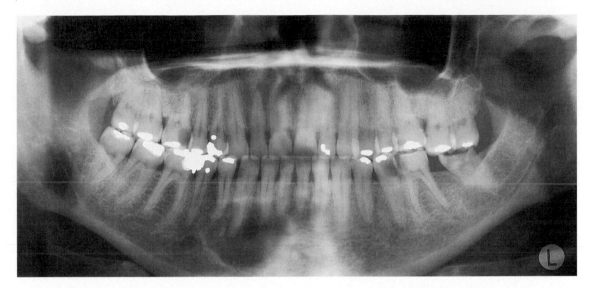

FIGURE 21-10 Panoramic tomogram showing restorations and a right mandibular defect. (Courtesy Kenneth Abramovitch.)

MAGNIFICATION RADIOGRAPHY

Magnification radiography is a technique used principally by vascular radiologists and neuroradiologists. Magnification radiography enhances the visualization of small vessels. Conventional radiography strives to minimize the object-to-image receptor distance (OID). Magnification radiography deliberately increases OID.

Magnification radiography uses the principles of magnification from Chapter 19. To obtain a magnified radiograph, the OID is increased, while the SID is held constant (Figure 21-11). The degree of magnification is given by the **magnification factor (MF)** as follows:

MAGNIFICATION FACTOR

$$MF = \frac{SID}{SOD} = \frac{Image\ size}{Object\ size}$$

---

where SID is the source-to-image receptor and SOD is the source-to-object distance.

Question: A magnified radiograph of the sella turcica is taken at 100 cm SID with the object positioned 25 cm from the image receptor. If the image of the sella turcica measures 16 mm, what is its actual size?

Answer: $MF = \dfrac{100}{(100 - 25)} = 1.33$

$$\frac{Image\ size}{Object\ size} = MF$$

$$Object\ size = \frac{Image\ size}{MF}$$

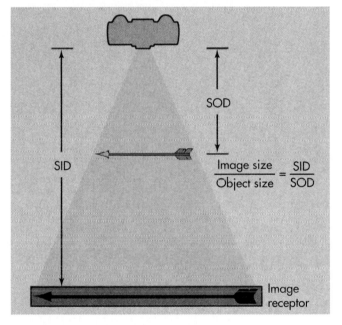

FIGURE 21-11 Principle of magnification radiography. The magnification factor is equal to the ratio of image size to object size.

$$= \frac{16}{1.33}$$

$$= 12.0\ mm$$

A small focal spot must be used for magnification radiography to help reduce the loss of image detail. The focal spot blur resulting from an unnecessarily large focal spot can destroy the diagnostic value of the magnified radiograph.

Usually, grids are not needed for magnified radiography. The large OID results in a significant air-gap so that much of the scatter radiation misses the image receptor. The larger the OID, the lower the amount of scatter radiation reaching the image receptor.

The principal disadvantage of magnification radiography, like so many specialized techniques, is increased patient dose. To obtain a magnification factor of 2, one must position the patient halfway between the x-ray tube and the image receptor. Recall that radiation intensity is related to the square of the distance, which suggests a fourfold increase in patient dose. In reality, most magnification radiographs result in only three times the normal patient dose because grids are not used.

SUMMARY

Although CT and MRI have replaced much of the plain-film tomographic examinations, tomography of the chest and kidneys is still frequently performed. The emphasis is generally on linear techniques with thin, 1 cm tomographic sections.

Zonography is defined as thick-slice tomography with a tomographic angle of less than 10 degrees. Panoramic tomography was originally developed for dental radiography but has found application in imaging the mandible and other facial structures.

The tomographic object plane contains the fulcrum, which is the imaginary pivot point from which the tube and image receptor move. The tomographic angle is the angle of movement and determines the tomographic section thickness. The principal advantage of tomography is improved radiographic contrast. By blurring the structures above and below the object plane, the contrast of the anatomy in the tomographic section is enhanced.

The two adjustments made by the radiologic technologist are the height of the fulcrum to determine the height of the object plane and the tomographic angle to determine the section thickness.

Magnification radiography is a technique used mainly for cardiovascular and interventional radiography.

All the alternative radiographic procedures discussed in this chapter have the disadvantage of increasing patient dose. As a result, it is important to take care when positioning patients and when selecting technical factors.

CHALLENGE QUESTIONS

1. Define or otherwise identify:
   a. OID
   b. Tomographic angle
   c. Zonography
   d. Magnification factor
   e. Fulcrum
   f. Object plane
   g. Tomographic layer
   h. SOD
   i. Section thickness
   j. Contrast resolution
2. Explain how tomography improves image contrast.
3. Describe the relationship between tomographic angle and tomographic section thickness.
4. List three common tomographic procedures and the approximate radiographic technique for each.

5. How can one tell if radiographic apparatus is capable of tomography?

6. What is the relationship among (a) x-ray tube, (b) object plane, (c) image receptor, (d) tomographic angle, and (e) tomographic section thickness during tomography?

7. Diagram linear tomography and identify the fulcrum, tomographic angle, object plane, image plane, grid position, film position, and image receptor.

8. What is the principal advantage to linear tomography?

9. What special equipment is required for magnification radiography?

10. Why is tomography necessary as an alternative to conventional radiographs?

11. What two imaging procedures have replaced most tomographic examinations?

12. What is the role of an air-gap in magnification radiography?

13. Describe the equipment alterations required for tomography.

14. Are linear structures that lie perpendicular to the tube motion more or less easily blurred?

15. What anatomic structures are best imaged using panoramic tomography.

16. Why does the x-ray tube move opposite the motion of the image receptor?

17. What is the relationship between grid lines and tomographic direction?

18. Given an SID of 100 cm, OID of 10 cm and an image size of 3.2 cm, what is the true object size?

19. The 4th lumbar vertebra is radiographed at an SID of 150 cm and an SOD of 50 cm. The width of L4 on the radiograph measures 72 mm. What is the true width of L4?

20. What is the major disadvantage of tomography and magnification radiography?

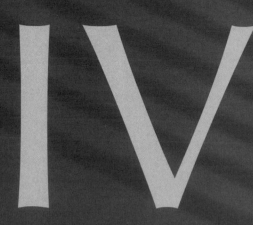

PART **IV**

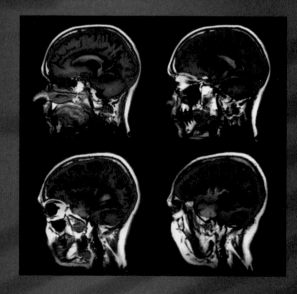

SPECIAL X-RAY IMAGING

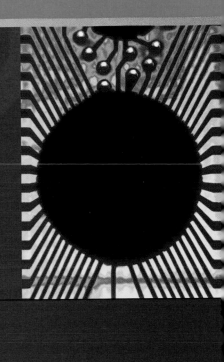

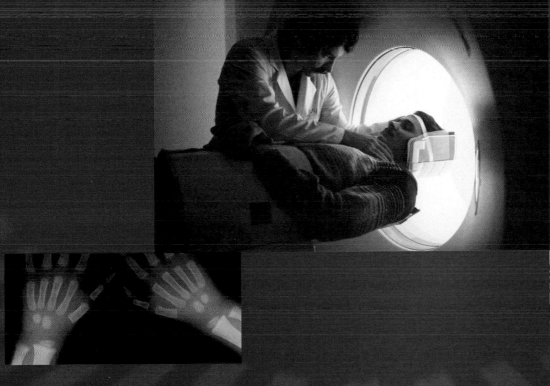

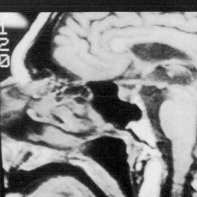

Mammography

OBJECTIVES

At the completion of this chapter, the student should be able to do the following:

1. Discuss the differences between soft tissue radiography and conventional radiography
2. Describe the anatomy of the breast
3. Identify the recommended intervals for self-examination and x-ray examination of the breast
4. Describe the unique features of a mammographic imaging system
5. Discuss the requirement for compression in mammography
6. Describe the image receptors used and spatial resolution obtained in mammography
7. Explain the differences between diagnostic and screening mammography

OUTLINE

BREAST CANCER is the second leading cause of death from cancer in women (lung cancer is first). Each year about 175,000 new cases of breast cancer are reported in the United States, with one quarter of these cases resulting in death. These statistics indicate that one of every eight women will develop breast cancer during her life.

It is widely thought that early detection of breast cancer leads to more effective treatment and fewer deaths. X-ray mammography has proved to be an accurate and simple method of detecting breast cancer but it is not simple to perform. The radiographer and support staff must have exceptional knowledge, skill, and caring.

The federal government has recently mandated regulations in the Mammography Quality Standards Act (MQSA), which sets standards for image quality, radiation dose, personnel qualifications, and examination procedures.

SOFT TISSUE RADIOGRAPHY

Radiographic examination of soft tissues, called **soft tissue radiography**, requires selected techniques that differ from those used in conventional radiography. These differences in technique are due to the substantial differences in the anatomy being imaged. In conventional radiography, the subject contrast is great because of the large differences in mass density and atomic number among bone, muscle, fat, and lung tissue.

In soft tissue radiography, only muscle and fat structures are imaged. These tissues have similar effective atomic numbers (see Chapter 12, Table 12-1) and similar mass densities (see Table 12-2). Consequently, soft tissue radiographic techniques are designed to enhance differential absorption in these very similar tissues.

A prime example of soft tissue radiography is **mammography**—radiographic examination of the breast. As a distinct type of radiographic examination, mammography was first attempted in the 1920s. Its development at that time was prevented by the era's lack of adequate equipment. In the late 1950s, Robert Egan renewed interest in mammography with his demonstration of a successful technique using low kVp, high mAs value, and direct film exposure.

In the 1960s, Wolf and Ruzicka showed that **xeromammography** was superior to direct film exposure at a much lower patient dose. Detail and contrast were much improved because of the spatial characteristic **edge enhancement,** the accentuation of the interface between different tissues. This property is frequently used in the postprocessing of digital images. Xeromammography was retired by 1990 because single screen-film mammography provided better images at even lower patient doses.

Mammography has undergone much change and development. It now enjoys widespread application thanks to the efforts of the American College of Radiology (ACR) volunteer accreditation program and the federally mandated Mammography Quality Standards Act (MQSA) enacted in 1991.

BASIS FOR MAMMOGRAPHY

The principal motivation for the continuing development and improvement of mammography is the high incidence of breast cancer. Breast cancer is the leading cancer in women. Unfortunately, lung cancer has passed breast cancer as the leading cause of cancer death in women because of the increasing use of tobacco.

Risk of Breast Cancer

Each year approximately 175,000 new cases of breast cancer are reported in the United States, and this number is growing. Several factors have been identified that increase a woman's risk of breast cancer (Box 22-1).

 One of every eight women will develop breast cancer.

Breast cancer is now a disease that is far from fatal. In 1995, The National Cancer Institute reported the first reduction in breast cancer mortality in 50 years, and this trend continues. With early mammographic diagnosis, more than 90% of patients are cured.

One important consideration in the overall efficacy of mammography is patient dose because radiation can cause breast cancer as well as detect it. However, considerable evidence shows that the mature breast in the screening age group has very low sensitivity to radiation-induced breast cancer. Radiation carcinogenesis (the induction of cancer) is discussed in Chapter 36.

The dose necessary to produce breast cancer is unknown; however, the dose experienced in mammography is well known and is covered in Chapter 40. This chapter concerns the imaging technique, equipment, and procedures used in mammography.

Types of Mammography

There are two different types of mammographic examination. **Diagnostic mammography** is performed on patients with symptoms or elevated risk factors. Two or three views of each breast may be required. **Screening mammography** is performed on asymptomatic women using a two-view protocol, usually medial lateral oblique and cranial caudad, to detect an unsuspected cancer.

Screening mammography in patients 50 years and older reduces cancer mortality. Screening women in the 40- to 50-year age group is also beneficial. Because younger women have potentially more years of life left, screening in this group results in more years of life saved.

The American Cancer Society recommends that women perform monthly breast self-examination, wherein a health care professional teaches a woman to check her breasts regularly for lumps, thickening of the skin, or any changes in size or shape. Table 22-1 relates the recommended intervals for breast self-examination and screening mammography.

The American Cancer Society also recommends annual breast examination by a physician and a baseline mammogram. A **baseline mammogram** is the first radiographic examination of the breasts usually obtained before age 40. Radiologists use it for comparison with all future mammograms.

The risk of radiation-induced breast cancer resulting from x-ray mammography has been given a lot of attention. Mammography is considered very safe and effective. The ratio of benefit (lives saved) to risk (deaths caused) is estimated at 700:1 to 1000:1.

BOX 22-1 Risk Factors for Breast Cancer

Age: the older you are, the higher the risk
Family history: mother, sister with breast cancer
Genetics: presence of BRCA1 or BRCA2 genes
Menstruation: onset before age 12
Menopause: onset after age 55
Prolonged use of **estrogen**
Late age at birth of first child or **no children**
Education: risk increases with higher education
Socioeconomics: risk increases with higher status

Breast Anatomy

The anatomy of the breast and its tissue characteristics make imaging difficult (Figure 22-1). The young breast is dense and more difficult to image because of glandular tissue. The older breast is more fatty and easier to image.

The normal breasts consist of three principal tissues: fibrous, glandular, and adipose (fat). In a premenopausal woman the fibrous and glandular tissues are structured into various ducts, glands, and connective tissues. These are surrounded by a thin layer of fat. The radiographic appearance of glandular and connective tissue is very dense.

Postmenopausal breasts are characterized by a degeneration of this fibroglandular tissue and an increase in the adipose tissue. Adipose tissue is less dense radiographically and requires less exposure.

 The tissue most sensitive to cancer by radiation is *glandular tissue.*

If a malignancy is present, it appears as a distortion of the normal ductal and connective tissue patterns. Approximately 80% of breast cancer is ductal and may have associated deposits of **microcalcifications** that appear as small grains of varying size. In terms of detecting breast cancer, microcalcifications smaller than approximately 500 μm are of interest. The incidence of breast cancer is highest in the upper lateral quadrant of the breast (Figure 22-2).

Because the mass density and atomic number of soft tissue components of the breast are so similar, conventional radiographic technique is useless. In the 70 to 100 kVp range, Compton scattering predominates with soft tissue; thus, differential absorption within soft tissues is minimal. Low peak kVp must be used to maximize the photoelectric effect and therefore enhance differential absorption.

Recall from Chapter 12 that x-ray absorption in tissue occurs principally by photoelectric effect and

TABLE 22-1   Recommended Intervals for Breast Examination

| | PATIENT AGE | | |
Examination	<40 Years	40–49 Years	≥50 Years
Self-examination	Monthly*	Monthly	Monthly
Physician physical examination	Annually†	Annually	Annually
X-ray mammography			
High risk	Baseline	Annually	Annually
Low risk	Baseline	Biannually	Annually

*Beginning at age 20.
†Beginning at age 35.

Compton effect. The degree of absorption is determined by the mass density and effective atomic number.

Absorption caused by differences in mass density is simply proportional to the mass density for both photoelectric and Compton effects. Absorption caused by differences in the atomic number, however, is directly proportional for Compton interactions and proportional to the cube of the atomic number for photoelectric interactions.

 At low x-ray energy, photoelectric absorption predominates over Compton scattering.

Therefore, x-ray mammography requires a low kVp technique. As kVp is reduced, however, the penetrability of the x-ray beam is also reduced, which in turn requires an increase in the mAs value.

If the peak kVp is too low, an inordinately high mAs value may be required, which could be unacceptable because of the increased patient dose. Technique factors of approximately 23 to 28 kVp are used as an effective compromise between the increasing dose at low kVp and reduced image quality at high peak kVp.

THE MAMMOGRAPHIC IMAGING SYSTEM

X-ray mammography became clinically acceptable with the introduction of molybdenum as target and filter (1966) and the dedicated, single-emulsion, screen-film image receptor (1972). By 1990, grid technique, emphasis on compression, high-frequency generators, and especially effective automatic exposure control (AEC) performance raised mammography to the level of excellence in breast imaging.

Conventional x-ray imaging systems are unacceptable for mammography, which requires specially designed, dedicated systems. Nearly all x-ray manufacturers now produce such systems. Figure 22-3 shows four popular models.

Dedicated mammographic imaging systems are designed for flexibility in patient positioning and have an integral compression device, low ratio grid, AEC, and microfocus x-ray tube. Desirable features of a dedicated mammography imaging system are given in Table 22-2.

High-Voltage Generation

All mammography imaging systems incorporate high-frequency generators (see Chapter 8). Such a generator accepts a single-phase input, which is rectified and capacitor-smoothed to produce a direct current (DC) voltage waveform.

This DC power is fed to an inverter circuit, which changes the power to high-frequency (typically 5 to 10 kHz) that is then capacitor-smoothed. The resulting

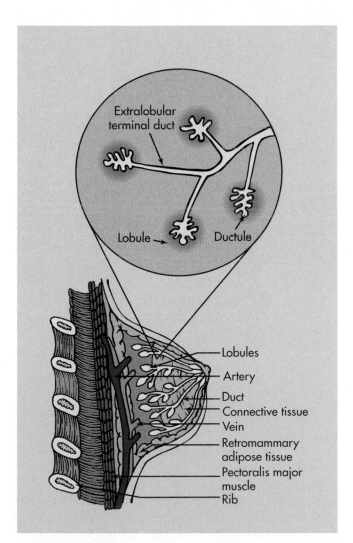

FIGURE 22-1 Breast architecture determines the requirements for x-ray imaging systems and image receptors.

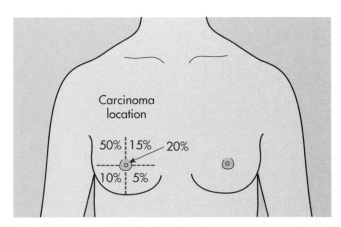

FIGURE 22-2 Approximate incidence of breast cancer by location within the breast.

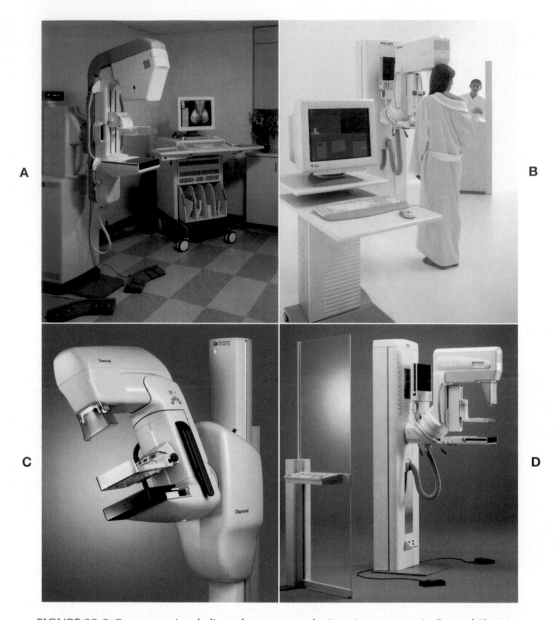

FIGURE 22-3 Representative dedicated mammography imaging systems. **A,** General Electric Senograph. (Courtesy General Electric Medical Systems.) **B,** Philips Mammo Diagnost. (Courtesy Philips Medical Systems.) **C,** Instrumentarium Alpha IQ. (Courtesy Instrumentarium Imaging.) **D,** Siemens Mammomat. (Courtesy Siemens Medical Systems.)

voltage ripple in the x-ray tube is approximately 1%, essentially constant potential.

Compared with earlier single- and three-phase mammography generators, high-frequency generators are smaller and less expensive to manufacture. They provide exceptional exposure reproducibility, which contributes to improved image quality.

Target Composition

Mammographic x-ray tubes are manufactured with either a tungsten (W), a molybdenum (Mo), or a rhodium (Rh) target. Figure 22-4 shows the x-ray emission spectrum from a tungsten target tube filtered with 0.5 mm Al operating at 30 kVp. Note that the bremsstrahlung spectrum predominates and that only the 12 keV char-

TABLE 22-2	Features of a Dedicated Mammography System for Use with Screen-Film
High-voltage generator	High frequency, 5–10 kHz
Target/filter	W/60 μm Mo
	Mo/30 μm Mo
	Mo/50 μm Rh
	Rh/50 μm Rh
kVp	20–35 kVp in 1 kVp increments
Compression	Low Z, auto adjust and release
Grids	Ratio of 3:1 to 5:1, 30 lines/cm
Exposure control	Automatic to account for tissue thickness, composition, and reciprocity law failure
Focal spot (large/small)	0.3 mm/0.1 mm
Magnification	Up to 2 ×
SID	50–80 cm

SID, Source-to-image receptor distance.

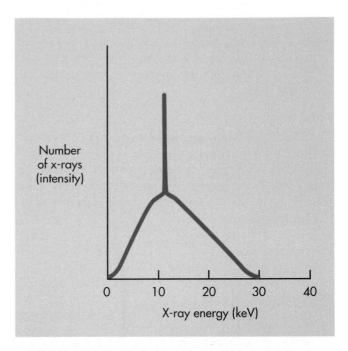

FIGURE 22-4 X-ray emission spectrum for a tungsten-target x-ray tube with a 0.5 mm Al filter operated at 30 kVp.

acteristic x-rays from L-shell transitions are present. These x-rays are all absorbed and contribute only to patient dose, not to the image.

 Tungsten L-shell x-rays are of no value in mammography because their 12 keV energy is too low to penetrate the breast.

The x-rays most useful for enhancing differential absorption in breast tissue and for maximizing radiographic contrast are those in the range of 17 to 24 keV. The tungsten target supplies sufficient x-rays in this energy range but also an abundance of x-rays above and below this range.

Figure 22-5 shows the emission spectrum from a molybdenum-target tube filtered with 30 μm of molybdenum; note the near absence of bremsstrahlung x-rays. The most prominent x-rays are characteristic, with energy of 19 keV resulting from K-shell interactions. Molybdenum has an atomic number of 42 compared with 74 for tungsten, and this difference is responsible for the differences in emission spectra.

The x-ray emission spectrum from a rhodium target filtered with rhodium appears similar to that from a molybdenum target (Figure 22-6). However, rhodium has a slightly higher atomic number ($Z = 45$) and therefore a slightly higher K-edge (23 keV) and more bremsstrahlung x-rays.

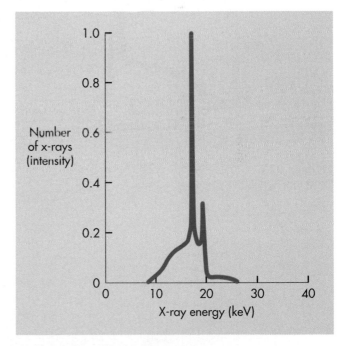

FIGURE 22-5 X-ray emission spectrum for a molybdenum-target x-ray tube with a 30 μm Mo filter operated at 26 kVp.

Bremsstrahlung x-rays are produced more easily in target atoms with high Z than in target atoms with low Z. Molybdenum and rhodium K-characteristic x-rays have energy corresponding to their respective K-shell electron binding energy. This is within the range of energy that is most effective for mammographic imaging.

All currently manufactured mammography imaging systems have target/filter combinations of Mo/Mo. Many are also equipped with Mo/Rh and Rh/Rh. Table 22-3 is an example of an appropriate mammographic technique chart.

Focal Spot

Focal-spot size is an important characteristic of mammography x-rays tubes because of the higher demands for spatial resolution. Imaging microcalcifications requires small focal spots. Mammography x-ray tubes usually have stated focal-spot sizes—large/small of 0.3/0.1 mm.

In general, the smaller the better; however, the shape of the focal spot is also important (Figure 22-7). A circular focal spot is preferred, but rectangular shapes are common. Manufacturers shape the focal spot through clever cathode design and focusing-cup voltage bias. The allowed variance is considerable for the stated nominal focal spot size, and therefore medical physics acceptance testing of focal-spot size or spatial resolution is essential.

In order to obtain such small focal-spot size and adequate x-ray intensity over the entire breast, manufacturers take advantage of the line-focus principle and tilting of the x-ray tube (Figure 22-8). The effective focal spots, 0.3/0.1 mm, are obtained with an approximate 23° anode angle and a 6° tube tilt. Normally, the cathode is positioned to the chest wall. This allows for easier patient positioning as well as smaller effective focal spots.

Tilting the x-ray tube to achieve smaller effective focal spots also ensures imaging of the tissue next to the chest wall (see Figure 22-8). When the tube is tilted, the central ray parallels the chest wall and no tissue is missed.

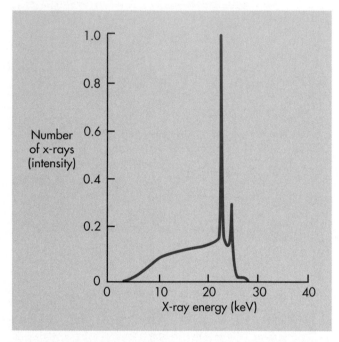

FIGURE 22-6 X-ray emission spectrum for a rhodium-target x-ray tube with a 50 μm Rh filter operated at 28 kVp.

TABLE 22-3	Mammographic Technique Chart	
Compressed Breast Thickness	**Target/Filter**	**kVp**
0–2 cm	Mo/Mo	24
3–4 cm	Mo/Mo	25, 26
5–6 cm	Mo/Rh	28
7–8 cm	Mo/Rh	32 or
7–8 cm	Rh/Rh*	30*

*To be used with systems that have Rh targets.

FIGURE 22-7 Pinhole camera images of (**A**) the circular focal spot of a mammography x-ray tube and (**B**) a double banana-shaped focal spot from a general-purpose x-ray tube. (Courtesy Donald Jacobson.)

Filtration

At the low kVp used for mammography, it is important that the x-ray tube window not attenuate the x-ray beam significantly. Therefore, dedicated mammography x-ray tubes have either a beryllium (Z = 4) window or a very thin borosilicate glass window. Most mammography x-ray tubes have inherent filtration in the window of approximately 0.1 mm Al equivalent. Beyond the window, the proper type and thickness of x-ray beam filtration must be installed.

 Under no circumstances is total beam filtration less than 0.5 mm Al equivalent.

If a tungsten target x-ray tube is used, it should have a molybdenum or rhodium filter. The purpose of each filter is to reduce the higher-energy bremsstrahlung x-rays. Some research has suggested that 50 μm rhodium (Z = 45) is a better filter for imaging thicker and denser breasts when the x-ray tube target is tungsten. Figure 22-9 shows the emission spectrum from a tungsten target tube designed for screen-film mammography filtered by either molybdenum or rhodium. The radiologic technologist selects the proper filter after determining the patient's breast characteristics.

The use of a filter of the same element as the x-ray tube target is designed to allow the k-characteristic x-rays to expose the breast while suppressing the higher- and lower-energy bremsstrahlung x-rays. Figure 22-10 shows this process of selective filtration in order to shape the x-ray beam with Mo/Mo.

The unfiltered Mo beam (Figure 22-10, *A*) has a prominent characteristic x-ray emission and substantial bremsstrahlung x-ray emission. The Mo filter has its k-absorption edge at the energy of the k-characteristic x-ray emission (Figure 22-10, *B*). The combination Mo/Mo target/filter results in an emission spectrum with suppressed bremsstrahlung and prominent characteristic x-ray emission (Figure 22-10, *C*).

If a Mo target x-ray tube is used, then Mo filtration of 30 μm or Rh filtration of 50 μm is recommended. These combinations provide the Mo characteristic x-rays for imaging along with the suppressed bremsstrahlung x-ray emission spectrum.

If a Rh target x-ray tube is used, it should be filtered with 25 μm Rh. This combination provides a slightly higher-quality x-ray beam of greater penetrability. The use of Rh as a target or filter is designed for thicker more dense breasts. Regardless of the x-ray tube target or filtration, the half-value layer is always very low.

Mammography x-ray tubes fabricated with a target of molybdenum-tungsten-rhodium alloy are also used. Such tubes emit a mixed radiation spectrum having the characteristics of each target element. When aluminum, molybdenum, or rhodium is selected as the filter, the

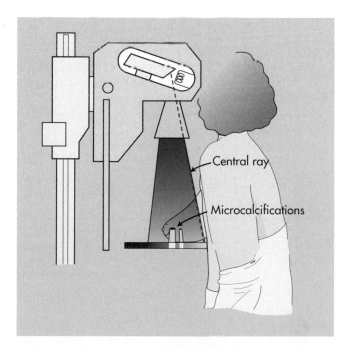

FIGURE 22-8 When the x-ray tube is tilted in its housing, the effective focal spot is small, the x-ray intensity is more uniform, and tissue against the chest is imaged.

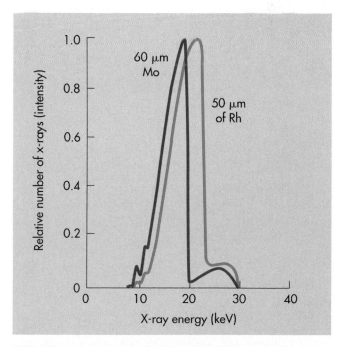

FIGURE 22-9 Emission spectrum from a tungsten-target x-ray tube filtered by molybdenum and rhodium.

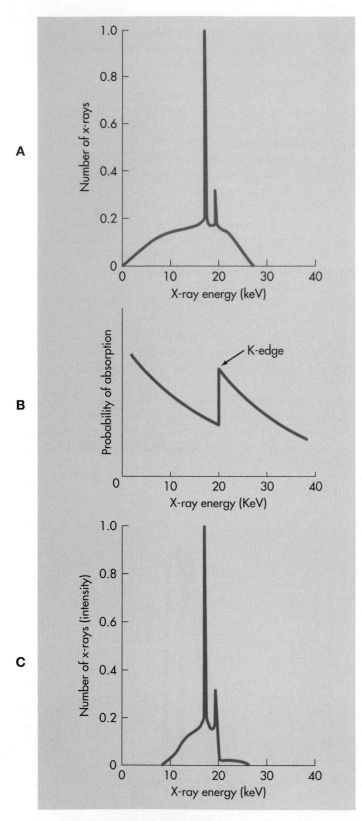

FIGURE 22-10 **A,** Molybdenum x-ray emission spectrum. **B,** The probability of x-ray absorption in molybdenum reduces bremsstrahlung x-rays while transmitting characteristic x-rays to make the x-ray beam more monoenergetic. **C,** Bremsstrahlung x-rays are suppressed and characteristic x-ray emission becomes prominent when a molybdenum target is filtered with molybdenum.

x-ray emission spectrum can be shaped to be compatible with the type of image receptor used and the patient's breast characteristics.

Many x-ray tubes designed specifically for mammography are stationary anode. Newer bi-angle and double-track anodes (one track is Mo and the other Rh) are rotating anode tubes.

Heel Effect

The heel effect is highly important to mammography. The conic shape of breasts should require that the radiation intensity near the chest wall be higher than that to the nipple side to ensure near-uniform exposure of the image receptor. This could be accomplished by positioning the cathode to the chest wall (Figure 22-11). In practice, this is not necessary because **compression** ensures imaging of a uniform thickness of tissue.

When the cathode is positioned to the chest wall, the spatial resolution of tissue near the chest wall is reduced because of the increased focal spot blur created by the larger effective focal-spot size. However, most manufacturers of dedicated mammography imaging systems use a relatively long source-to-image receptor distance (SID), 60 to 80 cm, with the cathode to the chest wall and the x-ray tube tilted. That is considered the best arrangement because the focal spot is made effectively smaller and tissue at the chest wall is imaged.

One consequence of the heel effect is the variation in focal-spot size over the image receptor. However, the use of long SID and vigorous compression makes this change in effective focal spot size clinically insignificant.

Compression

Compression is important in many aspects of conventional radiology but is particularly important in mammography. Vigorous compression offers several advantages (Figure 22-12). A compressed breast is of more uniform thickness, and therefore the optical density of the image is more uniform. Tissues near the chest wall are less likely to be underexposed, and tissues near the nipple are less likely to be overexposed.

 Vigorous compression must be used in x-ray mammography.

When vigorous compression is used, all tissue is brought closer to the image receptor and focal-spot blur is reduced. Compression also reduces absorption blur and scatter radiation. All dedicated mammographic x-ray imaging systems have a built-in stiff compression device that is parallel with the surface of the image receptor. Vigorous compression of the breast is necessary for the best image quality.

Image quality is improved with vigorous compression as summarized in Table 22-4. Compression immobilizes the breast and therefore reduces motion blur.

Compression spreads out the tissue and thus reduces superimposition of tissue structures.

Compression results in thinner tissue and therefore less scatter radiation and improved contrast resolution. The overall result of this improved image quality is improved ability to detect small, low-contrast lesions and high-contrast microcalcifications because of **improved spatial resolution.** Additionally, vigorous compression results in **lower patient dose.**

 Compression improves spatial resolution and contrast resolution.

Although it may be difficult for patients to understand, compression of the breast is essential for a quality mammogram. The optimum degree of compression is unknown; however, the more vigorous the compression, the better the image and the lower the dose, but the higher the patient discomfort. Skilled mammographers attempt to compress the breast until it is "taut" or "just less than painful," whichever occurs first.

Grids

Grids are routinely used in mammography. Although mammographic image contrast is high because of the low kVp used, it is not high enough. Many systems now

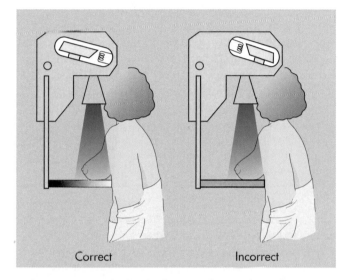

Correct   Incorrect

FIGURE 22-11 The heel effect can be used to advantage in mammography by positioning the cathode toward the chest wall to produce a more uniform optical density.

TABLE 22-4	Advantages of Vigorous Compression
Effect	**Result**
Immobilization of breast	Reduced motion blur
Uniform thickness	Equal optical density on mammogram
Reduced scatter radiation	Improved contrast resolution
Shorter OID	Improved spatial resolution
Thinner tissue	Reduced radiation dose

OID, Object-to-image receptor distance.

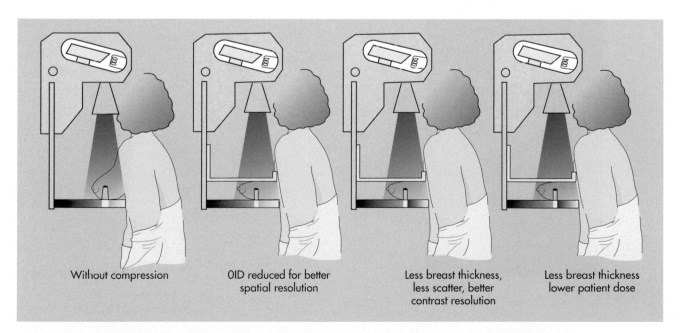

Without compression   OID reduced for better spatial resolution   Less breast thickness, less scatter, better contrast resolution   Less breast thickness lower patient dose

FIGURE 22-12 Compression in mammography has three principal advantages: improved spatial resolution, improved contrast resolution, and lower patient dose.

use moving grids with a ratio of 4:1 to 5:1 focused to the SID to increase image contrast. Grid frequencies of 30 to 50 lines/cm are typical.

Use of such grids does not compromise spatial resolution but it does increase patient dose. The use of a 4:1 ratio grid approximately doubles the patient dose compared with nongrid contact mammography. However, the dose is acceptably low and the improvement in contrast is significant.

A unique grid developed specifically for mammography is the high-transmission cellular (HTC) grid (Figure 22-13). This grid has the clean-up characteristics of a crossed grid by reducing scatter radiation in two directions rather than the one direction of a linear or focused grid. The HTC grid has copper as grid strip material and air for the interspace, and its physical dimensions result in a 3.8:1 grid ratio.

Automatic Exposure Control

Phototimers for mammography are designed to measure not only x-ray intensity at the image receptor but also x-ray quality. These phototimers are called *automatic exposure control (AEC) devices*, and they are positioned after the image receptor to minimize the object-to-image receptor distance (OID) and improve spatial resolution (Figure 22-14). Two types are used: ionization chamber or a solid-state diode. Each type has multiple detectors or a single detector, which can be positioned along the chest wall/nipple axis. Some AEC devices incorporate many detectors to cover the entire breast.

The detectors are filtered differently so that the AEC can estimate the beam quality after passing through the breast. This allows an assessment of breast composition and selection of proper target/filter combination. Thick, dense breasts are imaged better with Rh/Rh; thin, fatty breasts are imaged better with Mo/Mo.

The AEC must be accurate to ensure reproducible images at low radiation dose. The AEC should be able to hold optical density within ±0.1 OD as voltage is varied from 23 kVp to 32 kVp and for breast thickness of 2 to 8 cm regardless of breast composition.

Magnification Mammography

Magnification techniques are frequently used in mammography, producing images up to twice the normal size. Magnification mammography requires special equipment such as microfocus tubes, adequate compression, and patient positioning devices. Effective focal-spot size should not exceed 0.1 mm.

 Magnification mammography should not be used routinely.

Standard mammograms are adequate for most patients, so magnification mammography is usually unnecessary. The purpose of magnification mammography is to investigate small suspicious lesions or microcalcifications seen on standard mammograms. The breast may not be completely imaged, and patient dose is approximately doubled.

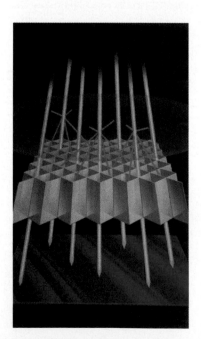

FIGURE 22-13 A high-transmission cellular grid designed specifically for mammography. (Courtesy Hologic Imaging.)

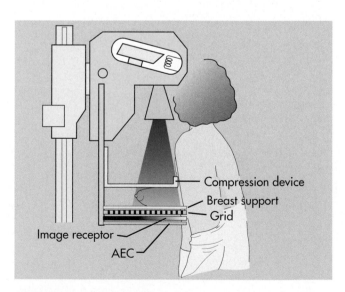

FIGURE 22-14 The relative position of the automatic exposure control (AEC) device.

SCREEN-FILM MAMMOGRAPHY

Four types of image receptors have been used for mammography: direct-exposure film, xeroradiography, screen-film, and digital detectors. Only screen-film and digital detectors are used today.

Radiographic intensifying screens and films have been specially designed for x-ray mammography. The films are single-emulsion and matched with a single back screen. This arrangement avoids light crossover. Tabular grain emulsion has been replaced by cubic grain emulsion in many films (Figure 22-15). The result is somewhat higher contrast, especially in the toe region, which is particularly useful in mammography.

Regardless of the type of film, it must be matched for the light emission of the associated intensifying screen. Special emulsions coupled with rare earth screen material are available.

The screen-film combination is placed in a specially designed cassette that has a low-Z front cover for low attenuation. The latching/spring mechanism is designed to produce especially good screen-film contact.

The use of the radiographic intensifying screen increases the speed of the imaging system significantly, resulting in a low patient dose. The use of screens also enhances the radiographic contrast compared with that from direct-exposure examination.

 The emulsion surface of the film must always be next to the screen, and the film must be on the x-ray tube side of the radiographic intensifying screen.

The position of the radiographic intensifying screen and film in the cassette is important (Figure 22-16). X-rays interact primarily with the entrance surface of the screen. If the screen is between the x-ray tube and the film, screen blur is excessive. If, on the other hand, the film is between the x-ray tube and the screen, with the emulsion side to the screen, spatial resolution is better.

Processing and viewing the mammogram are critical stages of mammography. These steps are discussed in Chapter 23, but when they are properly conducted, image receptor speeds can reach approximately 200. This results in an average glandular dose of 50 to 100 mrad (0.5 to 1.0 mGy$_t$). Image receptor contrast—the average gradient—is approximately 3.5.

DIGITAL MAMMOGRAPHY

Recent developments of digital radiographic image receptors have special applications in digital mammography. The image receptors that are currently under development for digital mammography are **charge-coupled devices (CCD)**, amorphous silicon-CsI, and amorphous selenium.

The CCD is an image receptor similar to that used in personal video camcorders. The result of military research, the CCD has found significant application in astronomy.

 The CCD is a solid-state device that converts visible-light photons to electrons.

As with screen-film mammography, the image-forming x-ray beam interacts with an intensifying screen. Here

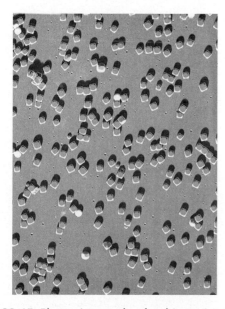

FIGURE 22-15 Photomicrograph of cubic grains in mammography film emulsions; the grains are 0.5 to 0.9 μm to produce higher contrast. (Courtesy Fujifilm Medical Systems.)

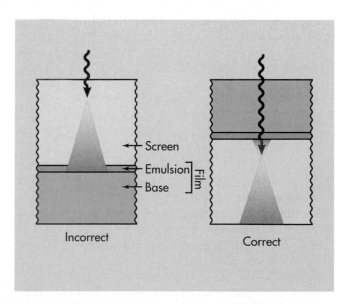

FIGURE 22-16 Correct way to load mammography film and position the cassette. Spatial resolution improves when the x-ray film is placed between the x-ray tube and the radiographic intensifying screen.

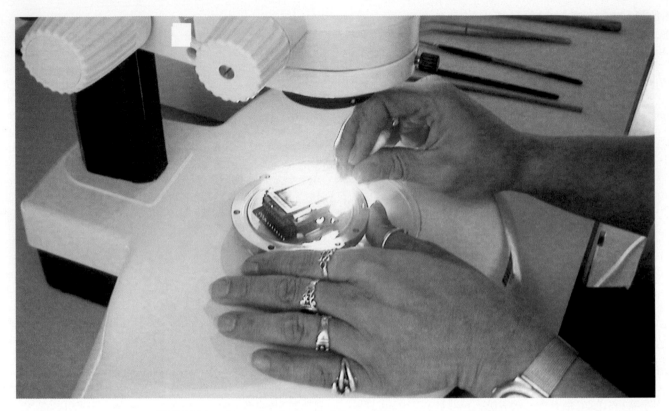

FIGURE 22-17 A charge coupled device (CCD). (Courtesy Swissray.)

the similarity ceases (Figure 22-17). The light from the intensifying screen is captured either by a fiber-optic bundle or a lens system and directed to the CCD. The electron signal is read in pixel fashion to form an image.

Because the CCD is small and has limited coverage, several may be coupled (Figure 22-18) in order to image the entire breast. Spatial resolution of 8 to 10 lp/mm is achievable. Although this does not come close to the 20 lp/mm available with screen-film, even 5 lp/mm with digital imaging seems adequate because of the enhanced contrast resolution available with postprocessing.

Direct or indirect x-ray capture, using amorphous selenium or silicon fabricated into thin film transistors (TFT), is also available for digital mammography. These devices are discussed in Chapter 27.

Most digital image receptors that are based on phosphor interaction use thallium-activated cesium iodide. This phosphor can be grown as parallel needle-like light pipes for improved spatial resolution.

Because these digital detectors are electronic, they produce electronic noise. The noise can be reduced by cooling the detector to improve contrast resolution. Digital detectors have image characteristics similar to that of screen-film except that the response to x-rays is linear (Figure 22-19).

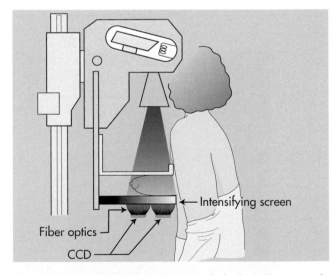

FIGURE 22-18 Multiple CCDs view light from the intensifying screen and convert the light to a digital image.

 The principal advantage of digital imaging is the ability to postprocess the image, resulting in enhanced contrast resolution.

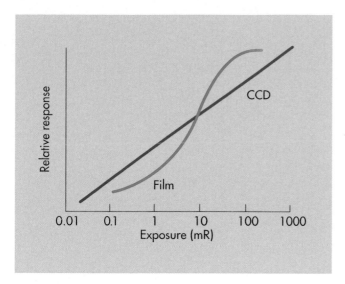

FIGURE 22-19 The response of a CCD is linear, not curvilinear as with screen-film.

The spatial resolution of any of these digital mammography images is limited by the discrete physical pixel size of the image receptor. Current pixel size ranges from approximately 40 μm to 100 μm, and this results in limiting spatial frequencies of 12.5 lp/mm and 5 lp/mm, respectively.

Chapter 27 provides a complete discussion of digital radiographic methods. Each method has potential application in digital mammography.

SUMMARY

Breast cancer is the leading cause of death in women between 40 and 50 years of age. This is a principal reason mammographic equipment and techniques have improved over the years and why the Mammography Quality Standards Act was instituted.

Anatomically, the breast consists of three different tissues: fibrous tissue, glandular tissue, and adipose tissue. Premenopausal women have breasts composed mainly of fibrous and glandular tissue surrounded by a thin layer of fat. These breasts are dense and difficult to image. In postmenopausal women, the glandular tissue turns to fat. Because of its predominant fatty content, the older breast is easier to image.

The mammographer must know the recommended intervals of breast self-examination, physician examination of the breasts, and mammographic examination for women of various age groups in order to advise such patients. Diagnostic x-ray mammography is often performed every 6 months on women who have an elevated risk of breast cancer or who have a known lesion.

Compression is an important factor in producing high-quality mammograms.

Radiographic imaging systems are specially designed for mammographic examination. Mammographic x-ray tube targets are tungsten, molybdenum, or rhodium. A low kVp is used in order to maximize radiographic contrast of soft tissue. The x-ray beam should be filtered with 30 to 60 μm of molybdenum or rhodium to accentuate the characteristic x-ray emission.

Small focal spots should be used for imaging microcalcifications because of the demand for increased spatial resolution. Moving grids and single-emulsion screen-film systems further increase radiographic contrast and image detail. AEC devices accommodate imaging of various sizes of breast tissue.

CHALLENGE QUESTIONS

1. Define or otherwise identify:
   a. Minimum filtration for mammography
   b. SID
   c. Adipose tissue
   d. Mammographic grid ratio
   e. Molybdenum
   f. AEC
   g. CCD
   h. Breast cancer incidence
   i. Mammography SID
   j. Characteristic x-radiation
2. Describe the anatomy of the breast, including the types of tissue and structural sizes.
3. Discuss changes in image quality and patient dose in mammography as kVp is increased.
4. Graphically compare the x-ray emission of a tungsten-target x-ray tube with a molybdenum-target x-ray tube operated at 28 kVp.
5. The electron binding energies for molybdenum are K-shell, 20 keV; L-shell, 2.6 keV; M-shell, 0.5 keV. What are the possible characteristic x-ray energies when operated at 28 kVp?
6. Discuss the influence of the heel effect on image quality in mammography.
7. Why should mammography be performed with an x-ray tube target of molybdenum or rhodium?
8. Draw the relationships among x-ray tube target, intensifying screen, film base, film emulsion, and patient for single-emulsion screen-film mammography.
9. How is soft tissue radiography different from conventional radiography?
10. What do the abbreviations ACR and MQSA refer to?
11. What is the difference between diagnostic and screening mammography?
12. List the recommended intervals for screening x-ray mammography.
13. Explain why mammography requires a low kVp technique.

14. List the advantages of mammographic compression.
15. Name the three materials used for mammographic x-ray tube targets.
16. What focal-spot sizes are used for mammography? Why?
17. What is the best target/filter combination for imaging dense breast tissue?
18. What grid ratio and grid frequency are used for mammography?
19. What feature of a dedicated mammography imaging system is important for imaging microcalcifications?
20. What is the purpose of tilting the mammography x-ray tube?

Mammography Quality Control

OBJECTIVES

At the completion of this chapter, the student should be able to do the following:

1. Define quality control and its relationship to quality assurance
2. List the members of the quality control team in radiology
3. Describe the role of the radiologist and the medical physicist in quality control
4. Itemize the mammographer's quality control duties on a weekly, monthly, and annual basis
5. List the processor quality control steps

OUTLINE

MAMMOGRAPHY HAS been a screening and diagnostic tool for many years but still faces challenges in producing high-quality mammographic images while keeping patient radiation dose low. A team that includes the radiologist, medical physicist, and mammographer works together using a quality control (QC) program to produce excellence in mammographic imaging. Each member of the team has specific tasks that relate to QC. This chapter identifies these responsibilities.

Chapter 31 details the specific evaluation and monitoring tests for any QC program. The discussion here centers on the various responsibilities of personnel and tasks specific to mammography QC.

QUALITY CONTROL TEAM

The American College of Radiology (ACR) and the Mammography Quality Standards Act (MQSA) have endorsed a QC program of specific duties required of the **radiologist,** the **medical physicist,** and the **mammographer** (Figure 23-1). Each of these individuals is important in ensuring the best available care with the least radiation exposure. This chapter discusses the responsibilities of each of these three positions but emphasizes the mammographer's duties.

Radiologist

The ultimate responsibility for mammography QC lies with the radiologist. These responsibilities often fall under the more broad area of **quality assurance (QA).** QA is an administrative program designed to fuse the different aspects of QC and to ensure that all activities are being carried out at the highest level. The radiologist is responsible for selecting qualified medical physicists and mammographers and overseeing the activities of these team members regularly.

 The radiologist's principal responsibility is supervision of the entire QA program.

Another responsibility of the radiologist is supervising patient communication and tracking. Quality patient care is the ultimate goal of any mammography facility, and the final responsibility for this goal lies with the radiologist. The level of any QA/QC program directly reflects the radiologist's attitude and appreciation for the

need of such a program. The MQSA mandates daily "clinical image evaluation" by the radiologist. Continuous Quality Improvement (CQI) is an extension of any QA/QC program, including administrative protocols for the continuous improvement of mammographic quality.

Medical Physicist

The role of the medical physicist as a member of the mammography QC team is multidimensional. One such aspect is QC evaluation of the physical equipment used to produce an image of the breast. This evaluation should be performed annually or whenever a major component has been replaced. The evaluation consists of a number of measurements and tests that are summarized in Box 23-1.

The medical physicist should understand how the different technical aspects of the imaging chain affect the resulting image and therefore be able to identify existing or potential image-quality problems. Occasionally, the medical physicist may pass information directly to the service engineer or serve as an intermediary between the facility and the service engineer. The aim of this portion of the QC program is to ensure that equipment functions properly to provide the highest-quality images with the lowest dose to the patient.

 The medical physicist's principal responsibility is an annual performance evaluation of the imaging systems.

Another role of the medical physicist is advising the mammographer. The medical physicist should understand all of the tests expected of the mammographer well enough to predict likely problems or complications.

An additional responsibility is evaluating the QC program on site at least annually. The medical physicist should review all procedures to ensure compliance with current recommendations and standards. The medical physicist should thoroughly review charts and records to check for compliance and to ensure that they are prepared properly and contain all necessary information.

The medical physicist is an integral part of the QC team, whose full cooperation and attention is expected. This very achievable goal involves a first-class QC program being maintained by a competent mammographer.

The mammographer must call the medical physicist whenever images or the imaging system changes substantially.

Mammographer

The mammographer is extremely important to a mammography QC program. The mammographer is the

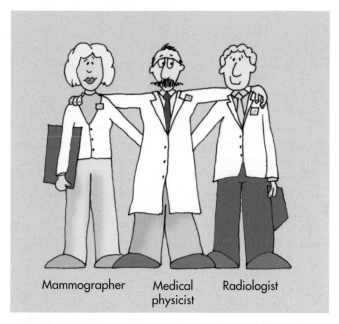

FIGURE 23-1 The three members of the mammography QC team.

BOX 23-1 Annual QC Evaluation to be Performed by the Medical Physicist

Mammographic unit assembly inspection
Collimation assessment
Evaluation of spatial resolution
kVp accuracy and reproducibility
Beam quality assessment (half-value layer)
Automatic exposure control performance assessment
Automatic exposure control reproducibility
Uniformity of screen speed
Breast entrance exposure
Average glandular dose
Image quality evaluation
Artifact evaluation
Radiation output intensity
Measurement of viewing conditions

TABLE 23-1	Elements of a Mammographic QC Program	
Task	**Minimum Frequency**	**Approximate Time to Carry Out Procedures (min)**
Darkroom cleanliness	Daily	5
Processor quality control	Daily	20
Screen cleanliness	Weekly	10
Viewboxes and viewing conditions	Weekly	5
Phantom Images	Weekly	30
Visual checklist	Monthly	10
Repeat analysis	Quarterly or 250 pts	60
Analysis of fixer retention in film	Quarterly	5
Conference with radiologist	Quarterly	45
Darkroom fog	Semiannually	10
Screen-film contact	Semiannually	80
Compression	Semiannually	10

Total annual time required for QC: 160 hrs.

---

most hands-on member of the QC team; being responsible for day-to-day QC and for producing and monitoring all control charts and logs for any trends that might indicate problems. In imaging facilities using several mammographers, one should be assigned the responsibility of **QC mammographer.**

The 12 specific QC tasks for which the mammographer is responsible may be broken into categories reflecting frequency of performance. Table 23-1 outlines these tasks and estimates the time each task requires.

QUALITY CONTROL PROGRAM

The mammographer's 12 tasks are well defined, with recommended performance standards for each of them. To maintain a thorough and accurate QC program, the mammographer must fully understand these tasks as well as the reasons for recommended performance standards.

Daily Tasks

Darkroom Cleanliness. The first task each day is to wipe the darkroom clean. Maintaining the cleanest possible conditions in the darkroom minimizes artifacts on mammograms (Figure 23-2). First, the floor should be mopped with a damp mop. Next, all unnecessary items should be removed from counter tops and work surfaces. A clean damp towel should be used to wipe off the processor feed tray and all counter tops and work surfaces.

If a passbox is present, it should be cleaned daily as well. Hands should be kept clean to minimize fingerprints and handling artifacts. Overhead air vents and safelights should be wiped or vacuumed weekly before the other cleaning procedures are performed. Even the ceiling tiles should be cleaned to prevent flaking.

 Daily cleaning of the darkroom reduces image artifacts.

Smoking, eating, or drinking in the darkroom is prohibited. Food or drink should not be taken into the darkroom at any time. There should be nothing on the counter top except for items used for loading and unloading cassettes because other objects would only collect dust. There should be no shelves above the counter tops in the darkroom as these also serve as sites for dust collection; such dust eventually falls onto work surfaces.

Processor QC. Before any films are processed, it should be verified that the processor chemical system is in accord with preset specifications. The first step in a processor QC program is establishing operating control levels. To begin, a new dedicated box of film should be set aside to carry out the future daily processor QC. The processor tanks and racks should be cleaned and the processor supplied with the proper developer replenisher, fixer, and developer starter fluids as specified by the manufacturer.

The developer temperature, as well as the developer and fixer replenishment rates, should also be set to the levels specified by the manufacturer. Never use a mercury thermometer. Should the thermometer break, mercury contamination could render the processor permanently useless.

Once the processor has been allowed to warm up and the developer is at the correct temperature and stable, testing may continue. In the darkroom, a sheet of control film should be exposed with a sensitometer (Figure 23-3). The sensitometric strip should always be processed in exactly the same manner. The least-exposed end is fed into the processor first. The same side of the feed tray is used, with the emulsion side down. The time between exposure and processing should be similar each day.

Next a densitometer is used to measure and record the optical densities (ODs) of each of the steps on the sensitometric strip. This process should be repeated each day for 5 consecutive days. The average OD is then determined for each step from the five different strips.

Once the averages have been determined, the step that has an average OD closest to 1.2, but not less than 1.2, should be found and marked as the **mid-density (MD)** step for future comparison. This is sometimes called the **speed index.**

Next, the step with an average OD closest to 2.2 and the step with an average OD closest to but not less than 0.5 should be found and marked for future comparison. The difference between these two steps is recorded as the **density difference (DD)**, which is sometimes called the **contrast index.**

Finally, the average OD from an unexposed area of the strips is recorded as the **base plus fog (B+F)**. The three values that have now been determined should be recorded on the center lines of the appropriate control chart. An example of a control chart is shown in Figure 23-4.

Once the control values have been established, the daily processor QC begins. At the beginning of each day, before any films are processed, a sensitometric strip should be exposed and processed according to the guidelines previously discussed. The MD, DD, and B+F are each determined from the appropriate predetermined steps and plotted on the control charts.

The MD is determined to evaluate the constancy of image-receptor speed. The DD is determined to evaluate the constancy of image contrast. These values are allowed to vary within 0.15 of the control values. If either value is out of this control limit, the point should be cir-

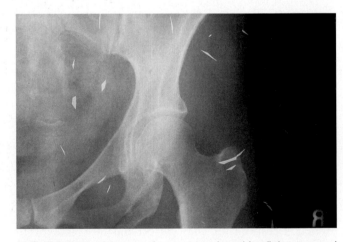

FIGURE 23-2 These specks were produced by flakes trapped between the film and screen. (Courtesy Linda Shields.)

cled on the graph, the cause of the problem corrected, and the test repeated.

 If the value of the MD or the DD cannot be brought within the 0.15 variance of control, *no clinical images should be processed.*

If either value falls ±0.1 outside the range of the control value, the test should be repeated. If the value continues to remain outside this range, the processor may be used for clinical processing but should be monitored closely while the problem is identified.

The B+F evaluates the level of fog in the processing chain. This value is allowed to vary within +0.03 of the control value. Anytime the value exceeds this limit, steps should be taken as described for the MD and DD values.

Weekly Tasks

Screen Cleanliness. Screens are cleaned to ensure that mammographic cassettes and intensifying screens are free of dust and dirt particles, which can resemble microcalcifications and may result in misdiagnoses. Radiographic intensifying screens should be cleaned using the material and methods suggested by the screen

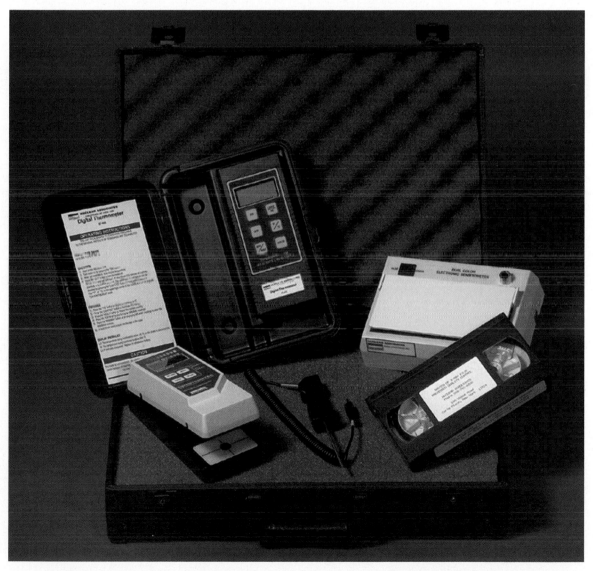

FIGURE 23-3 Processor QC kit, including a sensitometer and densitometer. (Courtesy Cardinal Health.)

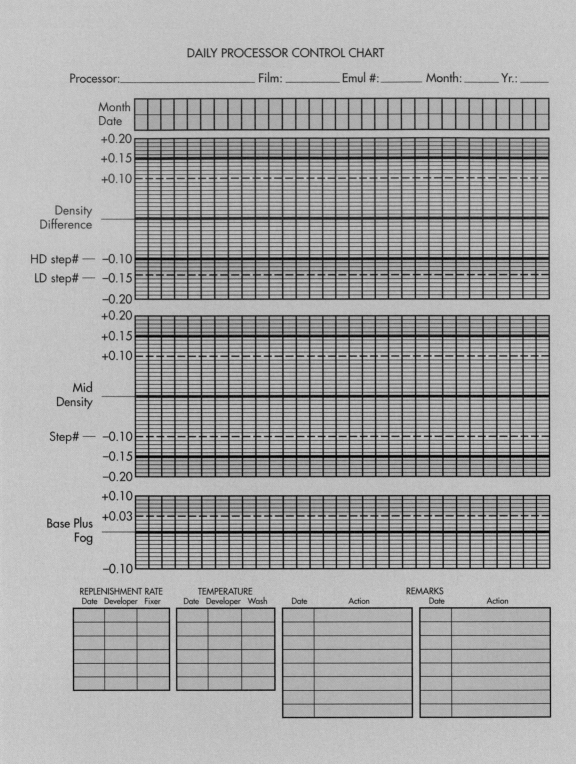

FIGURE 23-4 An example of the type of processor QC record that should be maintained for each processor.

manufacturer. If a liquid cleaner is used, screens should be allowed to air dry while standing vertically, as shown in Figure 23-5, before the cassettes are closed or used. If compressed air is used, the air supply should be checked to ensure that no moisture, oil, or other contaminants are present.

 If dust or dirt artifacts are ever noticed, the screens should be cleaned immediately.

Each screen cassette combination should be clearly labeled. The identification should be on the exterior of the cassette, as well as on a lateral border of the screen, so it will be legible on the processed film. This enables the mammographer to identify specific screens that have been found to contain artifacts.

Viewboxes and Viewing Conditions. Viewboxes and viewing conditions must be maintained at an optimal level. Viewbox surfaces should be cleaned with window cleaner and soft paper towels, ensuring that all marks have been removed.

The viewboxes should be visually inspected for uniformity of luminance and to ensure that all masking devices are functioning properly. Room illumination levels should be visually checked as well to ensure that the room is free of bright light and that the viewbox surface is free of reflections.

Any marks that are not easily removed require an appropriate cleaner that will not damage the viewbox. If the viewbox luminance appears to be nonuniform, all of the interior lamps should be replaced. Mammography viewboxes have considerably higher luminance levels than conventional viewboxes. A luminance of at least 3000 nit (candela per square meter) is required.

All mammograms and mammography test images should be completely **masked** for viewing so that no extraneous light from the viewbox enters the viewer's eyes. Masking can be provided simply by cutting black paper to the proper size (Figure 23-6). Commercially adjustable masks are available.

Ambient light in the area of the viewbox should also be diffuse and reduced to approximately that reaching the eye through the mammogram. Sources of glare must be removed and surface reflections eliminated.

Phantom Images. Phantom images are taken to ensure optimal OD, contrast, uniformity, and image quality of the x-ray imaging system and film processor. A standard film and a cassette designated as the *control* or *phantom cassette* should be used to take an image of an MQSA accreditation phantom.

The phantom should be placed on the image receptor assembly so that its edge is aligned with the chest wall edge of the image receptor as shown in Figure 23-7. The compression device should be brought into contact with the phantom and the automatic exposure control (AEC) sensor should be positioned in a location that will be used for all future phantom images.

The technique selected for imaging the phantom should be the same that is used clinically for a 50% fatty/50% dense, 4.5 cm compressed breast. When the exposure is made, the time or mAs value is recorded. The film should then be processed just like a clinical mammogram.

A densitometer is used to determine the OD for the density disk and for the background immediately adjacent to the density disk. The time or mAs value recorded earlier, the background OD, and the DD should be plotted on a phantom image control chart such as the one shown in Figure 23-8.

FIGURE 23-5 The proper way to dry screens after cleaning is to position them vertically. (Courtesy Linda Joppe.)

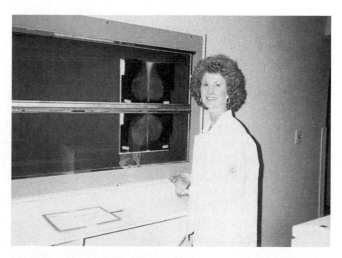

FIGURE 23-6 Mammograms must be masked for proper viewing. (Courtesy Lois Depouw.)

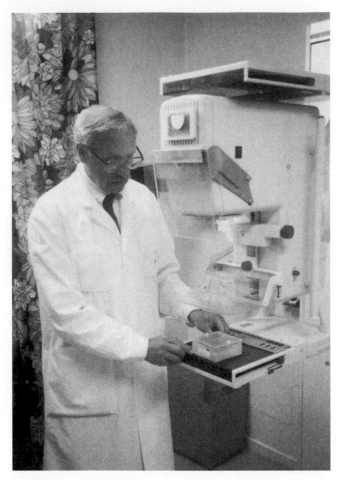

FIGURE 23-7 Analysis of an image of the ACR mammography phantom by a medical physicist scores the detection limits of the system for fibrils, microcalcifications, and nodules. (Courtesy Art Haus.)

The exposure time or mAs value should stay within a range of ±15%. The background OD of the film should be approximately 1.4, with an allowed range of ±0.2. A good target value is approximately 1.6. The DD should be approximately 0.4, with an allowed range of ±0.05. However, this is defined for 28 kVp, so slightly different ODs should be expected at other peak kVps.

The next step is to score the phantom image. This involves determining the number of fibers, speck groups, and masses visible in the phantom image. The ACR accreditation phantom and its image are shown in Figure 23-9. These results should also be plotted on the phantom image control chart.

Scoring the objects requires that they always be counted from the largest object to the smallest, with each object group receiving a score of 1.0, 0.5, or zero. A **fiber** may be counted as 1.0 if its entire length is visible at the correct location and with the correct orienta-

tion. A fiber may be given a score of 0.5 if at least half of its length is visible at the correct location and with the correct orientation. The score is zero if less than half of the fiber is visible.

A **speck group** may be counted as a full point if four or more of the six specks are visible with a magnifying glass. A score of 0.5 may be given to a speck group if at least two of the six specks are visible. If less than two specks in group are visible, the score is zero.

A **mass** may be counted as a full point if a density difference is visible at the correct location with a generally circular border. A score of 0.5 may be given to a mass if a density difference is visible at the correct location but the shape is not circular. If there is only a hint of a density difference, the score is zero.

Next, the magnifying glass is used to check the image for nonuniform areas or artifacts (Figure 23-10). If any artifacts that resemble the phantom objects are found, they should be subtracted from the score given for that object. Never subtract below the next full integer point. For example, if a score of 3.5 or 4 was given, the score cannot be subtracted below 3.

The score of phantom objects counted on subsequent phantom images for each type object should not decrease by more than 0.5. The minimum number of objects required to pass ACR accreditation is four fibers, three speck groups, and three masses.

Phantom images should be taken after equipment installation to determine the control values of the phantom objects for future comparison. Phantom images should also be taken after the imaging equipment undergoes any maintenance.

When the phantom image results in any of the factors exceeding the control values, the cause should be investigated and corrected as soon as possible. The phantom images should always be viewed by the same person, on the same mammography viewbox, under the same viewing conditions, using the same type of magnifier used for mammograms, and at the same time of day.

Monthly Tasks

Visual Checklist. The visual check (1) ensures that the imaging system lights, displays, and mechanical locks and detents are functioning properly and (2) confirms the optimal level of the equipment's mechanical rigidity and stability (Figure 23-11).

The mammographer should review all the items on the list and indicate the condition of each. If a particular piece of equipment has a feature that does not appear on the checklist, the feature should be added. This helps to ensure patient safety, high-quality images, and operator convenience. If any item on the list fails visual inspection, immediate steps should be taken to remedy the problem. The checklist should be dated and initialed.

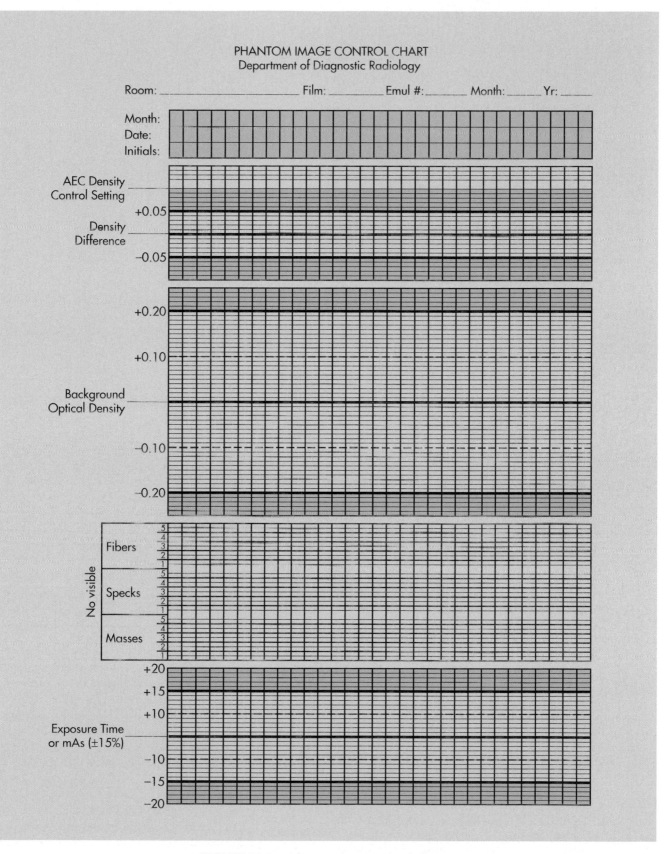

FIGURE 23-8 A phantom image control chart.

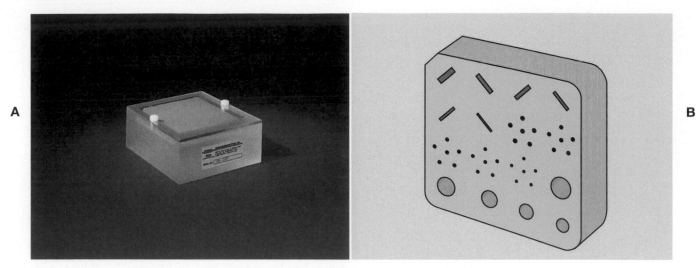

FIGURE 23-9 A, The ACR accreditation phantom. **B,** Its images are shown. (Courtesy Gammex RMI.)

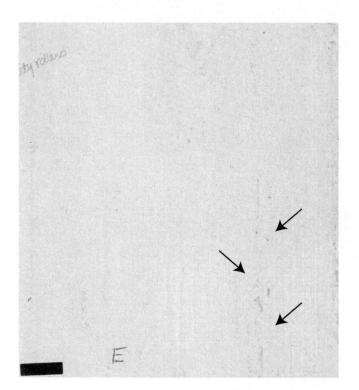

FIGURE 23-10 These really gross artifacts are caused by processor rollers that have not been cleaned. (Courtesy Cristl Thompson.)

Quarterly Tasks

Repeat Analysis. This is a procedure to determine the number and cause of repeated mammograms. Repeat analysis also identifies ways to improve efficiency, reduce costs, and reduce unnecessary patient dose. Such evaluations are valid only if patient volume is at least 250 examinations.

To begin the analysis, all presently rejected films should be discarded so that the analysis starts at zero. A complete inventory of the remaining film supply is taken, and all rejected films are collected for the next quarter. If the workload is low, the repeat analysis is continued until 250 patient examinations have been performed. The rejected films are sorted into different categories, such as poor positioning, patient motion, too light, and the other categories shown on the reject analysis form in Figure 23-12.

Next, the total number of films repeated should be counted, as should the total number of films exposed. The repeat rate is computed as follows:

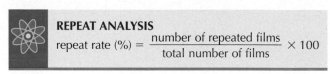

REPEAT ANALYSIS

$$\text{repeat rate (\%)} = \frac{\text{number of repeated films}}{\text{total number of films}} \times 100$$

The repeat rate for each category is determined by dividing the number of repeated films in a given category by the total number of repeats. The overall repeat rate should be ≤2%, as should the rates for each category. If there is a high overall rate or if a single category is higher than the others, the problem should be investigated. *All films repeated should be included in the analysis,* not just those rejected by the radiologist.

Question: A mammographic service examined 327 patients during the third calendar quarter of 2000. A total of 719 films were exposed during this period, 8 of which were repeats. What is the repeat rate?

Answer: repeat rate $= \dfrac{8}{719} \times 100 = 1.1\%$

MAMMOGRAPHY QC VISUAL CHECKLIST

Room #:_____ Tube: _____

Month: J F M A M J J A S O N D

C-ARM	SID indicator or marks												
	Angulation indicator												
	Locks (all)												
	Field light												
	High-tension cable/other cables												
	Smoothness of motion												
CASSETTE HOLDER	Cassette lock (small and large)												
	Compression device												
	Compression scale												
	Amount of compression: automatic manual												
	Grid												
CONTROL BOOTH	Exposure control												
	Observation window												
	Panel switches/lights/meters												
	Technique charts												
OTHER	Cones												
	Cleaning solution												
	Pass = √ Month:												
	Fail – X Date:												
	Not applicable = NA R.T.												

FIGURE 23-11 This checklist contains items that the mammographer should inspect monthly.

Analysis of Fixer Retention in Film. This task determines the amount of residual fixer in the processed film. The result is used as an indicator of archival quality.

One sheet of unexposed film is processed. Next, one drop of residual hypo test solution should be placed on the emulsion side of the film and allowed to stand for 2 minutes. The excess solution should be blotted off and the stain compared with a hypo estimator, which comes with the test solution. Use a white sheet of paper as background.

The matching number from the hypo estimator should be recorded. The comparison should be made immediately after blotting because a prolonged delay allows the spot to darken.

The hypo estimator provides an estimate of the amount of residual hypo in grams per square meter. If the comparison results in an estimate of more than 0.05 g/m^2, the test must be repeated. If elevated residual hypo is then indicated, the source of the problem should be investigated and corrected. Figure 23-13 shows the result from one such test.

MAMMOGRAPHY REPEAT ANALYSIS		
From _____ To _____		
Cause	Number of films	Percentage of repeats
1. Positioning		
2. Patient motion		
3. Light film		
4. Dark film		
5. Black film		
6. Static		
7. Fog		
8. Incorrect patient I.D., or double exposure		
9. Mechanical		
10. Miscellaneous		
11. Good film (no apparent problem)		
12. Clear film		
13. Wire localization		
14. Q.C.		

	Totals	
Rejects (all; 1-14)	%	
Repeats (1-11)	%	

Total film used	

FIGURE 23-12 Examination repeat analysis form.

Semiannual Tasks

Darkroom Fog. Darkroom fog analysis ensures that darkroom safelights and other sources of light inside and outside of the darkroom do not fog mammographic films. Fog results in a loss of contrast and hence a loss of diagnostic information. This test should also be performed for a new darkroom and any time safelight bulbs or filters are changed.

Safelight filters should be checked to ensure that they are those recommended by the film manufacturer and that they are not faded or cracked. The wattage and distance of the bulbs from work surfaces should also be checked against the recommendations of the film manufacturer.

Next, all lights should be turned off for 5 minutes, allowing the eyes to adjust to the darkness. Then the door, passbox, processor, and ceiling should be checked for light leaks. Light leaks are often visible from only one perspective, so you may have to move around the darkroom. Any leaks should be corrected before proceeding.

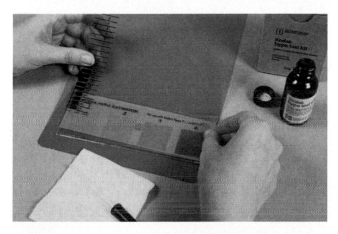

FIGURE 23-13 Analysis to determine the amount of fixer retained on the film. (Courtesy Eastman Kodak.)

If fluorescent lights are present, they should be turned on for at least 2 minutes and then turned off. A piece of film should then be loaded into the phantom cassette in total darkness. Now, a phantom image should be taken as previously described. The film should be taken to the darkroom and placed emulsion side up on the countertop, one half of the image (left or right) being covered with an opaque object. The safelights should then be turned on for 2 minutes with the half-covered film on the counter top.

After 2 minutes, the film should be processed and the OD measured very near both sides of the line separating the covered and uncovered portions of the film. The difference in the two ODs represents the amount of fog created by the safelights or by fluorescent-light afterglow. This value should be recorded.

The level of this type of fog should not exceed 0.05 OD. Excessive fog levels should be investigated to find the source and take corrective action. The background OD (unfogged) of the phantom should be in the range specified previously (1.4 to 1.6).

Screen-Film Contact. Screen-film contact is evaluated to ensure that close contact is maintained between the screen and the film in each cassette. Poor screen-film contact results in image blur, again causing a loss of diagnostic information in the mammogram.

New cassettes should always be tested before being placed into service. All cassettes and screens should be completely cleaned and allowed to air dry for at least 30 minutes before being loaded with film for this test. After loading, the cassettes should be allowed to sit upright for 15 minutes to allow any trapped air to escape.

The cassette to be tested should *be placed on top of the cassette holder assembly* with the test tool placed directly on top of the cassette. An appropriate test tool is made of copper wire mesh with a grid density of at least 40 wires per inch (Figure 23-14). The compression pad-

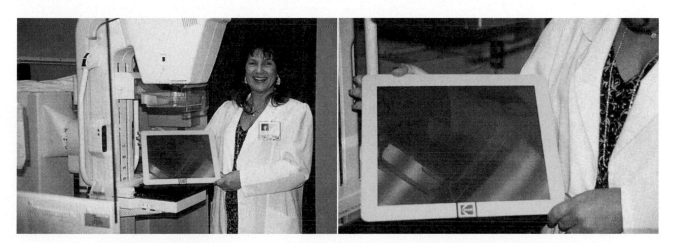

FIGURE 23-14 Wire mesh test tool for evaluating mammographic screen-film contact. (Courtesy Susan Sprinkle Vincent.)

dle should be raised as high as possible. A manual technique of approximately 26 kVp should be selected, which results in an OD between 0.7 and 0.8 near the chest wall. The exposure time should be at least 500 ms.

A piece of acrylic should be placed between the x-ray tube and cassette if the stated parameters cannot be met under normal circumstances. If acrylic is used, it should be placed as close as possible to the x-ray tube to reduce the scatter radiation reaching the cassette.

The film should be processed regularly and viewed from a distance of at least 3 feet. Dark areas on the film indicate poor screen-film contact (Figure 23-15). Any cassettes with poor screen-film contact should be cleaned and tested again. If the poor contact persists at the same spot, the problem should be investigated and the cassette removed from service until the problem is corrected.

Compression. Observation of compression ensures that the mammographic system can provide adequate compression in the manual and power-assisted modes for an adequate amount of time. This analysis must also show that the equipment does not allow excessive compression.

To check the compression device, a towel, tennis balls, or similar cushioning material is placed on the cassette holder assembly, followed by a flat bathroom scale centered under the compression device. Another towel should be placed over the scale without covering the readout area (Figure 23-16). The compression device should be engaged automatically until it stops, the degree of compression should be recorded, and the device should then be released.

The procedure should be repeated using the manual drive, again recording the compression. Never exceed 40 pounds of compression in the automatic mode. If such excess is possible, the equipment should be recalibrated so that 40 pounds of compression cannot be exceeded. Both modes should be able to compress between 25 and 40 pounds and hold this compression for at least 15 s. If either mode fails to reach these levels, the equipment should be properly adjusted.

Firm compression is absolutely necessary for high-quality mammography. Compression reduces the thickness of tissue that the x-rays must penetrate and thus reduces scatter radiation, resulting in increased image contrast at reduced patient dose. Compression improves spatial resolution by reducing focal-spot blur and patient motion. Finally, compression serves to make the thickness of the breast more uniform, resulting in a more uniform OD and making the image easier to read.

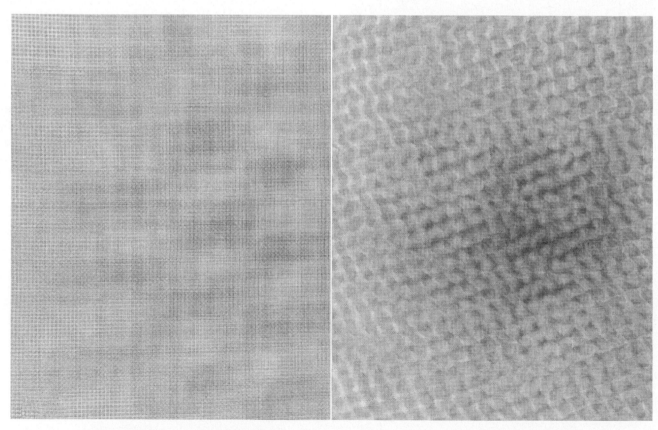

FIGURE 23-15 Images of a high-frequency wire mesh phantom showing **(A)** good and **(B)** poor screen-film contact. (Courtesy Sharon Glaze.)

Nonroutine Tasks

Film Crossover. When a new box of film must be opened and dedicated for processor QC, the old film must be crossed over, a very difficult and time-consuming activity. More detailed sources should be studied before attempting this exercise.

Five strips from each of the old and new boxes of film should be exposed and processed at the same time. The OD should be read on each film for the three predetermined steps and the B+F. The five values for each of the old and the new set of films are then averaged for each of the predetermined steps.

The difference between the old and new values of MD, DD, and B+F should be determined and the control chart control values adjusted to the new values. If the B+F of the new film exceeds the B+F of the old film by more than 0.02, the cause should be investigated and remedied.

The use of strips exposed with the sensitometer more than an hour or two before processing is unacceptable because these strips may be less sensitive to changes in the processor. The proper combination of film, processor, chemistry, developer temperature, immersion time, and replenishment rate should be used as recommended by the film manufacturer. QC should also be performed on the densitometer, sensitometer, and thermometer to maintain their proper calibrations. A log of these evaluations should be maintained.

SUMMARY

QC in mammography is part of an overall evaluation analysis and includes performance monitoring, record keeping, and evaluation of results. The three QC team members are the radiologist, who has specific duties of administration and tracking diagnostic results; the medical physicist, who examines and monitors the performance of imaging equipment; and the mammographer, who performs many tests and evaluations involving equipment, processing, and mammographic images.

The many duties and responsibilities of the QC mammographer are listed by time intervals. Daily routines include maintaining darkroom cleanliness and performing processor QC. Processor QC includes sensitometry and densitometry as well as daily graphing of the results.

Weekly routines include cleaning intensifying screens and viewbox illuminators, producing phantom images, and performing equipment checks.

Repeat analysis, based on at least 250 mammographic examinations, should occur four times a year. A repeat rate of ±2% is required. Greater repeat rates should be investigated. Also, an archival check of film quality is performed quarterly.

Semi-annually, the darkroom fog check is conducted and screen-film contact tests are performed. Finally, the compression test is done using a bathroom scale under the compression paddle. Compression should never exceed 40 lbs of pressure. The automatic and manual modes should compress between 25 and 40 lbs of compression for 15 s. Annually, the medical physicist evaluates the mammography imaging system.

CHALLENGE QUESTIONS

1. Define or otherwise identify:
   a. Quality assurance (QA)
   b. CQI
   c. Mammography phantom
   d. Density difference
   e. Repeat rate
   f. Crossover
   g. NIT
   h. densitometer
   i. Average glandular dose
   j. MQSA

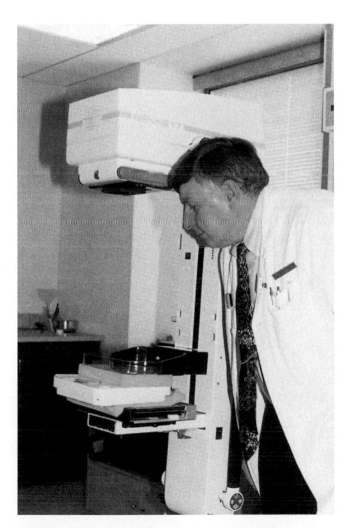

FIGURE 23-16 Testing breast compression with a conventional bathroom scale. (Courtesy Edward Nickoloff.)

2. List two aspects of the radiologist's duties involving mammographic QC.
3. What is the most time-consuming task of the mammographic QC radiographer?
4. Which member of the QC team tracks positive diagnoses?
5. Which member of the QC would notice a temperature error in the developer solution?
6. What do the fibrils of the ACR accreditation phantom simulate?
7. Describe how to clean radiographic intensifying screens. How often is this task performed?
8. Explain how mammographic viewboxes are different from conventional viewboxes.
9. What is masking?
10. What are the three objects on the mammographic phantom?
11. Describe the process of scoring phantom objects.
12. How do you check for light leaks in the darkroom?
13. What is the acceptable fog value for 2 minutes of safelight exposure of film?
14. Describe the device used to check screen-film contact.
15. What is the maximum pressure allowed for the compression device?
16. How do you ensure darkroom cleanliness?
17. What is the speed index and how is it determined?
18. What is the minimum required luminance of a mammography viewbox?
19. When producing phantom images, what technique should be used?
20. Show how to compute repeat rate.

Fluoroscopy

OBJECTIVES

At the completion of this chapter, the student should be able to do the following:

1. Discuss the development of fluoroscopy
2. Explain visual physiology and its relationship to fluoroscopy
3. Describe the components of an image intensifier
4. Calculate brightness gain and identify its units
5. List the approximate kVp levels for common fluoroscopic examinations
6. Discuss the role of the television monitor and television image in forming the fluoroscopic image

OUTLINE

THE PRIMARY FUNCTION of the fluoroscope is to provide real-time viewing of anatomic structures. Dynamic studies are examinations that show the motion of circulation or the motion of hollow internal structures.

During fluoroscopy, the radiologist generally uses contrast media to highlight the anatomy. The radiologist then views a continuous image of the internal structure while the x-ray tube is energized. If the radiologist observes something during the fluoroscopic examination and would like to preserve that image for further study, a radiograph called a *spot film* can be taken with little interruption of the dynamic examination.

The recent introduction of computer technology into fluoroscopy and radiography increases the training and performance demands placed on radiologic technologists. This chapter presents the basic principles of computerized imaging; Chapters 27-30 explain the emerging role of computer science in radiology in greater depth.

AN OVERVIEW

Since Thomas A. Edison invented the fluoroscope in 1896, it has been a valuable tool in the practice of radiology. The fluoroscope is primarily used for dynamic studies. During fluoroscopy, the radiologist views a continuous image of the motion of internal structures while the x-ray tube is energized.

 The fluoroscope is used for examining moving internal structures and fluids.

A radiologist may observe something that he or she would like to preserve for later study; in this case, a permanent image can be made with little interruption of the examination. One such method is known as a spot film, a small static image on a small-format image receptor. Cineradiography, video imaging, and digital images are other examples.

Fluoroscopy is actually a rather routine type of x-ray examination except for its application in the visualization of vessels, called **angiography**. The two main areas of angiography are neuroradiology and vascular radiology. As with all fluoroscopic procedures, spot-film radiographs can also be obtained.

These areas of angiography are now known as interventional radiology.

Figure 24-1 presents the layout of a fluoroscopic imaging system. The x-ray tube is usually hidden under the patient table. The image intensifier and other image detection devices are set over the patient table. Some fluoroscopes have the x-ray tube over the patient table and the image receptor under the patient table. Some fluoroscopes are operated remotely from outside the x-ray room. There are many different arrangements for fluoroscopy, and the radiologic technologist must become familiar with each.

During image-intensified fluoroscopy, the radiologic image is displayed on a television monitor. The image-intensifier tube and the television chain are described later in the chapter.

During fluoroscopy, the x-ray tube is operated at less than 5 mA; contrast this with a radiographic examination, in which the x-ray tube current is measured in hundreds of mA. Despite the lower mA, however, the patient dose is considerably higher during fluoroscopy than it is in radiographic examinations because the x-ray beam exposes the patient for a considerably longer time.

The kVp of operation depends entirely on the section of the body being examined. Fluoroscopic equipment allows the radiologist to select an image brightness level that is subsequently maintained automatically by varying the kVp, mA, or sometimes both. Such a feature of the fluoroscope is called **automatic brightness control (ABC)**.

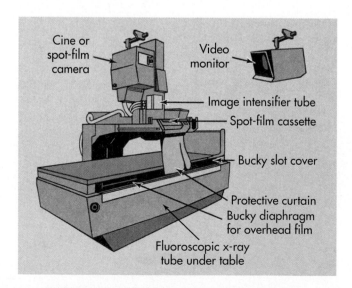

FIGURE 24-1 Fluoroscope and associated parts.

SPECIAL DEMANDS OF FLUOROSCOPY

Fluoroscopy is a dynamic process; thus, the radiologist must adapt to moving images that are sometimes dim. This requires some knowledge of image illumination and visual physiology.

Illumination

The principal advantage of image-intensified fluoroscopy over earlier fluoroscopy is the increased image brightness. Just as it is much more difficult to read a book in dim illumination than in bright illumination, it is much harder to interpret a dim fluoroscopic image than a bright one.

Illumination levels are measured in units of lamberts (L) and millilamberts (mL) (1 L = 1000 mL). It is not necessary to know the precise definition of a lambert; its importance lies in demonstrating the wide range of illumination levels over which the human eye is sensitive. Figure 24-2 lists some approximate illumination levels for familiar objects. Radiographs are visualized under illumination levels of 10 to 1000 mL; image-intensified fluoroscopy is performed at similar illumination levels.

Human Vision

The structures in the eye responsible for the sensation of vision are called **rods** and **cones**. Figure 24-3 is a cross-section of the human eye, identifying its principal parts and its appearance on MRI. Light incident on the eye must first pass through the **cornea**, a transparent protective covering, and then through the **lens**, where the light is focused onto the **retina**.

Between the cornea and the lens is the **iris**, which behaves like the diaphragm of a photographic camera to control the amount of light admitted to the eye. In the presence of bright light, the iris contracts and allows only a small amount of light to enter. During low-light conditions, such as a darkened movie theater, the iris dilates (that is, it opens up) and allows more light to enter. In digital fluoroscopes, a functionally similar iris lies between the image-intensifier tube and the television camera tube.

When light arrives at the retina, it is detected by the rods and the cones. Rods and cones are small structures; there are more than 100,000 of them per square millimeter of retina. The cones are concentrated at the center of the retina in an area called the **fovea centralis**. Rods, on the other hand, are most numerous on the periphery of the retina. There are no rods at the fovea centralis.

The rods are sensitive to low light levels and are stimulated during dim light situations. The threshold for rod vision is approximately 10^{-6} mL. Cones, on the other hand, are less sensitive to light; their threshold is only approximately 10^{-2} mL, but they are capable of responding to intense light levels, whereas rods cannot.

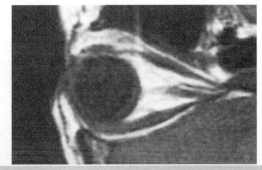

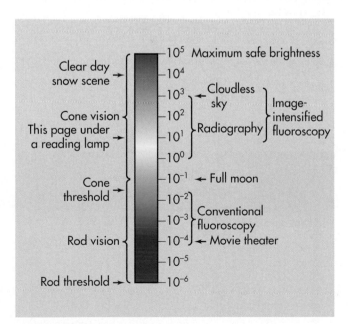

FIGURE 24-2 The range of human vision is wide; it covers eleven orders of magnitude.

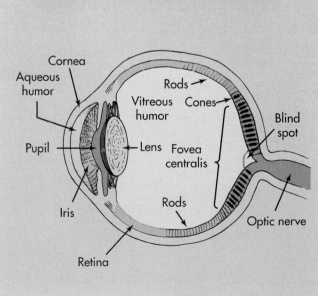

FIGURE 24-3 The human eye's appearance on a magnetic resonance image and the parts responsible for vision. (Courtesy Helen Schumpert).

Consequently, cones are used primarily for daylight vision, called **photopic vision,** and rods are used for night vision, called **scotopic vision.** This aspect of visual physiology explains why dim objects are more readily viewed if they are not looked at directly. Astronomers and radiologists are familiar with the fact that a dim object is best viewed peripherally, where rod vision predominates.

Cones perceive small objects much better than rods do. This ability to perceive fine detail is called **visual acuity.** Cones are also much better at detecting differences in brightness levels. This property of vision is called **contrast perception.** Furthermore, cones are sensitive to a wide range of wavelengths of light. Cones perceive color, but rods are essentially colorblind.

FLUOROSCOPIC TECHNIQUE

During fluoroscopy, maximum image detail is desired; this requires high image brightness. The image intensifier was developed principally to replace the conventional fluorescent screen, which had to be viewed in a darkened room and then only after 15 minutes of dark adaptation (Figure 24-4). The image intensifier raises the illumination into the cone-vision region, where visual acuity is greatest.

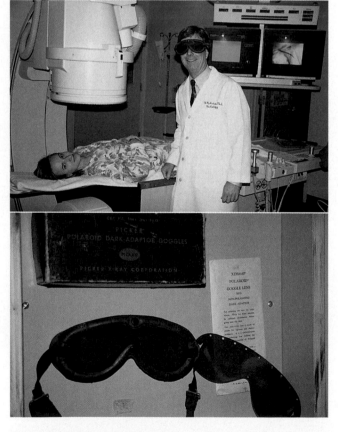

FIGURE 24-4 Red goggles were used to dark adapt for conventional screen fluoroscopy. This radiologist is back to the future. (Courtesy Ben Archer.)

The brightness of the fluoroscopic image depends primarily on the anatomy being examined, the kVp, and the mA. The patient's anatomy cannot be controlled by the radiologic technologist; fluoroscopic kVp and mA can.

The influence of kVp and mA on fluoroscopic image quality is similar to their influence on radiographic image quality. Generally, high kVp and low mA are preferred.

The precise fluoroscopic technique is determined by the training and experience of the radiologist and radiologic technologist. Table 24-1 relates representative fluoroscopic peak kilovoltage for several common examinations. The fluoroscopic mA is not given because this value varies according to patient characteristics and the response of the ABC system.

IMAGE INTENSIFICATION
Image-Intensifier Tube

The image-intensifier tube is a complex electronic device that receives the image-forming x-ray beam and converts it into a visible-light image of high intensity. Figure 24-5 is a rendition of an x-ray image-intensifier tube. The tube components are contained within a glass or metal envelope that provides structural support but more importantly maintains a vacuum. When installed, the tube is mounted inside a metal container to protect it from rough handling and breakage.

X-rays that exit the patient and are incident on the image intensifier tube are transmitted through the glass envelope and interact with the **input phosphor,** which is cesium iodide (CsI). When an x-ray interacts with the input phosphor, its energy is converted into visible light; this is similar to the effect of radiographic intensifying screens.

The CsI crystals are grown as tiny needles and tightly packed in a layer of approximately 300 μm (Figure 24-6). Each crystal is approximately 5 μm in diameter. This re-

TABLE 24-1	Representative Fluoroscopic and Spot-Film kVp for Common Examinations	
Examination	**kVp**
Gall bladder	65–75
Nephrostogram	70–80
Myelogram	70–80
Barium enema (air contrast)	80–90
Upper gastrointestinal	100–110
Small bowel	110–120
Barium enema	110–120

sults in microlight pipes with little dispersion and improved spatial resolution.

The next active element of the image intensifier tube is the **photocathode,** which is bonded directly to the input phosphor with a thin, transparent adhesive layer. The photocathode is a thin metal layer usually composed of cesium and antimony compounds that respond to stimulation of input phosphor light by the emission of electrons.

 The photocathode emits electrons when illuminated by the input phosphor.

This process is known as **photoemission.** The term is similar to **thermionic emission,** which refers to electron emission following heat stimulation. Photoemission is electron emission following light stimulation.

It takes many light photons to cause the emission of one electron. The number of electrons emitted by the photocathode is directly proportional to the intensity of light reaching it. Consequently, the number of electrons emitted is proportional to the intensity of the incident image-forming x-ray beam.

The image intensifier tube is approximately 50 cm long. A potential difference of about 25,000 V is maintained across the tube between photocathode and anode so that the electrons produced by photoemission will be accelerated to the anode.

The anode is a circular plate with a hole in the middle to allow the electrons through to the **output phosphor,** which is just the other side of the anode, and is usually made of zinc cadmium sulfide. The output phosphor is where the electrons interact and produce light.

For the image pattern to be accurate, the electron path from the photocathode to the output phosphor must be precise. The engineering aspects of maintaining proper electron travel are called **electron optics** because the pattern of electrons emitted from the large cathode end of the image intensifier tube must be reduced to the small output phosphor.

The devices responsible for this control, called **electrostatic focusing lenses,** are located along the length of the image-intensifier tube. The electrons arrive at the output phosphor with high kinetic energy and contain the image of the input phosphor in minified form.

The interaction of these high-energy electrons with the output phosphor produces a considerable amount of light is produced. Each photoelectron that arrives at the output phosphor produces 50 to 75 times as many light photons as were necessary to create it. The entire sequence of events from initial x-ray interaction to output image is summarized in Figure 24-7. This ratio of the number of light photons at the output phosphor to the number of x-rays at the input phosphor is the **flux gain.**

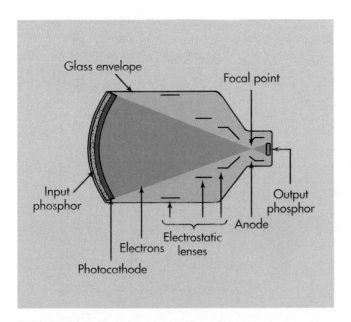

FIGURE 24-5 The image-intensifier tube converts the pattern of the x-ray beam into a bright visible light image.

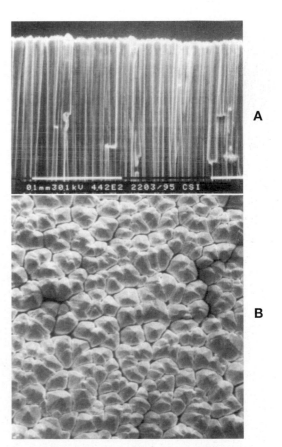

FIGURE 24-6 Cesium iodide crystals are grown as linear filaments and packed tightly as shown in these photomicrographs. **A,** Cross section. **B,** Face. (Courtesy Philips Medical Systems.)

FLUX GAIN

$$\text{Flux gain} = \frac{\text{number of output light photons}}{\text{number of input x-ray photons}}$$

The increased illumination of the image is due to the multiplication of the light photons at the output phosphor compared with the x-rays at the input phosphor and the image minification from input phosphor to output phosphor. The ability of the image intensifier to increase the illumination level of the image is called its **brightness gain.** The brightness gain is simply the product of the **minification gain** and the **flux gain.**

BRIGHTNESS GAIN

Brightness gain = minification gain × flux gain

The minification gain is the ratio of the square of the diameter of the input phosphor to the square of the diameter of the output phosphor. Output phosphor size is fairly standard at 2.5 or 5 cm. Input phosphor size varies from 10 to 35 cm and is used to identify image intensifier tubes.

MINIFICATION GAIN

$$\text{Minification gain} = \left(\frac{d_i}{d_o}\right)^2$$

where d_i = diameter of input phosphor
d_o = diameter of output phosphor

Question: What is the brightness gain for a 17 cm image intensifier tube having a flux gain of 120 and a 2.5 cm output phosphor?

Answer:
$$\text{Brightness gain} = \frac{17^2}{2.5^2} \times 120$$
$$= 46 \times 120$$
$$= 5520$$

The brightness gain of most image intensifiers is 5000 to 30,000, and it decreases with tube age and use. As an image intensifier ages, patient dose increases in order to maintain brightness. Ultimately, the image intensifier must be replaced.

Brightness gain is now defined as the ratio of the illumination intensity at the output phosphor, measured in candela per meter squared (cd/m²), to the radiation intensity incident on the input phosphor, measured in milliroentgens per second (mR/s). This quantity is called the **conversion factor** and is approximately 0.01 times the brightness gain. Conversion factor is the proper quantity for expressing the intensification.

CONVERSION FACTOR

$$\text{Conversion factor} = \frac{\text{output phosphor illumination (cd/m}^2)}{\text{input exposure rate (mR/s)}}$$

Image intensifiers have conversion factors of 50 to 300. This corresponds to brightness gains of 5000 to 30,000.

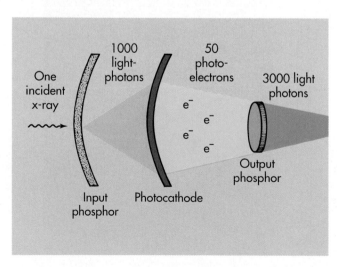

FIGURE 24-7 In an image-intensifier tube, each incident x-ray that interacts with the input phosphor results in a large number of light photons at the output phosphor. The image intensifier shown here has a gain of 3000.

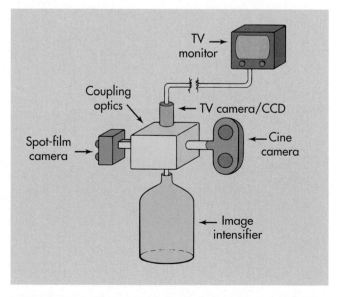

FIGURE 24-8 Some possible modes of operation with an image intensifier tube. *CCD,* Charge coupled device.

Figure 24-8 demonstrates some of the modes of operation that can be accommodated with the image-intensifier tube. Fluoroscopic images are viewed on a television monitor. The spot-film camera uses 105 mm film. The cineradiography camera is used almost exclusively in cardiac catheterization, but the use of digital images is growing.

Scatter radiation in the form of x-rays, electrons, and particularly light can reduce the contrast of image-intensifier tubes through a process called **veiling glare**. A veiling glare signal is produced behind a lead disc positioned on the input phosphor. Veiling glare is depicted in Figure 24-9. Advanced II tubes have output phosphor designs to reduce veiling glare.

Multifield Image Intensification

Most image intensifiers are of the multifield type. These multifield image intensifiers provide for considerably more flexibility for all fluoroscopic examinations and are standard components in digital fluoroscopy. Dual field tubes come in various sizes, but perhaps the most popular is the 25 cm/17 cm (25/17) design. Trifield tubes of 25/17/12 or 23/15/10 are also used.

These numeric dimensions refer to the diameter of the input phosphor of the image-intensifier tube. The operation of a typical multifield tube is illustrated by the 25/17 type shown in Figure 24-10. In the 25 cm mode, the photoelectrons from the entire input phosphor are accelerated to the output phosphor.

When switched to the 17 cm mode, the voltage on the electrostatic focusing lenses increases, which causes the electron focal point to move further from the output phosphor. Consequently, only electrons from the center 17 cm diameter of the input phosphor are incident on the output phosphor.

The principal result of this change in focal point is to reduce the field of view and thereby magnify the image. Use of the smaller dimension of a multifield image intensifier tube always results in a magnified image, with a magnification factor in direct proportion to the ratio of the diameters. A 25/17 tube operated in the 17 cm mode produces an image that is 1.5 times larger than the image produced in the 25 cm mode.

Question: How magnified is the image of a 25/17/12 image intensifier in the 12 cm mode compared with the 25 cm mode?

Answer: $MF = \dfrac{25}{15} = 2.1$ magnification

This magnified image comes at a price. In the magnified mode, the minification gain is reduced and there are

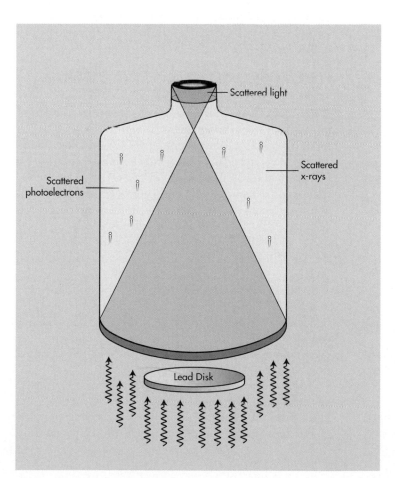

FIGURE 24-9 Veiling glare reduces contrast of an image intensifier tube.

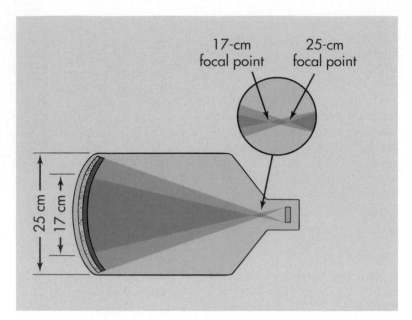

FIGURE 24-10 A 25/17 image-intensifier tube produces a magnified image in 17 cm mode.

fewer photoelectrons incident on the output phosphor. A dimmer image results.

To maintain the same level of brightness, the x-ray tube mA is increased by the ABC, which increases the patient dose. The increase in dose is approximately equal to the ratio of the area of the input phosphor used, or [$25^2 \div 12^2 \sim 4.4$], the dose obtained in the wide field of view mode.

Question: A 23/15/10 image intensifier tube is used in the 10 cm mode. How much higher is the patient dose in this mode compared with the 23 cm mode?

Answer: $23^2/10^2 = 5.3$ times as high!

This increase in patient dose results in better image quality. The patient dose is higher because more x-rays per unit area are required to form the image. This results in lower noise and improved **contrast resolution.**

MAGNIFICATION MODE RESULTS IN

Better spatial resolution

Better contrast resolution

Higher patient dose

The portion of any image resulting from the periphery of the input phosphor is inherently unfocused and suffers from **vignetting,** a reduction in brightness at the periphery of the image.

Because only the central region of the input phosphor is used in the magnification mode, **spatial resolution** is also improved. In the 25 cm mode, a CsI image-intensifier tube can image approximately 0.125 mm objects (4 lp/mm); in the 10 cm mode, the resolution is approximately 0.08 mm (6 lp/mm).

The concept of spatial resolution as measured in line pairs per millimeter is discussed in Chapter 15 and more completely in Chapter 29. At this stage, it is sufficient to know that good spatial resolution is associated with a higher lp/mm value.

FLUOROSCOPIC IMAGE MONITORING
Television Monitoring

When a **television monitoring system** is used, the output phosphor of the image intensifier tube is coupled directly to a television camera tube. The **vidicon** (Figure 24-11) is the television camera tube most often used in television fluoroscopy. It has a sensitive input surface that is the same size as the output phosphor of the image-intensifier tube. The television camera tube converts the light image from the output phosphor of the image intensifier into an electrical signal that is sent to the television monitor, where it is reconstructed as an image on the television screen.

A significant advantage of television monitoring is that brightness level and contrast can be controlled electronically. With television monitoring, several observers can view the fluoroscopic image at the same time. It is even common to place monitors outside the examination room for others to observe.

Television monitoring also allows for storage of the image in its electronic form for later playback and image manipulation. Television monitoring is an essential part of the digital fluoroscopic equipment described in Chapter 28.

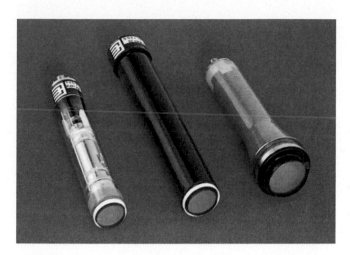

FIGURE 24-11 These three variations of a vidicon television camera tube have a diameter of approximately 1 inch and a length of 6 inches. The right tube uses electrostatic rather than electromagnetic electron beam deflection. (Courtesy Marconi Medical Systems.)

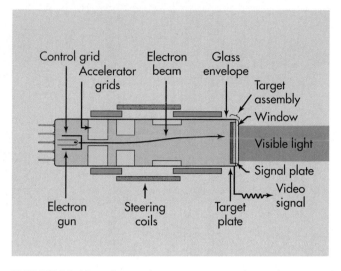

FIGURE 24-12 Vidicon television camera tube and its principal parts.

Television Camera. The television camera consists of a cylindrical housing, approximately 15 mm in diameter by 25 cm in length, which contains the heart of the television camera tube. It also contains electromagnetic coils for properly steering the electron beam inside the tube. A number of such television camera tubes are available for television fluoroscopy, but the **vidicon** and its modified version, the **Plumbicon,** are used most often.

Figure 24-12 shows a typical vidicon. The **glass envelope** serves the same function that it does for the x-ray tube: to maintain a vacuum and provide mechanical support for the internal elements. The internal elements are the cathode, its **electron gun,** assorted **electrostatic grids,** and a **target assembly** that serves as an anode.

The electron gun is a heated filament that supplies a constant electron current by thermionic emission. These electrons are formed into an electron beam by the control grid, which also helps to accelerate the electrons to the anode.

The electron beam is further accelerated and focused by additional electrostatic grids. The size of the electron beam and its position is controlled by external electromagnetic coils known as deflection coils, focusing coils, and alignment coils.

At the anode end of the tube the electron beam passes through a wire mesh-like structure and interacts with the target assembly. The target assembly consists of three layers sandwiched together. The outside layer is the **face plate** or **window,** the thin part of the glass envelope. Coated on the inside of the window is a thin

layer of metal or graphite, called the **signal plate.** The signal plate is thin enough to transmit light yet thick enough to efficiently conduct electricity. Its name derives from the fact that it conducts the video signal out of the tube into the external video circuit.

A photoconductive layer of antimony trisulfide is applied to the inside of the signal plate. This layer is called the **target** or **photoconductive layer,** and the electron beam interacts with the layer. Antimony trisulfide is photoconductive because, when illuminated, it conducts electrons; when dark, it behaves as an insulator.

The mechanism of the target assembly is complex but can be described briefly as follows. When light from the output phosphor of the image-intensifier tube strikes the window, it is transmitted through the signal plate to the target.

If the electron beam is incident on the same part of the target at the same time, some of its electrons are conducted through the target to the signal plate and conducted from there out of the tube as the video signal. If that area of the target is dark, no video signal is produced. The magnitude of the video signal is proportional to the intensity of light (Figure 24-13).

Coupling to the Image Intensifier. Image intensifiers and television camera tubes are manufactured so that the output phosphor of the image-intensifier tube is the same diameter as the window of the television camera tube, usually 2.5 or 5 cm. Two methods are commonly used to attach, or **couple,** the television camera tube or charge-coupled device (CCD) to the image-intensifier tube (Figure 24-14).

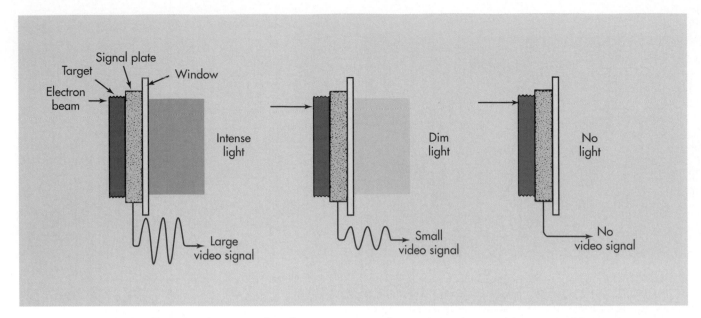

FIGURE 24-13 The target of a television camera tube conducts electrons, creating a video signal only when illuminated.

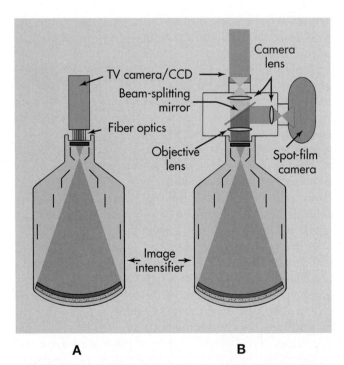

A   **B**

FIGURE 24-14 Television camera tubes and charge coupled devices (CCD) are coupled to an image-intensifier tube in two ways. **A,** Fiber optics. **B,** Lens system.

The simplest method is to use a bundle of **fiber optics.** The fiber optics bundle is only a few millimeters thick and contains thousands of glass fibers per square millimeter of cross-section. One advantage of this type of coupling is its compact assembly, making it easy to move the image-intensifier tower. This coupling is also rugged and can withstand relatively rough handling.

The principal disadvantage is that it cannot accommodate auxiliary imaging devices such as cine or photospot cameras. This type of coupling requires cassette-loaded spot films.

To accept a cine or photospot camera, **lens coupling** is required. This type of coupling results in a much larger assembly that should be handled with care. It is absolutely essential that the lenses and mirror remain precisely adjusted. Malposition results in a blurred image.

The **objective lens** accepts the light from the output phosphor and converts it into a parallel beam. When recording an image on film, this beam is interrupted by a **beam-splitting mirror** so that only a portion is transmitted to the television camera; the remainder is reflected to a film camera. Such a system allows the fluoroscopist to view the image while it is being recorded.

Usually, the beam-splitting mirror is retracted from the beam when a film camera is not in use. Both the television camera and the film camera are coupled to lenses that focus the parallel light beam onto the film and target of the respective cameras. These **camera lenses** are the most critical elements in the optical chain in terms of alignment. Although the lenses are shown as simple convex lenses, it should be understood that each is a compound lens system consisting of several separate lens elements.

Television Monitor. The video signal is amplified and transmitted by cable to the television monitor, where it is transformed back into a visible image. The television

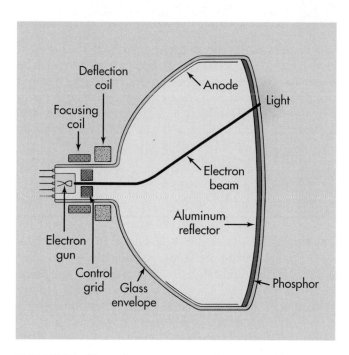

FIGURE 24-15 A television picture tube (CRT) and its principal parts.

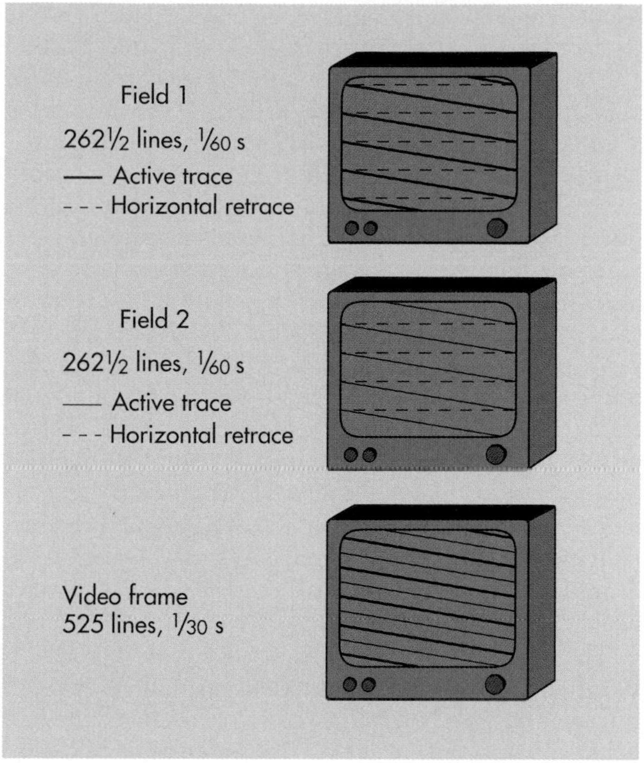

Field 1
262½ lines, ⅟₆₀ s
—— Active trace
--- Horizontal retrace

Field 2
262½ lines, ⅟₆₀ s
—— Active trace
--- Horizontal retrace

Video frame
525 lines, ⅟₃₀ s

FIGURE 24-16 A video frame is formed from a raster pattern of two interlaced video fields.

monitor forms one end of a closed-circuit television system. The other end is the television camera tube.

There are two immediately obvious differences between closed-circuit television fluoroscopy and a home television set: no audio and no channel selection. There are usually only two controls that the radiologic technologist manipulates: contrast and brightness.

The heart of the television monitor is the **television picture tube,** or cathode ray tube (CRT) (Figure 24-15). It is similar to the television camera tube in many ways: glass envelope, electron gun, and external coils for focusing and steering the electron beam. It is different from a television camera tube in that it is much larger and its anode assembly consists of a fluorescent screen and graphite lining.

The video signal received by the picture tube is **modulated;** that is, its magnitude is directly proportional to the light intensity received by the television camera tube. Unlike the television camera tube, the electron beam of the television picture tube varies in intensity according to the modulation of the video signal.

The intensity of the electron beam is modulated by a **control grid,** which is attached to the electron gun. This electron beam is focused onto the output fluorescent screen by the external coils. There, the electrons interact with an output phosphor and produce a burst of light.

The phosphor is composed of linear crystals aligned perpendicularly to the glass envelope to reduce **lateral dispersion.** It is usually backed by a thin layer of aluminum, which transmits the electron beam but reflects the light.

Television Image. The image on the television monitor is formed in a complex way, but it can be described rather simply. It involves transforming the visible light image of the output phosphor of the image intensifier tube into an electrical video signal that is created by a constant electron beam in the television camera tube. The video signal then **modulates** the electron beam of the television picture tube and transforms that electron beam into a visible image at the fluorescent screen of the picture tube.

Both electron beams, the constant one of the television camera tube and the modulated one of the television picture tube, are finely focused pencil beams that are precisely and synchronously directed by the external electromagnetic coils of each tube. The beams are synchronous because they are always at the same position at the same time and move in precisely the same fashion.

The movement of these electron beams produces a **raster pattern** on the screen of a television picture tube (Figure 24-16). Although the following discussion relates to a picture tube, remember that the same electron-beam pattern is occurring in the camera tube.

The electron beam begins in the upper left corner of the screen and moves to the upper right corner, creating a line of varying intensity of light as it moves. This is called an **active trace.** The electron beam then is **blanked,** or turned off, and it returns to the left side of the screen as shown. This is the **horizontal retrace.**

There follows a series of active traces followed by horizontal retraces until the electron beam is at the bottom of the screen. This is much like the action of a word-processing secretary who types a line of information (the active trace): the cursor returns (the horizontal retrace) and continues this sequence to the bottom of the page. Whereas the secretary completes a page, the electron beam completes a **television field.**

The similarity stops there, however, because the secretary would continue word processing. The electron beam is blanked again and undergoes a **vertical retrace** to the top of the screen.

The electron beam now describes a second television field, the same as the first except that each active trace lies between two adjacent active traces of the first field. This movement of the electron beam is called **interlace,** and two interlaced television fields form one **television frame.**

In the United States, power is supplied at 60 Hz; therefore, there are 60 television fields per second and 30 television frames per second. This is fortunate because the flickering of home movies (shown at 16 frames per second) or old-time movies does not appear on the television image. Flickering is not detectable by the human eye at rates above approximately 20 frames per second. At a frame rate of 30 per second, each frame is 33 ms long.

Video monitoring uses a rate of 30 frames per second.

In the television camera tube, as the electron beam reads the optical signal, the signal is erased. In the television picture tube, as the electron beam creates the television optical signal, it immediately fades; hence the term "fluorescent screen." Therefore, each new television frame represents 33 ms of new information.

Standard broadcast and closed circuit televisions are called 525-line systems because they have 525 lines of active trace per frame. Actually, there are only about 480 lines per frame because of the time required for retracing. Other special purpose systems have 875 or 1024 lines per frame and therefore have better **spatial resolution.** These high-resolution systems are particularly important for digital fluoroscopy.

For a 23 cm image intensifier, a 525-line TV system provides a spatial resolution of approximately 1 lp/mm; a 1024-line system provides 2 lp/mm.

The **vertical resolution** is determined by the number of scan lines. The **horizontal resolution** is determined by **bandpass.** Bandpass is expressed in frequency (Hz) and describes the number of times per second that the electron beam can be **modulated.** A 1 MHz bandpass would indicate that the electron-beam intensity could be changed a million times each second.

The higher the bandpass, the better the horizontal resolution.

The objective of television designers is to create a television frame having equal horizontal and vertical resolution. Commercial television systems have a bandpass of about 3.5 MHz. Those used in fluoroscopy are approximately 4.5 MHz; 1000-line high-resolution systems have a bandpass of approximately 20 MHz.

The television monitor remains the weakest link in image-intensified fluoroscopy. A 525-line system has approximately 2 lp/mm spatial resolution, but the image intensifier is good to about 5 lp/mm. Therefore, to take advantage of the superior resolution of the image intensifier, the image must be recorded on film through an optically coupled photographic camera.

Image Recording

The conventional **cassette-loaded spot film** is one method used with image-intensified fluoroscopes. The spot film is positioned between the patient and the image intensifier (Figure 24-17).

During fluoroscopy the cassette is parked in a lead-lined shroud so that it is not unintentionally exposed. When a cassette spot-film exposure is desired, the radiologist must actuate a control that properly positions the cassette in the x-ray beam and changes the operation of the x-ray tube from low fluoroscopic mA to high radiographic mA. Sometimes it takes the rotating anode a second or two to be energized to a higher speed.

The cassette-loaded spot film is masked by a series of lead diaphragms to allow several image formats. When the entire film is exposed at one time, it is called "one-on-one." When only half of the film is exposed at a time, two images result—"two-on-one." Four-on-one and six-on-one modes are also available, with the images becoming successively smaller.

Use of cassette-loaded spot film requires a higher patient dose, and the pre-exposure delay is sometimes a

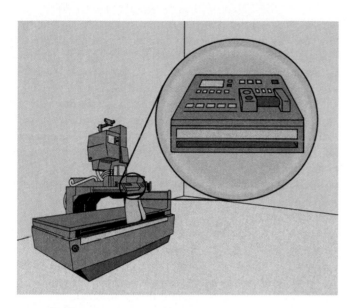

FIGURE 24-17 The cassette loaded spot film is positioned between the patient and the image intensifier.

TABLE 24-2	Cassette Spot Versus Photospot	
	Cassette Spot	**Photospot**
Spatial resolution	8 lp/mm	5 lp/mm
Frame rate	1/s	12/s
Patient ESE	200 mR	100 mR

nuisance. Cassette-loaded spot films, however, do provide a familiar format for the radiologist and produce high image quality.

The **photospot camera** is similar to a movie camera except that it exposes only one frame when activated. It receives its image from the output phosphor of the image-intensifier tube and therefore requires less patient exposure than the cassette-loaded spot film. The photospot camera does not require significant interruption of the fluoroscopic examination and avoids the additional heat load on the x-ray tube associated with cassette-loaded spot films.

The photospot camera uses film sizes of 70 and 105 mm. As a general rule, **the larger film format results in better image quality but at increased patient dose.** Even with 105 mm spot films, however, the patient dose is only approximately half of that with cassette-loaded spot films.

The trend in spot filming is to use the photospot camera. The photospot camera provides adequate image quality without interruption of the fluoroscopic examination and at a rate of up to 12 images per second. (Table 24-2).

SUMMARY

The original fluoroscope, invented by Edison, had a zinc-cadmium sulfide screen placed in the x-ray beam directly above the patient. The radiologist stared directly into the screen and viewed a faint yellow-green fluoroscopic image. It was not until the 1950s that the image intensifier was developed.

In the past, fluoroscopy required radiologists to adapt their eyes to the dark before the examination. Under dim viewing conditions, the human eye uses rods for vision, which have low visual acuity. The image from today's fluoroscope is bright enough to be perceived by cone vision. Cone vision has superior visual acuity and contrast perception. When viewing the fluoroscopic image, the radiologist is able to see fine anatomic detail and differences in brightness levels of anatomic parts.

The image intensifier is a complex device that receives the image-forming x-ray beam, converts it to light and increases the light intensity for better viewing. The input phosphor converts the x-ray beam into light. When stimulated by light, the photocathode then emits electrons and the electrons are accelerated to the output phosphor.

The following relationships define several characteristics of image-intensified fluoroscopy:

$$\text{Flux gain} = \frac{\text{Number of output light photons}}{\text{Number of input x-ray photons}}$$

$$\text{Minification gain} = \frac{(\text{Diameter of input phosphor})^2}{(\text{Diameter of output phosphor})^2}$$

$$\text{Brightness gain} = \text{minification gain} \times \text{flux gain}$$

Brightness gain is also expressed as the conversion factor:

$$\text{Conversion factor} = \frac{\text{Output phosphor illumination (candella/meter}^2)}{\text{Input exposure rate (mR/s)}}$$

The fluoroscopy television camera is attached to the image intensifier with a lens coupling to accommodate a cine or a spot-film camera. When recording an image on film, a beam-splitting mirror separates the beam so that only a portion is transmitted to the television camera and the remainder is reflected to a spot-film camera.

CHALLENGE QUESTIONS

1. Define or otherwise identify:
   a. Photopic vision
   b. Automatic brightness control
   c. Visual acuity
   d. Flux gain
   e. Angiography
   f. Vidicon
   g. Photoemission
   h. Bucky slot cover
   i. Spot-film camera sizes
   j. Modulation
2. Draw a diagram showing the relationship between the x-ray tube, the patient table, and the image intensifier.
3. What is the difference between rod and cone vision? With which is visual acuity greater?
4. What is the approximate peak kilovoltage for the following fluoroscopic examinations: barium enema, gallbladder, and upper gastrointestinal?
5. Draw a cross-section of the human eye and label the cornea, lens, and retina.
6. Explain the difference between photoemission and thermionic emission.
7. Diagram the image-intensifier tube, label its principle parts, and discuss the function of each.
8. A 23 cm image-intensifier has an output phosphor size of 2.5 cm and a flux gain of 75. What is its brightness gain?
9. What is vignetting?
10. Why is the television monitor considered the weakest link in image-intensified fluoroscopy?
11. What is the primary function of the fluoroscope?
12. Who invented the fluoroscope in 1896? What was the phosphor used on that original fluoroscopic screen?
13. What determines the image frame rate in video fluoroscopy?
14. What limits the vertical resolution and horizontal resolution of a video monitor?
15. Does spatial resolution change when viewing in the magnification mode compared to the normal mode?
16. What is meant by a trifield image intensifier?
17. Draw the approximate raster pattern for a conventional video monitor.
18. When switching the image intensifier from 15 cm mode to 25 cm mode, what happens to patient dose and contrast resolution?
19. Trace the path of information carrying elements in a fluoroscopic system from incident x-rays to video image.
20. What is the principal difference between a standard video system for fluoroscopy and a high-resolution system?

Interventional Radiology

OBJECTIVES

At the completion of this chapter, the student should be able to do the following:

1. Describe the measures used to provide radiation protection for patients and personnel during interventional radiology
2. Describe the reasons why minimally invasive (percutaneous) vascular procedures often are more beneficial than traditional surgical procedures
3. Discuss the advantages that nonionic (water-soluble) contrast media offer over ionic contrast media
4. Identify the risks of arteriography
5. Describe the special equipment in the interventional suite

OUTLINE

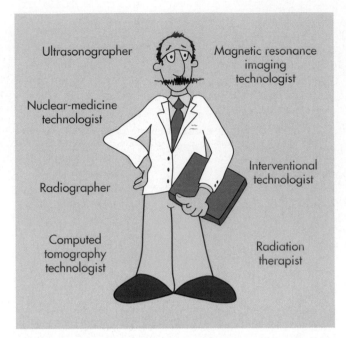

FIGURE 25-1 A radiologic technologist can specialize in many types of imaging modalities.

TABLE 25-1	Representative Procedures Conducted in an Interventional Radiology Suite
Imaging Procedures	**Interventional Procedures**
Angiography	Stent placement
Aortography	Embolization
Arteriography	Intravascular stent
Cardiac catheterization	Thrombolysis
Myelography	Balloon angioplasty
Venography	Atherectomy
	Electrophysiology

Isn't it interesting how advances in technology are accompanied by changes in terminology? We made radiographs with x-rays because that is how Roentgen named them. X is the mathematical symbol for unknown, which is how Roentgen viewed his discovery.

As imaging technology has developed, so has our identity. First we were called x-ray operators, then technicians, and now radiologic technologists or, more specifically, radiographers. A radiologic technologist can be a radiographer, a nuclear medicine technologist, or another imaging technologist (Figure 25-1).

In the same way that radiologic technology has become more precisely divided into disciplines, so has our imaging task. We used to do **special procedures,** such as pneumoencephalography, myelography, and neuroangiography. The rapid development of vascular imaging and aggressive therapeutic intervention through vessels has resulted in rooms and equipment designed especially for **interventional radiologic procedures.** The radiologic technologists involved are **interventional radiologic technologists.**

TYPES OF INTERVENTIONAL PROCEDURES

Interventional radiologic procedures began in the 1930s with **angiography;** needles and contrast media were used to enter and highlight an artery. In the early 1960s, Mason Jones pioneered **transbrachial selective coronary angiography**—entering select coronary arteries through an artery of the arm.

Also during the 1960s, transfemoral angiography—entering an artery in the thigh—of selective visceral, heart, and head arteries was developed. Melvin Judkins introduced coronary angiography, and Charles Dotter introduced visceral angiography.

Angiography refers to the opacification of vessels by injection of contrast media. **Angioplasty, thrombolysis, embolization, vascular stents,** and **biopsy** are interventional therapeutic procedures conducted in and through vessels. Table 25-1 lists the types of imaging and interventional procedures likely to be conducted in an interventional radiologic suite.

BASIC PRINCIPLES
Arterial Access

In 1953, Sven Ivar Seldinger described a method of arterial access using a catheter. The Seldinger needle is an 18-gauge hollow needle with a stylet. Once the Seldinger needle is inserted into the femoral artery and pulsating arterial blood returns, the stylet is removed.

A guidewire is then inserted through the needle into the arterial lumen. With the guidewire in the vessel, the Seldinger needle is removed and a catheter is threaded onto the guidewire. Under fluoroscopic view, the catheter is then advanced along the guidewire.

The common femoral artery is most often accessed for arterial access in angiography. The common femoral artery can be palpated by locating the pulse in the groin below the inguinal ligament, which passes between the symphysis pubis and the anterior superior iliac spine.

Guidewires

Guidewires allow the safe introduction of the catheter into the vessel. Once the catheter is in place, the guidewire allows the radiologist to position the catheter within the vascular network.

Guidewires are fabricated of stainless steel and contain an inner core wire tapered at the end to a soft, flexible tip. The core wire prevents loss of sections of the wire should it break. The trailing end of the guidewire is stiff and allows the guidewire to be pushed and twisted so that the catheter can be positioned in the chosen vessel.

Conventional guidewires are 145 cm long. Catheters overlaying the guidewire are usually 100 cm long or less. Guide wires are additionally categorized by length to the beginning of the tapered tip, configuration of the tip, stiffness of the guidewire, and coating. They are coated with a hydrophilic material so that the catheter slides over the wire more easily. This also makes the guide wires more resistant to thrombus (blood clot) and easier to irrigate while they are in the vascular system.

The J-tip for guidewires is a variation of the tip configuration initially designed for use in atherosclerotic vessels that are filled with plaques. The J-tip deflects off edges of plaques and helps prevent subintimal dissection of the artery. The coatings on guidewires are materials designed to reduce friction and include Teflon, heparin coatings, and more recently hydrophilic polymers. The latter type is called a **glide wire**, which represents a major technologic advance in interventional radiology.

Catheters

Just like guidewires, catheters are designed in many different shapes and sizes. Usually, catheter diameter is categorized in French (Fr) sizes, with 3 Fr equaling 1 mm in diameter. Figure 25-2 illustrates four common catheter shapes. The shaped tip of the catheter is required for selective catheterization of openings into specific arteries.

The H1 or headhunter tip designed by Vincent Hinck is used for the femoral approach to the brachiocephalic vessels. The Simmons catheter is highly curved for approach to sharply angled vessels and was also designed for cerebral angiography but was later adopted for visceral angiography. The C2 or Cobra catheter has an angled tip joined to a gentle curve and is used for introduction into celiac, renal, and mesenteric arteries.

Pigtail catheters have side holes for ejecting contrast media into a compact bolus. A catheter with side holes is fenestrated and helps reduce a possible whiplash ef-

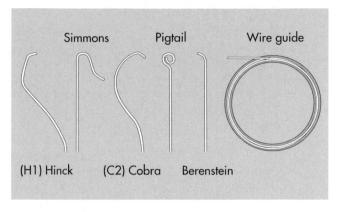

FIGURE 25-2 Typical catheter shapes.

fect. The jet effect is minimized with the curved pigtail, which prevents injury to the vessel.

Once the catheter is introduced into the vessel, the guidewire is removed. The catheter must then immediately be flushed to prevent clotting of blood within the catheter. Heparinized saline is generally used to flush catheters.

After catheter placement, a test injection is performed under fluoroscopy before static imaging to check that the catheter tip is not wedged and is in the correct vessel. Injection rates of the automatic power injector are gauged by the test flow speed.

Contrast Media

Vessels under investigation in angiography are injected with radiopaque contrast media. Initially, ionic iodine compounds have been used for contrast injections; however, nonionic contrast media have largely replaced the ionic agents. Because of their low concentration of ions (low osmolality), physiologic problems and adverse reactions are reduced for a patient undergoing angiographic injection.

Patient Preparation and Monitoring

Before angiography, the radiologist visits the patient to establish rapport and to explain the procedure and its risks. A history and physical examination are necessary to assess the patient's medical history for allergies and other conditions to conclude whether a procedure is indicated and which route is optimal. Orders are written for intravenous hydration and a diet of clear liquids. The patient may be premedicated in the interventional radiologic suite to reduce anxiety.

During the procedure, monitoring by electrocardiography, automatic blood pressure measurement, and pulse oximetry is mandatory. The code or "crash" cart for life-threatening emergencies must be accessible. After the procedure, when the catheter is removed, the femoral puncture site must be manually compressed. The patient is then instructed to remain immobile for several hours after the angiographic procedure while vital signs are monitored and the puncture site inspected.

Risks of Arteriography

The most common complication relating to catheter angiography is continued bleeding at the puncture site. Of course, there is also risk of reaction to the contrast media, and there are risk factors related to kidney failure. Minimization of these risks requires a complete patient medical examination and the taking of surgical and allergy histories before any angiographic procedure can be done. Although uncommon, serious adverse reactions related to blood clot formation or catheter or guidewire penetrating injury can occur.

INTERVENTIONAL RADIOLOGY SUITE

Unlike radiography and fluorography, interventional radiology requires a suite of rooms (Figure 25-3). The procedure room itself should not be less than 20 ft along any wall and not less than 500 ft². Such a size is required to accommodate the extent of equipment required and the large number of people involved in most procedures.

The procedure room normally has at least three means of access. Patient access should be through a door wide enough to accommodate a bed. Access to the central room does not normally require a door. An open passageway is adequate. Doors interfere with personnel movement.

The procedure room should be finished with consideration for maintaining a clean and sterile environment. The floor, walls, and all counter cabinet surfaces must be smooth and easily cleaned.

The control room should be large, perhaps 100 ft². Ideally, this room should communicate directly with the viewing areas.

Personnel

A radiographer can specialize in many different fields. The radiographer who specializes in interventional radiography requires additional skills. The American Registry of Radiologic Technologists offers an examination in cardiovascular and interventional radiography. Once the examination is passed, the radiographer may add (CV) after the RT (R).

There may be two or three radiographers in the interventional radiography suite as well as the interventional radiologist and a radiology nurse, who carefully monitors the patient. During procedures that require the patient to be highly medicated, an anesthesiologist may also be present.

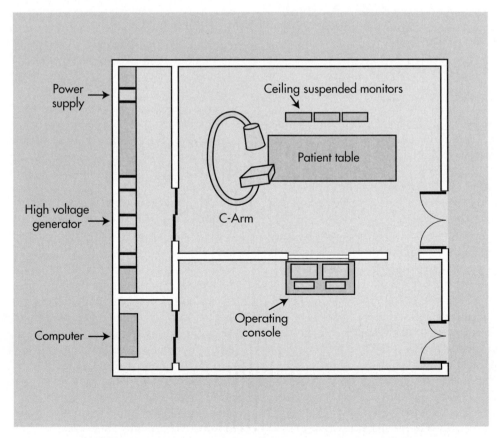

FIGURE 25-3 Typical layout for an interventional radiology suite.

Equipment

The x-ray apparatus for an interventional radiologic suite is generally more massive, flexible, and expensive than that required for conventional radiographic and fluoroscopic imaging. Advanced radiographic and fluoroscopic equipment is required (Figure 25-4). Generally, two ceiling track-mounted radiographic x-ray tubes are required, with an image intensified fluoroscope mounted on a C or an L arm.

X-Ray Tube. The x-ray tube used for interventional radiologic procedures has a small target angle, a large-diameter massive anode disk, and cathodes designed for magnification and serial radiography. Table 25-2 describes the specifications for such an x-ray tube.

A small focal spot of not greater than 0.3 mm is necessary for the spatial-resolution requirements of small-vessel magnification radiography. Neuroangiography can be performed in contrast-filled vessels as small as

1 mm with typical selection of geometric factors and careful patient positioning.

When using a source-to-image receptor distance (SID) of 100 cm and an object-to-image receptor distance (OID) of 40 cm, the radiographer can take advantage of the air gap to improve image contrast. A 0.3 mm focal spot results in a focal-spot blur of 0.2 mm.

Question: A left cerebral angiogram is performed with a 0.3 mm focal spot at 100 cm SID. The artery to be imaged is 20 cm from the image receptor. What is the magnification factor and focal-spot blur?

Answer: $MF = \dfrac{100 \text{ cm SID}}{80 \text{ cm SOD}} = 1.25$

$$FSB = 0.3 \left(\frac{20 \text{ OID}}{80 \text{ SOD}} \right) = 0.075 \text{ mm}$$

TABLE 25-2	Specifications for a Typical Interventional X-Ray Tube	
Feature	**Size**	**Why**
Focal spot	1.0 mm/0.1 mm	Large for heat load; small for magnification radiography
Disc size	15 cm diameter, 5 cm thick	To accommodate heat load
Power rating	80 kW	For rapid sequence, serial radiography
Anode heat capacity	1 MHU	To accommodate head load

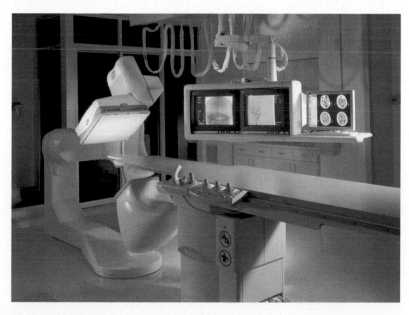

FIGURE 25-4 X-ray imaging apparatus in a typical interventional radiology suite. (Courtesy Philips Medical Systems.)

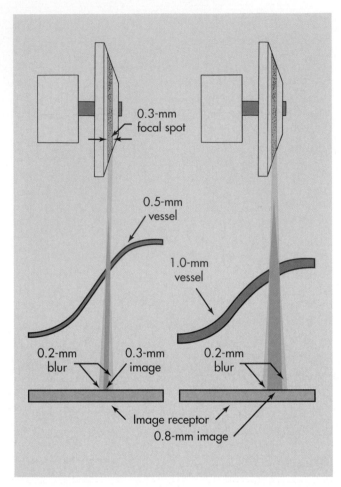

FIGURE 25-5 For a given geometry, such as this one that results in 0.5 mm focal-spot blur, the vessels must be twice the size of the focal-spot blur.

Spatial resolution for this procedure can be approximated by multiplying the focal spot blur by 2. Figure 25-5 shows geometry that results in 0.5 mm focal-spot blur images of a 10 mm vessel. A 0.5 mm vessel will be too blurred to be seen. Any vessel larger than 1.0 mm will be imaged.

All of the other essential characteristics of an interventional x-ray tube are based on required tube loading. The size and construction of the anode disk determines the anode heat capacity, which in turn influences the power rating. An x-ray tube with a minimum 80 kW rating and 1 MHU heat capacity is required.

High-Voltage Generator. High-frequency generators are increasingly popular in all x-ray examinations including interventional radiologic procedures. However, some interventional radiologic procedures require higher power than may be available with high-frequency

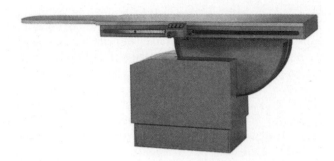

FIGURE 25-6 Typical interventional radiology patient couch with a floating, rotating, and tilting top. (Courtesy of Odelft Corporation.)

generators. High-voltage generators with three-phase, 12-pulse power capable of at least 100 kW with low ripple are needed for such high power requirements.

Patient Couch. Whereas most general fluoroscopy imaging systems have a tilt-table, interventional radiologic imaging systems do not. General fluoroscopy often requires head-down and head-up tilting of the patient for manipulation of contrast media. Imaging techniques such as myelography requires a tilt-couch; therefore, such procedures are common in general fluoroscopy.

Other imaging and interventional procedures do not require a tilt-couch. They use a stationary patient couch with a floating or moveable tabletop (Figure 25-6). Controls for couch positioning are located on the side of the table and duplicated on a floor switch. The floor switch is necessary to accommodate patient positioning while maintaining a sterile field.

The patient couch may also have a computer-controlled **stepping** capability. This feature is necessary to allow imaging from the abdomen to the feet after a single injection of contrast media. An additional requirement of this stepping feature is the ability to preselect the time and position of the patient couch to coincide with the image receptor.

Image Receptor. Three different types of image receptors are used in interventional radiologic procedures. The cinefluorographic camera is used during cardiac catheterization. The serialographic changer was the principal image receptor for many years, but digital fluoroscopy has now made these devices obsolete (see Chapter 28). Photofluorographic cameras (Figure 25-7) have been previously described (see Chapter 24).

Cinefluorographic Camera (Cine). In cinefluorography the television camera tube is replaced with a movie camera that records the image on film for later playback. Cinefluorography is used most often in cer-

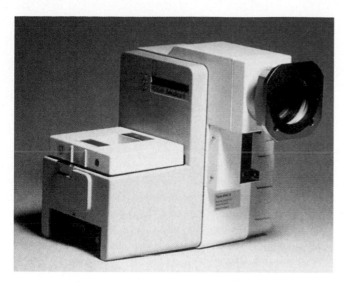

FIGURE 25-7 This 105 mm photofluorographic spot-film camera captures images from the output phosphor of an image intensifier in either single or rapid serial fashion. (Courtesy Odelft Corporation.)

tain angiographic procedures, especially those associated with cardiac catheterization. The patient dose is much higher than that required for recording images electronically but the image quality is better.

Both 16 and 35 mm film movie cameras are used for cinefluorography. The 35 mm film format requires more patient exposure than the 16 mm film format, but the projected image is larger.

Cine cameras are driven by **synchronous motors** controlled by the frequency of the line voltage, which is 60 Hz. Therefore they have frame rates of 7.5, 15, 30, and 60 frames per second. The higher the frame rate, the higher the radiation dose. High frame rates are necessary for cardiac studies, but 7.5 frames per second may be adequate for other examinations.

Cinefluorographic systems are **synchronized.** That is, the x-ray tube is energized only during the time when the cine film is in position for exposure. The x-ray tube is not energized during the time between frames when the film is advancing because this would result in considerably excessive and unnecessary patient exposure.

Charge-Coupled Device (CCD). CCDs are photosensitive silicon chips that are rapidly replacing the television camera tube in the fluoroscopic chain. CCDs look like computer chips and can be used anywhere that light is to be converted to a digital video image. CCDs are covered more completely in Chapter 28.

SUMMARY

Angiography refers to the many ways of imaging contrast-filled vessels. In 1953 Sven Ivan Seldinger described a method of arterial access that uses an 18-gauge hollow needle with a stylet. Using a guidewire and catheter, radiologists can access the vascular network without surgery. The common femoral artery is most often used for arterial access in angiography.

Catheter tip designs vary widely, and each is used for specific arteries. The contrast media used are generally nonionic, which reduces the incidence of physiologic problems and adverse reactions in patients undergoing angiographic procedures. During the procedure, the patient's vital signs must be carefully monitored. The most common risk to patients is continued bleeding at the puncture site.

The typical interventional radiologic x-ray tube is designed for magnification, high resolution, and massive heat loads. The patient couch is a floating tabletop with a stepping capability to automatically allow imaging from abdomen to feet after a single injection of contrast media.

Cine cameras with 16 or 35 mm frames are used in cardiac imaging procedures. Serial changers or digital imaging is generally used for interventional procedures. With both serial changers and digital imaging, power injection of contrast media and imaging are synchronized to optimize visualization of the vessel of interest.

CHALLENGE QUESTIONS

1. Define or otherwise identify:
   a. Contrast media
   b. Arteriography
   c. Contrast media
   d. Seldinger catheter
   e. Catheter
   f. Guidewire
   g. Arterial dissection
   h. Biplane imaging
   i. Tilt-couch
   j. Fenestrated
2. Describe cardiac catheterization.
3. What is the Seldinger method for arterial access?
4. What is the most common artery used for arterial access in angiography?
5. Why is a guidewire used for arterial access of catheters?
6. List four types of catheters and the vessels for which they are designed.
7. Name two reasons why the radiologist visits the patient before an interventional radiologic procedure.
8. What is the most common problem patients encounter after an interventional radiologic procedure?
9. What are thrombolysis and embolization?
10. What is the required heating capacity of the interventional x-ray tube?

11. Name the titles and describe the duties of the team of personnel who work in the interventional radiologic suite.
12. List the focal-spot requirements for the interventional x-ray tube. For what procedure is the small focal spot used?
13. What does it mean when the patient couch has a stepping capability?
14. Name the frame rates for a cine camera.
15. What are the frame rates for the cut-film serial changer?
16. Discuss how subtraction films are obtained during an interventional radiologic procedure.
17. Why are some catheters fenestrated?
18. How does osmolarity affect the action of a contrast agent?
19. What is the recommended minimum size for an interventional radiologic suite?
20. What initials may an ARRT with a specialty in interventional radiology place as a title postscript?

Introduction to Computer Science

OBJECTIVES

At the completion of this chapter, the student should be able to do the following:

1. Discuss the history of computers and the role of the transistor
2. Explain the difference between a microcomputer, a minicomputer, and a mainframe computer
3. List and define the components of computer hardware
4. Define "bit," "byte," and "word" as used in computer terminology
5. Contrast the two classifications of computer programs: systems software and applications programs
6. List and explain various computer languages
7. Discuss four computer processing methods

OUTLINE

History of Computers
Anatomy of a Computer
    Hardware
    Software
Processing Methods
    Batch Processing
    On-Line Systems
    Time-Sharing Systems
    Real-Time Systems

TODAY, THE word *computer* refers to the personal computer (PC), primarily responsible for the explosion in computer applications. In addition to scientific, engineering, and business applications, the computer has become evident in everyday life. For example, we know computers are involved in video games, automatic teller machines (ATMs), and highway toll systems. Other everyday uses include supermarket checkouts, ticket reservation centers, industrial processes, touch-tone telephone systems, traffic lights, and automobile ignition systems.

Computer applications in radiology also continue to grow. The first large-scale radiology application was computed tomography (CT). Magnetic resonance imaging (MRI) and diagnostic ultrasonography use computers much as CT imaging systems do. Computers control x-ray generators and radiographic control panels, making digital fluoroscopy and digital radiography routine. Telecommunication systems have provided for the development of teleradiology—the transfer of images and patient data to remote locations for interpretation and filing. Teleradiology has also changed the way human resources are allocated for these tasks.

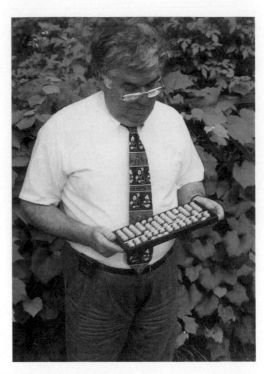

FIGURE 26-1 The abacus is the earliest calculating tool. (Courtesy Robert J. Wilson.)

HISTORY OF COMPUTERS

The earliest calculating tool, the abacus (Figure 26-1), was invented thousands of years ago in China and is still used in some parts of Asia. In the 17th century, two mathematicians, Blaise Pascal and Gottfried Leibniz, built mechanical calculators using pegged wheels that could perform the four basic arithmetic functions of addition, subtraction, multiplication, and division.

In 1842, Charles Babbage designed an analytical engine that performed general calculations automatically. Herman Hollerith designed a tabulating machine to record census data in 1890. The tabulating machine stored information as holes on cards that were interpreted by machines with electrical sensors. Hollerith's company later grew to become IBM.

In 1939, John Atansoff and Clifford Berry designed and built the first electronic digital computer.

The first general-purpose modern computer was developed in 1944 at Harvard University. Originally called the Automatic Sequence Controlled Calculator (ASCC), it is now known simply as the Mark I. It was an electromechanical device and was exceedingly slow and prone to malfunction.

The first general-purpose **electronic computer** was developed in 1946 at the University of Pennsylvania by J. Presper Eckert and John Mauchly at a cost of $500,000. This computer, called **ENIAC** (**E**lectronic **N**umerical **I**ntegrator **A**nd **C**alculator), contained over 18,000 vacuum tubes that failed at an average of 1 every 7 minutes (Figure 26-2). Neither the Mark I nor the ENIAC had their instructions stored in a memory device.

In 1948, scientists led by William Shockley at the Bell Telephone Laboratories developed the transistor. A transistor is an electronic switch that alternately allows or does not allow electronic signals to pass. It made possible the development of the "stored-program" computer and thus the continuing explosion in computer science.

The transistor allowed Eckert and Mauchly, of the Sperry-Rand Corporation, to develop **UNIVAC** (**UNIV**ersal **A**utomatic **C**omputer), which appeared in 1951 as the first commercially successful general-purpose, stored-program electronic digital computer.

Computers have undergone four generations of development distinguished by the technology of their electronic devices. First-generation computers were vacuum tube devices (1939–1958). Second-generation computers, which became generally available in about 1958, were based on individually packaged transistors.

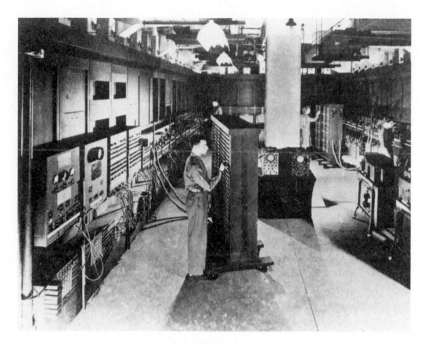

FIGURE 26-2 The ENIAC computer occupied an entire room. It was completed in 1946 and is recognized as the first all-electronic, general-purpose digital computer. (Courtesy Sperry-Rand Corporation.)

Third-generation computers used integrated circuits (IC). Integrated circuits consist of many transistors and other electronic elements fused onto a chip, a tiny piece of semiconductor material, usually silicon. They were introduced in 1964. The microprocessor was developed in 1971 by Ted Hoff of Intel Corporation.

The fourth generation of computers, which first appeared in 1975, was an extension of the third generation and incorporated large scale integration (LSI), now replaced by very–large-scale integration (VLSI), which places millions of circuit elements on a chip less than 1 cm in size (Figure 26-3).

 The word *computer* refers to any general-purpose, stored-program electronic digital computer.

The word computer today identifies the PC to most of us (Figure 26-4). This device is made of both electronic and electromechanical components. General-purpose identifies a computer as able to solve a variety of problems. This is unlike special-purpose computers, which are designed for a particular singular task, such as control of an assembly-line robot or an automobile ignition switch.

All modern computers are stored-program because they have their instructions (programs) and data stored in their memory. These stored-program computers are laid out so that the sequence of steps to be followed dur-

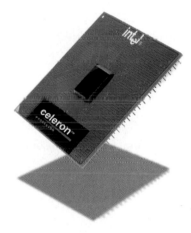

FIGURE 26-3 This Celeron microprocessor incorporates over 1 million transistors on a chip of silicon less than 1 cm on a side. (Courtesy Intel.)

ing any calculation is preestablished. Electronic implies that the computer is powered by electrical (transmits power) and electronic (transmits information) devices, rather than by a mechanical device.

Today, digital computers have replaced analog computers and the word *digital* is almost synonymous with *computer.* A timeline showing the evolution of computers shows how rapidly this technology is advancing (Figure 26-5).

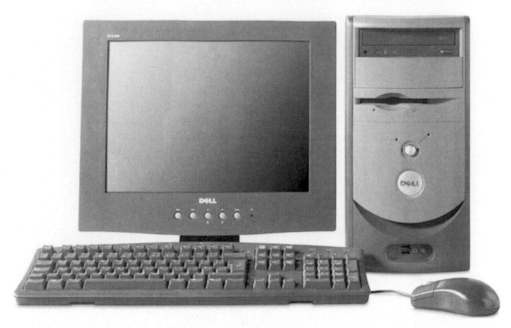

FIGURE 26-4 Today's personal computer has exceptional speed capacity flexibility. There are numerous applications in radiology. (Courtesy Dell Computer Corporation.)

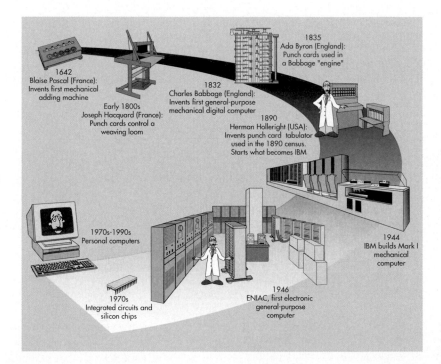

FIGURE 26-5 A timeline showing the evolution of today's computer.

 Analog refers to a continuously varying quantity; a *digital* system uses only two values that vary discretely through coding.

The difference between analog and digital is illustrated in Figure 26-6, which shows two kinds of watches. An analog watch is mechanical and has hands that move continuously around a dial face. A digital watch contains a computer chip and indicates time with numbers.

Analog and digital meters are used in many commercial and scientific applications. Digital meters are easier to read and can be more precise.

Computers are distinguished from calculators by their functionality. Most calculators can handle only

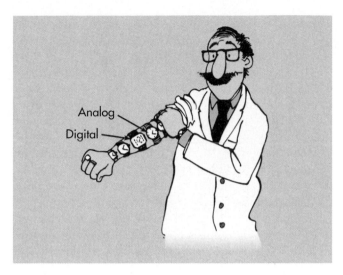

FIGURE 26-6 Two styles of wristwatches demonstrate analog versus digital.

arithmetic functions, whereas computers can handle arithmetic and **logic functions:** "do," "if," "then," and "else." However, new technology has brought us advanced calculators with graphing and limited programming abilities. Now, calculators can execute logic functions, solve equations, draw lines, and transmit data to or from other calculators or computers by cords or infrared beams.

 Logic functions evaluate an intermediate result and perform subsequent computations depending on that result.

Computers are also often classified according to size, processing speed, and storage capacity. Distinguishing these types has become more difficult as technology improves, but they are defined as the following categories: supercomputers, mainframe computers, workstations, microcomputers, and microcontrollers.

Supercomputers are the fastest and highest-capacity computers, containing hundreds to thousands of microprocessors. They are often used for research in fields such as weather forecasting, oil exploration, and mathematics.

Mainframe computers are fast, mid- to large-size, large-capacity systems that also have multiple microprocessors. They can support a few hundred to thousands of users and are found in airlines, banks, universities, and government.

Workstations were introduced in the early 1980s and are powerful desktop systems, often used by scientists and engineers. They are often connected to larger computer systems to transfer and share data and information.

Microcomputers, best known as PCs, also include electronic organizers and personal data assistants (PDAs), such as palmtop and hand-held systems.

Microcontrollers are tiny computers installed in "smart" appliances like microwave ovens and calculators.

A radiographic operating console is controlled by a microcomputer that can analyze and control many characteristics of an examination. For example, when body part, size of patient, and image receptor are selected, the microcomputer logically selects the proper radiographic technique.

ANATOMY OF A COMPUTER

There are two principal parts to a computer, hardware and software, each of which has several components. The **hardware** is everything about the computer that is visible—the nuts, bolts, and chips of the system that form the central processing unit (CPU) and the various input/output devices. Hardware is usually categorized according to which operation it performs. These operations are input processing, memory, storage, output, and communications.

The **software** is invisible. It consists of the computer programs that tell the hardware what to do and how to store and manipulate data.

Hardware

Input. Input hardware includes keyboards, pointing devices, and source–data entry devices. A keyboard includes the standard typewriter keys, used to enter words and numbers and specialized keys or function keys that enter specific commands. Digital fluoroscopy (Chapter 28) uses function keys for masking, reregistration, and time-interval-difference imaging.

 Input hardware converts data into a form that the computer can use.

A **mouse** is a pointing device that the user rolls on a desktop or mouse pad to direct a pointer on the computer's display screen. High-end systems often use an optical mouse, which does not roll. The pointer is a symbol, often an arrow, that selects items from lists and menus or positions the cursor on the screen. The **cursor** indicates the insertion point on the screen where data may be entered.

A **trackball** is a variant of the mouse, usually found in laptop computers. A **joystick** is a pointing device used primarily in video games and computer-aided design systems. Special joysticks are also available for people with certain disabilities.

Touchpads are small, rectangular devices that allow the user to control the cursor with a finger. A light pen connects by a wire to a computer display and, when pressed to the screen, identifies that screen position to the computer.

Pen-based systems use a penlike instrument to input handwriting and marks into a computer. Pen-based systems are being used in hospitals to enter comments into patient records.

Source–data entry devices include scanners, fax machines, imaging systems, audio and video devices, electronic cameras, voice-recognition systems, sensors, and biologic input devices. **Scanners** translate images of text, drawings, or photographs into a digital format recognizable by the computer. **Bar-code readers,** which translate the vertical, black-and-white striped codes on retail products into digital form, are a type of scanner.

An **audio input device** translates analog sound into digital format. Similarly, video images, such as those from a VCR or camcorder, are digitized by a special video card that can be installed in a computer. The newest cameras and video recorders capture images in digital format that can easily be transferred to computer for immediate access.

Voice-recognition systems add a microphone and audio sound card to a computer and can convert speech into digital format. Radiologists are beginning to use these systems to produce rapid diagnostic reports and send findings to remote locations by teleradiology.

Sensors collect data directly from the environment and transmit it to a computer. Sensors are used to detect things like wind speed or temperature.

Human biology input devices detect specific movements and characteristics of the human body. Security systems that identify a person through a fingerprint or retinal vascular pattern are examples of these devices.

Processing

In large computers, such as mainframes, the processing hardware is the central processing unit or CPU. In microcomputers, it is often referred to as the *microprocessor*. Figure 26-7 is a photomicrograph of the Pentium microprocessor manufactured by the Intel Corporation. The Pentium processor is designed for large, high-performance, multiuser or multitasking systems.

 The electronic circuitry that does the actual computations and the memory that supports this are together called the *processing hardware* or *processor.*

A computer's processor (CPU) consists of a **control unit** and an **arithmetic/logic unit** (**ALU**). These two components and all other components are connected by an electrical conductor called a **bus** (Figure 26-8). The control unit tells the computer how to carry out software instructions, which direct the hardware to perform a task. The control unit directs data to the arithmetic/

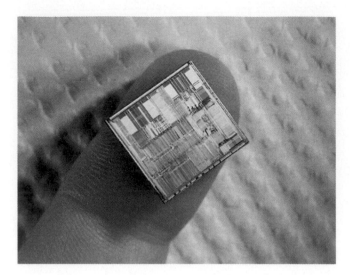

FIGURE 26-7 The width of the conductive lines in this microprocessor chip is 1.5 μm. (Courtesy Intel.)

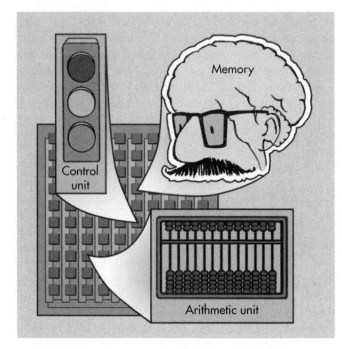

FIGURE 26-8 The central processing unit (CPU) contains a control unit, an arithmetic unit, and sometimes memory.

logic unit or to memory. It also controls data transfer between main memory and the input and output hardware (Figure 26-9).

The speed of these tasks is determined by an internal system clock. The faster the clock, the faster the processing. Microcomputer processing speeds are usually defined in megahertz (MHz), where 1 MHz equal 1 million cycles per second. Today's microcomputers commonly run at up to several gigahertz (GHz; 1 GHz = 1000 MHz).

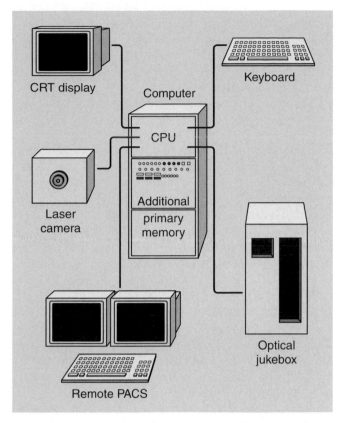

FIGURE 26-9 The control unit is a part of the central processing unit and is directly connected with additional primary memory and various input/output devices.

Workstations, microcomputers, and mainframes measure processing speed as MIPS (millions of instructions per second). Speeds can range from 100 MIPS in a workstation to 1200 MIPS (1.2 BIPS) in a mainframe. Supercomputer processing is measured in flops (floating-point operations per second) and is represented as megaflops (mflops), gigaflops, and teraflops, which correspond to millions, billions, and trillions of flops, respectively.

The ALU performs arithmetic or logic calculations, temporarily holds the results until they can be transferred to memory, and controls the speed of these operations. The speed of the ALU is also controlled by the system clock.

Memory. Computer memory is distinguished from storage by its function. Memory is more active, whereas storage is more archival. This active storage is also referred to as memory, primary storage, internal memory, or random access memory (RAM). *Random access* means data can be stored or accessed at random from anywhere in main memory in approximately equal amounts of time, regardless of where the data is located.

RAM contents are temporary and RAM capacities vary widely in different computer systems. RAM capac-

ity is usually expressed as megabytes (MB), gigabytes (GB), or terabytes (TB), referring to millions, billions, or trillions of characters stored.

 Main memory is the working storage of a computer.

RAM chips are manufactured using CMOS (complementary metal-oxide semiconductor) technology. These chips are arranged as single-line memory modules (SIMMS).

There are two types of RAM, dynamic RAM (DRAM) and static RAM (SRAM). DRAM chips are more widely used, although SRAM chips are faster. SRAM retains its memory even if power to the computer is lost, but it is more expensive than DRAM and requires more space and power.

Special high-speed circuitry areas called registers are also found in the control unit and ALU. Registers are contained in the processor and hold information that will be used immediately. Main memory is located outside of the processor and holds material that will be used "a little bit later."

Read-only memory (ROM) contains information supplied by the manufacturer, called "firmware," and cannot be written on or erased. One of the ROM chips contains instructions that tell the processor what to do when the system is first turned on and the "bootstrap program" is initiated. Another ROM chip helps the processor transfer information between the screen, printer, and other peripheral devices to make sure all units are working correctly. These instructions are called ROM BIOS (basic input/output system). ROM is also one of the factors in making a "clone" PC; for instance, to be a true IBM clone, a computer must have the same ROM BIOS as an IBM computer.

There are three variations of ROM chips that are used in special situations; PROM, EPROM, and EEP-ROM. PROM (programmable **read-only memory**) chips are blank chips that a user, with special equipment, can write programs to. Once the program is written, it cannot be erased.

EPROM (erasable programmable **read-only memory**) chips are like PROM chips except that the contents are erasable using a special device that exposes the chip to ultraviolet light. EEPROM (**electronically erasable programmable read-only memory**) can be reprogrammed using special electron impulses.

The motherboard or system board is the main circuit board in a system unit. This board contains the microprocessor, any coprocessor chips, RAM chips, ROM chips, other types of memory, and expansion slots, which allow additional circuit boards to be added.

All main memory is addressed; that is, each memory location is designated by a unique label in which a character of data or part of an instruction is stored during processing. Each address is similar to a post office address that allows the computer to access data at specific places in memory without disturbing the rest of memory.

A sequence of memory locations may contain steps of a computer program or a string of data. The control unit keeps track of where the current program instructions are stored, which allows the computer to read or write data to other memory locations, then return to the current address for the next instruction.

All data processed by a computer pass through main memory. The most efficient computers, therefore, have enough main memory to store all data and programs needed for processing.

Usually secondary memory is required, though, in the form of diskettes and hard disk drives. Secondary memory functions like a filing cabinet—you store data there until you need to retrieve it.

Once the appropriate file has been retrieved, it is copied into primary memory, where the user works on it. An old version of the file remains in secondary memory while the copy of the file is being edited/updated. When the user is finished with the file, it is taken out of primary memory and returned to secondary memory (the filing cabinet), where the updated file replaces the old file.

The word file is used to refer to a collection of data or information that is treated as a unit by the computer. Each computer file has a unique name, and PC-based file names have extension names added after a period. For example, .DOC is added by a word processing program to files containing word processing documents (i.e., REPORT.DOC).

Common file types are program files, which contain software instructions; data files, which contain data, not programs; image files, which contain digital images; audio files, containing digitized sound; and video files, which contain digitized video images.

Storage. To understand storage hardware, it is necessary to understand the terms used to measure the capacity of storage devices. A **bit** describes the smallest unit of measure, a binary digit 0 or 1. Bits are combined into groups of 8 bits, called a **byte.**

A byte represents one character, digit, or other value. A kilobyte represents 1024 bytes. A megabyte (MB) is approximately 1 million bytes and often reflects capacities of microcomputers. A gigabyte (GB) is approximately 1 billion bytes and is used to measure the capacity of microcomputer hard disk drives and the main memory of mainframes and some supercomputers. A **terabyte** (TB) is approximately 1 thousand billion bytes and is used to describe the memory capacity of some supercomputers.

 Storage is an archival form of memory.

The most common types of secondary storage devices are tape, diskette, hard disk, and optical disk. Magnetic tape used to be a common storage medium for large computer systems but is now used primarily on large systems for backup and archiving historical records, such as patient images.

Magnetic tape has a polyester base and is coated on one side with iron oxide. When the coated side is magnetized, it becomes the recording medium. The tape is fed across the read-write heads of a reel-to-reel tape system.

The write head produces a small magnetic field when an electric current is passed through it. The magnetic field reverses when the direction of the current is reversed. The two binary digits, 0 and 1, are then easily represented by these changes in the current. When the magnetic field produced by the head interacts with the magnetic coating of the tape, it magnetizes a small spot on the coating.

When a tape is to be read, a series of tiny magnetic fields move rapidly past the read head. As each field contacts the read head, it produces an electric current. The direction of the current depends on the direction of the magnetic field, causing the recorded information to be retrieved. This entire process is based on electromagnetic induction (Chapter 7).

A diskette or floppy disk stores data and programs as magnetized spots on a round, flat piece of mylar plastic. The diskette is removable from the computer and is housed in a square plastic case to protect it from damage. "Floppy" refers to the fact that the disk in the plastic case is flexible, not rigid.

The most common size of a diskette is 3½ inches in diameter. Data are recorded on a diskette in rings called tracks, which are invisible, closed concentric rings. The number of tracks on a diskette is called TPI, or tracks per inch. The higher the TPI, the more data a diskette can hold.

Each track is divided into sectors, which are invisible sections used by the computer for storage reference. The number of sectors on a diskette varies according to the recording density, which refers to the number of bits per inch that can be written to the diskette.

Diskettes are also defined as either high-density (HD) or extended density (ED). A high-density 3½ inch diskette can store 1.44 MB, and ED diskettes can store 2.8 MB. A **disk drive** is the device that holds, spins, reads data from, and writes data to a diskette.

In contrast to diskettes, hard disks are thin, rigid glass or metal platters. Each side of the platter is coated with a recording material that can be magnetized. Hard disks are tightly sealed in a hard disk drive and data can be recorded on both sides of the disk platters. In microcomputers, hard disk drives are usually built into the system and are not removable.

Compared with diskettes, hard disks can have thousands of tracks per inch and up to 64 sectors. Storage systems that use several hard disks use the cylinder method to locate data (Figure 26-10). Hard disks have greater capacity and speed than diskettes.

Microcomputer hard disk drives can typically hold up to 10 GB. Hard disks allow quicker data access because a hard disk spins several times faster than a diskette. These advantages explain why hard disks are often used in radiologic imaging procedures.

The hard disk technology for large computer systems is allowing users to access large databases of information through organizations such as CompuServe and America Online. Secondary storage devices for large computers consist of removable packs of fixed disk drives.

A removable hard disk system is composed of 6 to 20 hard disks aligned one above the other in a sealed hard disk unit. The capacity of these units extends into the terabytes.

Fixed disk drives are high-speed, high-capacity disk drives that are sealed in their own cabinets. A mainframe computer might have up to 100 of these drives attached to it.

A RAID (redundant array of inexpensive disks) system consists of two or more disk drives in a single cabinet that collectively act as a single storage system. RAID systems have greater reliability because if one disk drive fails, others can take over.

Optical disks, also called laser disks, are removable disks that data are written to and read from using laser technology. A small laser is used to make "pits" in the disk and later to read them.

The most familiar form of optical disk is the compact disk (CD) used in the music industry. A single CD-ROM (compact disk—read-only memory) can typically hold 6250 MB of data. CD-ROM drives used to handle only one disk at a time, but now there are multidisk drives called "jukeboxes" that can handle up to 100 disks. In an all-digital radiology department, the optical disk jukebox would replace the film file room.

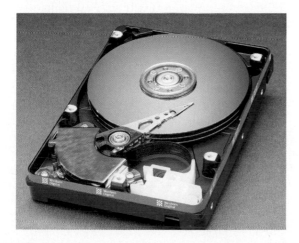

FIGURE 26-10 This disk drive reads all formats of optical compact disks and reads, erases, writes, and rewrites to a 650-MB optical cartridge. (Courtesy Western Digital.)

CD-R (compact disk—recordable) is a CD format that allows users with CD-R drives to write data, only once, onto a specialized disk that can then be read by a standard CD-ROM drive. An example of this technology is the Photo CD system, developed by Eastman Kodak, which allows photographs taken with a 35-millimeter camera to be stored digitally on an optical disk.

Erasable optical disks called CDE or CD-RW allow users to erase data and use the disk over and over again. These drives are much more durable than magnetic hard drives and they are widely used.

Another technology, the DVD-ROM (digital versatile disk—read-only memory), is an optically readable digital disk that can store up to 20 GB of data. DVD provides better audio and video quality and, in computers, can provide record and rewrite capabilities.

Output. Common output devices are display screens and printers. Other devices include plotters, multifunction devices, and audio output devices.

The output device that people use the most is the display screen or monitor. The cathode ray tube (CRT) is a vacuum tube used as a display screen in a computer or video display terminal (VDT). Softcopy is the term that refers to the output seen on a display screen.

Flat-panel displays (liquid crystal displays [LCD]) are thinner, lighter, and consume less power than CRTs. These displays are made of two plates of glass with a substance in between them that can be activated in different ways.

 Output hardware consists of devices that translate computer information into a form that humans can understand.

A terminal is an input/output device that uses a keyboard for input and a display screen for output. Terminals are either dumb or intelligent.

A dumb terminal cannot do any processing on its own; it is used only to input data or receive data from a main or host computer. Airline clerks at ticketing and check-in counters are usually connected to the main computer system through dumb terminals.

An intelligent terminal has built-in processing capability and RAM but does not have its own storage capacity. Most radiologic applications use intelligent terminals.

A printer prints characters, symbols, or graphics on paper. This printed output is often called hardcopy. Printers are categorized by the manner in which the print mechanism physically contacts the paper to print an image. Impact printers have direct contact with the paper; nonimpact printers do not.

An impact printer forms characters or images by striking a print hammer or print wheel against an inked ribbon. Impact printers are used less and less frequently, but some systems continue to use dot-matrix printers.

Dot-matrix printers can print draft quality or near-letter quality, at speeds up 300 characters per second. Another type of impact printer is a high-speed line printer, used with large computer systems. Line printers can print an entire line of characters at once, rather than one character at a time, at speeds of up to 3000 lines per minute.

Nonimpact printers are the most frequently used printers today. The two types of nonimpact printers used with microcomputers are laser printers and ink-jet printers.

A laser printer operates similarly to a photocopying machine. Images are created with dots on a drum, treated with a magnetically charged inklike substance called toner, and then transferred from drum to paper.

Laser printers produce crisp images of text and graphics, with resolution ranging from 300 dots per inch (dpi) to 1200 dpi and in color. They can print up to 32 text-only pages per minute for a microcomputer and more than 120 pages per minute for a mainframe. Laser printers have built-in RAM chips to store output from the computer, ROM chips that store fonts, and their own small, dedicated processor.

Ink-jet printers also form images with little dots. These printers electrically charge small drops of ink that are then sprayed onto the page. Ink-jet printers are quieter and less expensive and can also print in color. Up to 20 pages per minute (ppm) for black text and 10 ppm for color images are available with even modestly priced ink-jet printers.

Other specialized output devices serve specific functions. For example, plotters are used to create documents like architectural drawings and maps. Multifunction devices deliver several capabilities like printing, imaging, copying, and faxing in one unit. Specialized audio output devices provide the ability to output speechlike sounds, distinctive sounds, such as beeps, and music.

Communications. Communications or telecommunications describes the transfer of data from a sender to a receiver across a distance. The practice of teleradiology involves the transfer of medical images as well as patient data.

Electric current, radiofrequency (RF), or light is used to transfer the data through a physical medium, which may be a cable, wire, or even the atmosphere. Many communications lines are still analog, and therefore a computer needs a modem (modulate/demodulate) to convert digital information into analog. The receiving computer's modem converts the analog information back into digital.

Teleradiology is the transfer of images and patient reports to remote sites.

Transmission speed is the speed at which a modem transmits data and is measured in bits per second (bps) or kilobits per second (kbps). In addition to modems, computers need communications software. Often this software is packaged with the modem, or it might be included as part of the system software.

Technology advances have allowed for the development of faster and faster communication devices. Cable modems connect computers to cable-TV systems that offer telecommunication services. Some cable providers are offering transmission speeds up to 1000 times faster than a basic telephone line.

Integrated services digital network (ISDN) transmits over regular phone lines up to five times faster than basic modems. Digital subscriber lines (DSL) transmit at speeds in the middle range of the previous two technologies. DSL also uses regular phone lines.

Telecommunications in the form of teleradiology is changing the way we allocate human resources to improve the speed of interpretation, reporting, and archiving of images and other patient data.

Software

All that has been described thus far regarding the computer has been hardware. Hardware refers to the fixed, visible components of the system. The CPU, all input/output devices, and other auxiliary or peripheral devices are hardware. But these are only half of the computer. The other half is software.

Software refers to the instructions written in a computer language that guide the computer through its designated operations.

Although the computer can accept and report alphabetic characters and numeric information in the decimal system, it operates in the binary system. In the decimal system, the system we normally use, 10 digits (0 to 9) are used. The word *digit* comes from the Latin for finger or toe. The origin of the decimal system is obvious (Figure 26-11).

Other number systems have been formulated to many other base values. The duodecimal system, for instance, has 12 digits. It is used to describe the months of the year and the hours in a day and night. Computers operate on the simplest number system of all, the binary number system. It has only two digits, 0 and 1.

Binary Number System. Counting in the binary number system starts with 0 to 1 and then counts over again (Table 26-1). There are only two digits, 0 and 1, and the computer performs all operations by converting alphabetic characters, decimal values, and logic functions to binary values.

Even the computer's instructions are stored in binary form. That way, although the binary numbers may be-

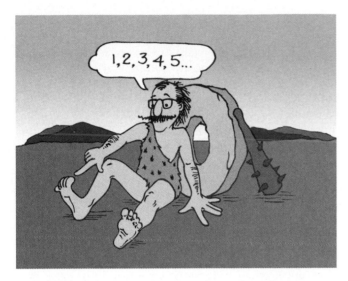

FIGURE 26-11 The origin of the decimal number system.

TABLE 26-1	Organization of Binary Number System	
Decimal Number	Binary Equivalent	Binary Number
0	0	0
1	2^0	1
2	$2^1 + 0$	10
3	$2^1 + 2^0$	11
4	$2^2 + 0 + 0$	100
5	$2^2 + 0 + 2^0$	101
6	$2^2 + 2^1 + 0$	110
7	$2^2 + 2^1 + 2^0$	111
8	$2^3 + 0 + 0 + 0$	1000
9	$2^3 + 0 + 0 + 2^0$	1001
10	$2^3 + 0 + 2^1 + 0$	1010
11	$2^3 + 0 + 2^1 + 2^0$	1011
12	$2^3 + 2^2 + 0 + 0$	1100
13	$2^3 + 2^2 + 0 + 2^0$	1101
14	$2^3 + 2^2 + 2^1 + 0$	1110
15	$2^3 + 2^2 + 2^1 + 2^0$	1111
16	$2^4 + 0 + 0 + 0 + 0$	10000

no 2^1 plus no 2^0 or 100 in binary form. Each time it is necessary to raise two to an additional power to express a number, the number of binary digits increases by one.

Just as we know the meaning of the powers of 10, it is necessary to recognize the powers of 2. Power of two notation is used in radiologic imaging to describe image size, image dynamic range (shades of gray), and image storage capacity.

Table 26-2 is a review of these power notations. Note the following similarity. In both power notations, the number of zeros to the right of 1 equal the value of the exponent.

Question: Express the number 193 in binary form.
Answer: 193 falls between 2^7 and 2^8. Therefore, it will be expressed as 1 followed by seven binary digits. Simply add the decimal equivalent of each binary digit from left to right:

Yes 2^7 = 1 = 128
Yes 2^6 = 1 = 64
No 2^5 = 0 = No 32
No 2^4 = 0 = No 16
No 2^3 = 0 = No 8
No 2^2 = 0 = No 4
No 2^1 = 0 = No 2
Yes 2^0 = 1 = 1
11000001 = 193

Question: What is the decimal value of the binary number 100110011?
Answer: Follow the previous process by first listing the binary number and then computing each power of 2.

1 = 2^8 Yes = 256
0 = 2^7 No = 0
0 = 2^6 No = 0
1 = 2^5 No = 32
1 = 2^4 Yes = 16
0 = 2^3 No = 0
0 = 2^2 No = 0
1 = 2^1 Yes = 2
1 = 2^0 Yes = 1
= 307

Digital images are made of discrete picture elements, **pixels,** arranged in a matrix (Chapter 27). The size of the image is described in the binary number system by power of two equivalents. Most images are either 256 × 256 (2^8) or 1024 × 1024 (2^{10}). The 1024 × 1024 matrix is used in digital fluoroscopy and digital radiography. Matrix sizes of 2048 × 2048 (2^{11}) and 4096 × 4096 (2^{12}) are being developed for digital radiography.

Bits, Bytes, and Words. In computer language, a single binary digit, 0 or 1, is called a **bit.** Depending on the microprocessor, a string of 8, 16, or 32 bits is manipulated simultaneously.

come exceedingly long, computation can be handled by properly adjusting the thousands of flip-flop circuits in the computer.

In the binary number system, 0 is 0 and 1 is 1, but there the direct relationship with the decimal number system ends. It ends at 1 because the 1 in binary notation comes from 2^0. Recall that any number raised to the zero power is 1, therefore 2^0 is 1.

In binary notation, the decimal number 2 is equal to 2^1 plus 0. This is expressed as 10. The decimal number 3 is equal to 2^1 plus 2^0 or 11 in binary form; 4 is 2^2 plus

The computer uses as many bits as necessary to express a decimal digit, depending on how it is programmed. The 26 characters of the alphabet and other special characters are usually encoded by 8 bits.

 To encode is to translate from ordinary characters to computer-compatible characters—binary digits.

Bits are often grouped into bunches of eight called **bytes.** Computer capacity is expressed by the number of bytes that can be accommodated. The most popular personal computers use 16- and 32-bit microprocessors with 20 gigabytes (GB) of memory.

One kilobyte (kB) is equal to 1024 bytes. Note that *kilo* is not metric in computer use. Instead, it represents 2^{10} or 1024. The minicomputers used in radiology have capacities measured in megabytes, where 1 MB = 1 kB $\times$ 1 kB = $2^{10} \times 2^{10} = 2^{20} = 1,048,576$ bytes.

Question: How many bits can be stored on a 64-kB chip?

Answer: $\dfrac{1024}{\text{kbytes}} \times 64 \text{ kbytes} \times \dfrac{8 \text{ bits}}{\text{bytes}} =$

$2^{10} \times 2^{6} \times$

$2^{3} = 2^{19} = 424,288 \text{ bits}$

Depending on the computer configuration, two bytes usually constitute a **word.** In the case of a 16-bit microprocessor, a word would be 16 consecutive bits of information that are interpreted and shuffled about the computer as a unit. Sometimes half a byte is called a "nibble" and two words is a "chomp!" Each word of data in memory has its own address.

Computer Programs. The sequence of instructions developed by a software programmer is called a *computer program*. It is useful to distinguish two classifications of computer programs: systems software and application programs.

Systems software consists of programs that make it easy for the user to operate a computer to its best advantage. Computer buffs describe efficient software as "user friendly."

Application programs are those written in a higher-level language expressly to carry out some user function. Most computer programs as we know them are application programs.

 Computer programs are the software of the computer.

A computer language described as higher level is one that approaches human language and thought processes. The lowest-level computer language is machine language—that is, the only language the computer understands, binary numbers.

Systems Software. The computer program most closely related to the system hardware is the operating system. The operating system is that series of instructions that organizes the course of data through the computer to the solution of a particular problem. It makes the computer's resources available to application programs.

Commands such as "run file" to begin a sequence or "save file" to store some information in secondary memory are typical of operating system commands. MAC-OS, Windows, and Unix are popular operating systems.

This type of program is usually developed by the computer manufacturer and may be stored in ROM in the CPU. Because the CPU recognizes instructions only in binary or machine language form, formulating the operating system is perhaps the most tedious of all computer programming tasks.

Computers ultimately understand only zeros and ones. To relieve humans from the task of writing programs in this form, other programs called *assemblers*, *compilers*, and *interpreters* have been written. These types of software provide a computer language to communicate between the language of the operating system and everyday language.

An assembler is a computer program that recognizes symbolic instructions such as "subtract (SUB)," "load (LD)," and "print (PT)" and translates them into the corresponding binary code. Assembly is the translation of a program written in symbolic, machine-oriented instructions into machine language instructions.

Compilers and interpreters are computer programs that translate an application program from its high-level language, such as BASIC, C++, or Pascal, into a form suitable for the assembler or into a form accepted directly by the CPU. Interpreters make program develop-

TABLE 26-2	Power of Ten, Power of Two, and Binary Notation	
Power of Ten	**Power of Two**	**Binary Notation**
$10^0 = 1$	$2^0 = 1$	1
$10^1 = 10$	$2^1 = 2$	10
$10^2 = 100$	$2^2 = 4$	100
$10^3 = 1000$	$2^3 = 8$	1000
$10^4 = 10,000$	$2^4 = 16$	10000
$10^5 = 100,000$	$2^5 = 32$	100000
$10^6 = 1,000,000$	$2^6 = 64$	1000000
	$2^7 = 128$	10000000
	$2^8 = 256$	100000000
	$2^9 = 512$	1000000000
	$2^{10} = 1024$	10000000000

ment easier because they are interactive. Compiled programs run faster because they create a separate machine language program.

Application Programs. Computer programs that are written by the computer manufacturer, a software manufacturer, or the users themselves to permit the computer to perform a specific task are called application programs. Examples are Lotus, Quicken, and Excel.

Application programs allow the user to print a mailing list, complete an income tax form, evaluate a financial statement, or reconstruct an image from an x-ray transmission pattern. They are written in one of many high-level computer languages and are then translated through an interpreter or compiler into a corresponding machine language program that is subsequently executed by the computer.

The diagram in Figure 26-12 illustrates the flow of the software instructions from turning the computer on to completing a computation. When the computer is first turned on, nothing is in its memory except a program called a bootstrap. This is frozen permanently in ROM. When the computer is started, it automatically runs the bootstrap program, which is capable of transferring the other necessary programs off the disk and into the computer memory.

The bootstrap program loads the operating system into primary memory, which in turn controls all subsequent operations. A machine language application program can likewise be copied from the disk into primary memory where the prescribed operations occur. After completion of the program, the results are transferred from primary memory to an output device under the control of the operating system.

Hexadecimal Number System. The hexadecimal number system is used by assembly-level applications. As you have seen, assembly language acts as a midpoint between the computer's binary system and the user's human language instructions. The set of hexadecimal numbers is 0, 1, 2, 3, 4, 5, 6, 7, 8, 9, A, B, C, D, E, F. Each of these symbols is used to represent a binary number or, more specifically, a set of four bits. Therefore, because it takes eight bits to make a byte, a byte can be represented by two hexadecimal numbers. The set of hexadecimal numbers corresponds to the binary numbers for 0 to 15, as shown in Table 26-3.

Computer Languages. High-level programming languages allow the programmer to write instructions in a form approaching human language, using words, symbols, and decimal numbers rather than the ones and zeros of machine language. A brief list of the more popular programming languages is given in Table 26-4. Using one of these high-level languages, a set of instructions can be written that will be understood by the system software and be executed by the computer through its operating system.

FORTRAN. The oldest language for scientific, engineering, and mathematical problems is FORTRAN (FORmula TRANslation). It was the prototype for today's algebraic languages, which are oriented toward

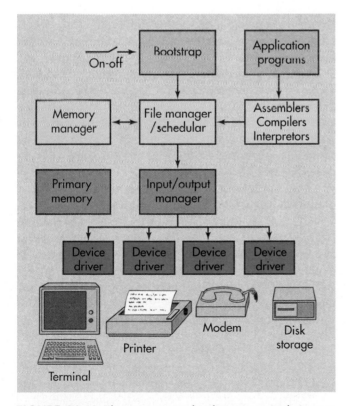

FIGURE 26-12 The sequence of software manipulations to complete an operation.

TABLE 26-3	The Hexadecimal Number System	
Decimal	**Binary**	**Hexadecimal**
0	0000	0
1	0001	1
2	0010	2
3	0011	3
4	0100	4
5	0101	5
6	0110	6
7	0111	7
8	1000	8
9	1001	9
10	1010	A
11	1011	B
12	1100	C
13	1101	D
14	1110	E
15	1111	F

TABLE 26-4	Programming Languages	
Language	**Date Introduced**	**Description**
FORTRAN	1956	First successful programming language; for solving engineering and scientific problems
COBOL	1959	Minicomputer and mainframe computer applications in business
ALGOL	1960	Especially useful in high-level mathematics
BASIC	1964	Most frequently used with microcomputers and minicomputers; science, engineering, and business applications
BCPL	1965	Development-stage language
B	1969	Development-stage language
C	1970	Combines the power of assembly language with the ease of use and portability of high-level language
Pascal	1971	High-level, general-purpose language; used for teaching structured programming
ADA	1975	Based on Pascal; used by the U.S. Department of Defense
VisiCalc	1978	First electronic spreadsheet
C++	1980	Response to complexity of C; incorporates object-oriented programming methods
QuickBASIC	1985	Powerful high-level language with advanced user features
Visual C++	1992	Visual language programming methods; design environments
Visual BASIC	1993	Visual language programming methods; design environments; advanced user-friendly features

computational procedures for solving mathematical and statistical problems.

Problems that can be expressed in terms of formulas and equations are sometimes called **algorithms.** An algorithm is a step-by-step process used to solve a problem, much like a recipe is to bake a cake, except the algorithm is more detailed—it would include instructions to remove the shell from the egg. FORTRAN was developed in 1956 by IBM in conjunction with some major computer users.

BASIC. Developed at Dartmouth College in 1964 as a first language for students, BASIC (Beginners All-purpose Symbolic Instruction Code) is an algebraic programming language. It is an easy-to-learn, interpreter-based language. BASIC contains a powerful arithmetic facility, several editing features, a library of common mathematical functions, and simple input and output procedures.

QuickBASIC. Microsoft developed BASIC into a powerful programming language that can be used for both commercial applications and quick, single-use programs. QuickBASIC's advanced features for editing, implementation, and decoding make it an attractive language for professional and amateur programmers.

COBOL. One high-level, procedure-oriented language designed for coding business data processing problems is COBOL (COmmon Business Oriented Language). A basic characteristic of business data processing is the existence of large files that are updated continuously. COBOL provides extensive file handling, editing, and report-generating capabilities for the user.

Pascal. Pascal is a high-level, general-purpose programming language developed in 1971 by Nicklaus Wirth of the Federal Institute of Technology at Zürich, Switzerland. A general-purpose programming language is one that can be put to many different applications. Currently, Pascal is the most popular programming language for teaching programming concepts, partly because its syntax is relatively easy to learn and closely resembles the English language in usage.

C, C++. C is considered by many to be the first modern "programmer's language." It was designed, implemented, and developed by real working programmers and reflects the way they approached the job of programming. C is thought of as a middle-level language because it combines elements of high-level languages with the functionality of an assembler (low-level) language.

In response to the need to manage greater complexity, C++ was developed by Bjarne Stroustrup in 1980, who initially called it "C with Classes." C++ contains the entire C language, as well as many additions designed to support object-oriented programming (OOP).

Once a program exceeds approximately 30,000 lines of code, it becomes so complex that it is difficult to grasp as one object. Therefore, OOP is a method of dividing up parts of the program into groups, or objects, with related data and applications, in the same way that a book is broken into chapters and subheadings to be more readable.

Visual C++, Visual Basic. Visual programming languages are the most recent languages and they are under continuing development. They are designed specifically for creating Windows applications. Although both Visual C++ and Visual Basic use their original respective programming language code structures, they both were developed with the same goal in mind: to create user-friendly Windows applications with minimal effort from the programmer.

In theory, the most inexperienced programmer should be able to create complex programs with visual languages. The idea is to have the programmer design the program in a design environment without ever really writing extensive code. Instead, the visual language creates the code to match the programmer's design.

Macros. Most spreadsheet and word processing applications offer built-in programming commands called *macros.* They work the same way as commands in programming languages and they are used to carry out user-defined functions or a series of functions in the application. One application that offers a very good library of macro commands is EXCEL, a spreadsheet. The user can create a command to manipulate a series of data by performing a certain series of steps.

Macros can be written or they can be designed in a fashion similar to that of visual programming. This process of designing a macro is called recording. The programmer turns the macro recorder on, carries out the steps he wants the macro to carry out, and stops the recorder. The macro now knows exactly what the programmer wants implemented and can run the same series of steps repeatedly.

Other program languages have been developed for other purposes. LOGO is a language designed for children. ADA is the official language approved by the U.S. Department of Defense for software development. It is used principally for military applications and artificial intelligence.

PROCESSING METHODS

Regardless of the operating software or the application programs in use, the essential modes of computer processing are batch, time-sharing, on-line, and real-time systems. The modes often operate together as interactive systems when short response time between issuing a command and receiving a response is of major importance.

Batch processing results in a relatively long turnaround time but aims at lowering computing costs; the other modes are more responsive and quicker.

Batch Processing

When a computer is performing operations on defined data without human input or intervention, the computer is said to be batch processing data. Depending on the amount of data involved and the operation, the computer could run by itself for weeks.

A batch operating system is the most widely used mode of processing with mainframe computers. The users submit the complete job, which includes the program, the data, and the control statements. After a relatively long time, tens of minutes to hours, the results are available.

Normally, the jobs in a batch are processed in sequence, one after the other. This method does not require the user to attend to the system once the batch has started. Batch processing can be handled by a remote job-entry (RJE) system in which users submit their batch jobs to a remote terminal connected to the computer by a cable or modem.

On-Line Systems

In an on-line system, certain transactions are processed immediately. In such a system, the users have multiple access terminals from which they may introduce one or a few of the transactions exclusively. The response comes within seconds. Examples of on-line systems include airline reservation systems, automatic bank tellers, and supermarket checkout systems.

Time-Sharing Systems

The goal of time-sharing systems is to provide the illusion of having the computer dedicated exclusively to each user. Several hundred users, with the maximum number depending on the system, may simultaneously interact with the computer.

The time between the user's sign-on and sign-off is called a *session.* During a typical session, the user does the following:

1. Signs onto the system by presenting a password
2. Enters a program under the control of a text editor
3. Usually saves this program under an assigned name
4. Has the program compiled
5. Runs the program

While the program is being run, the user may interact with it. For example, the user may request the result of a partial execution of a program or the computer may make a request of the user and then proceed based on the result. This type of system is in use in most large research and development institutions where multiple user groups must be accommodated.

Real-Time Systems

Real-time systems are most often designed as special-purpose operating systems to provide for fast management of the system hardware. This is the case in most radiologic imaging. The processing of the incoming data (e.g., from the detectors of a CT imager) is completed in a matter of seconds at the most.

Real-time systems often use special-purpose, high-speed hardware to perform computationally intensive tasks like image reconstruction and filtering. Pipeline processors work like an assembly line. Different parts of the data are processed by different parts of the processor at the same time. The data move through the processor ("down the pipe") and are fully processed by the time they reach the output. Array processors perform the same computations in parallel on many items of data at once.

SUMMARY

The word *computer* is used as an abbreviation for any general-purpose, stored-program electronic digital device. "General-purpose" means the computer can solve problems. "Stored-program" means the computer has instructions and data stored in its memory. "Electronic" means the computer is powered by electrical and electronic devices. "Digital" means that the "data" are in discrete values.

There are two principal parts of a computer: the hardware and the software. The hardware is the computer's nuts and bolts. The software is the computer's programs, which tell the hardware what to do.

There are several types of hardware: central processing unit (CPU), control unit, arithmetic unit, memory units, input and output devices, video terminal display, secondary memory devices, printer, and modem.

The basic parts of the software are the bits, bytes, and words. In computer language, a single binary digit, either 0 or 1, is called a *bit*. Bits grouped in bunches of eight are called *bytes*. Computer capacity is expressed in bytes or megabytes.

Computers have a specific language to communicate commands in the software systems and programs. Computers operate on the simplest number system of all—the binary system. There are only two digits, 0 and 1. The computer performs all operations by converting alphabetic characters, decimal values, and logic functions into binary values. There are other computer languages, allowing the programmer to write instructions in a form approaching human language.

CHALLENGE QUESTIONS

1. Define or otherwise identify:
   a. Logic function
   b. Central processing unit
   c. Modem
   d. Character generator
   e. Byte
   f. Operating system
   g. Bootstrap
   h. Algorithm
   i. BASIC
2. Name three operations in diagnostic imaging departments that are computerized.
3. The acronyms ASCC, ENIAC, and UNIVAC stand for what titles?
4. What is the difference between a calculator and a computer?
5. Explain the differences between the microcomputer, the minicomputer, and the mainframe computer.
6. What are the two principal parts of a computer and the distinguishing features of each?
7. List and define the several parts of computer hardware.
8. Define bit, byte, and word as used in computer terminology.
9. Distinguish systems software from applications programs.
10. List several types of computer languages.
11. What is the difference between a CD and a DVD?
12. A memory chip is said to have 256 MB of capacity. What is the total bit capacity?
13. What is high-level computer language?
14. What computer language was the first modern programmers' language?
15. List and define the four computer processing methods.
16. What type of computer is used by the U.S. Census Bureau?
17. Describe a CPU. Include its three principal parts and their functions.
18. What input/output devices are commonly used in radiology?
19. Convert the decimal number 147 into binary form.
20. Convert the binary number 110001 into decimal form.

Digital Radiography

OBJECTIVES

At the completion of this chapter, the student should be able to do the following:

1. Discuss the use of digital modalities in today's imaging department
2. Relate the research and development of digital imaging
3. Explain the characteristics of digital images, specifically image matrix and dynamic range
4. Discuss the components and use of a digital radiography system
5. Explain the picture archiving and teleradiology systems used in diagnostic imaging departments

OUTLINE

CONVENTIONAL RADIOGRAPHIC imaging systems have worked well for over a century, providing increasingly better diagnostic images. However, conventional radiology has limitations.

Screen-film radiographic images require processing time that can delay the completion of the examination. Once an image is obtained, there is very little that can be done to enhance the information content. When the examination is complete, the images are in the form of hardcopy film that must be cataloged, transported, and stored for future review. Furthermore, such images can be viewed only in a single geographic location at a time.

Another and perhaps more severe limitation is the noise inherent in these images. Radiography uses a large rectangular area beam of x-rays. The Compton-scattered portion of the image-forming x-ray beam increases with increasing field size. That increases the noise of the radiographic image and severely degrades contrast resolution.

These limitations can be overcome somewhat by incorporating computer technology into diagnostic x-ray imaging. This chapter introduces the current technology of digital radiography. Digital fluoroscopy is covered in the next chapter.

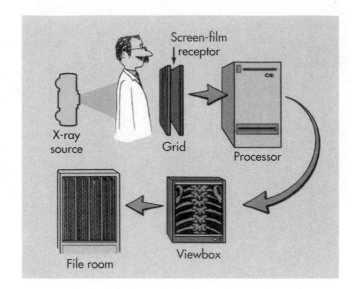

FIGURE 27-1 The imaging chain in conventional radiography.

DIGITAL IMAGES

Medical imaging is undergoing revolutionary change at this time. Since Roentgen's discovery of x-rays, until recently, anatomic images have been obtained in basically the same fashion. Now, that is changing and changing very rapidly.

A conventional radiographic image is made like a shadowgraph, using an area beam of x-rays that forms an image pattern after transmission through the patient. The image receptor, a screen-film combination, is a device that records this transmitted image directly. Figure 27-1 diagrams the imaging chain for conventional radiography.

Radiography uses a large area beam of x-rays.

Digital imaging techniques are applied to computed tomography (CT), diagnostic ultrasonography, nuclear medicine, magnetic resonance imaging (MRI), digital radiography (DR), and digital fluoroscopy (DF). DR and DF are under continuing development and increasing clinical application. As our computer technology advances, so will digital x-ray imaging.

Standard nomenclature for identifying the methods of obtaining digital radiographic images has not yet been uniformly adopted. Terms such as **computed radiography (CR)**, **scan beam digital radiography**, **direct digital radiography (DDR)**, **digital radiography (DR)**, and others appear frequently.

In the following discussions, *digital radiography* refers to the images produced with either a fan x-ray beam intercepted by a linear array of radiation detectors or an area x-ray beam intercepted by a photostimulable phosphor plate or a direct-capture solid-state device.

Advent of Digital Radiography

Practical DR imaging equipment was limited until sufficient computer technology became available to process the large quantities of data generated. Advanced microprocessors and semiconductor memory made DR technology possible. Initial activity, begun in the early 1970s, followed two independent approaches and became a clinical reality by 1980.

DR has enjoyed a path of development influenced by a number of different investigators. One approach, developed in the late 1970s to complement CT, uses a narrow fan beam of x-rays that intercepts a linear array of radiation detectors. This is commonly referred to as scanned projection radiography (SPR). The signal from each detector is computer manipulated to reconstruct an image.

A second approach to DR was developed by Fuji, also in the late 1970s, and has been advanced and marketed by a number of x-ray companies. It is referred to as *computed radiography* (CR) and uses a photostimulable phosphor as the image receptor and an area beam. Newer imaging systems have been introduced based on direct-capture solid-state devices, such as selenium, silicon, and thin-film transistors (TFT) as the image receptor.

Image Characteristics

The image obtained in DR is like that obtained in conventional radiography where x-rays form a latent image directly on the image receptor, which must be chemically developed into a visible image. With DR, x-rays form an electronic latent image on a radiation detector. That latent image is then electronically developed by a computer, converted into a **matrix** of numeric values, and temporarily stored in memory.

Image Matrix. The term *image matrix* refers to a layout of cells in rows and columns. Each cell corresponds to a specific location in the image. The value of the cell represents the brightness or intensity at that location.

Figure 27-2 shows a 10 × 10 matrix of cells, a 5 × 5 matrix of cells, a 5 × 5 matrix of numbers in imaginary cells, and the associated image (Figure 27-3). Each digital image consists of a matrix of cells having various brightness levels on the video monitor. The brightness of a cell is determined by the computer-generated number stored in that cell.

Each cell of the image matrix is called a **pixel** (picture element). In digital x-ray imaging, the value of the pixel determines pixel brightness. The value is relative and defines the image contrast.

In CT imaging, the numeric value of each pixel is a CT number or Hounsfield unit (HU). The value of the HU can be manipulated to judge the composition of the tissue represented. In MRI, diagnostic ultrasonography, and nuclear medicine, the numeric value of the pixel also has a relationship to the composition of the tissue imaged (Table 27-1).

The size of the image matrix is determined by characteristics of the imaging equipment and by the capacity of the computer. Matrix size may be selected by the operator. Digital imaging systems provide image matrix sizes of 64 × 64 and 4096 × 4096. Table 27-2 summarizes these image matrices.

For the same field of view (FOV), *spatial resolution* will be better with a larger image matrix.

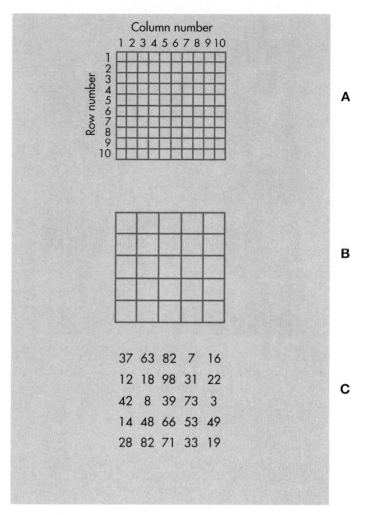

FIGURE 27-2 A matrix is an arrangement of columns and rows. Three matrices are shown. **A,** A 10 × 10 matrix of cells. **B,** A 5 × 5 matrix of cells. **C,** A 5 × 5 matrix of numbers in imaginary cells.

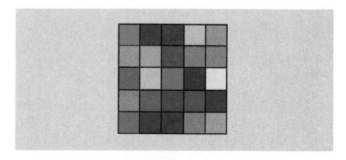

FIGURE 27-3 Associated image of the matrix in Figure 27-2, C.

Question: How many pixels are contained in an image matrix described as 256 × 256?

Answer: 256 × 256 = 65,536

Figure 27-4 illustrates the influence of matrix size on image quality. A 64 × 64 image matrix appears definitely

TABLE 27-1	Pixel Value as a Function of Tissue Characteristics for Several Types of Imaging
Image Modality	**Tissue Characteristic**
Radiography/ fluoroscopy	Atomic number, mass density
Computed tomography	Atomic number, mass density
Nuclear medicine	Radionuclide uptake
Diagnostic ultrasonography	Interface reflectivity
Magnetic resonance	Proton density, spin relaxation

TABLE 27-2	Image Matrix Size for Various Imaging Modalities
Modality	**Matrix Size**
Nuclear medicine	64×64
Diagnostic ultrasonography	128×128
Computed tomography	256×256
Magnetic resonance imaging	512×512
Digital radiography	1024×1024
Computed radiography	2048×2048
	4096×4096

"boxy," whereas a 512×512 image is a good representation of the original analog image. A 1024×1024 image is nearly indistinguishable from the original.

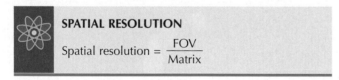

SPATIAL RESOLUTION

$$\text{Spatial resolution} = \frac{\text{FOV}}{\text{Matrix}}$$

The size of the image matrix and the FOV determine the spatial resolution for digital images, such as CT, MRI, and digital ultrasonography.

 Spatial resolution in digital imaging is limited by the size of a pixel.

The future for total digital imaging is dictated by the requirements of chest imaging. There has been much effort to define these requirements. With a 14×14 inch chest image as the standard, the accepted minimum spatial resolution requires an image matrix size of 2048×2048. Less than that and spatial resolution is unacceptably poor.

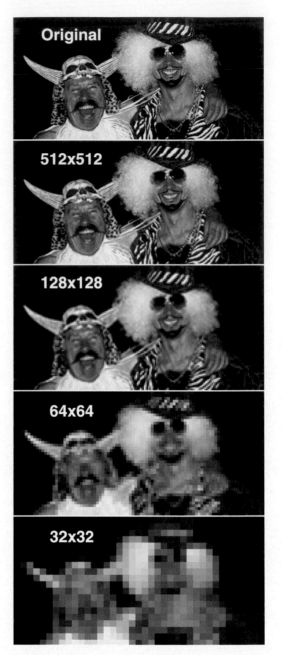

FIGURE 27-4 This Zulu king and his Mardi Gras consort (actually Louisiana radiologic technologists) posed to illustrate the improvement in spatial resolution with larger matrix size. The 512×512 matrix is an acceptable rendition of the original. At a 32×32 matrix, the students became true blockheads. (Courtesy Robert Malone.)

Question: What is the pixel size for a 14×14 inch digital image reconstructed on a 2048×2048 matrix?

Answer: 14 in $\times$ 25.4 mm/in = 355.6 mm

$$\frac{355.6 \text{ mm}}{2048 \text{ pixels}} = 0.17 \text{ mm/pixel}$$

Question: When the pixel size is 0.17 mm, what is the associated spatial frequency (see Chapter 29)?

Answer: 1 pixel = 0.17 mm

therefore, 1 line pair (lp) = 2 × 0.17 mm

= 0.35 mm

$$\text{therefore, spatial resolution} = \frac{1}{0.35 \text{ mm/lp}}$$

= 2.9 lp/mm

Dynamic Range. An imaging system that could display only black or white would have a dynamic range of 2^1 or 2. Such an image would be very high contrast but would display very little information unless it were a printed page.

Although the actual value of each pixel is important, the range of values is extremely important in determining the final image. This is especially true for subtraction techniques.

> The range of values over which a system can respond is called its *gray-scale range* or *dynamic range.*

Dynamic range is described as the number of shades of gray that can be represented. The maximum number of shades of gray that can be represented by a digital imaging system is the numeric range of each pixel or "bit depth." The actual dynamic range may be less than the bit depth.

The dynamic range of the human eye is approximately 2^5 or 32 shades of gray stretching from white to black. The dynamic range of the x ray beam as it exits the patient is in excess of 2^{10}. Although we cannot visualize such a dynamic range, a computer with sufficient capacity can.

The larger the dynamic range, the more gradual will be the gray scale representing the range from maximum x-ray intensity to minimum x-ray intensity. The greater the dynamic range, therefore, the better the contrast resolution.

Digital x-ray imaging systems are characterized by their dynamic range, which is limited by the capacity of the computer and the software. Most use an 8-, 10-, or 12-bit dynamic range, meaning a 2^8, 2^{10}, or 2^{12} dynamic range. The digital form is displayed as an image matrix, where each pixel is capable of a range of 2^8 (0 to 255), 2^{10} (0 to 1023), or 2^{12} (0 to 4095).

> For acceptable contrast resolution on radiographic CT and MRI images, a 12-bit dynamic range is required.

Figure 27-5 illustrates the effect of dynamic range on the appearance of the image. Clearly, a system with low dynamic range is high contrast but only over a limited

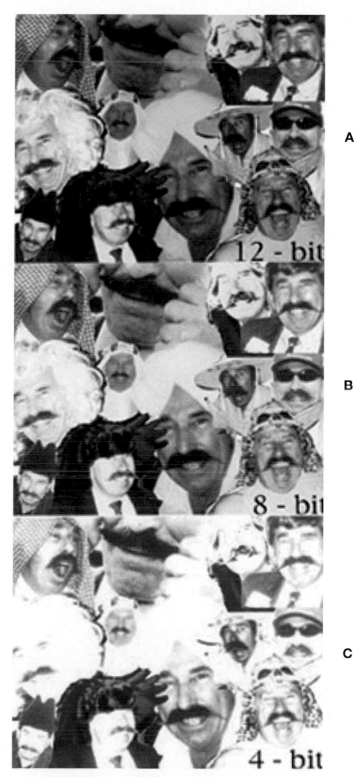

FIGURE 27-5 This image of Texan cultural people of the world illustrates the concept of dynamic range. **A,** 12-Bit dynamic range. **B,** 8-Bit dynamic range. **C,** 4-Bit dynamic range. (Courtesy David Gee.)

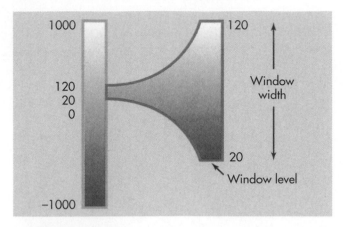

FIGURE 27-6 Windowing a digital image controls the image contrast and optical density (brightness).

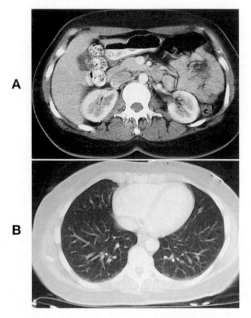

FIGURE 27-7 The selection of window level depends on the anatomy imaged. **A,** Soft tissue of the abdomen requires a low window level (level 50, width 400). **B,** The lung fields require a negative window level (level −500, width 1500). (Courtesy Nancy Adams.)

portion of the image. High dynamic range allows for wide image latitude.

The contrast of a region of interest (ROI) of the image can be enhanced if the computer system has sufficient dynamic range. When a subtraction examination is undertaken, the information contained in the final image is far greater for a system with high dynamic range.

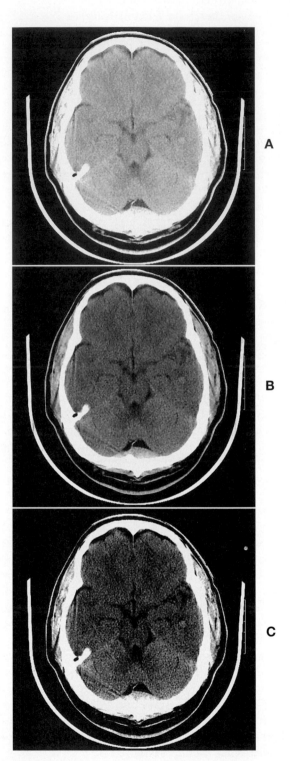

FIGURE 27-8 These brain images show the loss of contrast with increasing window width. **A,** Level 40, width 40. **B,** Level 40, width 100. **C,** Level 40, width 160. (Courtesy Mike Enrique.)

Often, the radiologic technologist is responsible for producing film images from the cathode ray tube (CRT) of proper optical density (OD) and contrast. This is done by using the computer to change the appearance of an image after it has been acquired through a technique called windowing.

A digital image with a 10-bit dynamic range contains 1024 gray values; however, the human eye can see only about 32 such shades. Modifying the image after it has been acquired, or postprocessing the image, allows the visualization of only a "window" of the entire dynamic range.

The two characteristics of the window are window level and window width (Figure 27-6). Window level identifies the type of tissue to be imaged. For instance, a CT window level of 50 best images abdominal tissue, whereas a window level of 500 best images lung tissue (Figure 27-7).

Window width determines the gray-scale rendition of that tissue, and therefore image contrast. The wider the window width, the longer will be the gray scale. Narrow window widths produce high contrast (Figure 27-8).

DIGITAL RADIOGRAPHY

DR is advancing along several approaches simultaneously. It differs from conventional radiography because film is not the image receptor.

Other types of radiation detectors whose electrical output is proportional to the radiation intensity are used. Initially, this output signal may be in analog form, but it is converted to digital form. The image is displayed on a monitor after computer processing.

Scanned Projection Radiography

Perhaps, the first clinically useful application of DR was a complement to CT developed by General Electric Medical Systems. This has come to be known as SPR. Basically, SPR involves the use of the existing CT gantry and computer to generate an image that looks surprisingly like a conventional radiograph (Figure 27-9).

This image is similar to a conventional radiographic image because there is superposition of tissues through the body. It differs from a conventional image in that it is virtually free of scatter radiation and is digital in form. The digital form of the image permits subtraction techniques as described for DF and provides for other types of image manipulation.

The basic components of an SPR system is an x-ray beam shaped into a fan by collimators that confine the beam to 0.5- to 10-mm thickness through an arc of 30 to 45 degrees (Figure 27-10). There are two collimators. The prepatient collimators shape the beam, reduce scatter radiation, and control patient dose. The postpatient

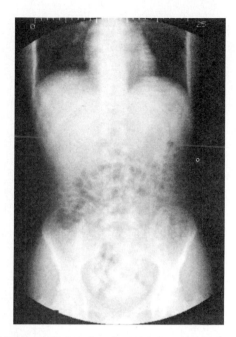

FIGURE 27-9 This digital radiograph is typical of scan projection radiographs obtained with computed tomography imaging systems. (Courtesy Larry Rothenberg.)

collimators further reduce scatter radiation and improve image contrast.

On passing through the patient and postpatient collimators, the image-forming x-rays are intercepted by a detector array. Each detector responds with a signal that is related to the attenuation due to the body part through which the x-ray beam passed. The response of the total detector array therefore represents an attenuation profile of that body section.

 The reduced scatter radiation of SPR results from the narrowness of the fan beam collimation and produces enhanced image contrast.

Another way to view the production of the high-contrast image in DR is to consider that the rejection of scattered x-rays reduces the noise in the image. Remember that Compton-scattered x-rays carry no useful information but simply contribute to the background noise of an image. Consequently, in SPR the radiographic contrast is high and the detection of low-contrast objects is better.

 In any imaging system, noise is the principal limitation to contrast resolution.

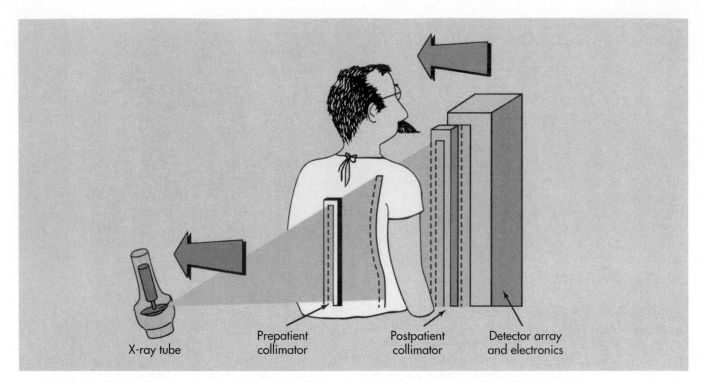

FIGURE 27-10 The components of a scanned projection radiography system. The source-detector assembly translates across the patient. (Courtesy Gary Barnes.)

The principal disadvantage with any DR system is its poor spatial resolution. Whereas a conventional screen-film system can image 100-μm objects, SPR can do no better than approximately 500 μm. Of course, this degree of resolution is adequate for most examinations. In DR, resolution is controlled principally by the design of the detector array and the speed with which the patient or x-ray beam is translated.

 The more detectors there are per degree of fan x-ray beam, the better the spatial resolution.

Fewer x-rays are detected as the speed of translation is increased, whether it be the translation of the patient through the x-ray beam or the translation of the beam across the patient. This restricts the resulting image quality by reducing contrast resolution.

To obtain enough profiles for a complete image, the source-detector assembly remains stationary and the patient is translated through the x-ray beam. Alternatively, the patient may remain stationary while the source-detector assembly translates. During translation, either the x-ray beam is pulsed or each detector is sampled intermittently. The sequential profiles obtained during translation are computer processed to form an image resembling a radiograph.

SPR designs based on patient translation are incorporated into most CT scanners. By proper positioning

of the source-detector array, one can obtain anterior-posterior, posterior-anterior, lateral, and oblique views. Dedicated DR systems use translation of the source-detector assembly across a stationary patient.

Source-Detector Assembly

An x-ray tube used for SPR must have a high heat capacity. A heat capacity in excess of 1 MHU is usually required. The requirement for a high heat capacity occurs because of two characteristics of the system: imaging time and detector efficiency. Usually, 20 to 50 cm of the patient is imaged at a translation speed of 1 to 2 cm/s. The detectors may not be intrinsically as efficient as a screen-film receptor and because of the precise beam collimation, few scattered x-rays reach the detectors. Consequently, techniques of 500 to 2000 mAs are required.

The solid-state scintillation detector array incorporates individual crystal-photodiode assemblies. Such an array usually presents an active area to the x-ray beam of 5 × 20 mm with a small interspace between detectors. This results in a limit to the number of detectors that can be used.

The scintillation crystal used is cadmium tungstate ($CdWO_4$), although bismuth germinate (BGO), cesium iodide (CsI), and sodium iodide (NaI) have also been used. The photodiode is a semiconductor material, usually silicon or germanium, whose output signal is proportional to the intensity of light incident on it.

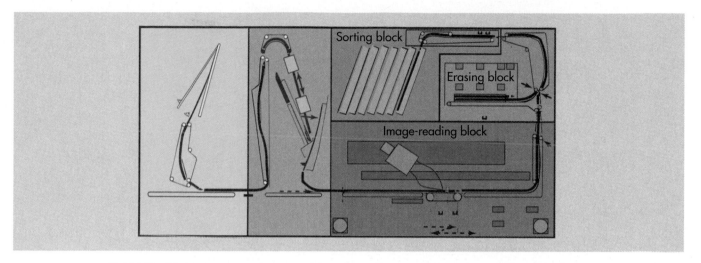

FIGURE 27-11 Process of computed radiography using photostimulable phosphors. (Courtesy Fuji Photo Company.)

Area Beam Versus Fan Beam

A principal limitation to the SPR mode of DR is the time required to obtain an image. In conventional radiography, a latent image is produced in a matter of milliseconds. When a fan beam is used in DR, an exposure of several seconds may be required, and this may increase image blur because of patient motion.

The image acquisition time in DR can be reduced by decreasing the translation time in SPR or by using the area beam. Providing an area beam is straightforward. It may be difficult, however, to fabricate an area image receptor that will retain the rapid response time required.

Three approaches are available for using an area beam in DR. CR has been used widely for 20 years. The use of tiled charge-coupled devices (CCDs) is another line of development. An assembly of solid-state detectors formed in matrix fashion can be used. The electronics associated with the enormous number of detectors required is quite sophisticated, and therefore the expense can be excessive.

Computed Radiography

Digital images can be acquired with a **photostimulable phosphor** as a solid-state image receptor in rectangular plate form, as shown schematically in Figure 27-11; this technique is termed *computed radiography*.

The image receptor resembles a conventional radiographic intensifying screen and is exposed in a cassette with conventional x-ray equipment. The active ingredient is europium-activated barium fluorohalide, which is energized when exposed to x-rays. The sensitivity is approximately equal to a 200-speed screen-film combination and can be much greater when contrast resolution is sacrificed. The latent image consists of valence electrons stored in high-energy traps.

The latent image is made manifest by exposure to a very small beam from a high-intensity laser. The laser beam causes the trapped electrons to return to the valence band with the emission of violet light. This phenomenon is called **light-stimulated phosphorescence** (see Chapter 15); it also is known as *stimulated luminescence*.

The violet emission is viewed by an ultrasensitive photomultiplier tube. The electronic signal, which is the output of the photomultiplier tube, is digitized and stored for subsequent display on a CRT or hard copy from a laser printer. Figure 27-12 is a cut-away schematic of a CR image processor.

The spatial resolution of CR is not quite as good as conventional radiography, but the contrast resolution is better because of image postprocessing. The latitude of the system is exceptional and for many examinations, patient dose is considerably less than par speed systems.

Charge-Coupled Device. CCDs are photosensitive silicon chips that are rapidly replacing the television camera tube in the fluoroscopic chain. CCDs are similar in appearance to a computer chip and can be used anywhere that light is to be converted to a digital video image.

Mammography and interventional radiology procedures were the first medical imaging applications to use CCDs. CCDs can serve as a wide-area detector for stationary radiography by converting x-rays into light using a fluorescent screen and focusing the light onto a CCD array by lenses or fiber optics. Figure 27-13 shows a flexible DR system based on CCDs viewing a CsI phosphor. A linear array of CCDs can serve as a narrow x-ray beam detector. CCDs are discussed more completely in Chapter 28.

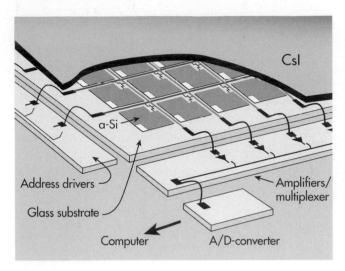

FIGURE 27-12 Direct capture digital radiographic images can be produced from the CsI phosphor light detected by the active matrix array (AMA) of silicon photodiodes.

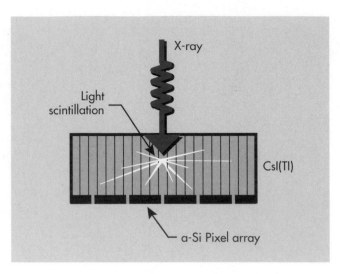

FIGURE 27-13 The CsI phosphor in digital radiography image receptors is in the form of crystalline channels for improved confinement of light dispersion.

Direct-Capture Radiography

In the late 1990s, two totally new approaches to direct-capture DR appeared. It is too early to tell which will prevail or whether the two approaches will complement each other.

Both direct-capture systems are based on TFTs fashioned as an active matrix array (AMA). The result is a flat-panel image receptor the size of conventional screen-film receptors.

The first demonstration of direct-capture radiography used a CsI scintillation phosphor coated over an AMA of amorphous silicon (a-Si) photodiodes. In the amorphous state, the silicon is easily coated on the AMA at controlled thickness.

 The term *amorphous* denotes a noncrystalline state of an otherwise crystalline material.

Image-forming x-rays interact with the CsI to produce light, which in turn interacts with the a-Si to produce a signal. The TFT stores the signal until readout, one pixel at a time.

The second approach does not use a phosphor coating. Image-forming x-rays interact directly with a thin layer of amorphous selenium (a-Se), creating electron hole-pairs (EHP; Figure 27-14). The EHP is the signal that charges the AMA of TFTs.

The advantage of the a-Se approach is that there is no spreading of light in the phosphor, and therefore spatial resolution is improved (Figure 27-15). On the other hand, the CsI phosphor has high detective quantum efficiency (DQE), and therefore results in lower dose.

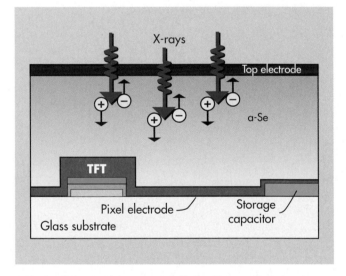

FIGURE 27-14 In this type of direct-capture digital radiography, electron-hole pairs are generated and detected by the active matrix array of thin-film transistors.

With both systems, the latent image is electronic, stored in the TFT array. This array is read sequentially from one TFT to another through precise electronic control (Figure 27-16).

The array of TFTs is such that each TFT and its x-ray detector represents a pixel. Consequently, spatial resolution again is limited by the pixel size. Available pixel size is limited to approximately 100 μm, which is equivalent to 5 lp/mm spatial resolution (Figure 27-17). Much smaller pixels are being developed.

Although the DQE, and therefore patient dose is determined principally by the atomic number of the detec-

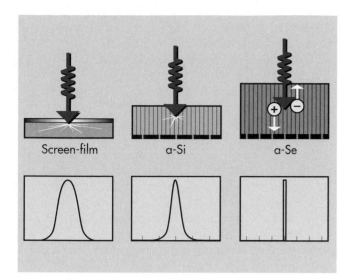

FIGURE 27-15 This represents the relative blur of a single x-ray interaction in three types of image receptors. CsI phosphor detection has better dose efficiency, whereas a-Se can provide better spatial resolution.

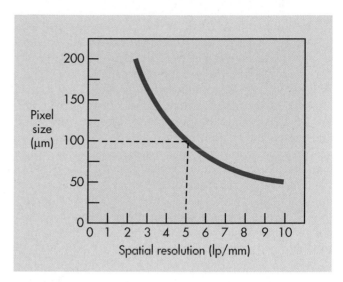

FIGURE 27-17 Digital radiography pixel size is approximately 100 μm^2, which results in limiting spatial resolution to 5 line pairs/mm.

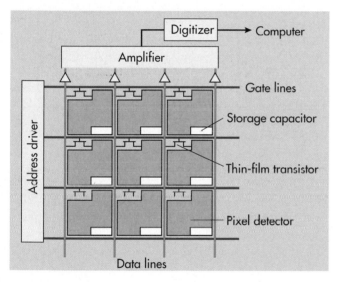

FIGURE 27-16 The active matrix array of pixels is read sequentially, one pixel at a time.

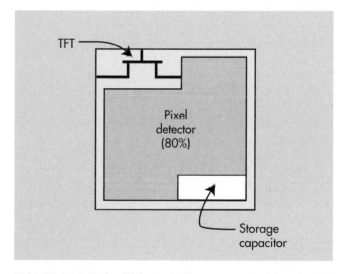

FIGURE 27-18 The fill factor is the percentage of the pixel element occupied by the sensitive image receptor.

tor ($Z_{CsI} = 55/53$, $Z_{Se} = 34$), the geometry of each pixel is also very important (Figure 27-18). A portion of the pixel face is occupied by electronic conductors and the TFT. The "fill factor" is the percentage of the pixel face that contains the x-ray detector. Fill factor is approximately 80%.

Direct-capture radiography has all of the advantages of other digital imaging techniques: postprocessing and a picture archiving and communication system. The future is very bright for this modality.

SUMMARY

Conventional radiography has several limitations. First, images require processing time that can delay completion of an examination. Second, once images are obtained, little can be done to enhance their information content. Third, distribution and storage of film images is slow and inefficient. Most important, however, is the noise inherent in conventional radiography and fluoroscopy because of Compton-scattered radiation from the x-ray beam.

Development of digital imaging equipment was stalled in the 1970s until microprocessor and semiconductor memory systems were developed in the 1980s that were capable of processing the large amount of data generated. Digital images are displayed as a matrix of pixels of various gray-scale values. Postprocessing allows the radiologic technologist to optimize the digital image for contrast resolution.

One type of DR uses a fan-shaped beam to reduce scatter and enhance radiographic contrast. The primary disadvantage of this type of DR is poor spatial resolution compared with screen-film radiography. The fan-shaped image-forming x-ray beam is intercepted by a detector array, which is either a gas-filled detector or a solid-state scintillation detector.

Wide-area digital detectors share the limitations that Compton-scattered radiation impose on conventional radiographs.

One wide-area image receptor is a solid-state plate. Barium-fluorohalide compounds are energized when exposed to x-rays. The spatial resolution of the digitized image is not as good as a screen-film image, but it does allow for postprocessing.

CHALLENGE QUESTIONS

1. Define or otherwise identify:
   a. Matrix
   b. Pixel
   c. Voxel
   d. Trackball
   e. Dynamic range
   f. Fan beam
   g. SPR
   h. FOV
   i. Windowing
   j. Amorphous
2. Define *image matrix*.
3. How many pixels are contained in an image whose matrix size is 256×256?
4. Define *windowing*, and explain window level and window width.
5. A digital image with a 10-bit dynamic range will contain how many gray-scale values?
6. Describe the process of recording an image with CR.
7. What are the postprocessing image enhancements that can be made on a digital image?
8. Explain what the dynamic range of values for digital imaging means.
9. What are the principal advantages of DR over conventional radiography?
10. What are the components of a scanned projection radiography system, and how is the image produced?
11. How does spatial resolution change with image matrix size and field of view?
12. What is meant by the term *fill factor* when applied to DR?
13. What is an electron-hole pair?
14. Why does DR have better contrast resolution than screen-film imaging?
15. How does a photostimulable phosphor work?
16. A DR image receptor has a pixel size of 80 μm. What is its limiting spatial resolution?
17. A dedicated DR chest imaging system has a 12-bit dynamic range. How many shades of gray can it render?
18. A 36×36 cm DR image receptor displays a 4096×4096 image. What is the size of each pixel?
19. A 512×512 image covers a 30-cm field of view. What is the pixel size?
20. Take the answer to the previous question and compute the limiting spatial resolution in line pairs per millimeter (lp/mm).

Digital Fluoroscopy

OBJECTIVES

At the completion of this chapter, the student should be able to do the following:

1. Describe the parts of a digital fluoroscopy system and their functions
2. Compute pixel size in digital fluoroscopy
3. Compare the use of a TV camera tube with a CCD
4. Outline the procedures for temporal subtraction and energy subtraction
5. Discuss the features of a picture archiving and communication system

OUTLINE

CONVENTIONAL FLUOROSCOPY produces a shadowgraph-type image on a receptor that is directly produced from the transmitted x-ray beam. Image intensifier tubes serve as the fluoroscopic image receptor. These tubes are usually electronically coupled to a television monitor for remote viewing, as described in Chapter 24. Figure 28-1 diagrams the components used in conventional fluoroscopy.

Digital fluoroscopy (DF) identifies a digital x-ray imaging system that produces a series of dynamic images obtained with an area x-ray beam and an image intensifier. The difference between conventional fluoroscopy and DF is the nature of the image and the manner in which it is digitized.

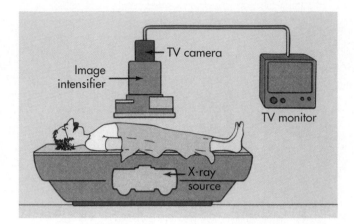

FIGURE 28-1 The imaging chain in conventional fluoroscopy.

The medical physics groups at the University of Wisconsin and the University of Arizona independently initiated studies of DF in the early 1970s. These studies were continued through the decade by the research and development groups of most x-ray equipment manufacturers.

The approach was to use fluoroscopic equipment while placing a computer between the television camera and the television monitor. The video signal from the television camera was routed through the computer, manipulated in various ways, and transmitted to the television monitor in a form ready for viewing.

The initial investigators of DF demonstrated that nearly instantaneous, high-contrast subtraction images could be obtained after intravenous injection of contrast media. Although the intravenous route is still widely used, intraarterial injections are also used with DF.

The advantages of DF over conventional fluoroscopy are the speed of image acquisition and postprocessing to enhance image contrast.

A 1024 × 1024 image matrix is sometimes described as a 1000-line system. In DF, the spatial resolution is determined both by the image matrix and by the size of the image intensifier. Spatial resolution is limited by pixel size.

DF PIXEL SIZE

$$\text{Pixel Size} = \frac{\text{Image intensifier size}}{\text{Matrix}}$$

Question: What is the pixel size of a 1000-line DF system operating in the 5-inch mode?

Answer: Five inches equals 127 mm (5 × 25.4 mm/inch). Therefore, the size of each pixel is

$$\frac{127 \text{ mm}}{1024} = 0.124 \text{ mm}$$

DIGITAL FLUOROSCOPY

A DF examination is conducted in much the same manner as a conventional fluoroscopic study. To the casual observer, the equipment is the same, but such is not the case (Figure 28-2). A computer has been added, as well as two monitors and a more complex operating console.

Figure 28-3 shows a representative operating console of a dedicated DF imaging system. It contains alphanumeric and special function keys in the left module for entering patient data and communicating with the computer. The right portion of the console contains additional special function keys for data acquisition and image display.

The module on the right also contains computer-interactive video controls and a pad for cursor and region of interest (ROI) manipulation. Other systems use a trackball, joystick, or mouse instead of the pad. Two monitors are used. The left monitor is used to edit patient and examination data and to annotate final images. The right monitor displays subtracted images.

High-Voltage Generator

During DF, the undertable x-ray tube actually operates in the radiographic mode. The tube current is measured in hundreds of mA instead of less than 5 mA, as in image-intensifying fluoroscopy.

This is not a problem, however. If the tube were energized continuously, it would fail because of thermal overloading and the patient dose would be exceedingly

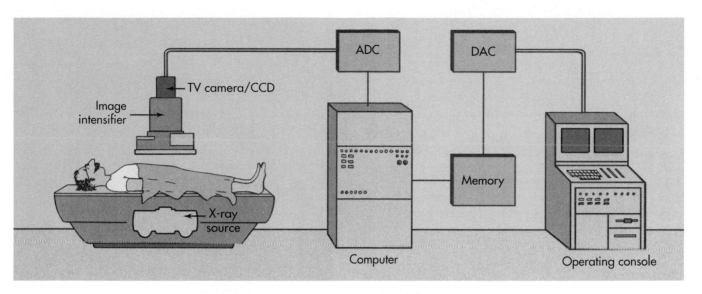

FIGURE 28-2 The components of a digital fluoroscopy system.

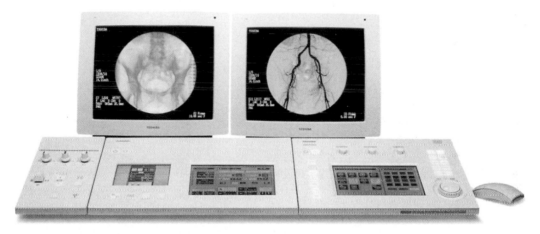

FIGURE 28-3 Operating console for a digital fluoroscopy system. (Courtesy Toshiba Medical Systems.)

high. Images from DF are obtained by pulsing the x-ray beam in a manner called *pulse-progressive fluoroscopy.*

 During DF, the x-ray tube operates in the radiographic mode.

Image acquisition rates of 1 per second to 10 per second are common in many examinations. Because it requires 33 ms to produce one video frame, x-ray exposures longer than that can result in unnecessary patient dose. That is a theoretical limit, however, and longer exposures may be necessary to ensure low noise and good image quality.

Consequently, the x-ray generator must be capable of switching on and off very rapidly. The time required for the x-ray tube to be switched on and reach the selected levels of kVp and mA is called the **interrogation time.** The time required for the x-ray tube to be switched off is the **extinction time.** DF systems must incorporate three-phase or high-frequency generators with interrogation and extinction times of less than 1 ms.

Charge-Coupled Device

The charge-coupled device (CCD) was developed in the 1970s for military applications, especially in night vision scopes. In the early 1980s, the CCD replaced the television camera tube in video systems. Today, CCDs are used in the home camcorder, commercial television, security surveillance, and astronomy (Figure 28-4).

The demands of medical imaging are much more rigorous than in these other applications. That is why the first fluoroscopic CCD did not appear until 1983.

The sensitive component of a CCD is a layer of crystalline silicon (Figure 28-5). When the silicon is illuminated, electrical charge is generated, which is then sampled, pixel by pixel, and manipulated to produce a digital image. The CCD is mounted on the output phosphor of the image intensifier tube and is coupled by fiber optics or a lens system (Figure 28-6).

The principal advantage to CCDs in most applications, such as a camcorder, is their small size and ruggedness. Their principal advantages for medical imaging are listed in Box 28-1.

The spatial resolution of a CCD is determined by its physical size and pixel count. Systems incorporating a 1024 matrix can produce images with 10 lp/mm. Television camera tubes can show spatial distortion in what is described as "pincushion" or "barrel artifact." There is no such distortion with a CCD.

The CCD has a higher sensitivity to light (DQE or detective quantum efficiency) and a lower level of electronic noise than a television camera. The result is higher signal-to-noise ratio (SNR) and better contrast resolution. These characteristics also result in substantially lower patient dose.

The response of the CCD to light is very stable. Warm-up of the CCD is not required. There is neither image lag nor blooming. It has essentially an unlimited lifetime and requires no maintenance.

Perhaps the single most important feature of CCD imaging is its linear response (Figure 28-7). Other image receptors have a sigmoid-shaped response, which makes it difficult to image either very dim or very bright objects. Information in the toe and shoulder region of such response is lost.

This linear response feature is particularly helpful for subtraction imaging. The result is improved dynamic range and better contrast resolution.

The next improvement in this type of imaging will probably be flat panel imagers composed of silicon pixel detectors (SPD). Such direct x-ray detectors exist in laboratories at this time. Perhaps at around the time all television camera tubes are replaced by CCDs, CCDs will begin to be replaced by SPDs!

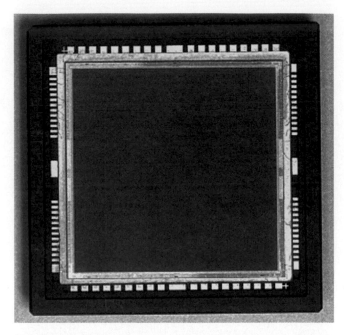

FIGURE 28-4 This charge-coupled device has 14 μm pixels arrayed in a 2048 × 2048 matrix and views the light output of an image intensifier tube. (Courtesy Apogee Instruments, Inc.)

Video System

The video system used in conventional fluoroscopy is usually a 525-line system. Such a system is adequate for DF, although higher spatial resolution can be obtained with 1000-line systems.

Conventional video, however, has two limitations that restrict its application in digital techniques. First, the interlaced mode of reading the target of the television camera can significantly degrade a digital image. Second, the conventional television camera tubes are relatively noisy. They have an SNR of about 200:1, whereas an SNR of 1000:1 is necessary for DF.

Interlaced Versus Progressive Mode. In Chapter 24, the method by which a conventional television camera tube reads its target assembly was described. That method was called an *interlaced mode,* where two fields of 262½ lines each were read in 1/60 s (17 ms) to form a 525-line video frame in 1/30 s (33 ms).

In DF, the camera tube reads in progressive mode. When reading the video signal in the progressive mode, the electron beam of the television camera tube sweeps the target assembly continuously from top to bottom in 33 ms (Figure 28-8).

The video image is similarly formed on the television monitor. There is no interlace of one field with another. This produces a sharper image with less flicker.

Signal-to-Noise Ratio. All analog electronic devices are inherently noisy. Because of heated filaments and voltage differences, there is always a very small electric

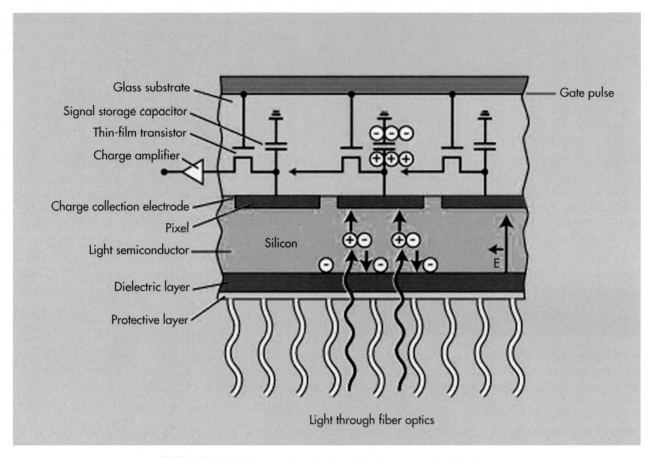

FIGURE 28-5 Cross-sectional view of a charge-coupled device.

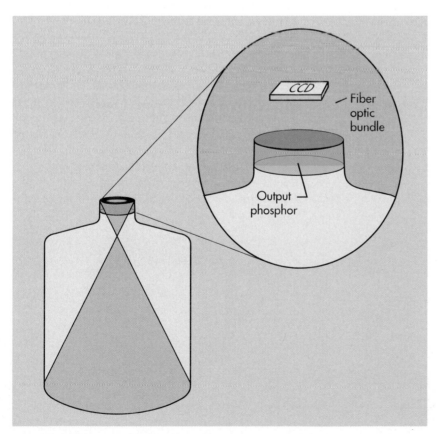

FIGURE 28-6 The manner in which a charge-coupled device can be coupled to the image intensifier tube.

current flowing in any circuit. This is called background electronic **noise**. It is similar to the noise (fog) on a radiograph in that it conveys no information and serves only to obscure the electronic **signal.**

Because conventional television camera tubes have an SNR of about 200:1, the maximum output signal will be 200 times greater than the background electronic noise. A SNR of 5:1 is minimally visible.

A SNR of 200:1 is not sufficient for DF because the video signal is rarely at maximum and lower signals become even more lost in the noise. This is especially true when subtraction techniques are used. Image contrast resolution is severely degraded by a system with a low SNR.

Figure 28-9 illustrates the difference between the output of a 200:1 SNR television camera tube and a 1000:1 tube. At 200:1, the dynamic range is less than 2^8, and at 1000:1 it is approximately 2^{10}. The tube with a 1000:1 SNR provides five times the useful information and is more compatible with computer-assisted image enhancement.

Computer

Minicomputers and microprocessors are used in DF. The capacity of the computer is an important factor in determining image quality, the manner and speed of image acquisition, and image processing and manipulation. Important characteristics of a DF system that are computer controlled are the **image matrix size, the system dynamic range,** and the **image acquisition rate.**

The output signal from the television camera tube is transmitted by cable to an **analog-to-digital converter (ADC).** The ADC accepts the continuously varying television camera output signal, the analog signal, and digitizes it.

To be compatible with the computer, the ADC must have the same dynamic range as the DF system. An 8-bit ADC would convert the analog signal into values between 0 and 255. A 10-bit ADC would be more precise, with an analog-to-digital conversion range from 0 to 2^{10} or 0 to 1023.

The output of the ADC is then transferred to main memory and manipulated so that a digital image in matrix form is stored. The dynamic range of each pixel, the number of pixels, and the method of storage determine the speed with which the image can be acquired, processed, and transferred to an output device.

If image storage is in primary memory, which is usually the case, then data acquisition and transfer can be as rapid as 30 images per second. In general, if the image matrix is doubled (e.g., from 512 to 1024), the image acquisition rate will be reduced by a factor of four.

A representative system might be capable of acquiring 30 images per second in the 512 × 512 matrix mode. However, if a higher spatial resolution image is required and the 1024 × 1024 mode is requested, then only 8 images per second can be acquired. This limitation on data transfer is imposed by the time required to

---

BOX 28-1 Advantages of Charge-Coupled Devices for Medical Imaging

High spatial resolution
High signal-to-noise ratio
High detective quantum efficiency (DQE)
No warm-up required
No lag or blooming
No spatial distortion
No maintenance
Unlimited life
Unaffected by magnetic fields
Linear response
Lower dose

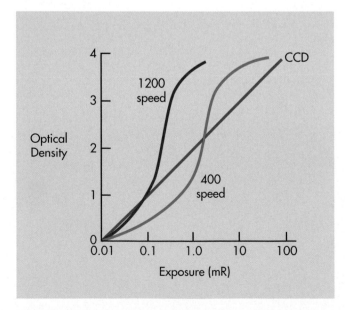

FIGURE 28-7 The response to light of a charge-coupled device is linear and can be electronically manipulated.

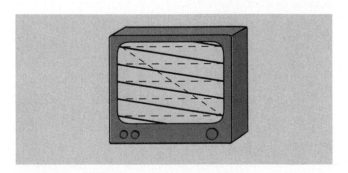

FIGURE 28-8 The progressive mode of reading a video signal.

conduct the enormous quantities of data from one segment of memory to another.

Image Formation

The principal advantages of DF examinations are the image subtraction techniques that are possible and the ability to visualize vasculature with a venous injection of contrast material. Unfortunately, an area beam must be used, which reduces image contrast because of the associated scatter radiation.

Image contrast, however, can be enhanced electronically. Image contrast is improved by subtraction techniques that provide instantaneous viewing of the subtracted image, during the passage of a bolus of contrast medium.

Digital fluoroscopy provides better contrast resolution by postprocessing image subtraction.

Temporal subtraction and energy subtraction are the two methods that receive attention in DF. Each has distinct advantages and disadvantages, and these are described in Table 28-1. Temporal subtraction techniques are most frequently used because of the high-voltage generator limitations in the energy subtraction mode. When the two techniques are combined, the process is called **hybrid subtraction**. Image contrast is enhanced still further by hybrid subtraction because of reduced patient motion between subtracted images.

Temporal Subtraction. Temporal subtraction refers to a number of computer-assisted techniques whereby an image obtained at one time is subtracted from an image obtained at a later time. If, during the intervening period, contrast material was introduced into the vasculature, the subtracted image will contain only the vessels filled with the contrast material. Two methods are commonly used: the **mask mode** and **time-interval difference mode (TID)**.

Mask Mode. A typical mask-mode procedure is diagramed in Figure 28-10. The patient is positioned under normal fluoroscopic control to ensure that the region of anatomy under investigation is within the FOV of the image intensifier.

A power injector is armed and readied to deliver 30 to 50 ml of contrast material at the rate of approximately 15 to 20 ml/s through a venous entry. If an arterial entry is chosen, 10 to 25 ml of diluted contrast material at 10 to 12 ml/s is typical.

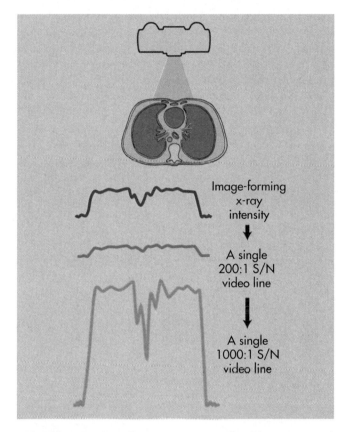

FIGURE 28-9 The information content of a video system with a high signal-to-noise ratio (SNR) is greatly enhanced. Shown here are a single video line through an object and the resulting signal at 200:1 and 1000:1 SNRs.

TABLE 28-1	Comparison of Temporal and Energy Subtraction
Temporal Subtraction	**Energy Subtraction**
A single kVp setting is used.	Rapid voltage switching is required
Normal x-ray beam filtration is adequate.	X-ray beam filter switching is preferred.
Contrast resolution of 1 mm at 1% is achieved.	Higher x-ray intensity is required for comparable contrast resolution.
Simple arithmetic image subtraction is necessary.	Complex image subtraction is necessary.
Motion artifacts are a problem.	Motion artifacts are greatly reduced.
Total subtraction of common structures is achieved.	Some residual bone may survive subtraction.
Subtraction possibilities are limited by number of images.	Many more types of subtraction images are possible.

The imaging apparatus is changed from the fluoroscopic mode to the DF mode. This requires an increase in x-ray tube current of 20 to 100 times the fluoroscopic mode and the activation of a program of pulse image acquisition.

 Mask mode results in successive subtraction images of contrast-filled vessels.

The injector is fired and after a delay of 4 to 10 s, before the bolus of contrast medium reaches the anatomic site, an initial x-ray pulsed exposure is made. The image

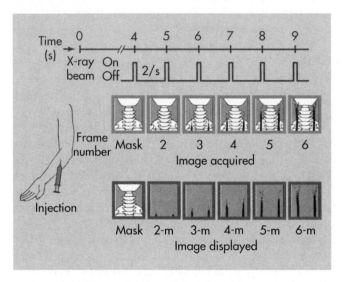

FIGURE 28-10 A schematic representation of mask-mode digital fluoroscopy.

obtained is stored in primary memory and displayed on video monitor A. This is the **mask image.**

This mask image is followed by a series of additional images that are stored in adjacent memory locations. While these subsequent images are being acquired, the mask image is subtracted from each with the result stored in primary memory. At the same time the subtracted image is displayed on video monitor B. Figure 28-11, *A* shows a preinjection mask lateral view of the base of the skull, an image following contrast injection (Figure 28-11, *B*), and a digital subtraction image obtained by subtracting the mask from the injection image (Figure 28-11, *C*).

The digital subtraction of the static object (the skull) allows a better analysis of the opacified arteries especially in their distal parts.

The subtracted images appear in real time and are then stored in memory. After the examination, each subtracted image can be recalled for closer examination.

As described here, each image was obtained from a 33-ms x-ray pulse. The time required for one video frame is 33 ms. Because the video system is relatively slow to respond and the video noise may be high, several video frames (usually four or eight) may be summed in memory to make each image. This process is called **image integration.** Although the process improves contrast resolution, it also increases patient dose because more image frames are acquired.

In mask-mode DF, the imaging sequence after acquisition of the mask can be manually controlled or preprogrammed. If preprogrammed, the computer controls the data acquisition in accordance with the demands of the examination.

To evaluate carotid flow, for example, after a brachial vein injection, the examiner could inject contrast media

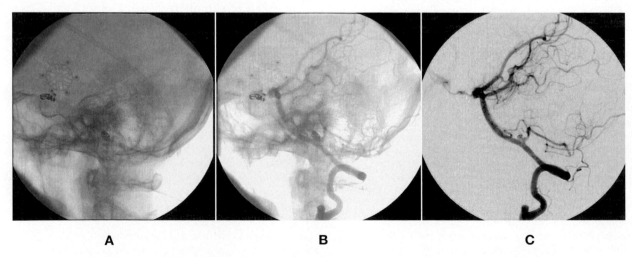

FIGURE 28-11 A, The preinjection mask. **B,** A postinjection image. **C,** Image produced when the preinjection mask is subtracted from the postinjection image. (Courtesy Charles Trihn.)

and acquire a mask image 2 s after the injection. After another 2-s delay, images are obtained at the rate of two per second for 3 s, one per second for 5 s, and one every other second for 14 s. If the computer capacity for acquiring images is sufficient, any combination of multiple delays and varying image acquisition rates is possible.

Remasking. If on subsequent examination the initial mask image is inadequate because of patient motion, improper technique, or any other reason, later images may be used as the mask image. A typical examination may require a total of 30 images in addition to the mask image.

If the intended mask image is technically inadequate and maximum contrast appears during the 15th image, a better subtraction image may be obtained by using image number 5 as the mask rather than image number 1. The examiner can even integrate several images (e.g.,

numbers four through eight) using the composite image as the mask. Unacceptable mask images can be caused by noise, motion, and technical factors.

Time-Interval Difference Mode. Some examinations call for each subtracted image to be made from a different mask and follow-up frame (Figure 28-12).

In a cardiac study, for example, image acquisition begins 5 s after injection at the rate of 15 images per second for 4 s. A total of 60 images is obtained in such a study. These images are identified as frame numbers 1 through 60. Each image is stored in a separate memory address as it is acquired.

If a TID of four images (268 ms) is selected, the first image to appear will be that obtained when frame one is subtracted from frame five. The second image will contain the subtraction of frame two from frame six, the third will contain the subtraction of frame three from frame seven, and so on.

FIGURE 28-12 The manner in which sequentially obtained images are subtracted in a time-interval difference study.

> TID mode produces subtracted images from progressive masks and following frames.

In real time, the images observed convey the flow of the contrast medium dynamically. Subsequent closer examination of each TID image shows it to be relatively free of motion artifacts but with less contrast than mask-mode imaging. As a result, TID imaging is principally applied in cardiac monitoring.

Figure 28-13 shows a typical digital subtraction angiogram (DSA) of the abdominal aorta. First a mask image *(A)* is obtained, then a post injection image *(B)*, and finally a subtracted image *(C)*.

Misregistration. If patient motion occurs between the mask image and a subsequent image, the subtracted

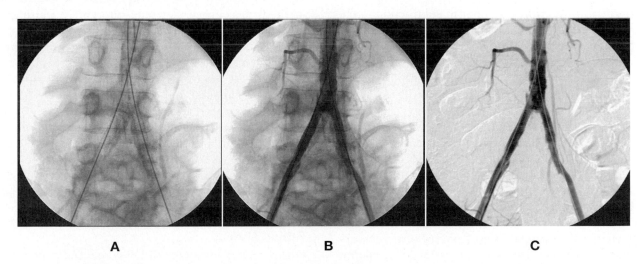

A   B   C

FIGURE 28-13 Digital subtraction angiography (DSA) of the aorto-iliac area revealing the details of the anomalies in the anastomosis region. (Courtesy Dick Fisher.)

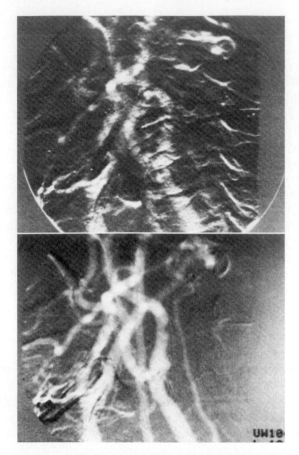

FIGURE 28-14 Misregistration artifacts. (Courtesy Ben Arnold.)

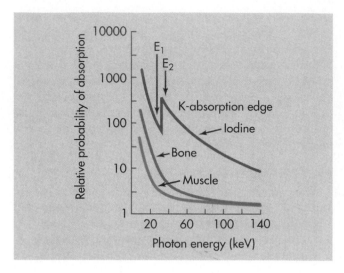

FIGURE 28-15 Photoelectric absorption in iodine, bone, and muscle.

image will contain **misregistration artifacts** (Figure 28-14). The same anatomy is not registered in the same pixel of the image matrix. This type of artifact can frequently be eliminated by **reregistration** of the mask, that is, by shifting the mask by one or more pixels so that **superimposition** of images is again obtained.

Energy Subtraction. Temporal subtraction techniques take advantage of changing contrast media during the time of the examination and require no special demands on the high-voltage generator. Energy subtraction uses two different x-ray beams alternately to provide a subtraction image resulting from differences in photoelectric interaction.

The basis for this technique is similar to that described in Chapter 15 for rare earth screens. It is based on the abrupt change in photoelectric absorption at the K edge of the contrast media compared with that for soft tissue and bone.

Figure 28-15 shows the probability of x-ray interaction with iodine, bone, and muscle as a function of x-ray energy. The probability of photoelectric absorption in all three decreases with increasing x-ray energy. At an energy of 33 keV, there is an abrupt increase in absorption in iodine and a modest decrease in soft tissue and bone.

This energy corresponds to the binding energy of the two K-shell electrons of iodine. When the incident x-ray energy is sufficient to overcome the K-shell electron binding energy of iodine, there is an abrupt and large increase in absorption. Graphically, this increase is known as the **K absorption edge.**

If monoenergetic x-ray beams of 32 and 34 keV could be used alternately, the difference in absorption in iodine would be enormous and the resulting subtraction images would have very high contrast. Such is not the case, however, because every x-ray beam contains a wide spectrum of energies.

Energy subtraction has the decided disadvantage of requiring some method of providing an alternating x-ray beam of two different emission spectra. Two methods have been devised—alternately pulsing the x-ray beam at 70 kVp and then 90 kVp, and introducing dissimilar metal filters into the x-ray beam alternately on a flywheel.

Hybrid Subtraction. Some DF systems are capable of combining temporal and energy subtraction techniques into what is called **hybrid subtraction** (Figure 28-16). Image acquisition follows the mask-mode procedure as previously described. Here, however, the mask and each subsequent image are formed by an energy subtraction technique. If patient motion can be controlled, hybrid imaging can theoretically produce the highest-quality DF images.

Patient Dose

One potential advantage to DF is reduced patient dose. DF images appear to be continuous, but in fact they are discrete. Most DF x-ray beams are pulsed to fill one or more 33-ms video frames; therefore, the fluoroscopic

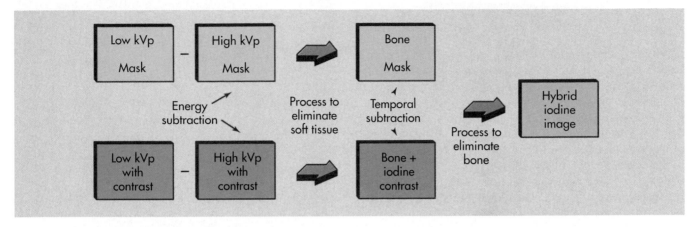

FIGURE 28-16 Hybrid subtraction involves temporal and energy subtraction techniques.

TABLE 28-2	Approximate Patient Dose in a Representative Fluoroscopic Examination		
		PATIENT DOSE	
Imaging Mode		**Conventional**	**Digital**
5 minutes' fluoroscopy		20 rad	10 rad
3 spot films—normal mode		0.6 rad	0.15 rad
3 spot films—mag 1 mode		1.0 rad	0.3 rad
2 spot films—mag 2 mode			0.35 rad
Total dose		21.6 rad	10.8 rad

dose rate is lower than that for continuous analog fluoroscopy even though the mA setting may be higher.

Static images with DF are also made with lower dose per frame than with a 100-mm spot film camera. Both the television camera tube and a CCD have higher sensitivity than the spot film. Table 28-2 compares a representative fluoroscopic study performed conventionally with one performed digitally.

Digital spot images are so easy to acquire that it is possible to make more exposures than is necessary. If the fluoroscopist gets carried away, any patient dose savings will disappear.

PICTURE ARCHIVING AND COMMUNICATION SYSTEM

Radiology is adopting digital imaging very rapidly. Estimates of the present level of digitally acquired images range up to 70%.

These digital images come from nuclear medicine, digital ultrasonography, digital subtraction angiography, computed tomography, and magnetic resonance imaging (MRI). Analog images, such as conventional radiographs, can be digitized using a device such as that shown in Figure 28-17. Such film digitizers are based on laser beam technology.

A picture archiving and communication system (PACS), when fully implemented, allows not only the acquisition but also the interpretation (soft copy) and storage of each medical image in digital form without resorting to film (hard copy). The projected efficiencies of time and cost are enormous. The four principal components of a PACS are the image acquisition system, the display system, the network, and the storage system.

Display System

The heart of a PACS display system is either the cathode ray tube monitor of a video workstation (Figure 28-18) or a solid-state flat panel display. To truly replace film viewing, each must be high resolution, at least 2048 × 2048. Current image matrices used with most digitally acquired images range from 256 × 256 to 1024 × 1024, which is considerably less than that required to equal the spatial resolution of film; however, PACS display stations are equipped with a keyboard and mouse control for the various image-processing modes.

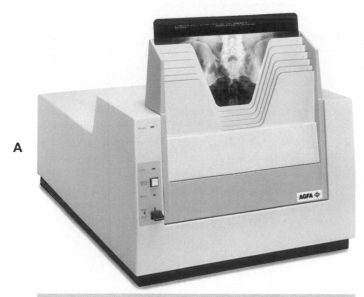

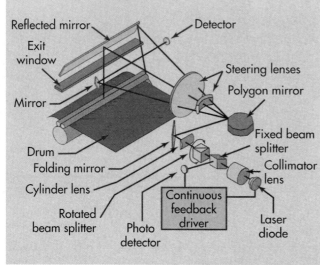

FIGURE 28-17 **A,** This film digitizer uses a laser beam to convert an analog radiograph into a digital image. (Courtesy Agfa.) **B,** The printing to film is similar to that of a laser printer. (Courtesy Imation.)

Some relaxation of the spatial resolution requirements of the workstation is allowed because of the electronic image processing modes that are available. The simplest example is the ability to pan and zoom and change the magnification of the displayed image. Image processing is possible because of the digital nature of the image and the interactive nature of the workstation.

Subtraction of one image from another emphasizes vascular structures. **Edge enhancement** is effective for fractures and small, high-contrast objects. **Windowing** is useful for amplifying soft tissue differences. **Highlighting** can be effective in identifying diffuse nonfocal disease. **Pan, scroll,** and **zoom** allow for careful visualization of precise regions of an image.

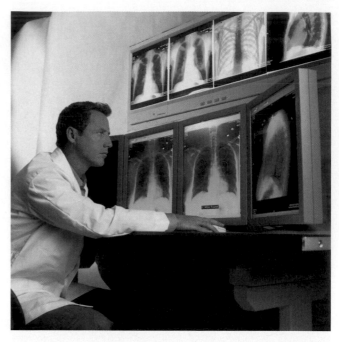

FIGURE 28-18 The picture archiving and communication system (PACS) workstation supports filmless digital image transfer by network. (Courtesy General Electric Medical Systems.)

To be truly effective, each of these image-processing modes must be quick and easy to use. This requires that each workstation be microprocessor-controlled and interact with each imaging device and the central computer. To provide for such interaction, a network is required.

Network

Computer scientists use the term *network* to describe the manner in which many computers can be connected to interact with one another. In a business office, for instance, each secretary might have a microprocessor-based workstation, which is interfaced with a central office computer, so that information can be transferred from one workstation to another or to and from the main computer memory.

In radiology, in addition to secretarial workstations, the network may consist of various types of images, PACS workstations, remote PACS workstations, a departmental mainframe, and a hospital mainframe (Figure 28-19). Each of these devices is called a **client** of the network. **Clients** are interconnected, usually by cable in a building, by telephone or cable television lines among buildings, and by microwave or satellite transmission to remote facilities.

The name **teleradiology** has been given to the process of remote transmission and viewing of images. To ensure adaptability between different types of radio-

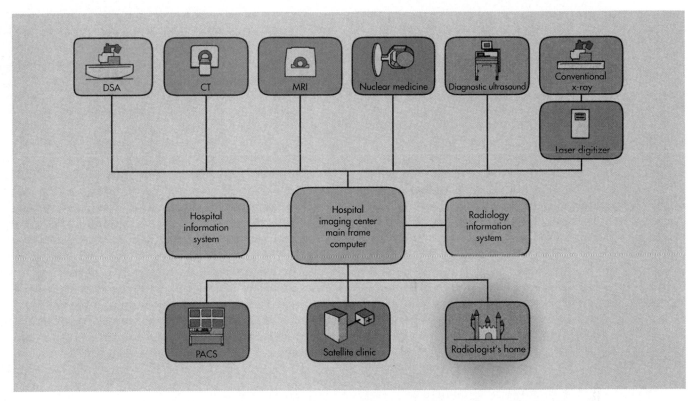

FIGURE 28-19 The picture archiving and communication system (PACS) network allows interaction among the various modes of data acquisition, image processing, and image archiving.

graphic equipment, the American College of Radiology (ACR), in cooperation with the National Electrical Manufacturers Association (NEMA), has produced a standard imaging and interface format called DICOM, for Digital Imaging and Communications in Medicine.

The network begins at the imaging system, where data are acquired in digital form. The images reconstructed from the data are processed at the console of the imaging system or transmitted to a PACS workstation for processing.

At any time, such images can be transferred to other clients within or outside the hospital. Instead of running films up to surgery for viewing on a viewbox, one simply transfers the image electronically to the PACS workstation in surgery.

When a radiologist is not immediately available for image interpretation, the image can be transferred to a PACS workstation in the radiologist's home. Essentially everywhere that film is required now, electronic images can be substituted. Time is essential when considering image manipulation, and therefore fast computers and networks with high bandwidth are required for this task.

These requirements are relaxed for the information management and database portion of PACS, which is the Radiology Information System (RIS). Such lower-priority RIS functions include message and mail utilities, calendar reporting, text data, and financial accounting and planning.

From the RIS workstation, any number of coded diagnostic reports can be initiated and transferred to a secretarial workstation for report generation. The secretarial workstation in turn can communicate with the main hospital computer for patient identification, billing, accounting, and interaction with other departments.

Similarly, a secretarial workstation at the departmental reception desk can interact with a departmental computer for scheduling of patients, technologists, and radiologists and for analysis of departmental statistics. Finally, at the completion of an examination, PACS allows for more efficient image archiving.

Storage System

One motivation for PACS is archiving. How often are films checked out from the file room and never returned? How many films disappear from jackets? How many jackets disappear? How often are films copied for clinicians? Just the cost of the hospital space to accommodate a film file may be sufficient to justify PACS.

Question: How much computer capacity is required to store an MRI examination consisting of 120 images, each with image matrix size of 256 × 256 and 256 shades of gray?

Answer:

Size of matrix		Shades of gray
256 × 256	×	256
256 × 256	×	8 bit
65,536	×	1 byte
		= 65,536 bytes

120 × 65,536 = 7,864,320 bytes or approximately 7.9 MB

Question: How much computer capacity is required to store a single chest image having a 4096 × 4096 matrix size and a 12-bit dynamic range (considered by most as minimally acceptable)?

Answer: This is a 4096 × 4096 matrix with 1024 shades of gray.

Size of matrix	Shades of gray
4096 × 4096	12 bit
16,777,216	1.5 byte
= 25,165,824 bytes	
or approximately 25 MB	

With PACS, a film file room is replaced by a magnetic or optical memory device. The future of PACS, however, depends on the continuing development of the optical disk. Optical disks can accommodate tens of gigabytes (GB) of data and images and, when stored in a "jukebox" (Figure 28-20), can accommodate terabytes (TB).

An entire hospital file room can be accommodated by a storage device the size of a desk. Electronically, images can be recalled from this archival system to any workstation in seconds.

SUMMARY

DF has added a computer, two monitors, and a complex control panel to conventional fluoroscopy equipment. The macrocomputers in DF control the image matrix size, the system dynamic range, and the image acquisition rate. Eight to 30 images per second can be acquired with DF depending on the image matrix mode.

Subtraction is a process of removing or masking all unnecessary anatomy from an image and enhancing only the anatomy of interest. With DF, subtraction is accomplished by either temporal or energy subtraction.

Digital processing can be used in diagnostic imaging departments for picture archiving and communication systems (PACS). The file room can be replaced by a magnetic or optical memory device about the size of a desk. Teleradiology is the remote transmission of digital images to workstations in other areas of the hospital or offsite.

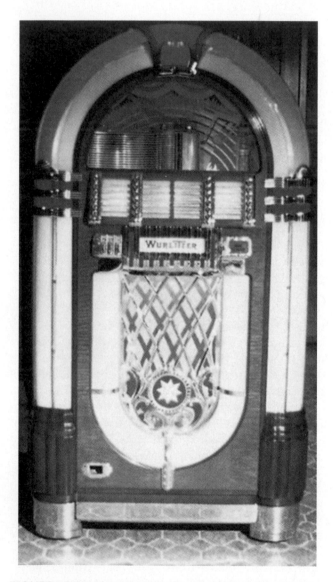

FIGURE 28-20 This 1946 Wurlitzer jukebox with its 78-rpm platters serves as a model for the optical disc jukebox of a picture archiving and communication system (PACS). (Courtesy Raymond Wilenzek.)

CHALLENGE QUESTIONS

1. Define or otherwise identify:
   a. Digital subtraction angiography
   b. Registration
   c. Interrogation time
   d. Hybrid subtraction
   e. CCD
   f. ROI
   g. Progressive video read
   h. Image Integration
   i. Node
   j. PACS

2. What are the principal advantages of DF over conventional fluoroscopy?
3. Describe the sequence of image acquisition in mask-mode fluoroscopy.
4. Describe the differences between a video system operating in the interlace mode and one operating in the progressive mode.
5. What is the reason that all electronic devices are inherently noisy?
6. Describe the process of energy subtraction.
7. What determines the spatial resolution of a DF system?
8. A DF system is operated in a 512×512 image mode with a 23-cm image intensifier. What is the size of each pixel?
9. The dynamic range of certain DF systems is described as being 12 bits deep. What does this mean?
10. What principally determines spatial resolution in digital imaging?
11. How much computer capacity is required to store 30 DF images having 12-bit dynamic range and a 1024×1024 matrix?
12. What is the pixel size of a 1000-line video system when the DF image intensifier is operated in the 12-cm mode?
13. Describe the equipment required to implement teleradiology.
14. What additional equipment is required to progress from conventional fluoroscopy to DF?
15. Discuss the patient dose implications associated with DF compared with conventional fluoroscopy.
16. How much time is required to acquire one video frame?
17. What x-ray energy (keV) would result in greatest contrast in digital subtraction angiography using an iodinated contrast agent ($E_6 = 33$ keV)?
18. What are some advantages to the use of a CCD instead of a TV camera tube?
19. How can misregistration artifacts be corrected?
20. Why is signal-to-noise ratio important in DF?

Computed Tomography

OBJECTIVES

At the completion of this chapter, the student should be able to do the following:

1. Discuss the concepts of transverse tomography, translation, and reconstruction of images
2. List and describe the various generations of computed tomography (CT) imaging systems
3. Relate the CT system components and their functions
4. Describe CT image characteristics of image matrix and Hounsfield unit
5. Review image reconstruction
6. Discuss image quality as it relates to spatial resolution, contrast resolution, noise, linearity, and uniformity

OUTLINE

THE COMPUTED TOMOGRAPHY (CT) imaging system is revolutionary. There is no ordinary image receptor, such as film or an image-intensifier tube. A well-collimated x-ray beam is directed on the patient and the attenuated image-forming radiation is measured by a detector whose response is transmitted to a computer.

After analyzing the signal from the detector, the computer reconstructs the image and displays the image on a monitor. The computer reconstruction of the cross-sectional anatomy is accomplished with mathematical equations (algorithms) adapted for computer processing.

To perform CT imaging effectively, the radiologic technologist must know something of the development of CT, the system components, and the characteristics of the CT image. These topics are presented in this chapter, along with a discussion of CT quality control.

The components necessary to construct a computed tomographic (CT) imaging system were available to medical physicists 20 years before Godfrey Hounsfield first demonstrated the technique in 1970. Hounsfield was a physicist/engineer with EMI, Ltd., the British company most famous for recording the Beatles, and both he and his company have received justifiably high acclaim.

Alan Cormack, a Tufts University medical physicist, shared the 1982 Nobel Prize in physics with Hounsfield. Cormack had earlier developed the mathematics now used to reconstruct CT images.

The CT imaging system is an invaluable radiologic diagnostic tool. Its development and introduction into radiologic practice have assumed an importance comparable with the Snook interrupterless transformer, the Coolidge hot-cathode x-ray tube, the Potter-Bucky diaphragm, and the image-intensifier tube. No other development in x-ray apparatus in the past 40 years is as significant.

One could argue correctly that magnetic resonance imaging (MRI) or diagnostic ultrasonography is equally as significant. However, neither is an x-ray procedure.

CT is revolutionary in that it does not record an image in the conventional way. There is no ordinary image receptor, such as film or an image-intensifier tube. A collimated x-ray beam is directed on the patient and the attenuated image-forming radiation is detected by a solid-state image receptor.

The computer analyzes the signal from the detector, reconstructs an image, and displays the image on a monitor. The computer reconstruction of the cross-sectional anatomy is accomplished with mathematical equations adapted for computer processing called **algorithms.**

The difference in operating characteristics and image quality is far greater over the range of CT imaging systems than for a comparable top-to-bottom range of conventional radiographic equipment. It is particularly important to perform a careful evaluation before purchasing a CT imaging system because of the many features now available. Scheduled preventive maintenance is a must.

PRINCIPLES OF OPERATION

When the abdomen is imaged with conventional radiographic techniques, the image is created directly on the film image receptor and is low in contrast principally because of scatter radiation. The image is also degraded because of superposition of all the anatomic structures in the abdomen.

For better visualization of an abdominal structure, such as the kidneys, conventional tomography can be used (Figure 29-1). In nephrotomography, the renal outline is distinct because the overlying and underlying tissues are blurred. In addition, the contrast of the in-focus structures has been enhanced. Yet, the image is still rather dull and blurred.

Conventional tomography is called **axial tomography** because the plane of the image is parallel with the long axis of the body and results in sagittal and coronal images. A CT image is a transaxial or **transverse** image. The image is perpendicular to the long axis of the body (Figure 29-2).

The precise methodology by which a CT imaging system produces a cross-sectional image is extremely complicated and requires a good knowledge of physics, engineering, and computer science. The basic principles, however, can be demonstrated if one considers the simplest of CT systems, consisting of a finely collimated x-ray beam and a single detector (Figure 29-3). The x-ray source and detector are connected so that they move synchronously.

When the source-detector assembly makes one sweep, or **translation,** across the patient, the internal structures of the body attenuate the x-ray beam according to their mass density and effective atomic number, as discussed in Chapter 12. The intensity of radiation detected varies according to this attenuation pattern and forms an intensity profile, or **projection** (Figure 29-4).

At the end of this translation, the source detector assembly returns to its starting position and the entire assembly **rotates** and begins a second translation. During the second translation, the detector signal will again be proportional to the x-ray beam attenuation of anatomic structures and a second projection will be described.

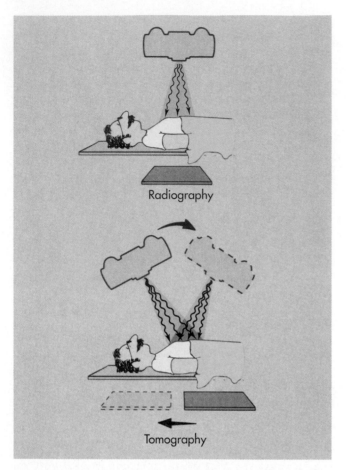

FIGURE 29-1 Equipment arrangement for obtaining a radiograph and a conventional tomograph.

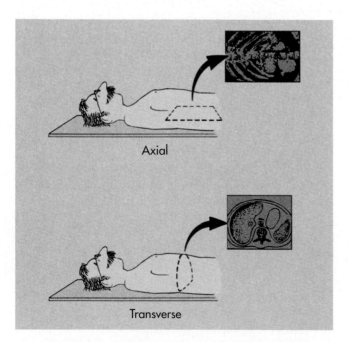

FIGURE 29-2 Conventional tomography results in an image that is parallel to the long axis of the body. CT produces a transverse image.

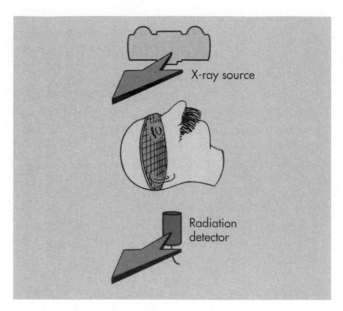

FIGURE 29-3 In its simplest form, a computed tomography imaging system consists of a finely collimated x-ray beam and a single detector, both moving synchronously in a translate–rotate mode.

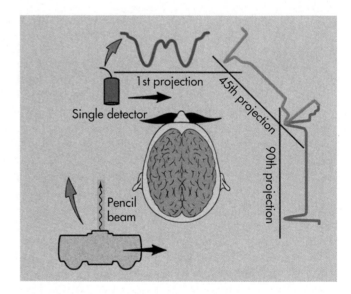

FIGURE 29-4 Each sweep of the source-detector assembly results in a projection, which represents the attenuation pattern of the patient profile.

If this process is repeated many times, a large number of projections is generated. These projections are not displayed visually but are stored in digital form in the computer. The computer processing of these projections involves the effective superimposition of each projection to **reconstruct** an image of the anatomic structures in that slice.

The superimposition of the projections does not occur as one might imagine. The detector signal during each translation is registered in increments with values as high as 1000. The value for each increment is related to the x-ray attenuation coefficient of the total path through the tissue. Through the use of simultaneous equations, a matrix of values is obtained that represents the cross-sectional anatomy.

OPERATIONAL MODES

First-Generation Imaging System

The previous description of a finely collimated x-ray beam and single detector assembly translating across the patient and rotating between successive translations is characteristic of **first-generation CT imaging systems**. The original EMI imaging system required 180 translations; each separated by a 1-degree rotation (Figure 29-5). It incorporated two detectors and split the finely collimated x-ray beam so two contiguous slices could be imaged during each procedure. The principal drawback to these systems was that nearly 5 minutes was required to complete one image.

 First-generation imaging system—translate–rotate, pencil beam, single detector, 5-minute imaging time.

Second-Generation Imaging System

First-generation CT imaging systems can be considered a demonstration project. They demonstrated the feasibility of the functional marriage of the source-detector assembly, the mechanical gantry motion, and the computer to produce an image.

Second-generation imaging systems were also of the translate–rotate type. These units incorporated the natural extension of the single detector to a multiple detector assembly intercepting a fan-shaped rather than a pencil-shaped x-ray beam (Figure 29-6).

One disadvantage to the fan beam is increased scatter radiation. This affects the final image in much the same way as in conventional radiography.

Another disadvantage is the increased intensity toward the edges of the beam because of body shape. This is compensated by use of a "bow tie" filter. The characteristic features of a second-generation CT imaging system are shown in Figure 29-7.

The principal advantage of the second-generation CT imaging system was speed. These imaging systems had 5 to 30 detectors in the detector assembly, and therefore shorter imaging times were possible. Because of the multiple detector array, a single translation resulted in the same number of data points as several translations with a first-generation CT imaging system. Consequently, each translation was separated by rotation increments of 5 degrees or more. With a 10-degree rotation

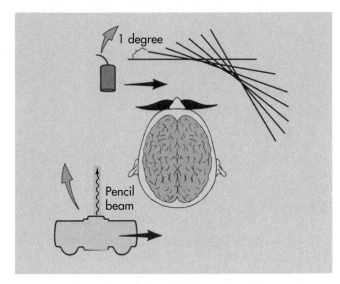

FIGURE 29-5 First-generation computed tomography imaging systems used a pencil-shaped x-ray beam and a single detector moving in the translate–rotate mode.

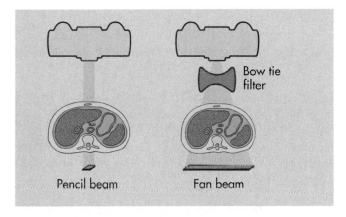

FIGURE 29-6 Profiles of two x-ray beams used in computed tomography imaging. With the fan-shaped beam, a bow-tie filter is sometimes used to equalize the radiation intensity reaching the detector array.

increment, only 18 translations would be required for a 180-degree image acquisition.

 Second-generation imaging system—translate–rotate, fan beam, detector array, 30-second imaging time.

Third-Generation Imaging System

The principal limitation of second-generation CT imaging systems was examination time. Because of the complex mechanical motion of translation–rotation and the

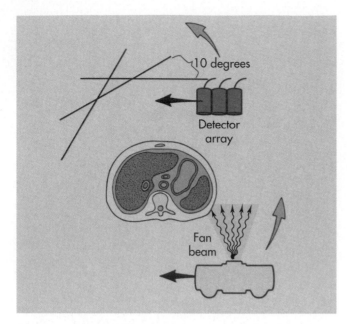

FIGURE 29-7 Second-generation computed tomography imaging systems operated in the translate–rotate mode with a multiple detector array intercepting a fan-shaped x-ray beam.

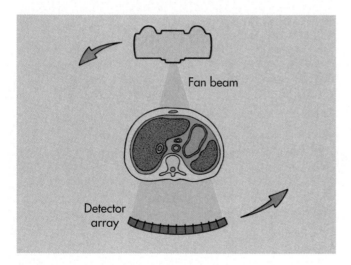

FIGURE 29-8 Third-generation computed tomography imaging systems operate in the rotate-only mode with a fan x-ray beam and a multiple detector array revolving concentrically around the patient.

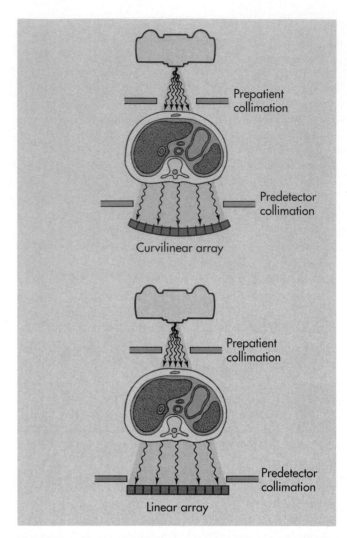

FIGURE 29-9 The linear detector array is characteristic of first- and second-generation computed tomography imaging systems; the curvilinear array is used in third- and fourth-generation imaging systems. The collimation is actually positioned on either side of the section imaged.

The third-generation CT imaging system uses a curvilinear array containing many detectors and a fan beam. The number of detectors and the width of the fan beam, between 30 and 60 degrees, are both substantially larger than for second-generation imaging systems. In third-generation CT imaging systems, the fan beam and detector array view the entire patient at all times.

The curvilinear detector array results in a constant source-to-detector path length, which is an advantage for good image reconstruction. This feature of the third-generation detector assembly also allows for better x-ray beam collimation to reduce the effect of scatter radiation. Figure 29-9 compares the detector assembly functions for second- and third-generation CT imaging systems.

enormous mass involved in the gantry, most units were designed for imaging times of 20 seconds or more. This limitation was overcome by **third-generation imaging systems.** In these imaging systems, the source and detector array are rotated about the patient (Figure 29-8). As rotate-only units, third-generation imaging systems can produce an image in less than 1 second.

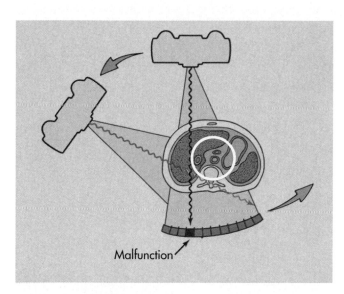

FIGURE 29-10 Ring artifacts can occur in third-generation computed tomography imaging systems because each detector views an anulus (ring) of anatomy during the examination.

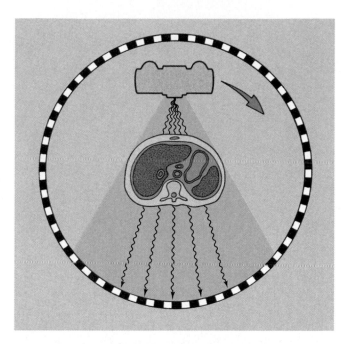

FIGURE 29-11 Fourth-generation computed tomography imaging systems operate with a rotating x-ray source and stationary detectors.

One of the principal disadvantages of third-generation CT imaging systems is the occasional appearance of ring artifacts. Should any single detector or bank of detectors malfunction, the acquired signal or lack thereof results in a ring on the reconstructed image (Figure 29-10). Software-corrected image reconstruction algorithms minimize such artifacts.

 Third-generation imaging system—rotate-rotate, fan beam, detector array, subsecond imaging time, ring artifacts.

Fourth-Generation Imaging System

The **fourth-generation** design for CT imaging systems incorporates a rotate–stationary configuration. The x-ray source rotates but the detector assembly does not.

Radiation detection is accomplished through a fixed circular array of detectors (Figure 29-11), which contains as many as 4000 individual elements. The x-ray beam is fan shaped with characteristics similar to those of third-generation fan beams. These units are capable of subsecond imaging times, can accommodate variable slice thickness through automatic prepatient collimation, and can provide the image manipulation capabilities of earlier imaging systems.

The fixed detector array of fourth-generation CT imaging systems does not result in a constant beam path from the source to all detectors, but it does allow each detector to be calibrated and its signal normalized dur-

ing each image, as was possible with second-generation imaging systems. Fourth-generation imaging systems are usually free of ring artifacts.

The principal disadvantage of fourth-generation CT imaging systems is patient dose, which is somewhat higher than with other types of imaging systems. The cost of these systems may be somewhat higher also because of the large number of detectors and their associated electronics.

Although many comparisons of image quality have been attempted, no generalizations are possible, and a clear decision regarding the best image is not likely. Much of the final image quality depends on the mathematics of image reconstruction, and these techniques are continually being refined.

 Fourth-generation imaging system—rotate–stationary, fan beam, detector array, subsecond imaging time.

Fifth-Generation Imaging System

Continuing developments in CT imaging system design promise further improvements in image quality at lower patient dose. Some incorporate novel motions of either the x-ray tube or the detector array, or both. Some involve patient motion as well. None of these designs has been acclaimed as the fifth-generation design, but spiral CT is the leading candidate.

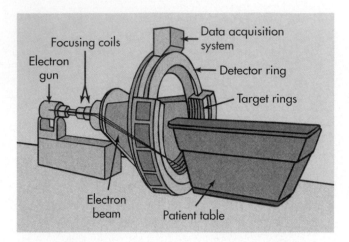

FIGURE 29-12 Electron beam computed tomography has no moving parts in the gantry.

Rotate–Nutate. Toshiba produced a novel extension of fourth-generation imaging systems. To maintain the x-ray source at the same distance from the patient as the detectors, the detector array nutated or wobbled as the x-ray source rotated.

Electron Beam CT. Electron beam CT (EBCT), a fundamentally different way to produce CT images, was pioneered by Imatron for cardiac imaging. The term "Heartscan" is used by many to describe this technique. EBCT is used to image all tissues, but especially when ultrafast imaging is required.

The EBCT consists of a **waveguide** to accelerate a focused electron beam onto a semicircular tungsten target through a bending magnet (Figure 29-12). Actually, there are four tungsten targets so that four tissue slices are imaged at the same time.

Nothing in the EBCT gantry moves except the electron beam. The tungsten target is fixed and so is the detector array. EBCT images are produced in as little as 50 ms.

SYSTEM COMPONENTS

It was convenient to classify the components of a conventional x-ray imaging system into three major subsystems: the x-ray tube, the generator, and the operating console. It also is convenient to identify the three major components of a CT imaging system: the gantry, the computer, and the operating console (Figure 29-13). Each of these major components has several subsystems.

Gantry

The gantry includes the x-ray tube, the detector array, the high-voltage generator, the patient support couch, and the mechanical support for each. These subsystems receive electronic commands from the operating console and transmit data to the computer for image production and postprocessing.

X-ray Tube. X-ray tubes used in CT imaging have special requirements. Although some operate at relatively low tube current, for many, the instantaneous power capacity must be high. The anode heating capacity must be at least several million heat units (MHU), and some tubes designed specifically for CT have 8 MHU capacity.

High-speed rotors are used in most for the best heat dissipation. Experience has shown that x-ray tube failure is a principal cause of CT imaging system malfunction and the principal limitation on sequential imaging frequency.

Focal spot size is also important in most designs, even though the CT image is not based on principles of direct projection imaging. CT imaging systems designed for high spatial resolution imaging incorporate x-ray tubes with a small focal spot.

X-ray tubes are energized differently, depending on the CT imaging system design. Third-generation CT imaging systems operate with either a continuous or a pulsed x-ray beam. Continuous x-ray beams at tube currents up to 400 mA are produced during the entire rotation. Pulsed x-ray beams at tube currents approaching 1000 mA are produced with pulse widths from 1 to 5 ms at pulse repetition rates of 60 Hz.

Detector Array. Early CT imaging systems had one detector. Modern CT imaging systems have multiple detectors in an array numbering up to tens of thousands in two general classifications: scintillation detectors and gas detectors.

Scintillation Detectors. Early scintillation detector arrays contained scintillation crystal–photomultiplier tube assemblies. These detectors could not be packed very tightly together and they required a power supply for each photomultiplier tube. Consequently, they have been replaced with scintillation crystal–photodiode assemblies.

Photodiodes convert light into electronic signal. They are smaller and cheaper, do not require a power supply, and are as efficient as other CT radiation detectors.

Sodium iodide (NaI) was the crystal used in the earliest imaging systems. This was quickly replaced by bismuth germanate ($Bi_4Ge_3O_{12}$ or BGO) and cesium iodide (CsI). Cadmium tungstate ($CdWO_4$) and special ceramics are the current crystals of choice. The concentration of scintillation detectors is an important characteristic of a CT imaging system that affects the spatial resolution of the system.

Scintillation detectors have high x-ray detection efficiency. Approximately 90% of the x-rays incident on the detector are absorbed and contribute to the output signal. It is now possible to pack the detectors so that the space between them is nil. Consequently, the overall detection efficiency approaches 90%.

Gas Detectors. Gas-filled detectors are also used in CT imaging systems (Figure 29-14). They are con-

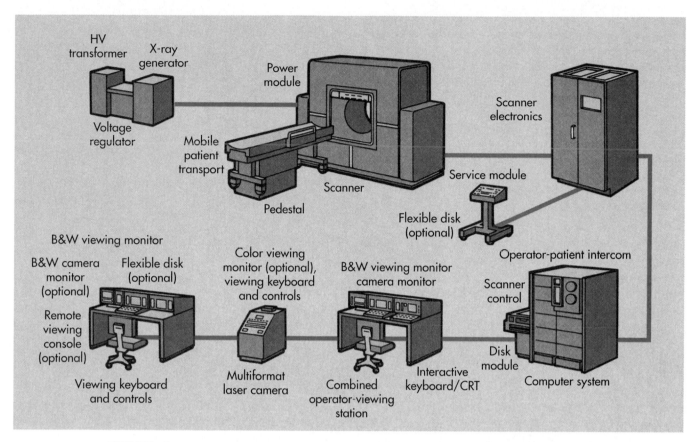

FIGURE 29-13 Components of a complete computed tomography imaging system. (Courtesy Philips Medical Systems.)

structed of a large metallic chamber with baffles spaced at approximately 1-mm intervals. The baffles are like grid strips and divide the large chamber into many small chambers.

Each small chamber functions as a separate radiation detector. The entire detector array is hermetically sealed and filled under pressure with a high atomic number inert gas, such as xenon or a xenon–krypton mixture. Ionization of the gas in each chamber is proportional to the radiation incident on the chamber and is detected in much the same way as the **ideal gas-filled detector** described in Chapter 39.

The intrinsic detection efficiency of a gas-filled detector is only approximately 45%; however, the detector interspace can be reduced so that very little of the face area of the detector assembly is not used. The geometric efficiency is diagrammed in Figure 29-15, which shows a comparison between the scintillation detector array and the gas detector array. Consequently, the overall total detection efficiency for a gas-filled detector array is approximately 45%. This contributes to increased patient dose and has resulted in abandonment of gas-filled detector arrays.

Collimation. Collimation is required during CT imaging for precisely the same reasons as in conventional radiography. Proper collimation reduces patient dose by re-

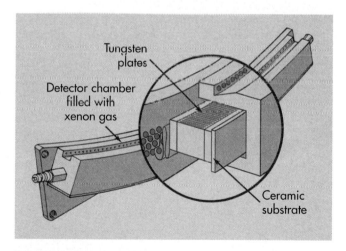

FIGURE 29-14 A gas-filled detector array features small detectors in high concentration with little interdetector dead space. (Courtesy General Electric Medical Systems.)

stricting the volume of tissue irradiated. More important, it enhances image contrast by limiting scatter radiation.

In conventional radiography there is only one collimator, which is mounted on the x-ray tube housing. In CT imaging, there are usually two collimators (Figure 29-16).

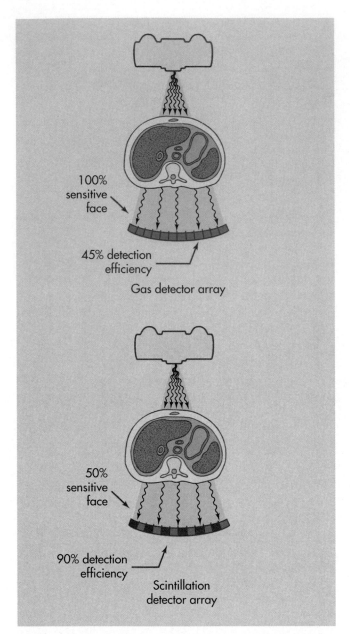

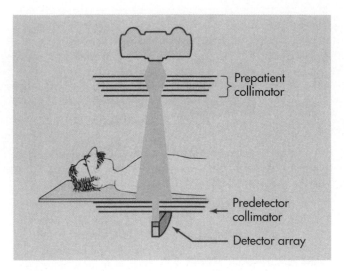

FIGURE 29-16 Computed tomography imaging systems incorporate both a prepatient collimator and a predetector collimator.

FIGURE 29-15 Overall detection efficiency of a gas-filled detector array is approximately equal to that of the scintillation detector array.

The **predetector collimator** restricts the x-ray beam viewed by the detector array. This collimator reduces the scatter radiation incident on the detector array and, when properly coupled with the prepatient collimator, defines the slice thickness, also called *sensitivity profile*. The predetector collimator reduces scatter radiation reaching the detector array and therefore improves image contrast.

The predetector collimator determines sensitivity profile and slice thickness.

High-Voltage Generator. All CT imaging systems operate on high-frequency power. This accommodates the higher x-ray tube rotor speeds and the instantaneous power surges characteristic of pulsed systems. Most manufacturers conserve space by mounting the high-voltage generator on the rotating wheel of the gantry.

Patient Positioning and Support Couch. In addition to supporting the patient comfortably, the patient couch must be constructed of low-Z material, such as carbon fiber, so that it does not interfere with x-ray beam transmission and patient imaging. It should be smoothly and accurately motor driven to allow precise patient positioning. This is particularly important during spiral CT.

When patient couch positioning is not exact, the same tissue can be imaged twice, doubling the dose, or missed altogether. The patient couch should be capable of automatic indexing so that the operator does not have to enter the examination room between each image. Such a feature reduces the examination time required for each patient.

One collimator is mounted on the x-ray tube housing or adjacent to it. This collimator limits the area of the patient that intercepts the useful beam, and thereby determines patient dose. This **prepatient collimator** usually consists of several sections so that a nearly parallel x-ray beam results.

Prepatient collimation determines dose profile and patient dose.

Computer

The computer is a unique subsystem of the CT imaging system. Depending on the image format, as many as 250,000 equations must be solved simultaneously; thus, a large computing capacity is required.

At the heart of the computer used in CT are the microprocessor and primary memory. These determine the time between the end of imaging and the appearance of an image, the **reconstruction time.** Subsecond reconstruction times are now common. The efficiency of an examination is greatly influenced by reconstruction time, especially when a large number of image slices are involved.

 Reconstruction time is the time from end of imaging to image appearance.

Many CT imaging systems use an **array processor** instead of a microprocessor for image reconstruction. The array processor does many calculations simultaneously and hence is significantly faster than the microprocessor.

Operating Console

CT imaging systems can be equipped with two or three consoles. One console is for the CT radiologic technologist to operate the imaging system. Another console may be available for a technologist to postprocess images for filming and filing. A third console may be available for the physician to view the images and manipulate image contrast, size, and general visual appearance.

The operating console contains meters and controls for selecting proper imaging technique factors, for proper mechanical movement of the gantry and patient couch, and for computer commands allowing image reconstruction and transfer. The physician's viewing console accepts the reconstructed image from the operator's console and displays it for viewing and diagnosis.

A typical operating console contains controls and monitors for the various technique factors (Figure 29-17). Operation is usually in excess of 120 kVp. The usual mA station is 100 mA if the x-ray beam is continuous and several hundred mA if it is a pulsed beam.

The thickness of the tissue slice to be imaged can also be adjusted. Nominal thicknesses are 1 to 10 mm, but some units provide slice thicknesses as thin as 0.5 mm for high-resolution imaging. Slice thickness is selected from the console by automatic collimator adjustment.

Controls are also provided for automatic movement and indexing of the patient support couch. This allows the operator to program for contiguous slices or for intermittent slices.

The operating console usually has two monitors. One is provided for the operator to annotate patient data on the image (e.g., hospital identification, name, patient number, age, sex) and to provide identification for each image (e.g., number, technique, couch posi-

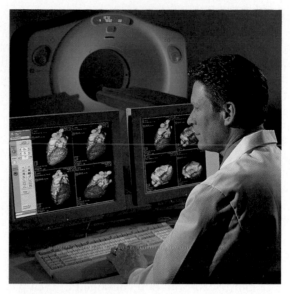

FIGURE 29-17 Operator's console for a computed tomography imaging system. (Courtesy General Electric Medical Systems.)

tion). The second monitor is provided for the operator to view the resulting image before transferring it to either hard copy or the physician's viewing console.

Physician's Viewing Console. Smaller, less expensive CT imaging systems may not have a physician's viewing console. If the workload is high and the system fully utilized, however, a physician's viewing console is essential so that patient images can be reviewed and reported without interfering with imaging operations. For maximum effectiveness, the physician's viewing console is supported by an independent computer.

This console allows the physician to call up any previous image and manipulate that image to optimize diagnostic information. The manipulative controls provide for contrast and brightness adjustments, magnification techniques, region of interest (ROI) viewing, and use of on-line computer software packages.

This software may include programs to generate plots of CT numbers along any preselected axis, computation of mean and standard deviation of CT values in an ROI, subtraction techniques, and planar and volumetric quantitative analysis. Reconstruction of images along coronal, sagittal, and oblique planes is also possible.

Image Storage. There are a number of useful image storage formats. CT imaging systems store current images on **disks,** and sometimes images are archived on magnetic tape. Removable hard disks are also used for archiving.

For later viewing and filing, CT images are sometimes recorded on film with a laser camera. Typical cameras use 14 × 17 inch films and can provide 1, 2, 4, 6, or 12 images to a film.

IMAGE CHARACTERISTICS

The image obtained in CT is unlike that obtained in conventional radiography. In radiography, x-rays form an image directly on the image receptor—the film. With CT imaging systems, the x-rays form a stored electronic image that is displayed as a matrix of intensities.

Image Matrix

The CT image format consists of many cells, each assigned a number and displayed as an optical density or brightness level on the monitor. The original EMI format consisted of an 80 × 80 matrix, for a total of 6400 individual cells of information. Current imaging systems provide matrices of 512 × 512, resulting in 262,144 cells of information.

Each cell of information is a **pixel** (picture element) and the numeric information contained in each pixel is a CT number or **Hounsfield Unit (HU)**. The pixel is a two-dimensional representation of a corresponding tissue volume (Figure 29-18).

The diameter of image reconstruction is called the **field of view (FOV)**. When the FOV is increased for a fixed matrix size, for example from 12 cm to 20 cm, the size of each pixel is increased proportionately. When the matrix size is increased for a fixed FOV, for example 512 × 512 to 1024 × 1024, pixel size is smaller.

PIXEL SIZE

$$\text{Pixel size} = \frac{\text{FOV}}{\text{Matrix size}}$$

Question: Compute the pixel size for the following characteristics of CT images used for brain scans:
a. FOV 20 cm, 120 × 120 matrix
b. FOV 20 cm, 512 × 512 matrix
c. FOV 36 cm, 512 × 512 matrix

Answer: a. $\dfrac{200 \text{ mm}}{120 \text{ pixels}} = 1.7 \text{ mm/pixel}$

b. $\dfrac{200 \text{ mm}}{512 \text{ pixels}} = 0.4 \text{ mm/pixel}$

c. $\dfrac{360 \text{ mm}}{512 \text{ pixels}} = 0.7 \text{ mm/pixel}$

The tissue volume is known as a **voxel** (volume element) and it is determined by multiplying the pixel size by the thickness of the CT image slice.

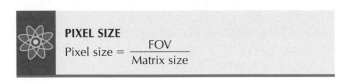

VOXEL SIZE

Voxel size (mm³) = pixel size (mm²) × slice thickness (mm)

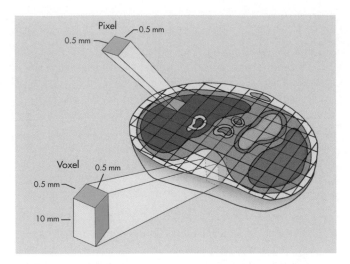

FIGURE 29-18 Each cell in a computed tomography image matrix is a two-dimensional representation (pixel) of a volume of tissue (voxel).

Question: If each of the three brain scans in the preceding question was conducted at a 5-mm slice thickness, what would be the respective voxel sizes?

Answer: a. (1.7 mm)² × 5 mm = 14.5 mm³
b. (0.4 mm)² × 5 mm = 0.8 mm³
c. (0.7 mm)² × 5 mm = 2.5 mm³

CT Numbers

Each pixel is displayed on the monitor as a level of brightness and on the photographic image as a level of optical density. These levels correspond to a range of CT numbers from −1000 to +1000 for each pixel. A CT number of −1000 corresponds to air, a CT number of +1000 corresponds to dense bone. A CT number of zero indicates water. Table 29-1 shows the CT values for various tissues along with respective x-ray linear attenuation coefficients.

The precise CT number of any given pixel is related to the x-ray attenuation coefficient of the tissue contained in the voxel. As discussed in Chapter 12, the degree of x-ray attenuation is determined by the average energy of the x-ray beam and the effective atomic number of the absorber and is expressed by the attenuation coefficient.

The value of a CT number is given by the following:

CT NUMBERS

$$\text{CT number} = k\left(\frac{\mu_t - \mu_w}{\mu_w}\right)$$

where μ_t is the attenuation coefficient of the tissue in the pixel under analysis, μ_w is the x-ray attenuation coefficient of water, and k is a constant that determines the scale factor for the range of CT numbers.

TABLE 29-1	CT Number for Various Tissues and X-Ray Linear Attenuation Coefficients (cm⁻¹) at Three kVp

		LINEAR ATTENUATION COEFFICIENT (CM⁻¹)		
Tissue	Approximate CT Number	100 kVp	125 kVp	150 kVp
Dense bone	1000	0.528	0.460	0.410
Muscle	50	0.237	0.208	0.184
White matter	45	0.213	0.187	0.166
Gray matter	40	0.212	0.184	0.163
Blood	20	0.208	0.182	0.163
Cerebrospinal fluid	15	0.207	0.181	0.160
Water	0	0.206	0.180	0.160
Fat	−100	0.185	0.162	0.144
Lungs	200	0.093	0.081	0.072
Air	1000	0.0004	0.0003	0.0002

This equation shows that the CT number for water is always zero because for water, $\mu_t = \mu_w$ so that $\mu_t - \mu_w = 0$. For the CT imaging system to operate with precision, detector response must continuously be calibrated so that water is always represented by zero.

 When k is 1000, the CT numbers are called Hounsfield Units.

Obviously, there is an enormous amount of information that is wasted when the actual dynamic range of the image is 2000 but it is displayed on a video screen or film at no more than 32 shades of gray. However, postprocessing with window and level adjustment allows the entire range to be made visible.

IMAGE RECONSTRUCTION

The projections acquired by each detector during CT are stored in computer memory. The image is reconstructed from these projections by a process called **filtered back projection.**

Here, the term **filter** refers to a mathematical function rather than a metal filter for the x-ray beam. This process is much too complicated to be discussed here, but a simple example helps explain how it works.

Imagine a box with two holes cut in each side (Figure 29-19). The box is divided into four cells labeled *a, b, c,* and *d,* and there is a Texas-sized cockroach in cell *c.* If we now cover the box and look through the four sets of holes, we can devise a way of determining precisely in which section the cockroach resides.

Let "1" represent the presence of the cockroach for each viewing. If one can see through a hole, two empty

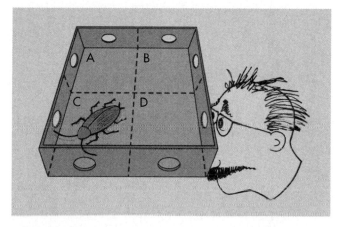

FIGURE 29-19 This four pixel matrix demonstrates the method for reconstructing a computed tomography image by back projection.

cells and the opposite hole, then obviously the cockroach is not there. We indicate the absence of the cockroach with "0." The path being viewed in Figure 29-19 can be represented symbolically as $c + d = 1$. Examining all possible paths show:

$$a + b = 0$$
$$c + d = 1$$
$$a + c = 1$$
$$b + d = 0$$

The result is four equations for which, if solved simultaneously, the solution is $c = 1$ and *a, b,* and $d = 0$.

In CT, we would have not four cells (pixels) but rather over 250,000. Consequently, CT image reconstruction requires the solution of over 250,000 simultaneous equations.

IMAGE QUALITY

The image quality of conventional radiographs is expressed in terms of spatial resolution, contrast resolution, and noise. These characteristics are relatively easy to describe but somewhat difficult to measure and express quantitatively.

Because CT images are composed of discrete pixel values, image quality is somewhat easier to characterize and quantitate. A number of methods are available for measuring CT image quality, and there are five principal characteristics that are numerically assigned. These are spatial resolution, contrast resolution, noise, linearity, and uniformity.

Spatial Resolution

If one images a regular geometric structure that has a sharp interface, the image at the interface will be somewhat blurred (Figure 29-20). The degree of blurring is a measure of the spatial resolution of the system and is controlled by a number of factors. Because the image of the interface is a visual rendition of pixel values, these values could be analyzed across the interface to arrive at a measure of spatial resolution.

Suppose the spine in Figure 29-20 was a square of material of a relatively high CT value (e.g., 1000). This would be a relatively high contrast interface. The CT numbers across the interface might have actual values, such as those shown in the object graph in Figure 29-20.

Because, however, the image is somewhat blurred owing to limitations of the CT imaging system, the expected sharp edge of CT values is replaced with a smoothed range of CT values across the interface. This smoothing results in reduced spatial resolution because of several features of the CT imaging system.

Spatial resolution is a function of pixel size: the smaller the pixel size, the better the spatial resolution. CT imaging systems allow reconstruction of images after imaging and this is a powerful way to affect spatial resolution. Focal spot size also plays a role, but it usually does not limit the system's spatial resolution.

Thinner slice thicknesses also allow better spatial resolution. Anatomy that does not lie totally within a slice thickness may not be resolved, an artifact called *partial volume*. Therefore, voxel size in CT also affects CT spatial resolution. The design of the prepatient and predetector collimation affects the level of scatter radiation and influences spatial resolution by affecting the contrast of the system.

The ability of the CT imaging system to reproduce with accuracy a high-contrast edge is expressed mathematically as the **edge response function (ERF)**. The measured ERF can be transformed into another mathematical expression called the **modulation transfer function (MTF)**. The MTF and its graphic representation are most often cited to express the spatial resolution of a CT imaging system.

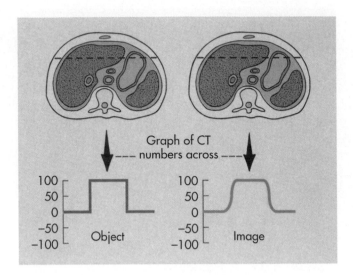

FIGURE 29-20 A computed tomography (CT) examination of a object organ with distinct borders results in an image with somewhat blurred borders. The actual CT number profile of the object is abrupt, whereas that of the image is smoothed.

Although the MTF is a rather complicated mathematical formulation, its meaning is not too difficult to represent. Consider, for instance, a series of bar patterns that are imaged by CT (Figure 29-21).

One bar and its equal-width interspace are called a **line pair (lp)**. The number of line pairs per unit length is called the **spatial frequency,** and for CT imaging systems it is expressed in line pairs per centimeter (lp/cm).

 A low spatial frequency represents large objects and a high spatial frequency represents small objects.

The image obtained from the low-frequency bar pattern will appear more like the object than the image from the high-frequency bar pattern. The loss in faithful reproduction with increasing spatial frequency occurs because of a number of limitations of the imaging system. Characteristics of the CT imaging system that contribute to such image degradation are collimation, detector size and concentration, mechanical-electrical gantry control, and the reconstruction algorithm.

In simplistic terms, the MTF is the ratio of the image to the object. If the image faithfully represents the object, the MTF of the CT imaging system would have a value of 1. If the image were simply blank and contained no information whatsoever about the object, the MTF would be equal to zero. Intermediate levels of fidelity result in intermediate MTF values.

In Figure 29-21, image fidelity is measured by the optical density along the axis of the image. At a spatial frequency of 1 lp/cm, for instance, the variation in optical

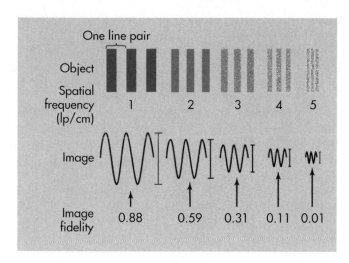

FIGURE 29-21 When a bar pattern of increasing spatial frequency is imaged, the fidelity of the image decreases. The tracing of optical density across the image reveals the loss of contrast.

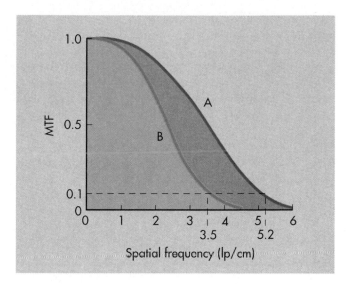

FIGURE 29-23 Modulation transfer function (MTF) curves for two representative computed tomography imaging systems. Imaging system *A* has higher spatial resolution than imaging system *B*.

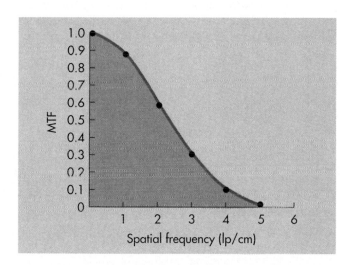

FIGURE 29-22 The modulation transfer function (MTF) is a plot of the image fidelity vs. spatial frequency. The six data points plotted here are from the analysis of Figure 29-21.

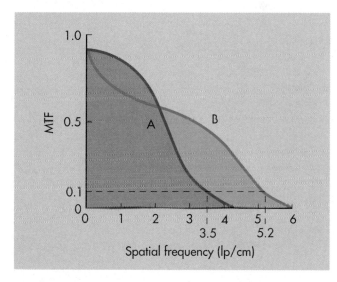

FIGURE 29-24 Imaging system *A* has better contrast resolution. Imaging system *B* has better spatial resolution.

density of the image is 0.88 times that of the object. At 4 lp/cm, it is only 0.1 or 10% that of the object. A graph of this ratio of image contrast to object contrast at each spatial frequency results in an MTF curve (Figure 29-22).

Figure 29-23 shows the MTF for two different CT imaging systems and illustrates how such curves should be interpreted. An MTF curve that extends farther to the right indicates higher spatial resolution, which means the imaging system is better able to reproduce very small objects. An MTF curve that is higher at low

spatial frequencies indicates better contrast resolution (Figure 29-24).

Obviously, MTF is a complex relationship because it relates the imaging capacity of the system for objects of various sizes. Most CT imaging systems are judged by the spatial frequency at an MTF equal to 0.1, sometimes called the **limiting resolution.** As shown in Figure 29-23, imaging system *A* has a 0.1 MTF at 5.2 lp/cm, whereas *B* can manage only 3.5 lp/cm. Therefore, *A* has better spatial resolution than *B*.

Although CT image resolution is most often expressed by the spatial frequency of the limiting resolution, it is easier to think in terms of the object size that can be reproduced. Figure 29-25 illustrates the relationship between spatial frequency and object size. The absolute object size that can be resolved by a CT imaging system is equal to one-half the reciprocal of the spatial frequency at the limiting resolution.

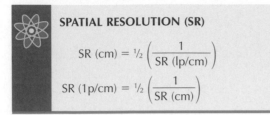

SPATIAL RESOLUTION (SR)

$$SR \ (cm) = \frac{1}{2} \left(\frac{1}{SR \ (lp/cm)} \right)$$

$$SR \ (1p/cm) = \frac{1}{2} \left(\frac{1}{SR \ (cm)} \right)$$

Question: A CT imaging system is said to be capable of 5 lp/cm resolution. What size object does this represent?

Answer: The reciprocal of 5 lp/cm = $(5 \ lp/cm)^{-1}$

$$= \frac{1}{5 \ lp/cm}$$

$$= \frac{1 \ cm}{5 \ lp}$$

$$= \frac{10 \ mm}{5 \ lp}$$

$$= \frac{2 \ mm}{lp}$$

Because a line pair consists of a bar and an interspace of equal width, 2 mm/lp represents a 1-mm object separated by a 1-mm interspace. The system resolution is therefore 1 mm.

Question: Currently, the best CT imaging systems have a limiting resolution of approximately 20 lp/cm. What object size does this represent?

Answer: The reciprocal of 20 lp/cm = $\dfrac{1}{20 \ lp/cm}$

$$= \frac{1 \ cm}{20 \ lp}$$

$$= \frac{10 \ mm}{20 \ lp}$$

$$= \frac{0.5 \ mm}{lp}$$

Therefore, the CT resolution is 0.25 mm.

Question: A CT imaging system can resolve a 0.65 mm high-contrast object. What spatial frequency does this represent?

Answer: 0.65 mm object + 0.65 mm interspace = 1.3 mm/lp

$$\frac{1}{1.3 \ mm/lp} = 0.77 \ lp/mm$$

$$= 7.7 \ lp/cm$$

Specially designed test objects are necessary for evaluating CT imaging system performance. Such test objects are usually fabricated from plastic of different densities in various shapes and configurations.

The important measures of imaging system performance that can be evaluated with test objects are artifact generation, contrast resolution, and spatial resolution. Figure 29-26, shows the four test sections of the phantom designed by the Physics Commission of the American College of Radiology to evaluate a number of CT image quality factors.

 The best possible spatial resolution for a CT image is the size of the pixel.

Although MTF and spatial frequency are used to describe CT spatial resolution, no imaging system can do better than the size of a pixel. In terms of line pairs, one line and its interspace require at least two pixels.

Contrast Resolution

The ability to distinguish one soft tissue from another without regard for size or shape is called **contrast resolution.** This is an area in which CT excels.

The absorption of x-rays in tissue is characterized by the x-ray linear attenuation coefficient. This coefficient, as we have seen, is a function of x-ray energy and the atomic number of the tissue. In CT, the amount of radiation penetrating the patient is determined also by the mass density of the body part.

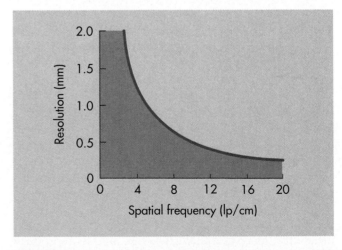

FIGURE 29-25 Increasing spatial frequency means smaller objects and better spatial resolution.

Consider the situation outlined in Figure 29-27, a fat–muscle–bone structure. Not only are the atomic numbers somewhat different (Z = 6.8, 7.4, and 13.8, respectively), but the mass densities are different (ρ = 0.91, 1.0, and 1.85 kg/m³, respectively). Although these differences are measurable, they are not imaged well in conventional radiography.

The CT imaging system is able to amplify these differences in subject contrast so that the image contrast is high. On computer reconstruction, the range of CT numbers for these tissues is approximately −100, 50, and 1000, respectively. This amplified contrast scale allows CT better to resolve adjacent structures that are similar in composition.

> Contrast resolution is superior in CT principally because of x-ray beam collimation.

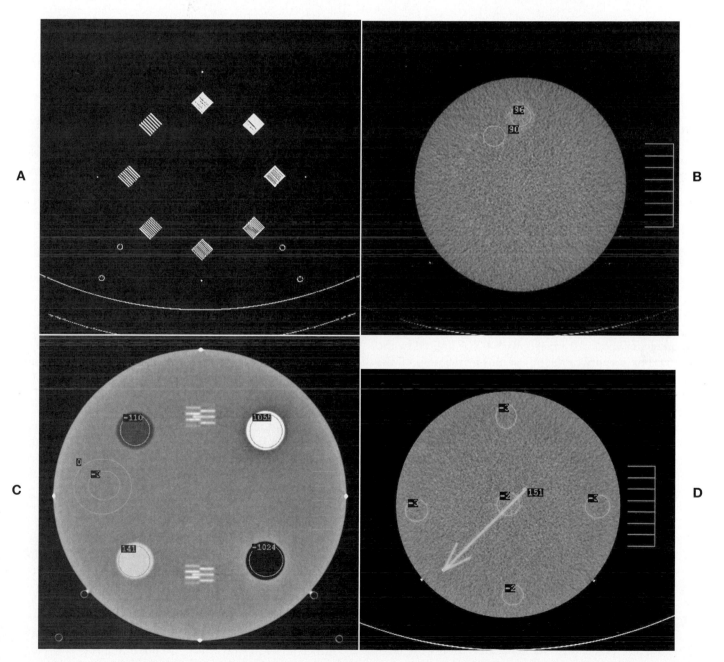

FIGURE 29-26 The phantom for evaluating computed tomography image quality contains test objects designed to measure spatial resolution **(A)**, contrast resolution **(B)**, linearity **(C)**, and other image quality factors **(D)**. (Courtesy American College of Radiology.)

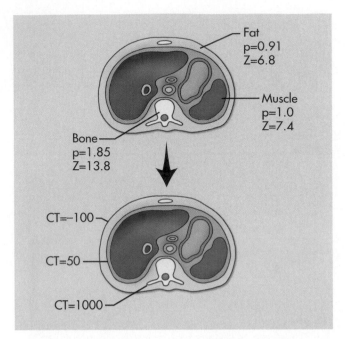

Fat
p=0.91
Z=6.8

Muscle
p=1.0
Z=7.4

Bone
p=1.85
Z=13.8

CT=-100

CT=50

CT=1000

FIGURE 29-27 There are not many differences in mass density and effective atomic number among tissues, but the differences are greatly amplified by computed tomography.

The contrast resolution provided by CT is considerably better than that available in conventional radiography principally because of the scatter radiation rejection of the prepatient and predetector collimators. The ability to image low-contrast objects with CT is limited by the size and uniformity of the object and by the **noise of the system.**

Noise

If a homogeneous medium such as water is imaged, each pixel should have a value of zero. Of course, this never occurs because the contrast resolution of the system is not perfect; therefore, the CT numbers may average zero but a range of values greater than or less than zero exists.

This variation in CT numbers above or below the average value is the **noise** of the system. If all pixel values were equal, noise would be zero.

A large variation of pixel values represents high image noise.

Noise is the percentage standard deviation of a large number of pixels obtained from a water bath image. It

should be clearly understood that noise depends on many factors:

1. kVp and filtration
2. Pixel size
3. Slice thickness
4. Detector efficiency
5. Patient dose

Ultimately it is patient dose, the number of x-rays used by the detector to produce the image, that controls noise.

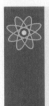

NOISE

$$\text{Noise } (\sigma) = \sqrt{\frac{\Sigma(x_1 - x)^2}{n - 1}}$$

where x_1 is each CT value, x is the average of at least 100 values, and n is the number of CT values averaged.

In statistics, noise is called a **standard deviation** and symbolized by σ.

Noise appears on the image as graininess. Low-noise images appear very smooth to the eye and high-noise images appear spotty or blotchy.

The resolution of low-contrast objects is limited by the noise of a CT imaging system.

Noise should be evaluated daily by imaging a 20-cm diameter water bath. All CT imaging systems have the ability to identify an ROI on the digital image and to compute the mean and standard deviation of the CT numbers in that ROI. When the radiologic technologist measures noise, the ROI must encompass at least 100 pixels. Such noise measurements should include five determinations—four on the periphery and one in the center.

The biggest tradeoff that is made in establishing CT imaging protocols is that between spatial resolution, noise, and patient dose. For example, if the slice thickness is reduced from 10 mm to 2 mm, the patient dose increases by a factor of five to maintain an acceptable level of noise.

Linearity

CT equipment must be frequently calibrated so that water is consistently represented by CT number zero and other tissues by their appropriate CT number. A check calibration that can be made daily uses the five-pin performance test object of the American Association of Physicists in Medicine (AAPM; Figure 29-28). The five pins are each made of a different plastic material with known physical and x-ray attenuation properties and are positioned in a water bath (Table 29-2).

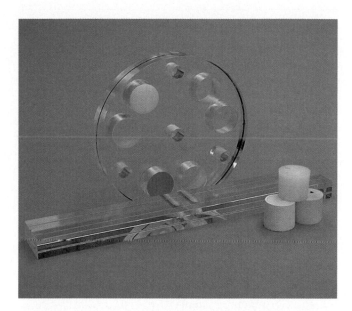

FIGURE 29-28 A version of the five-pin test object designed by the American Association of Physicists in Medicine. The attenuation coefficient for each pin is known precisely and the CT number computed. (Courtesy Nuclear Associates.)

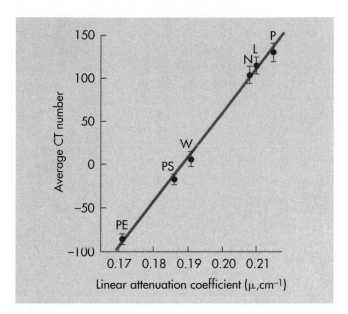

FIGURE 29-29 Computed tomography (CT) linearity is acceptable if a graph of average CT number versus the linear attenuation coefficient is a straight line passing through 0 for water.

TABLE 29-2	Characteristics of the Five-Pin AAPM Phantom			
Material		**Density (g/cm³)**	**Linear Attenuation Coefficient (cm⁻¹) at 60 keV**	**CT Number**
Polyethylene	C_2H_4	0.94	0.185	−85
Polystyrene	C_8H_8	1.05	0.196	−85
Nylon	$C_6H_{11}NO$	1.15	0.222	100
Lexan	$C_{16}H_{14}O$	1.20	0.223	115
Plexiglas	$C_5H_8O_2$	1.19	0.229	130
Water	H_2O	1.00	0.206	0

After imaging this test object, the CT number for each pin should be recorded and its mean value and standard deviation plotted (Figure 29-29). The plot of CT number versus linear attenuation coefficient should be a straight line passing through CT number 0 for water.

A deviation from **linearity** is an indication of misalignment or malfunction of the CT imaging system. A minor deviation would result in inaccurate CT number generation but would probably not significantly affect the visual image. Such a minor deviation, however, could greatly affect quantitative CT (QCT) analysis of tissue, the determination of tissue composition based on CT number.

Uniformity

When a uniform object such as a water bath is imaged, each pixel should have the same value because each pixel represents precisely the same object. Furthermore, if the CT imaging system is properly adjusted, that value should be zero. Because the CT imaging system is an extremely complicated electronic mechanical device, however, such precision is not consistently possible. The CT value for water may drift from day to day or even from hour to hour.

At any time a water bath is imaged, the pixel values should be constant in all regions of the reconstructed image. Such a characteristic is called **spatial uniformity**.

Spatial uniformity can be tested easily with an internal software package that allows the plotting of CT numbers along any axis of the image as a histogram or as a line graph. If all the values of the histogram or line graph are within two standard deviations of the mean value ($\pm 2\sigma$), the system is said to exhibit acceptable spatial uniformity. X-ray beam hardening may cause a decrease of CT numbers so that the middle of the image appears darker than the periphery. This is the "cupping" artifact, and it can be clearly demonstrated by imaging the water bath inside a Teflon rim to simulate bone.

SUMMARY

The CT imaging system does not record an image in a conventional way. The collimated x-ray beam is directed to the patient, the attenuated image-forming x-ray beam is measured by a detector, the signal from the detector is measured by a computer, the image is reconstructed in the computer, and, finally, the image is displayed on a television or flat-panel monitor.

CT acquires transverse images, which are sections of anatomy perpendicular to the long axis of the body. The internal structures of the body attenuate the x-ray beam according to their mass density and atomic number, and the resulting intensity projection is one of many used to reconstruct an image. All data from the projections are processed in digital form.

The resulting computer image is an electronic matrix of intensities. The matrix size is usually 512×512 pixels. Each pixel contains numeric information called a CT number or a Hounsfield unit. The pixel is a two-dimensional representation of a corresponding tissue volume voxel.

The voxel is determined by multiplying the pixel size by the thickness of the CT image slice. A CT number of -1000 corresponds to air. A number of $+1000$ corresponds to dense bone. A CT number of zero indicates water.

Contrast resolution of the CT imaging system is excellent because of scatter radiation reduction due to x-ray beam collimation. The ability to image low-contrast anatomy is limited by the noise of the system. System noise is determined by the number of x-rays used by the detector to produce the image.

The system components are similar in all CT imaging systems. There is the gantry, the x-ray tube, the detector assembly, collimation (prepatient and postpatient), the patient couch, and the computer.

CT technologists and medical physicists routinely monitor performance of the CT imaging system.

CHALLENGE QUESTIONS

1. Define or otherwise identify:
   a. Algorithm
   b. Transverse image
   c. Projection
   d. Detection efficiency
   e. Prepatient collimation
   f. Spatial frequency
   g. Hounsfield unit
   h. Image matrix
   i. MTF
   j. Noise
2. Name the individual who first demonstrated CT in 1970.
3. List the advantages and disadvantages of a fourth-generation CT imaging system.
4. What are the components the gantry portion of the CT imaging system?
5. What are the special requirements of the x-ray tube used in CT imaging?
6. Discuss the spacing and concentration of scintillation detectors on the CT imaging system.
7. Why is collimation so important in CT imaging?
8. Describe the two collimators used in CT imaging.
9. What material makes up the patient support couch?
10. Why must the CT computer be very fast and of large capacity?
11. What is the voxel size of a CT imaging system with a 320×320 matrix size, a 20-cm reconstruction diameter, and 0.5-cm slice thickness?
12. What device controls the slice thickness of a CT imaging system?
13. What kilovolt peak level is usually used for CT imaging?
14. Explain the mathematics of the CT image reconstruction process.
15. What is the blurring of high-contrast interfaces called?
16. A CT imaging system can resolve a 0.65-mm high-contrast object. What spatial frequency does this represent?
17. A fourth-generation CT imaging system has 720 detectors and a 30-degree fan beam. How many detectors will be in the beam at any given time?
18. A test pattern has a spatial frequency of 8 lp/cm. What is the width of line?
19. The CT computer must be maintained under what environmental conditions?
20. What does the term *CT linearity* describe?

Spiral Computed Tomography

OBJECTIVES

At the completion of this chapter, the student should be able to do the following:

1. Explain the spiral imaging principles of interpolation, pitch, index, and section sensitivity
2. Discuss the design features that make spiral computed tomography (CT) possible
3. Recognize the differences between step-and-shoot and spiral CT x-ray tubes
4. Describe the technique selection for spiral CT
5. Discuss the concept of Z-axis resolution
6. Describe multislice CT
7. List the advantages and limitations of spiral CT

OUTLINE

N 1989, SPIRAL computed tomography (CT) was introduced with great promise. The term spiral—some call it *helical*—was coined because it is the apparent motion of the x-ray tube during the image.

The future of medicine is changing as fast as newspaper headlines. Cost containment and limited reimbursement for high-tech studies such as CT and magnetic resonance imaging (MRI) are part of the future of health care. For CT to grow or at least survive, it had to provide more information than other imaging modalities in a cost-effective, time-efficient manner.

Spiral CT has emerged as a new and improved diagnostic tool. Spiral CT provides improved imaging of anatomy compromised by respiratory motion. Spiral CT is particularly good for the chest, abdomen, and pelvis. Spiral CT also has the ability to perform conventional transverse imaging for regions of the body where motion is not a problem, such as the head, spine, and extremities.

This chapter introduces the physical principles of spiral CT and multislice spiral CT. Special imaging system design features and image characteristics are reviewed. The slinky toy is an example of a spiral (Figure 30-1); so is the structure of the DNA molecule (see Chapter 33).

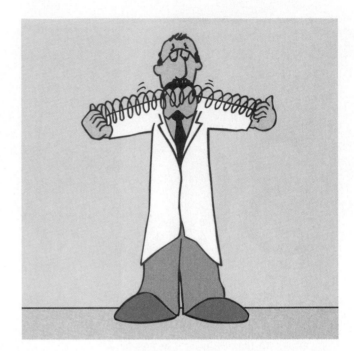

FIGURE 30-1 A slinky toy is a common example of a spiral.

IMAGING PRINCIPLES

Actually, the spiral motion in spiral CT is not like a slinky toy; it just appears that way. Figure 30-2 shows the difference.

When the examination begins, the x-ray tube rotates continuously. While the x-ray tube is rotating, the couch moves the patient through the plane of the rotating x-ray beam. The x-ray tube is energized continuously, data are collected continuously, and an image can then be reconstructed at any desired z-axis position along the patient (Figure 30-3).

Interpolation Algorithms

The ability to reconstruct an image at any z-axis position is possible because of a mathematical process called **interpolation.** Figure 30-4 presents a graphic representation of interpolation and **extrapolation.** If one wishes to estimate a value between known values, that is interpolation; if one wishes to estimate a value beyond the range of known values, that is extrapolation.

During spiral CT, image data are received continuously, as shown by the data points in Figure 30-5, *A*. When an image is reconstructed as in Figure 30-5, *B*, the plane of the image does not contain enough data for reconstruction. Data in that plane must be estimated by interpolation.

Data interpolation is performed by a special computer program called an **interpolation algorithm.** The first interpolation algorithms used 360-degree linear interpolation (Figure 30-6). The plane of the reconstructed image was interpolated from data acquired one revolution apart.

The interpolation algorithm is called *linear* because it assumed a straight-line relationship between the two known data points. The result of interpolation is a transverse image nearly identical with that of conventional CT.

When these images are formatted into sagittal and coronal views, prominent blurring can occur compared with conventional CT reformatted views. The solution to the blurring problem is interpolation of values separated by 180 degrees, half a revolution of the x-ray tube. This results in improved z-axis resolution and greatly improved reformatted sagittal and coronal views.

Different types of interpolation algorithms have been developed—simple linear interpolation and higher-order interpolation. The disadvantage of the 180-degree interpolation algorithms is increased image noise compared with 360-degree interpolation algorithms and conventional CT imaging.

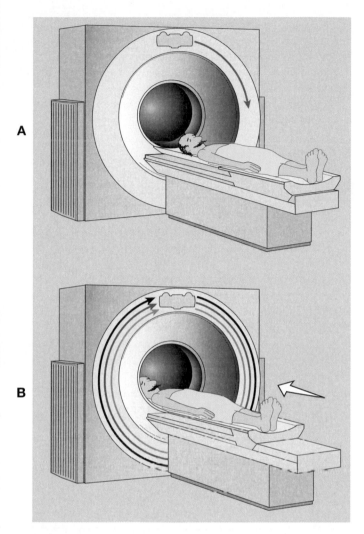

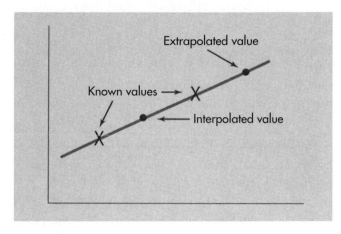

FIGURE 30-4 Interpolation estimates a value between two known values. Extrapolation estimates a value beyond known values.

FIGURE 30-2 The movement of the x-ray tube is not spiral **(A)**. It just appears that way because the patient moves through the plane of rotation during imaging **(B)**.

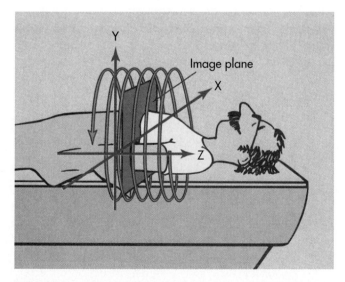

FIGURE 30-3 Transverse images can be reconstructed at any plane along the z-axis.

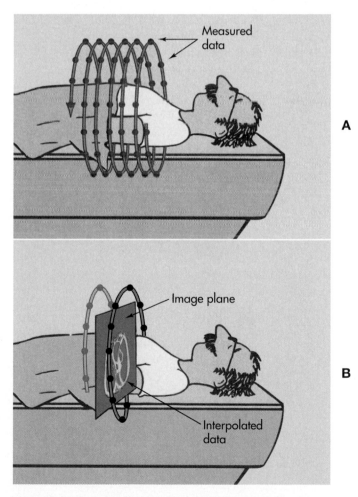

FIGURE 30-5 **A,** During spiral computed tomography, image data are continuously sampled. **B,** Interpolation of data is performed to reconstruct the image in any transverse plane.

This noise is not bothersome, but use of some higher-order interpolation algorithms can produce what is called a "breakup" artifact at high-contrast interfaces, such as bone–soft tissue. The breakup artifact has a stair-step appearance.

Linear interpolation at 180 degrees improves z-axis resolution.

Pitch

In addition to improved sagittal and coronal reformatted views, 180-degree interpolation algorithms allow imaging at a pitch greater than one. Spiral pitch ratio, referred to simply as **pitch,** is the relationship between the patient couch movement and x-ray beam collimation.

SPIRAL PITCH RATIO

$$\text{Pitch} = \frac{\text{Couch movement each } 360°}{\text{Slice thickness}}$$

Pitch is expressed as a ratio, such as 0.5:1, 1.0:1, 1.5:1, or 2:1. A pitch of 0.5:1 results in overlapping images and higher patient dose. A pitch of 2:1 results in extended imaging and reduced patient dose.

Question: During a 360-degree x-ray tube rotation, the patient couch moves 8 mm. Section collimation is 5 mm. What is the pitch?

Answer: $\dfrac{8 \text{ mm}}{5 \text{ mm}} = 1.6{:}1$

Increasing pitch above 1:1 increases the volume of tissue that can be imaged in a given time. This is the prin-

ciple advantage of spiral CT, the ability to image a larger volume of tissue in a single breathhold. This is particularly helpful in CT angiography, radiation therapy treatment planning, and imaging of uncooperative patients.

The relationship between the volume of tissue imaged and pitch is given as follows:

VOLUME IMAGING

Tissue imaged = collimation × pitch × imaging time

Table 30-1 shows this relationship for a fixed imaging time and fixed section thickness.

Question: How much tissue will be imaged if collimation is set to 8 mm, imaging time is 25 s, and the pitch is 1.5:1?

Answer: Tissue imaged = 8 mm × 25 s × 1.5
= 300 mm
= 30 cm

What if the gantry rotation time is not 360 degrees in 1 second? In such a situation, the volume of tissue imaged becomes:

VOLUME IMAGING

$$\text{Tissue imaged} = \frac{\text{Collimation} \times \text{Pitch} \times \text{Image time}}{\text{Gantry rotation time}}$$

If the gantry rotation time is reduced to 0.5 seconds, Table 30-1 is changed to Table 30-2 With such fast spi-

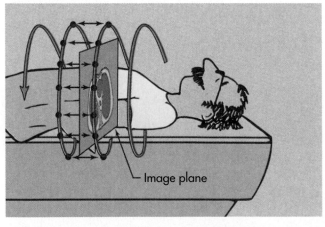

FIGURE 30-6 Interpolation between data points 360 degrees apart was the earliest spiral computed tomography reconstruction algorithm.

TABLE 30-1	Tissue Imaged With Changing Pitch			
Section thickness (mm)	10	10	10	10
Imaging time (s)	30	30	30	30
Pitch	1.0:1	1.3:1	1.6:1	2.0:1
Tissue imaged (cm)	30	39	48	60

TABLE 30-2	Tissue Imaged With Changing Pitch and a Gantry Rotation Time of 0.5 s		
Section thickness (mm)	10	10	10
Scan time (s)	30	30	30
Gantry rotation time (s)	0.5	0.5	0.5
Pitch	1.0:1	1.5:1	2.0:1
Tissue imaged (cm)	60	90	120

ral CT available, whole-body imaging is now possible within a single breathhold.

Question: How much tissue will be imaged with 5-mm collimation, a pitch of 1.6:1, and a 20-s image time at a gantry rotation time of 2 s?

Answer: Tissue imaged $= \dfrac{5 \text{ mm} \times 1.6 \times 20 \text{ s}}{2 \text{ s}}$

$$= 80 \text{ mm}$$
$$= 8 \text{ cm}$$

Question: One wishes to image 40 cm of tissue in 25 s with a slice thickness of 8 mm. If the gantry rotation time is 1.5 s, what should be the pitch?

Answer: Pitch $=$

$$\dfrac{\text{Tissue image} \times \text{Gantry rotation time}}{\text{Collimation} \times \text{Image time}}$$

$$= \dfrac{400 \text{ mm} \times 1.5 \text{ s}}{8 \text{ mm} \times 25 \text{ s}}$$

$$= \dfrac{600}{200}$$

$$= 3.0:1$$

Unfortunately, when the pitch exceeds approximately 2.0:1, the z-axis resolution is very poor because of a wide section sensitivity profile (SSP).

Sensitivity Profile

Consider the SSP of a 10-mm section obtained with a conventional CT imaging system (Figure 30-7). If properly collimated, it will have a **full width at half maximum (FWHM)** of 10 mm. The FWHM is as diagrammed in Figure 30-7, the width of the profile at one half of its maximum value. Some report SSP as full width at tenth maximum (FWTM).

At a pitch of 1:1, the SSP is only approximately 10% wider than in conventional CT (Figure 30-8). However, at a pitch of 2:1, the SSP is approximately 40% wider, and at a pitch of 3:1, the SSP soars.

Pitch influences SSP in the same way that the interpolation algorithm does. The z-axis resolution is worse for a 360-degree interpolation algorithm compared with a 180-degree interpolation algorithm because the SSP is wider (Figure 30-9).

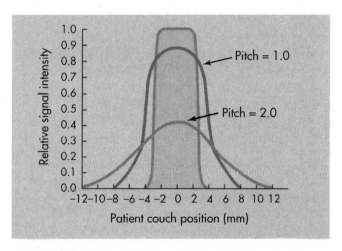

FIGURE 30-8 The section sensitivity profile for spiral computed tomography widens as pitch is increased.

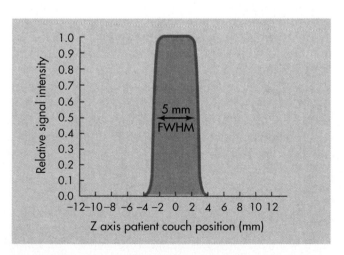

FIGURE 30-7 The section sensitivity profile (SSP) for a conventional computed tomography imaging system is nearly rectangular and is identified by its full width at half maximum (FWHM).

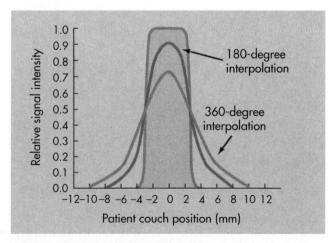

FIGURE 30-9 The section sensitivity profile is wider for 360-degree interpolation than for 180-degree interpolation.

IMAGING SYSTEM DESIGN

Spiral CT is made possible by **slip-ring** technology. Continuing development of advanced imaging protocols is also due to improvements in the x-ray tube, the high-voltage section, and the detector array.

Slip-Ring Technology

Slip rings are electromechanical devices that conduct electricity and electric signals through rings and brushes from a rotating surface onto a fixed surface. One surface is a smooth ring and the other a ring with brushes that sweep the smooth ring (Figure 30-10). Spiral CT is made possible by the use of slip-ring technology, which allows the gantry to rotate continuously without interruption.

Step-and-shoot CT imaging is performed with a pause between each gantry rotation. During the pause, the patient couch is moved and the gantry may be rewound to a starting position.

In a slip-ring gantry system, power and electric signals are transmitted through stationary rings within the gantry, eliminating the need for electrical cables that make continuous rotation impossible.

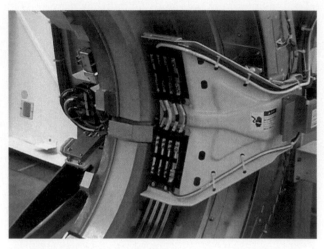

FIGURE 30-10 Slip rings and brushes electrically connect the components on the rotating gantry with the rest of the computed tomography imaging system. (Courtesy Toshiba Medical Systems.)

 Slip rings make spiral CT possible.

There are two slip-ring designs in spiral CT imaging systems, the **disk** and the **cylinder.** The disk design incorporates concentric conductive rings in the plane of rotation. The cylindrical design has the conductive rings lying parallel to the axis of rotation, forming a cylinder.

The brushes that transmit power to the gantry components glide in contact grooves on the stationary slip ring. Composite brushes made of conductive material (e.g., silver graphite alloy) are used as a sliding contact. The rings should last the life of the imaging system. The brushes have to be replaced every year or so during preventive maintenance.

There are usually three slip rings on a gantry. One provides high-voltage power to the x-ray tube and high-voltage generator. A second provides low-voltage power to control systems on the rotating gantry. The third slip ring transfers digital data from the rotating detector array. Some designs now use radiofrequency (RF) for data transfer.

The design of the high-voltage slip ring differs among manufacturers. One approach generates the high voltage off the gantry. In this design, the slip ring must be sealed to insulate the transfer of up to 150 kVp.

An alternate approach transfers a low voltage onto the rotating gantry, where it is increased to the desired kVp. This requires the design of inverters and transformers to produce that high voltage, yet be compact enough to fit on the rotating gantry. Intermediate between these two approaches are hybrid designs. Figure 30-11 shows how compact a rotating gantry must be.

X-Ray Tube

In step-and-shoot CT, the x-ray tube is energized for one rotation, usually 1 s, every 6 to 10 s. This allows the tube to cool between images. Spiral CT places a considerable thermal demand on the x-ray tube. The x-ray tube is energized up to 60 s continuously.

Because of the continuous rotation and energization of the x-ray tube for longer exposure times, higher power levels must be sustained. High heat capacity and high cooling rates are trademarks of x-ray tubes designed for spiral CT.

Most systems use an x-ray tube with two focal spots. The small spot is used for high-resolution examination and the large spot is used for high-technique studies of large anatomy.

Spiral CT x-ray tubes are very large. They have an anode heat storage capacity of 8 MHU or more. They have anode-cooling rates of approximately 1 MHU per minute because the anode disk has a larger diameter and it is thicker, resulting in much greater mass.

The limiting characteristic is focal-spot design and heat dissipation. The small focal spot must be especially robust in design. Manufacturers design **focal-spot cooling algorithms** to predict the focal-spot thermal state and to adjust mA setting accordingly. The x-ray tube in Figure 30-12 is designed especially for spiral CT. This x-ray tube is expected to last for at least 50,000 exposures, the approximate x-ray tube life for conventional CT.

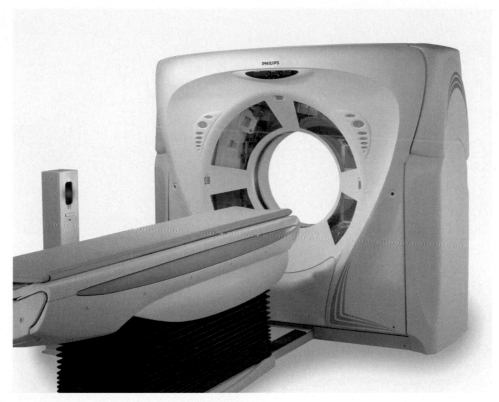

FIGURE 30-11 The gantry of this spiral computed tomography imaging system contains a high-voltage generator, x-ray tube, detector array, and assorted control systems. (Courtesy Philips Medical Systems.)

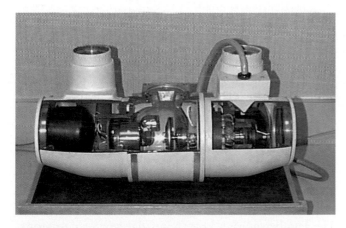

FIGURE 30-12 This x-ray tube is designed especially for spiral computed tomography. It has a 15-cm diameter disk, 5 cm thick with an anode heat capacity of 6.5 MHU. (Courtesy Marconi Medical Systems.)

X-Ray Detectors

The efficiency of the x-ray detector array reduces patient dose, allows faster imaging time, and improves image quality by increasing signal-to-noise ratio. Detector array design is especially critical for spiral CT. The total

detection efficiency for solid state arrays is approximately 80%.

High-Voltage Generator

The design constraints placed on the high-voltage generator are the same as those for the x-ray tube. In a properly designed spiral CT imaging system the two should be matched to maximum capacity. Approximately 50 kW power is necessary.

Designing such a high-voltage generator to fit onto the rotating gantry is indeed a challenge. Designing the insulated high-voltage slip rings is an equal challenge. Both design requirements have been adequately met.

TECHNIQUE SELECTION

The radiologist and radiologic technologist have more decisions to make and more work to do for spiral CT. The principal advantage to spiral CT is the ability to image a large volume of anatomy in one breathhold. However, the patient's ability at breathholding determines the image parameters selected.

The volume of tissue imaged is determined by the examination time, couch travel, pitch, and collimation.

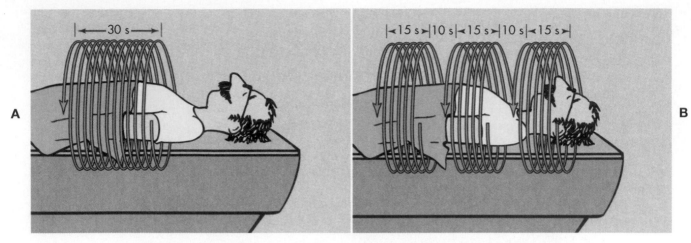

FIGURE 30-13 **A,** Most spiral computed tomography examinations can be completed in a single breathhold. **B,** When patient breathing is limited, a skip-scan technique must be selected.

In addition, rotation time, reconstruction algorithm, reconstruction index, and skip scan delay must be selected.

Examination Time

Most spiral CT imaging systems can perform up to 60 s continuously. Most patients can breathhold 40 s. Some can breathhold only 20 s. Therefore, if 45 s of imaging is required, as shown in Figure 30-13, *A,* it may be necessary to skip image (Figure 30-13, *B*) with a 10-s interscan delay to allow the patient to breathe.

Z-axis Resolution

Depending on the spatial resolution requirements of the examination, the z-axis resolution must be specified by technique selection. Longitudinal (z-axis) resolution is determined by several technique factors that must be preselected.

 Transverse resolution is determined by the reconstruction matrix and field of view.

When high z-axis resolution is required, thin-section collimation is selected. High z-axis resolution also requires selection of low-pitch, slow-couch motion, and 180-degree interpolation reconstruction.

 Z-axis resolution is determined by SSP, interpolation algorithm, and pitch.

TABLE 30-3	Representative Technique Factors for Imaging Lung Nodules and Renal Parenchyma	
	Lung Nodules	**Renal Parenchyma**
Slice thickness (mm)	2 mm	10 mm
Pitch	1.0:1	2.0:1
Couch movement (mm)	2 mm	5 mm
Gantry rotation (s)	1.0	1.5

Examinations requiring high z-axis resolution are those attempting to image small structures, such as lung calcifications and contrast-filled arteries (i.e., CT angiography). Normal resolution would be required for organ imaging, such as liver, spleen, and kidneys. Table 30-3 provides representative technique factors for high-resolution and normal-resolution spiral CT examinations.

To ensure the required anatomy is covered, a chart such as that shown in Table 30-4 should be constructed. The number in each box shows the length of anatomy to be imaged. A different table would be assembled for each image time.

Image Reconstruction

For high-resolution imaging, 180-degree interpolation is required. Transverse images or longitudinally reformatted images, or both, may be required. If a longitudinally reformatted image is required, a decision among **volume-rendered, surface-rendered,** or **CT angiography** may be required.

TABLE 30-4	Comparison of Image Characteristics and Patient Dose Between Conventional Computed Tomography and Spiral Computed Tomography			
			SPIRAL CT PITCH	
	Conventional Single-Slice CT	**0.5:1**	**1.0:1**	**2.0:1**
Relative z-axis resolution for a 10-mm slice	10 mm	9 mm	10 mm	12 mm
Relative image noise	1.0	0.8	1.0	1.3
Relative patient dose	1.0	2.0	1.0	0.5

MULTISLICE COMPUTED TOMOGRAPHY

In the early 1990s, the Israeli company El Scint introduced an improvement to spiral CT—the use of two detector arrays to produce two spiral slices in the time previously required for one slice (Figure 30-14). The advantages were obvious: imaging the same anatomy in half the time or imaging twice the anatomy in the same time. The latter proved to be more important.

By the end of the millennium, every CT vendor had developed and marketed multislice CT imaging systems. The are two principal distinguishing features of these multislice CT imaging systems. First, instead of a detector array, multislice CT requires several parallel detector arrays containing thousands of individual detectors (Figure 30-15). Second, energizing such a large detector array for large-volume imaging quickly requires a very fast, large-capacity computer.

Multislice Detector Array

After the initial demonstration of dual-slice imaging, detector arrays providing up to 16 image slices simultaneously have been developed. The following discussion assumes four image slices for simplicity.

The simplest approach to multislice imaging is four detector arrays, each of equal width. This design is shown in Figure 30-16 with a beam pitch of 2.0:1—the x-ray beam width is half the patient couch movement. The width of each detector array is 0.5 mm, resulting in four slices of 0.5-mm width.

The design of such a CT imaging system usually allows the detected signals from adjacent arrays to be combined to produce two slices of 1-mm width or one slice of 2-mm width (Figure 30-17). Wider slice imaging results in better contrast resolution at the same mA setting because the detected signal is larger.

This improvement in contrast resolution is accompanied by a slight reduction in spatial resolution because of increased voxel size. Alternatively, a larger tissue volume can be imaged with original contrast resolution at a reduced mA setting.

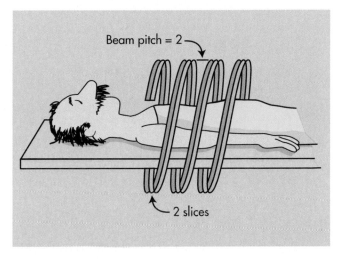

FIGURE 30-14 Dual detector arrays allow twice as much tissue volume to be imaged with no loss of image quality.

 Wider multislices allow more tissue volume to be imaged.

An alternate approach to four-slice imaging is shown in Figure 30-18. This design uses eight detector arrays of different widths. By combining adjacent arrays, one can obtain four 0.5-mm slices, four 1-mm slices, four 2-mm slices, or four 4-mm slices (Figure 30-19).

 Smaller detector size results in better spatial resolution.

Another design uses 32 detector arrays, each 0.5-mm wide, resulting in a total width of 16 mm. This design produces four contiguous slices, ranging from 0.5 mm each to 4 mm each (Figure 30-20). This design allows even better z-axis resolution.

The principal disadvantage is the reduced spatial resolution due to the larger detector size. With this type of

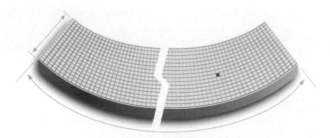

FIGURE 30-15 This multidetector array contains 16 rows of 912 individual detectors, each 1.25 mm wide (14,592 detectors). (Courtesy General Electric Medical Systems.)

design, some of the lost spatial resolution can be regained by the use of an additional predetector collimator (Figure 30-21).

The disadvantage to this approach is that the detector's geometric efficiency is reduced, resulting in wasted x-rays. The patient dose is increased because this mode of imaging requires higher mA to produce the same signal intensity.

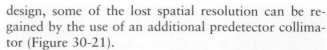

Higher-resolution multislice spiral CT results in higher patient radiation dose.

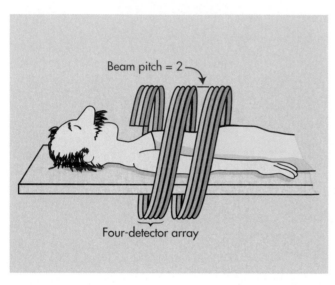

FIGURE 30-16 A four-detector array with a beam pitch of 2.0 covers eight times the tissue volume of single-slice spiral computed tomography.

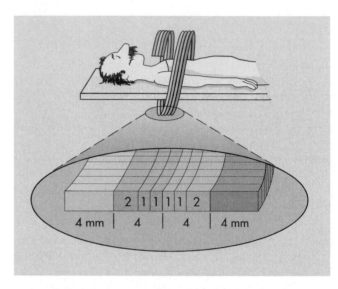

FIGURE 30-18 An asymmetric eight-detector array designed to provide four slices.

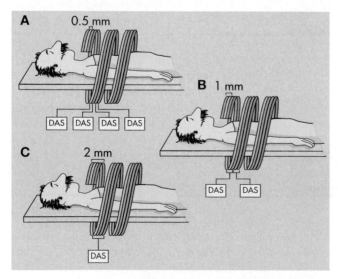

FIGURE 30-17 A four-detector array allows change of slice thickness to be made. **A,** Four slices of 0.5 mm each. **B,** Two 0.5-slices can be combined to make two 1-mm slices. **C,** Four 0.5-mm slices can be combined to make one 2-mm slice. *DAS,* Data acquisition system.

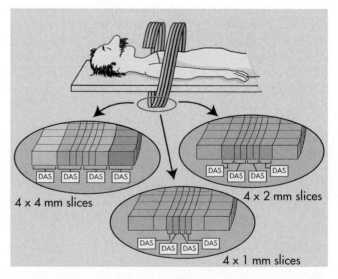

FIGURE 30-19 The asymmetric eight-detector array provides a choice of slice thickness by switching the data acquisition system.

Data Acquisition System

The signal from each individual radiation detector of a multislice spiral CT imaging system is connected to a computer-controlled electronic amplifier and switching device called a *data acquisition system* (DAS). It is the DAS that selects the detector combinations for signal summation (Figure 30-22).

Multislice Pitch

Spiral CT pitch as identified earlier is designed to convey information on image characteristics and patient dose. These relationships are reviewed in Table 30-4.

Pitch in multislice spiral CT must be stated differently because the entire width of the multidetector array or at least of those rows of detectors used for a particular imaging task intercepts the collimated x-ray cone beam (Figure 30-23). In fact, there are two designations for pitch in multislice spiral CT.

Beam pitch relates patient translation per 360-degree revolution to the width of the x-ray cone beam. For example, if all of the detectors of a 16-detector array are used, each of which is 1.25 mm in width, then when the patient couch translates 20 cm the beam pitch is 1.0 because the beam width is also 20 cm (Figure 30-24).

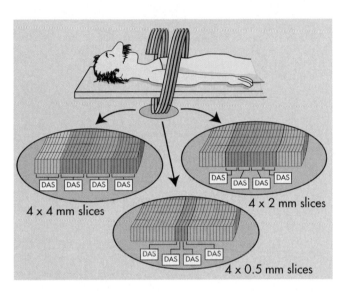

FIGURE 30-20 A 32-detector array where each detector row is of equal width and a 4-channel data acquisition system. Z-axis resolution or tissue volume can be emphasized.

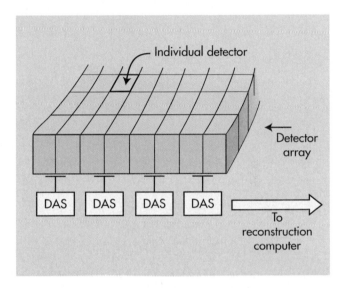

FIGURE 30-22 The data acquisition system selects combinations of detector arrays for various slice thicknesses.

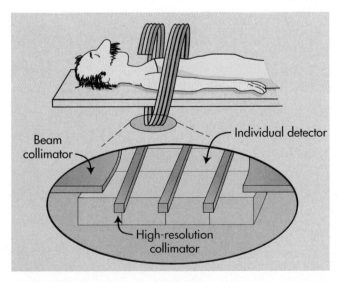

FIGURE 30-21 Additional predetector collimation is used to produce higher spatial resolution.

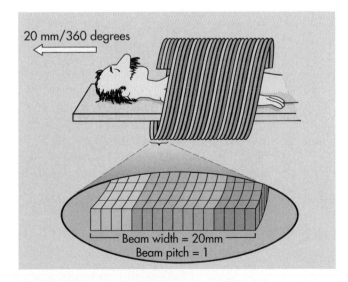

FIGURE 30-23 A 16-detector array collimated to a 20-mm beam width resulting in a beam pitch of 1.0.

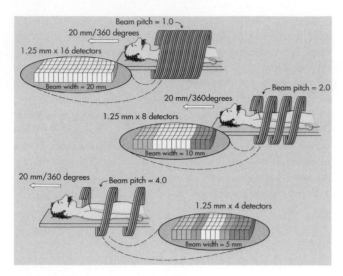

FIGURE 30-24 Beam pitch is the patient couch movement divided by x-ray cone beam width.

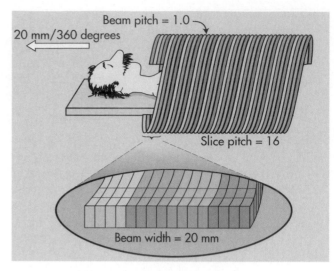

FIGURE 30-25 Slice pitch is not as important in spiral computed tomography as beam pitch.

If only the central rows of detectors are used, the x-ray cone beam width is collimated to 10 cm. Now, if the patient couch translates 20 cm, an extended spiral with a beam pitch of 2.0 is observed.

Question: The beam width during multislice spiral CT is 8 mm. If the patient couch moves 16 mm per revolution, what is the beam pitch?

Answer: $\text{Beam pitch} = \dfrac{\text{Patient movement}/360°}{\text{Beam width}}$

$= 16 \text{ mm}/8 \text{ mm}$

$= 2.0{:}1$, an extended spiral

Slice pitch has the same formulation as beam pitch except the denominator is the slice thickness rather than the beam width. For example, if the central 4 detectors of a 16-detector array, each of which is 1.25 mm in width, are selected and the patient couch translates 20 cm, the slice pitch is 16:1 and the beam pitch 4:1. If the patient couch translates only 10 cm, the slice pitch would be 8:1 and the beam pitch 2:1 (Figure 30-25).

Question: The slice width of a multislice spiral CT examination is 0.5 mm. If the patient couch moves 8 mm per revolution, what is the slice pitch?

Answer: $\text{Slice pitch} = \dfrac{\text{Patient movement per } 360°}{\text{Slice width}}$

$= 8 \text{ mm}/0.5 \text{ mm}$

$= 16{:}1$, a *very* extended spiral

Slice pitch does not have much application in multislice spiral CT because all except the outer rows of detectors are within the beam width. The outermost detector rows are also within the beam width unless the predetector collimators are not properly adjusted (Figure 30-26).

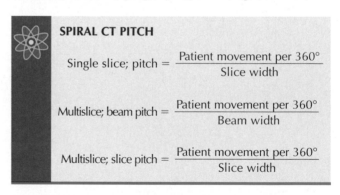

SPIRAL CT PITCH

Single slice; pitch $= \dfrac{\text{Patient movement per } 360°}{\text{Slice width}}$

Multislice; beam pitch $= \dfrac{\text{Patient movement per } 360°}{\text{Beam width}}$

Multislice; slice pitch $= \dfrac{\text{Patient movement per } 360°}{\text{Slice width}}$

In practice, the beam pitch for multislice spiral CT is usually 1.0. Because multiple slices are obtained and z-axis location and reconstruction width can be selected after imaging, overlapping images are unnecessary. Because of the multislice capability, more slices are acquired per unit time. This results in a much larger volume of tissue imaged, and hence extended spirals (beam pitch (1.0).

Slice Acquisition Rate

Multislice spiral CT results in 4, 8, or 16 slices being acquired in the same time previously required for a single slice. The slice acquisition rate (SAR) is one measure of the multislice spiral CT imaging system's efficiency.

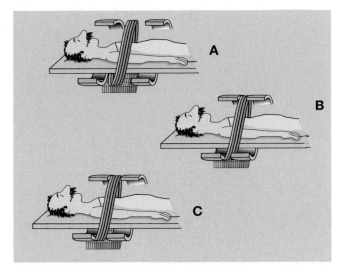

FIGURE 30-26 Improper collimation in multislice spiral computed tomography can result in excessive patient dose. **A,** Wide collimation, high dose. **B,** Narrow collimation, inadequate image. **C,** Proper collimation, normal dose and image quality.

SLICE ACQUISITION RATE

$$SAR = \frac{\text{Slices acquired per } 360°}{\text{Rotation time}}$$

Question: An eight-element multidetector array is used for 0.5-s multislice imaging. What is the SAR?

Answer: $SAR = \dfrac{\text{Slices acquired per } 360°}{\text{Rotation time}}$

$$= \frac{8}{0.5} = 16 \text{ slices/s}$$

Tissue Volume Covered

The principal advantage of multislice spiral CT is that a larger volume of tissue that can be imaged. At the limit, it is now possible to image the entire body—from head to toe—in a single breathhold. Although it is a volume of tissue that is being imaged, this volume is represented by the z-axis coverage as follows:

Z-AXIS COVERAGE (Z)

$$Z = (N/R) \times W \times T \times B$$

where

N = Number of slices acquired

R = Rotation time

W = Slice width

T = Imaging time

B = Beam pitch

Z-AXIS COVERAGE (Z)

$$Z = SAR \times W \times T \times B$$

where

SAR = Slice acquisition rate

Question: An eight-slice multislice examination is obtained with a 12-mm x-ray beam and a 20-s examination at 0.5-s per revolution. What z-axis coverage is obtained? The patient couch translates 6 mm each revolution.

Answer: $Z = (N/R) \times W \times T \times B$

where N = 8

R = 0.5 s

W = 1.5 mm (12 ÷ 8 = 1.5)

T = 20 s

B = 0.5 (6 ÷ 12 = 0.5)

$Z = (8/0.5) \times 1.5 \times 20 \times 0.5$

$= 30$ cm

IMAGE CHARACTERISTICS

Image quality in spiral CT, as measured by spatial resolution and contrast resolution, is comparable with that of step-and-shoot CT. Because the number of detectors, detector spacing, and number of projections in the image plane are usually the same as those in step-and-shoot CT, **in-plane resolution** is the same.

However, although the SSP is worse in spiral CT, there can be notable improvement in the z-axis spatial resolution because there are no gaps in the data. Reconstructed images can even overlap.

 With spiral CT, image reconstruction can be made at any position along the z-axis.

Overlapping Images

Consider the calcified lung nodule in Figure 30-27. With conventional step-and-shoot CT, the nodule may be missed if it lies at an interface between image slices. By moving the transverse image reconstruction along the z-axis, the nodule can be brought into the midsection with an accompanying improvement in contrast resolution.

In addition to overlapping transverse images for improved contrast resolution, spiral CT excels in three-dimensional **multiplanar reformation (MPR)**. Transverse images are stacked to form a three-dimensional data set, which can be rendered as an image in several ways. Three three-dimensional MPR algorithms are most frequently used: **maximum intensity projection (MIP), shaded surface display (SSD),** and **shaded volume display (SVD).**

Maximum Intensity Projection

MIP reconstructs an image by selecting the highest-value pixels along any arbitrary line through the data

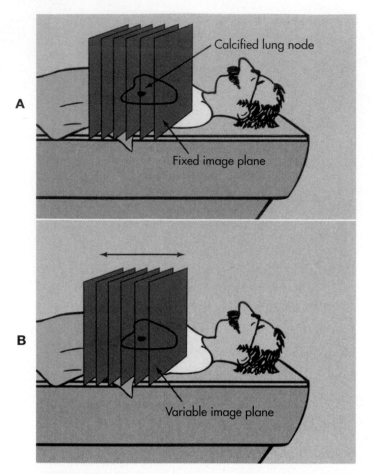

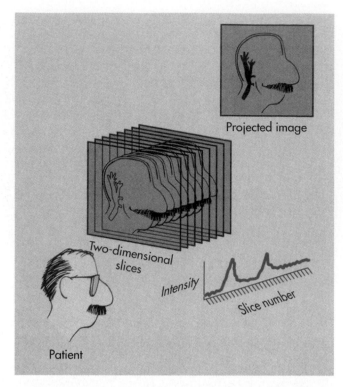

FIGURE 30-28 A maximum intensity projection reconstruction creates a three-dimensional image from multislice two-dimensional data sets. The result is a computed tomographic angiogram.

FIGURE 30-27 A very small structure, such as this lung nodule **(A)**, is poorly imaged by step-and-shoot computed tomography (CT) if the nodule is at the section interface. With spiral CT **(B)**, image reconstruction can be performed so that the nodule is totally within the slice.

set and exhibiting only those pixels (Figure 30-28). MIP images are widely used in CT angiography (CTA) because they can be reconstructed very quickly.

Only approximately 10% of the three-dimensional data points are used. The result can be a very high-contrast three-dimensional image of contrast-filled vessels (Figure 30-29). On most computer workstations, the image can be rotated to show striking three-dimensional features.

MIP is the simplest form of three-dimensional imaging. It provides excellent differentiation of vasculature from surrounding tissue but lacks vessel depth because superimposed vessels are not displayed. This is accommodated somewhat by image rotation. Small vessels that pass obliquely through a voxel may not be imaged because of partial volume averaging.

Shaded Surface Display

SSD is a computer-aided technique borrowed from computer-aided design and manufacturing applications. It was initially applied to bone imaging (Figure 30-30). SSD identifies a narrow range of values as belonging to the object to be imaged and displays that range. The range displayed appears as an organ surface that is determined by operator-selected values.

The computer capacity required for SSD is comparatively modest. Surface boundaries can be made very distinctive, and the image appears very three-dimensional (Figure 30-31).

SSD does appear somewhat shallow in depth because structures inside or behind the surface are not shown. For example, vessels within a renal capsule or thrombus within a vessel are not displayed. Shaded surface display is very sensitive to the operator-selected pixel range, which can make imaging of actual anatomic structures difficult.

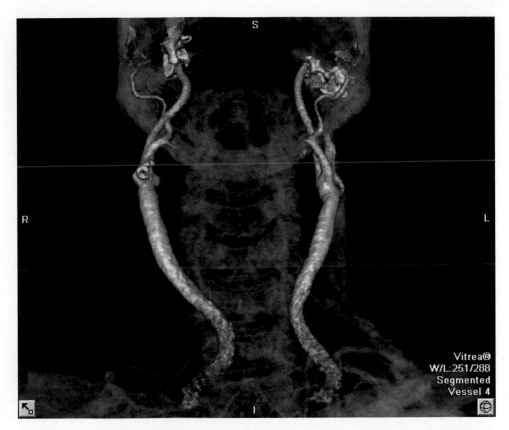

FIGURE 30-29 This carotid CT was reconstructed from a 16-slice spiral CT. (Courtesy Vital Images, Inc.)

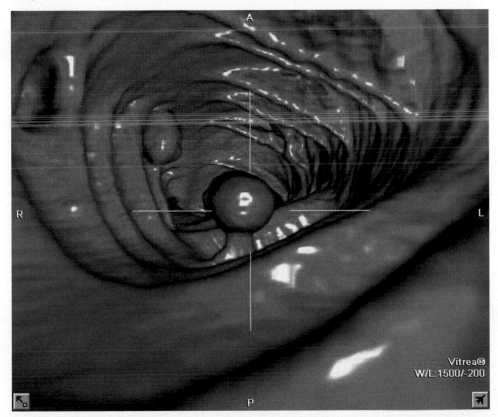

FIGURE 30-30 Shaded surface image obtained during virtual colonoscopy reconstructed from a 16-slice spiral CT data set. (Courtesy Vital Images, Inc.)

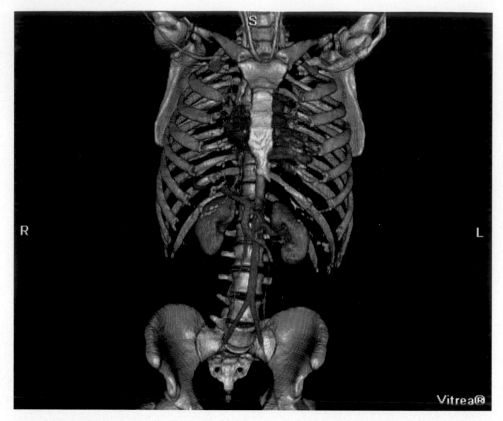

FIGURE 30-31 Volume-rendering display of the trunk. This image can be rotated for 3D visualization. (Courtesy Vital Images, Inc.)

TABLE 30-5	Features of Spiral Computed Tomography	
	What	**How/Why**
Advantages	No motion artifacts	Removes respiratory misregistration
	Improved lesion detection	Reconstructs at arbitrary z-axis intervals
	Reduced partial volume	Reconstructs at overlapping z-axis intervals
		Reconstructs smaller than image interval
	Optimized intravenous contrast	Data obtained during peak of enhancement
		Reduces volume of contrast agent
	Multiplanar images	Higher-quality reconstruction
	Improved patient throughput	Reduces imaging time
Limitations	Increased image noise	Needs bigger x-ray tubes
	Reduced z-axis resolution	Increases with pitch
	Increased processing time	More data, more images

ADVANTAGES AND LIMITATIONS OF SPIRAL COMPUTED TOMOGRAPHY

The advantages and limitations of spiral CT are summarized in Table 30-5.

SUMMARY

Spiral CT has following advantages over conventional CT: (1) motion blur is reduced, so there are fewer motion artifacts; (2) there is reduced imaging time; (3) there is reduced partial volume artifact; and (4) a larger volume of tissue can be imaged. These improvements allow CT to compete with the contrast resolution and three-dimensional versatility of MRI.

When the examination begins, the x-ray tube rotates continuously and the patient couch moves through the plane of the rotating beam. The data collected is reconstructed at any desired z-axis position by interpolation.

Spiral scan pitch ratio is the relationship between the patient couch movement and the x-ray beam collimation. Increasing the pitch above 1:1 increases the volume of tissue that can be imaged and at a reduced patient dose.

Spiral CT is made possible by slip-ring technology. Slip rings are electromechanical devices that conduct electric power and signals through brushes across a rotating surface onto a fixed surface. Slip-ring technology allows the gantry to rotate continuously.

The need for the x-ray tube to be energized for longer periods demands higher power levels in the spiral CT x-ray tube. Solid-state detector arrays with an overall detection efficiency of approximately 80% are preferred.

The volume of tissue imaged is determined by examination time, couch travel, pitch, and collimation. In addition, rotation time, reconstruction algorithm, reconstruction interval, and skip scan delay must be selected.

There is improvement in z-axis spatial resolution with spiral CT because there are no gaps in data and reconstruction images can even overlap. In addition, spiral CT excels in three-dimensional multiplanar reformation (MPR).

CHALLENGE QUESTIONS

1. Define or otherwise identify:
    a. Contrast resolution
    b. MIP
    c. Interpolation
    d. Section sensitivity profile
    e. Reformatted images
    f. Z-axis resolution
    g. Spiral pitch ratio
    h. DAS
    i. Full-width at half maximum
    j. Slip ring
2. Discuss the special computer program called the *interpolation algorithm.*
3. Explain the term "linear interpolation at 180 degrees."
4. Write the formula for the spiral scan pitch ratio.
5. What is the volume of tissue imaged with section thickness of 10 mm, scan time of 30 s, and pitch of 1.6:1?
6. What is the formula for tissue imaged as a function of scan time and gantry rotation time?
7. When imaging 40 cm of tissue in 25 s with a slice thickness of 8 mm, what would be the pitch if the gantry rotation time is 1.5 s?
8. Explain how slip-ring technology contributed to the development of spiral CT.
9. What special characteristics are required of the spiral CT x-ray tube?
10. Why is the solid-state detector array preferred over the gas-filled detector?
11. The volume of tissue imaged in spiral CT is determined by which technique selections?
12. Which examination requires high z-axis resolution?
13. Define multiplanar reformation (MPR).
14. List the limitations of spiral CT imaging.
15. What is the principal advantage of spiral CT over MRI?
16. What type of high-voltage generator is used for spiral CT?
17. A 10-s spiral CT examination is conducted with a 1.5:1 pitch and 5-mm collimation. How much tissue is imaged?
18. Why is a spiral CT pitch greater than 2:1 rarely used?
19. What happens to section sensitivity profile as pitch is increased?
20. What determines in-plane spatial resolution?

Quality Control

OBJECTIVES

At the completion of this chapter, the student should be able to do the following:

1. Define quality assurance and quality control
2. List the 10-step quality assurance model used in hospitals
3. Name the three steps of quality control
4. Describe the quality-control tests and schedule for radiographic systems
5. Discuss the quality-control tests and schedule for fluoroscopy
6. Explain the quality-control process for conventional tomography and computed tomography
7. Discuss processor quality control

OUTLINE

E VERY FIELD of medicine and every hospital department is required to develop and conduct programs that ensure the quality of patient care and management. Diagnostic imaging departments are leaders in promoting quality patient care.

This chapter discusses the properties of quality assurance and quality control, emphasizing radiographic and fluoroscopic imaging systems. Processor quality control is covered thoroughly in Chapter 23 and therefore is only reviewed here.

Two areas of activity are designed to ensure the best possible diagnosis at an acceptable radiation dose and with minimum cost. These areas are **quality assurance (QA)** and **quality control (QC).** There is still some confusion about the use of these terms, but responsible organizations are developing clearer definitions. Both programs rely heavily on proper record keeping.

QUALITY ASSURANCE

Healthcare organizations often adopt formal, structured QA models. The Joint Commission on Accreditation of Healthcare Organizations (JCAHO) promotes "The Ten-Step Monitoring and Evaluation Process." This QA program uses a 10-step process to resolve identified patient care problems. To make sure a healthcare organization is committed to providing high-quality services and care, accrediting agencies encourage the adoption of QA models such as that recommended by the JCAHO (see Box 31-1).

Quality assurance deals with people.

A program of QA monitors proper patient scheduling, reception, and preparation. Is the scheduled examination appropriate for the patient and, if so, has the patient been properly instructed prior to examination?

QA also involves image interpretation. Did the patient's ultimate disease or condition agree with the radiologist's diagnosis? This is called **outcome analysis.** Was the report of the diagnosis promptly prepared, distributed, and filed for subsequent evaluation? Was the clinician or patient properly informed in a timely fashion? All of these QA activities require attention from the imaging team, but they are principally the responsibility of the radiologist.

QUALITY CONTROL

Quality control (QC) is more tangible and obvious than QA. A program of QC is designed to ensure that the radiologist is provided with an optimal image resulting from good equipment performance.

Quality control deals with instrumentation and equipment.

QC begins with the x-ray equipment used to produce the image and continues with the routine evaluation of the image-processing facilities. QC concludes with a dedicated analysis of each image to identify deficiencies and artifacts (along with their cause) and to minimize reexamination.

Each new piece of radiologic equipment, whether it is x-ray producing or image processing, should be acceptance tested prior to clinical application. The acceptance test must be done by someone other than the manufacturer's representative because it is designed to show that the equipment is performing within the manufacturer's specifications.

With use, the performance characteristics of all such equipment changes and may deteriorate. Consequently, periodic monitoring of equipment performance is required. On most systems, annual monitoring is satisfactory unless a major component, such as an x-ray tube, has been replaced.

When periodic monitoring shows that equipment is not performing as it was intended, maintenance or repair is necessary. Preventive maintenance usually makes repair unnecessary.

An acceptable QC program has three steps: acceptance testing, routine performance monitoring, and maintenance.

As with QA, QC is a team effort, but QC is principally the responsibility of the medical physicist. In private offices, clinics, and hospitals the medical physicist establishes the QC program and oversee its implementation at a frequency determined by the activity of the institution.

In a large medical center hospital where the medical physicist is a member of the professional staff, he or she performs many of the routine activities and supervises other activities. With the help of the QC technologist and radiologic engineers, the medical physicist sees that all necessary monitoring measurement and observations are performed.

In addition to patient care, there are other reasons for conducting a QC program in radiology. Our litigious society demands QC records. Some insurance carriers pay for services only from facilities with an approved QC program. The JCAHO will not place its seal of approval on facilities that do not have an ongoing QC program. Most states, through their Department of Health and with guidance from the Council of Radiation Control Program Directors (CRCPD), require QC by regulation.

The nature of a QC program is determined somewhat by the characteristics of the image produced. Table 31-1 summarizes the characteristic features of most imaging systems. Usually, the QC program focuses on the strengths of the image to ensure that those strengths are maintained.

RADIOGRAPHIC QUALITY CONTROL

Organizations such as the American College of Medical Physics and the American Association of Physicists in Medicine (AAPM) have developed guidelines for QC programs in radiography as well as other imaging modalities.

Table 31-2 presents the essentials of such a program, the recommended frequency of evaluation, and the tolerance limit for each assessment. Figure 31-1 shows a medical physicist preparing dosimetry equipment for QC measurements.

Filtration

Perhaps the most important patient protection characteristic of a radiographic unit is filtration of its x-ray beam. State statutes require that general-purpose radiographic units have a minimum total filtration of 2.5 mm Al.

TABLE 31-1	Characteristics of Various Diagnostic Imaging Systems				
Procedure	Spatial Resolution	Contrast Resolution	Temporal Resolution	Signal-to-Noise Ratio	Artifacts
Radiography	E	F	E	E	F
Mammography	E	G	G	E	F
Fluoroscopy	G	F	E	G	F
Digital R&F	G	E	G	G	G
Computed tomography	F	E	G	F	G
Magnetic resonance imaging	F	E	G	F	F
Ultrasonography	F	G	G	G	F
Nuclear medicine	F	G	F	F	F

E = excellent; G = good; F = fair.

TABLE 31-2	Elements of a Quality Control Program for Radiographic Systems		
	Measurement	Frequency*	Tolerance
	Filtration	Annually	$\geq$2.5 mm Al
	Collimation	Semiannually	$\pm$2% SID
	Focal-spot size	Annually	$\pm$50%
	Calibration of kVp	Annually	$\pm$10%
	Exposure timer accuracy	Annually	$\pm$5% > 10 ms
			$\pm$20% $\leq$ 10 ms
	Exposure linearity	Annually	$\pm$10%
	Exposure reproducibility	Annually	$\pm$5%

*Evaluation should follow any major equipment modification.

It is normally not possible to measure filtration directly, so one resorts to a measurement of the half-value layer (HVL) of the x-ray beam as described in Chapter 12. The measured HVL must meet or exceed that value shown in Table 31-3 for the total filtration to be considered adequate. Filtration should be determined annually or at any time following a change in the x-ray tube or tube housing.

Collimation

The x-ray field must coincide with the light field of the variable-aperture light-localizing collimator. If these fields are misaligned, intended anatomy will be missed and unintended anatomy irradiated. Adequate collimation can be determined with any of a number of test tools designed for that purpose (Figure 31-2).

Misalignment must not exceed ±2% of the source-to-image receptor distance (SID).

Most systems today are equipped with **positive beam-limiting (PBL)** collimators. These devices are automatic collimators that sense the size of the image receptor and adjust the collimating shutters to that size.

Since different sizes of image receptors must be accommodated, the PBL function must be evaluated for all possible receptor sizes. With a PBL collimator, the x-ray beam must not be larger than the image receptor except in the override mode.

Distance and centering indicators must be accurate to within 2% and 1% of the SID, respectively. The distance indicator can be checked simply with a tape measure. The location of the focal spot usually is marked on the x-ray tube housing. Centering is checked visually for the light field and with markers for the exposure field.

Question: The distance from the Bucky tray to the dot on the x-ray tube housing indicating focal-spot position is measured at 98.4 cm. The automatic distance indications show 100 cm SID. Is this acceptable?

Answer: $\dfrac{100 - 98.4}{100} = \dfrac{1.6}{100} = 1.6\%$, yes

TABLE 31-3	Minimum Half-Value Layer (HVL) Required to Ensure Adequate X-Ray Beam Filtration				
		OPERATING KVP			
Minimum HVL (mm Al)	30	50	70	90	120
Single-phase	0.3	1.2	1.6	2.6	3.6
Three-phase/high frequency	0.4	1.5	2.0	3.1	4.2

FIGURE 31-1 Medical physicist preparing for QC measurements. (Courtesy Louis Wagner.)

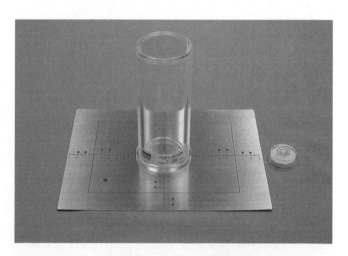

FIGURE 31-2 A test tool for monitoring the coincidence of the x-ray beam and light field. (Courtesy Nuclear Associates.)

Focal-Spot Size

The spatial resolution of a radiographic imaging system is principally determined by the focal-spot size of the x-ray tube. When new equipment or a replacement x-ray tube is installed, the focal-spot size must be measured (Figure 31-3).

 Three tools are used for measurement of focal-spot size: the pinhole camera, the star pattern, and the slit camera.

The pinhole camera is difficult to use and requires excessive exposure time. The star pattern is easy to use but has significant limitations for focal-spot sizes less than 0.3 mm. The standard for measurement of effective focal-spot size is the slit camera.

The fabrication of an x-ray tube is an exceptionally complex process. Specification of focal-spot size depends not only on the geometry of the tube but also on the focusing of the electron beam. Consequently, vendors are permitted a substantial variance from their advertised focal-spot sizes (see Table 10-2).

Focal-spot size should be evaluated annually or whenever an x-ray tube is replaced.

An acceptable alternative to focal-spot size measurement is using a line-pair test tool to determine limiting spatial frequency.

kVp Calibration

The radiologic technologist selects kVp for every examination. The radiologic technologist goes to exceptional lengths to determine the appropriate kVp therefore, the x-ray generator should be properly calibrated.

A number of methods are available to evaluate the accuracy of kVp. Today, most medical physicists use one of a number of devices based on filtered ion chambers or filtered photodiodes (Figure 31-4). Other methods that use voltage diodes and oscilloscopes are more accurate but require an exceptional amount of time.

The kVp calibration should be evaluated annually or whenever high-voltage generator components have changed significantly. In the diagnostic range, any change in peak kilovoltage affects patient dose. A variation in kVp of approximately 3% is necessary to affect image optical density and radiographic contrast.

 The measured kVp should be within ±10% of the indicated kVp.

Exposure Timer Accuracy

Exposure time is operator selectable on most radiographic consoles. Although many radiographic systems are phototimed or controlled by mAs, exposure time is still the responsibility of the radiologic technologist. This parameter is particularly responsible for patient dose and image optical density.

There are a number of ways to assess exposure timer accuracy. Most medical physicists use one of several commercially available products that measure exposure time based on the irradiation time of an ion chamber or photodiode assembly (Figure 31-5).

 Exposure timer accuracy should be within ±5% of the indicated time for exposure times greater than 10 ms.

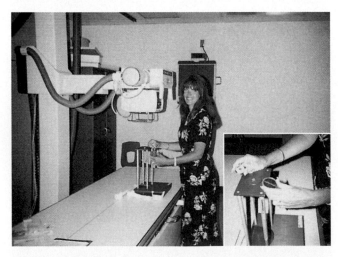

FIGURE 31-3 The pinhole camera, star pattern, and slit camera may be used to measure focal-spot size. (Courtesy Teresa Rice.)

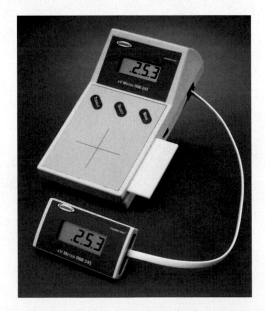

FIGURE 31-4 High-voltage (kVp) and other generator functions can be evaluated with compact test devices. (Courtesy Gammex RMI.)

The accuracy of the exposure timer should be assessed annually or more frequently if a component of the operating console or the high-voltage generator has undergone major repairs. An accuracy of ±20% is acceptable for exposure times of 10 ms or less.

Automatic exposure control (AEC) must also be evaluated. These devices are designed to provide a constant optical density regardless of tissue thickness, composition, or **failure of the reciprocity law** (see Chapter 18). AEC systems are evaluated by exposing an image receptor through various thicknesses of aluminum or acrylic. Regardless of the material thickness and the absolute exposure time, the optical density of the processed image should be constant.

Insertion of a lead filter allows one to adequately assess the functioning of the backup timer. If the phototimer fails, the backup timer should terminate the exposure at 6 s or 600 mAs, whichever occurs first.

Exposure Linearity

Many combinations of mA and exposure time produce the same mAs value. The ability of a radiographic unit to produce a constant radiation output for various combinations of mA and exposure time is called **exposure linearity.**

 Exposure linearity must be within ±10% for adjacent mA stations.

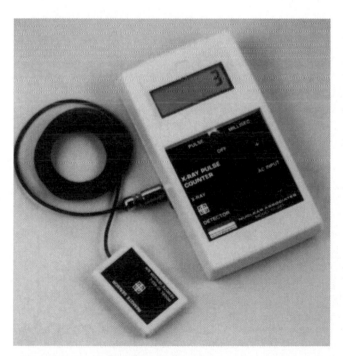

FIGURE 31-5 Device for measuring the accuracy of an exposure timer. (Courtesy Nuclear Associates.)

Exposure linearity is determined by a precision radiation dosimeter that measures radiation intensity at various combinations of mA and exposure time. Suppose, for example, that one were to choose 10 mAs for the evaluation of the combinations of mA and exposure time shown in Table 31-4. Each of these combinations would be energized, and radiation intensity would be measured.

When evaluated in this fashion, the radiation output for adjacent mA stations **should be within ±10%.** Exposure linearity should be evaluated annually or following any significant change or repair of the operating console or high-voltage generator.

This method of assessing exposure linearity is not valid if the exposure timer is inaccurate. Consequently, most would hold exposure time constant and vary only the mA. Under these conditions, the mR/mAs value **should be within** ±10% between adjacent mA stations.

Question: The following data is obtained to evaluate exposure linearity. Are the mA stations correctly calibrated?

Exposure Time	mA	mR
100 ms	50	29
100 ms	100	61
100 ms	200	109
100 ms	400	236

Answer:

mA	mR/mAs	% Difference
50	5.8	$\dfrac{6.1 - 5.8}{5.8} \times 100 = +5.2\%$, OK
100	6.1	$\dfrac{5.5 - 6.1}{6.1} \times 100 = -9.8\%$, OK
200	5.5	$\dfrac{4.8 - 5.5}{5.5} \times 100 = -13\%$, **UNACCEPTABLE**
400	4.8	

TABLE 31-4	Exposure Time and mA Combinations Equal to 10 mAs
Exposure Time (ms)	**mA**
1000	10
400	25
200	50
100	100
50	200
25	400
13	800
10	1000
8	1200

Exposure Reproducibility

When selecting the proper kVp, mA, and exposure time for a given examination, the radiologic technologist rightfully expects the image optical density and contrast to be optimal. If any or all of these technique factors are changed and then returned to the previous value, radiation exposure should be precisely the same. The radiation exposure should be **reproducible.**

 Sequential radiation exposures should be reproducible to within ±5%.

Two methods are available to evaluate exposure reproducibility; both rely on a precision radiation dosimeter. First, one can make a series of at least three exposures at the same technique factors, having changed the technique controls between each exposure. If the result is not reproducible, it is usually so because of error in the kVp control. Second, one can select a combination of technique factors and hold them constant for a series of 10 exposures.

Mathematical formulas can be used to determine reproducibility in both instances. These formulas basically require that the output radiation intensity not vary by more than ±5%.

Radiographic Intensifying Screens

Intensifying screens require periodic attention to minimize the appearance of artifacts. Screens should be cleaned with a soft, lint-free cloth and a cleaning solution provided by the manufacturer. The frequency of cleaning depends on the workload in the department but certainly should not be less than every other month.

Screen-film contact should be evaluated once or twice a year. This is done by radiographing a wire mesh pattern and analyzing the image for areas of blur (see Figures 23-14, 23-15). Should blur appear, the felt or foam pressure pad under the screen should be replaced. If that does not correct the problem, the cassette should be replaced.

Protective Apparel

All protective aprons, gloves, and gonadal shields should be radiographed or fluoroscoped annually for defects. If there are cracks, tears, or holes, the apparel may require replacement (Figure 31-6).

Film Illuminators

Viewbox illumination should be photometrically analyzed annually. This is done with an instrument called a **photometer** by measuring light intensity at several areas of the illuminator (Figure 31-7). This intensity should be at least 1500 cd/m² and should not vary by more than ±10% over the surface of the illuminator. If a bulb requires replacement, all bulbs should be replaced in that illuminator and matched to the type of bulbs in adjacent illuminators.

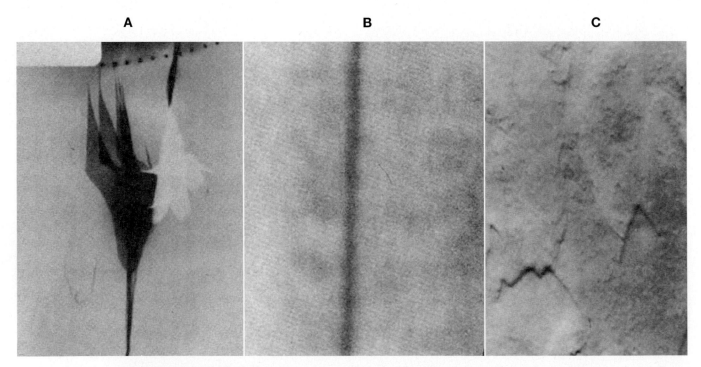

A   B   C

FIGURE 31-6 Radiographs of mistreated protective aprons showing bunching of the lead **(A)** from folding and tearing, a low density area in a new apron **(B)**, and cracking patterns in an apron **(C).** (Courtesy Sharon Glaze.)

FLUOROSCOPY QUALITY CONTROL

Fluoroscopic examination can result in high patient dose. The entrance skin exposure (ESE) for an adult averages 3 to 5 R/min (30 to 50 mGy$_a$/min) during fluoroscopy and can result in a skin dose of 10 rad (100 mGy$_t$) for many fluoroscopic examinations. For interventional procedures, a skin dose of 100 rad (1 Gy$_t$) is not uncommon but should be avoided if possible.

Approximate patient dose can be ensured through the performance of proper QC measurements. Some measurements may be required more frequently after significant changes in the operating console, high-voltage generator, or x-ray tube.

Exposure Rate

Federal law and most state statutes require that under normal operation the ESE rate shall not exceed 10 R/min (100 mGy$_a$/min). For interventional procedures, the fluoroscope may be equipped with a high level control, which allows an ESE up to 20 R/min (200 mGy$_a$/min). Unlimited exposure rates are permitted for recorded fluoroscopy, such as cineradiography.

Measurements are made with a calibrated radiation dosimeter to ensure that these levels are not exceeded. Lucite, aluminum, copper, and lead filters are required to determine the adequacy of any automatic brightness stabilization (ABS) system.

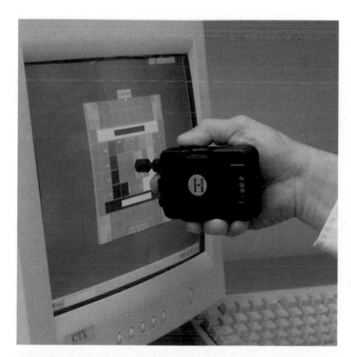

FIGURE 31-7 Measuring luminance of a CRT screen with a photometer. (Courtesy Nuclear Associates.)

Spot-Film Exposures

There are two types of spot-film devices, both of which must be evaluated for radiation exposure and proper collimation. Proper exposure of the **cassette spot film** depends on the kVp, mAs value, and sensitivity characteristics of the screen-film combination. ESEs for such a spot-film device vary widely (Table 31-5). The values reported in this table were obtained with a 10:1 grid using a 400 speed image receptor. Nongrid exposures are approximately half of the values reported here.

 An ESE of approximately 200 mR may be assumed for a cassette spot film.

The use of photofluorospot images is more routine. These images use less film, require less personnel interaction, and are produced with a lower patient dose. Photofluorospot images are recorded on film from the output phosphor of an image-intensifier tube.

In addition to the factors that affect cassette spot films, photofluorospot images depend on characteristics of the image intensifier, particularly the diameter of the input phosphor. Table 31-6 shows representative ESE for two input phosphor sizes and no grid. They are substantially lower than those with cassette spot films.

As the active area of the input phosphor of the image-intensifier tube is increased, patient dose is reduced in approximate proportion to the change in the diameter of the input phosphor. Use of a grid during photofluorospot imaging approximately doubles the ESE.

 An ESE of approximately 100 mR may be assumed for a photofluorospot.

Question: A photofluorospot image is made at 80 kVp in the 15 cm mode without a grid, as seen in Table 31-6. The measured ESE is 50 mR. What would be the expected ESE if the 25 cm mode were used?

TABLE 31-5	Extrance Skin Exposure with Cassette-Loaded Spot Film
kVp	**Entrance Skin Exposure (mR)**
60	450
70	270
80	170
90	150
100	130

Answer:
$$\frac{x}{50} = \frac{15}{25}$$
$$x = 50 \left(\frac{15}{25}\right)$$
$$= 30 \text{ mR}$$

Automatic Exposure Systems

All fluoroscopes are equipped with some sort of automatic brightness control (ABC), or automatic exposure control (AEC). Each system functions like the phototimer of a radiographic imager, producing constant image brightness on the video monitor regardless of the thickness or composition of the anatomy. These systems tend to deteriorate or fail with use.

 Fluoroscopic ABC should be evaluated annually.

TABLE 31-6	Entrance Skin Exposure with Photofluorospot Imagers	
	ESE (MR)	
kVp	**15 cm II**	**25 cm II**
60	90	50
70	65	35
80	50	30
90	40	25
100	30	20

Performance monitoring of an ABC is conducted by determining that the radiation exposure to the input phosphor of the image-intensifier tube is constant regardless of patient thickness. With a test object in place, the image brightness on the video monitor should not change perceptibly when various thicknesses of patient-stimulating material are inserted in the beam. The input exposure rate to the image-intensifier tube is measured and should be in the range of 10 to 40 μR/s (0.1 to 0.4 μGy$_a$/s).

The test object used for ACR accreditation is shown in Figure 31-8. This test object tracks ABC versus tissue thickness and assesses spatial resolution, contrast resolution, and contrast detail.

TOMOGRAPHY QUALITY CONTROL

In addition to the evaluations performed in the course of QC of a radiographic system, several additional measurements are required for those systems that can also perform conventional tomography.

Precise performance standards do not exist for conventional tomography. QC measurements are designed to ensure that the characteristics evaluated remain constant.

Patient exposure should be measured for the most frequent type of tomographic examinations. Table 31-7 is a sample of the results from a three-phase system and six representative tomographic examinations.

The geometric characteristics of a tomogram can be evaluated with any of a number of test objects designed for this use. Agreement between the indicated section

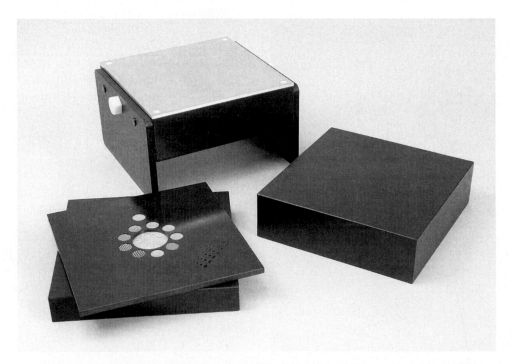

FIGURE 31-8 American College of Radiology radiographic/fluoroscopic accreditation phantom. (Courtesy American College of Radiography/CIRS.)

level and the measured level should be within ±5 mm. When incrementing from one tomographic section to the next, the section level should be accurate to within ±2 mm. Constancy of ±1 mm from one QC evaluation to the next should be achieved.

TABLE 31-7	Exposure Technique and Entrance Skin Exposure During Conventional Tomographic Examination

Examination	Technique (kVp/mAs)	Entrance Skin Exposure (mR)
Temporomandibular joint	90/300	2300
Cervical spine	76/200	1300
Thoracic and lumbar spine	78/250	1700
Chest	110/8	70
Intravenous pyelogram	70/300	1800
Nephrotomogram	74/350	2200

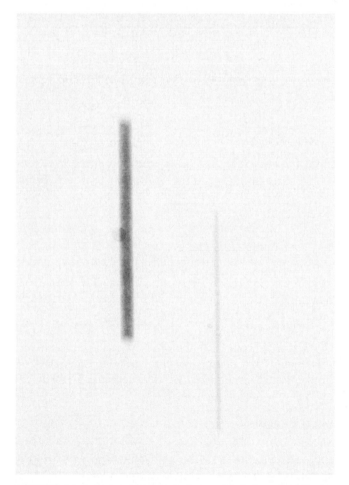

FIGURE 31-9 Images of a pinhole in a lead attenuator during linear tomography. The larger pinhole image shows modest staggering motion, resulting in varied optical density. (Courtesy Sharon Glaze.)

Section uniformity is evaluated by imaging a hole in a lead sheet. The optical density of the image tracing of the hole should be uniform with no perceptible variations, no gaps, and no overlaps (Figure 31-9).

COMPUTED TOMOGRAPHY QUALITY CONTROL

Computed tomography (CT) imagers are subject to all the misalignment, miscalibration, and malfunction difficulties of conventional x-ray imagers. They have the additional complexities of the multimotional gantry, the interactive console, and the associated computer.

Each of these subsystems increases the risk of drift and instability, which could result in degradation of image quality. Consequently, a dedicated QC program is essential for each CT imaging system. Such a program includes daily, weekly, monthly, and annual monitoring in addition to an ongoing preventive maintenance program.

Table 31-8 identifies the measurements and their required frequencies for an adequate QC program for a CT imaging system. Figure 31-10 shows a popular test object for CT measurements. The measurements specified for an annual performance should also be conducted on all new equipment and on all existing equipment following replacement or repair of a major component.

Noise and Uniformity

A 20 cm waterbath should be imaged weekly; the average value for water should be within ±10 HU of zero. Furthermore, the uniformity across the image should not vary by more than ±10 HU from center to periphery.

Nearly all CT imaging systems easily meet these performance specifications. If a system is used for quantitative CT, however, then tighter specifications may be appropriate. When performing this assessment, one should change one or more of the following: the CT scan parameters, the slice thickness, the reconstruction diameter, and the reconstruction algorithm.

Linearity

Linearity is assessed with an image of the AAPM five-pin insert. Analysis of the values of the five pins should show a linear relationship between the Hounsfield unit and electron density. The coefficient of correlation for this linear relationship should be at least 0.96%, or 2 standard deviations.

This assessment should be conducted semiannually. It is particularly important for systems used for quantitative CT, which requires precise determination of the value of tissue in Hounsfield units.

Spatial Resolution

Monitoring spatial resolution is the most important component of this QC program. Constant spatial resolution ensures proper performance of not only the detector array and reconstruction electronics but also the mechanical components.

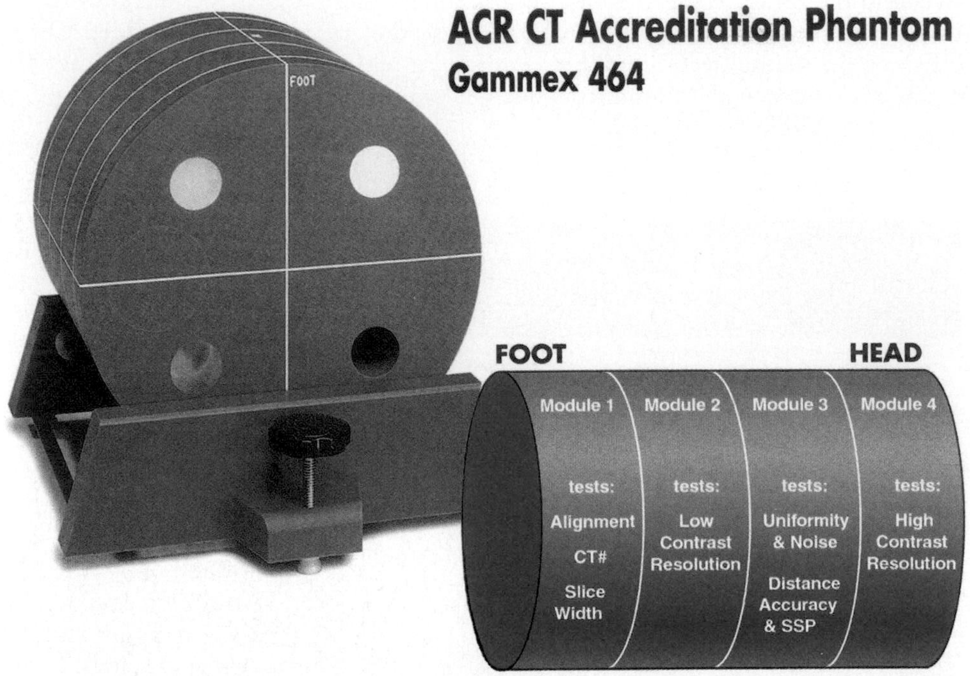

ACR CT Accreditation Phantom
Gammex 464

FIGURE 31-10 This CT test object is used to evaluate noise, spatial resolution, contrast resolution, slice thickness, linearity, and uniformity. (Courtesy American College of Radiology/Gammex RMI.)

TABLE 31-8	Elements of a Quality Control Program for Computed Tomography		
Measurement	**Frequency***	**Tolerance**	
Noise	Weekly	±10 HU	
Uniformity	Weekly	±10 HU	
Linearity	Semiannually	±2 σ	
Spatial resolution	Semiannually	20%	
Contrast resolution	Semiannually	5 mm at 0.5%	
Slice thickness	Semiannually	≥ 5 mm, 1 mm; <5 mm, 0.5 mm	
Couch incrementation	Semiannually	±2 mm	
Laser localizer	Semiannually	±1 mm	
Patient dose	Annually	Within manufacturer's specifications	
Dose profile	Annually	±10%	

*Evaluation should follow any major equipment modification.

Spatial resolution is assessed by imaging a wire or an edge to get the point-spread function or edge-response function, respectively. These functions are then mathematically transformed to obtain the modulation transfer function (MTF).

However, determining the MTF requires considerable time and attention. Most medical physicists find it acceptable to image a bar pattern or hole pattern. Spatial resolution should be assessed semiannually and should be within the manufacturer's specifications.

Contrast Resolution

CT excels as an imaging modality because of its superior contrast resolution. The performance specifications of the various CT imaging systems differ from one manufacturer to another and from one model to another, depending on the design of the imaging system. All CT imaging systems should be capable of resolving 5 mm objects at 0.5% contrast.

Contrast resolution should be assessed semiannually. It is done with any one of a number of low-contrast test objects with the built-in analytical schemes available on all CT imagers (Figure 31-11).

Slice Thickness

Slice thickness (sensitivity profile) is measured with a specially designed test object that incorporates a ramp, spiral, or step wedge. This assessment should be semiannual; the slice thickness should be within 1 mm of the intended slice thickness for a thickness of 5 mm or

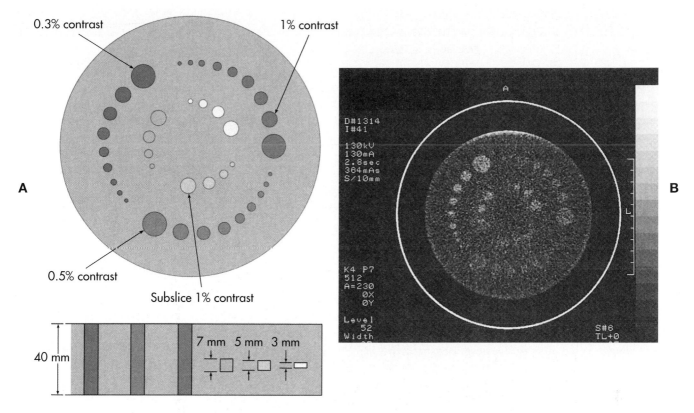

FIGURE 31-11 Schematic drawing **(A)** of a low-contrast CT test object and **(B)** its image. This test object is designed especially for spiral CT. (Courtesy Phantom Laboratory.)

greater. For an intended slice thickness of less than 5 mm, the acceptable tolerance is 0.5 mm.

Couch Incrementation

With the automatic maneuvering of the patient through the CT gantry, the patient must be precisely positioned. This evaluation should be done monthly. During a clinical examination with a patient-loaded couch, note the position of the couch at the beginning and at the end of the examination using tape measure and a straightedge on the couch rails. Compare this with the intended couch movement. It should be within ±2 mm.

Laser Localizer

Most CT imaging systems have internal and/or external laser localizing lights for patient positioning. The accuracy of these lasers can be determined with any number of specially designed test objects. Their accuracy should be assessed at least semiannually; this is usually done at the same time as the evaluation of couch incrementation.

Patient Dose

No recommended limits are specified for patient dose during CT examination. Furthermore, dose varies considerably according to the scan parameters. High-

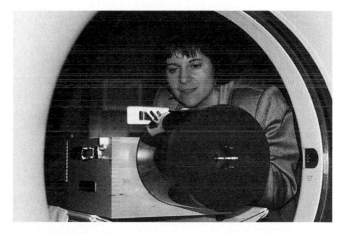

FIGURE 31-12 Medical physics evaluation of CT performance requires a number of measurements using specially designed test objects. (Courtesy Cynthia McCollough.)

resolution imaging requires a higher dose. Multislice CT imagers can lead to even higher doses.

When a fixed technique is used, patient dose should not vary by more than ±10% from one assessment to the next. Such an assessment should be semiannual or should follow replacement of the x-ray tube.

TABLE 31-9	Quality Control Program for Radiographic Processor	
Activity	**Procedure or Item**	**Schedule**
Processor cleaning	Cross-over racks	Daily
	Entire rack assembly and processing ranks	Weekly
Scheduled maintenance	Observation of belts, pulleys, and gears	Weekly
	Lubrication	Weekly or monthly
Processor monitoring	Planned parts replacement	Regularly
	Check developer temperature	Daily
	Check wash-water temperature	Daily
	Check replenishment tanks	Daily
	Sensitometry and densitometry	Daily

Patient dose is specified as **computed tomography dose index (CTDI)** and can be monitored with specially designed pencil ionization chambers or thermoluminescent dosimeters. In addition to patient dose, dose profile also must be measured for the most common slice thicknesses. Figure 31-12 illustrates these measurements in progress.

PROCESSOR QUALITY CONTROL

QC in any activity refers to the routine and special procedures developed to ensure that the final product is of consistently high quality. QC in diagnostic radiology requires a planned continuous program of evaluation and surveillance of radiologic equipment and procedures.

When applied to automatic processing, such a program involves periodic cleaning, system maintenance, and daily monitoring. Table 31-9 lists an appropriate processor QC program.

Processor Cleaning

The first automatic processor had a dry-to-drop time of 7 min. Soon this was shortened to 3 min by what are known as double-capacity processors. Processing time was reduced further with the fast-access system, which is today's popular 90 s processor. Such a processor can handle up to 500 films per hour but to do so it requires a high concentration of processing chemistry, a high development temperature (95°F [35°C]), and a developer immersion time of 22 s.

The wash water temperature should be 87°F (31°C). Earlier automatic processors were supplied with hot and cold water, so the wash temperature was primarily controlled through a mixing valve. Current processors are supplied with only cold water, and temperature is maintained with a thermostatically controlled heater.

This rapid activity, carried on at high temperature with concentrated chemistry, tends to wear and corrode the mechanism of the transport system and contaminate the chemistry with processing sludge. This may lead to a deposit of sludge and debris on the rollers, which can severely affect film quality and cause artifacts if the processor is not properly cleaned at appropriate intervals.

In most facilities, cleaning is conducted weekly; records of such cleaning should be maintained. The cleaning procedure is rather simple. One removes the transport and crossover racks and cleans them in the processing tanks.

This takes no more than a few minutes and pays great dividends in reduced processor wear and the consistent production of high-quality radiographs that are artifact free. When reassembled, sensitometric levels must be reestablished.

Processor Maintenance

As with any electromechanical device, maintenance is essential. If equipment is not properly maintained the processor may fail when least expected or when the workload is heaviest. There are three types of maintenance programs that should be a part of the QC program for an automatic processor.

Scheduled maintenance refers to routine procedures, usually weekly or monthly. Such maintenance includes observation of all moving parts for wear; adjustment of all belts, pulleys, and gears; and application of proper lubrication to minimize wear. During processor lubrication, it is especially important to keep the lubricant off of your hands, thereby keeping it away from film and rollers and, of course, out of processor chemistry.

Preventive maintenance is a planned program of parts replacement at regular intervals. Preventive maintenance requires that a part be replaced before it fails. Such a program should avoid unexpected downtime.

Nonscheduled maintenance is, of course, the worst kind. A failure in the system that necessitates processor repair is a nonscheduled event. A proper program of scheduled maintenance and preventive maintenance keeps nonscheduled maintenance to a minimum.

Processor Monitoring

At least once per day, processor operation should be observed and certain measurements recorded. The temperature of the developer and wash water should be noted. The developer and fixer replenishment rates should be observed and recorded.

The replenishment tanks should be checked to determine whether the floating lids are properly positioned and whether fresh chemistry is needed. It is often appropriate to check the pH and specific gravity of the developer and fixer solutions. Residual hypo should be determined.

A sensitometric strip should be passed through the processor and fog, speed, and contrast should then be appropriately measured and recorded. Most film suppliers provide forms and assistance to establish and conduct a program of processor monitoring. The written record of the results of such a program is important.

The processor monitoring described in Chapter 23 for the dedicated mammography processor can be applied to all other processors in the health care facility.

SUMMARY

In diagnostic imaging, Quality assessment involves the assessment and evaluation of patient care. Quality control is the measurement and performance evaluation of imaging equipment. Both processes ensure that the radiologist is provided with an optimal image for proper diagnosis.

The QA/QC team includes radiographers, management and secretarial personnel, the equipment manufacturer's representative, the medical physicist, radiologic engineers, and radiologists. The JCAHO does not accredit health care facilities unless proper QA and QC programs are evident.

The three steps of QC are (1) acceptance testing, (2) routine performance evaluation, and (3) error correction. Radiographic QC evaluates filtration, collimation, focal-spot size, kVp, timers, linearity, and reproducibility.

Intensifying screens are evaluated regularly for cleanliness and screen-film contact. All lead apparel is checked for cracks, tears, and holes. Finally, viewboxes or film illuminators are examined for intensity and cleanliness.

Because fluoroscopy leads to the highest patient dose of all x-ray procedures, fluoroscopic equipment is evaluated regularly for exposure rate. Under federal law, the ESE shall not exceed 10 R/min unless the fluoroscope has a high level control.

Conventional tomography section sensitivity is evaluated regularly. Each of the subsystems of CT is regularly checked for misalignment and miscalibration.

Radiographic processor QC is essential for optimal image quality. Sensitometry and densitometry are important daily functions of the QC radiographer.

CHALLENGE QUESTIONS

1. Define or otherwise identify:
   a. Quality assurance
   b. Required x-ray beam filtration
   c. CT linearity
   d. Outcome analysis
   e. Minimum half-value layer
   f. CRCPD
   g. JCAHO 10-step program
   h. CT section sensitivity
   i. Exposure linearity
   j. Quality control
2. List and explain the theory behind the JCAHO QA program used in hospitals.
3. Discuss the three steps of quality control for radiographic equipment.
4. Name the people on the diagnostic imaging QC team.
5. How is filtration measured in radiographic equipment?
6. Why are proper x-ray beam alignment and collimation important?
7. What are the limits for radiographic misalignment?
8. What are three QC tools used to measure focal-spot size?
9. What is the permitted variation of radiographic reproducibility?
10. What test is performed on intensifying screens and cassettes to check that there is proper screen-film contact?
11. What products are used to clean intensifying screens?
12. How often should lead apparel be checked for protective integrity?
13. What is the average entrance skin exposure during a fluoroscopic examination?
14. Describe the process of monitoring the spatial resolution in a CT imager.
15. List and briefly describe the eight parts of CT quality control.
16. What is the importance of preventive maintenance for a radiographic processor?
17. A high-frequency radiographic imaging system requires how much x-ray beam filtration?
18. What is the allowed radiographic collimator misalignment?
19. When should defective protective apparel be discarded?
20. Which procedure results in less patient radiation dose: cassette-loaded spot films or 105 mm photofluorospot images?

Image Artifacts

OBJECTIVES

At the completion of this chapter, the student should be able to do the following:

1. Visually identify the radiographic artifacts shown in this chapter
2. List and discuss the three categories of artifacts
3. Explain the causes of exposure artifacts
4. Describe the types of artifacts caused during film processing
5. Discuss how improper handling and storage of film can cause artifacts

OUTLINE

FOR STUDENT radiographers, one of the most interesting areas of study is the identification of image artifacts. Most schools have an extensive film file of artifacts, from pi lines to necklaces on chest radiographs. It is fun to identify such artifacts and their cause.

However, artifacts need to be prevented. Identification of the artifact and its cause is critical for quality control (QC). It is important for every radiographer to be alert to artifacts and their origin.

The cause of the artifact must be removed to prevent the same problem in subsequent radiographs. Finally, records of artifacts must be kept to indicate trends; for example, if sludge artifacts show up more than once before processor cleaning, consider cleaning the processor more frequently.

Artifacts are undesirable optical densities or blemishes on a radiograph or any other medical image. An artifact is something in the image that looks like it was created by the object but was in fact created by the process.

Artifacts can interfere with the visualization of anatomic structures and lead to misdiagnoses. Artifacts can be controlled when their cause is identified. There are generally three areas in which radiographic artifacts occur: exposure, processing, and handling. Figure 32-1 provides a classification of the artifacts one is likely to see in conventional screen-film radiography.

 An artifact is any irregularity on an image that is not caused by the proper shadowing of tissue by the primary x-ray beam.

EXPOSURE ARTIFACTS

Exposure artifacts are generally associated with the manner in which the radiographer conducts the examination. Incorrect screen-film match, poor screen-film contact, warped cassettes, and improper positioning of the grid can all lead to such artifacts.

Improper patient position, patient motion, double exposure, and incorrect radiographic technique can result in very poor images that some would call artifacts. Such examples of poor technique have been shown to result in the largest number of repeat examinations.

Improper preparation of the patient can lead to disturbing artifacts (Figure 32-2). However, they will never occur when the radiologic technologist properly instructs and prepares the patient.

Double exposures are also avoidable. When radiographers mix-up cassettes, double exposures can occur, which then requires repeat examination.

A radiograph with motion appears blurred. The patient may have moved or may not have breathed according to the radiographer's instructions. Clear instructions are required to encourage understanding and cooperation in patients.

 Exposure artifacts are usually easy to detect and correct.

Positioning errors can cause artifacts. If the patient is placed under the x-ray tube when the tube is not centered to the table or Bucky tray, grid cutoff artifacts may occur.

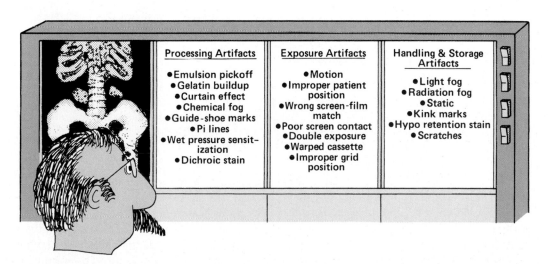

Processing Artifacts	Exposure Artifacts	Handling & Storage Artifacts
•Emulsion pickoff •Gelatin buildup •Curtain effect •Chemical fog •Guide-shoe marks •Pi lines •Wet pressure sensitization •Dichroic stain	•Motion •Improper patient position •Wrong screen-film match •Poor screen contact •Double exposure •Warped cassette •Improper grid position	•Light fog •Radiation fog •Static •Kink marks •Hypo retention stain •Scratches

FIGURE 32-1 Artifact classification.

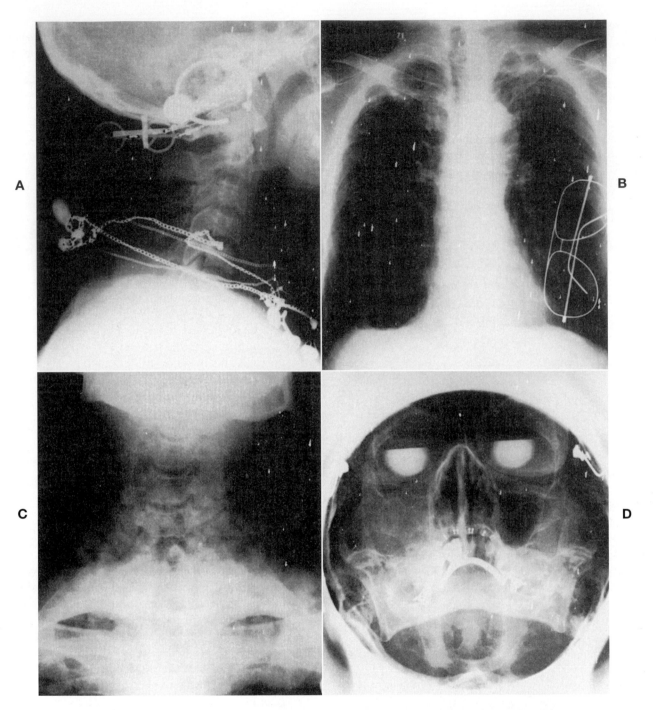

FIGURE 32-2 A, Lateral cervical spine of a patient with a "Mr. T starter set." **B,** The patient's glasses were not removed from the shirt pocket. **C,** The ice bag under the neck was not removed during this AP cervical spine. **D,** This Waters view was properly coned but the bifocals, earrings, and dental apparatus should have been removed. (Courtesy Paul Laudicina.)

Artifacts can occur if the wrong film is loaded into a cassette. If high-contrast, single-emulsion mammography film is loaded into a radiographic cassette, an unexpected image results. Cassettes that have not been checked for proper screen-film contact cause a smoothness in the area of poor contact, which obscures detail and constitutes an artifact.

When one is trying to locate an object that has been swallowed, it is not an artifact. On the other hand, if such an object appears on an image unexpectedly, it is an artifact. Table 32-1 summarizes the exposure artifacts discussed here.

The same errors that cause exposure artifacts in screen-film radiography also cause artifacts in digital radiography (DR). DR is more tolerant of incorrect exposure technique, but under- and overexposure can still produce artifacts (Figure 32-3).

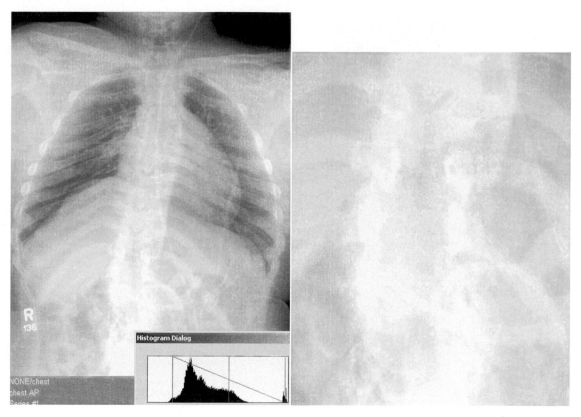

FIGURE 32-3 Underexposure in DR causes a loss of contrast in dense anatomy as well as a grainy appearance. (Courtesy Charles Willis.)

TABLE 32-1	Common Exposure Artifacts
Appearance on Radiographic Film	**Cause**
Unexpected foreign objects such as jewelry	Improper patient preparation
Double exposure	Reuse of cassettes already exposed
Blur	Improper patient movement, including breathing
Grid cutoff artifacts	Improper patient positioning
Obscured detail	Poor screen-film contact

PROCESSING ARTIFACTS

Any number of artifacts can be produced during processing. Most are pressure-type artifacts caused by the transport system of the processor. Pressure-type artifacts usually sensitize the emulsion and appear as higher optical density (OD). Those that scrape or remove emulsion appear as lower OD.

 Processing artifacts are eliminated with a proper processor QC program and frequent cleaning.

Table 32-2 summarizes the processing artifacts discussed here as well as some other common artifacts.

Roller Marks

Guide-shoe marks occur when the guide shoes in the turn-around assembly of the processor are sprung or improperly positioned (Figure 32-4). If the guide shoe is before the developer, the ridges in the guide shoes press against the film, sensitize it, and leave a characteristic mark. Guide-shoe marks can be found on the leading edge or the trailing edge of the film parallel to the direction of film travel through the processor.

Pi lines occur at 3.1416 inch (π) intervals because of dirt or a chemical stain on a roller, which sensitizes the emulsion. Because the rollers are 1 inch in diameter, 3.1416 inches represent one revolution of a roller and the artifact appears perpendicular to the film's direction of travel through the processor. Figure 32-5 is an example of pi lines appearing on the same film.

Dirty Rollers

Dirty or warped rollers can cause **emulsion pick-off** and **gelatin buildup,** which results in **sludge** deposits on the film. These artifacts usually appear as sharp areas of either increased or reduced OD. Occasionally, particles of sludge are transported through the processor and are actually dried on the film in the dryer.

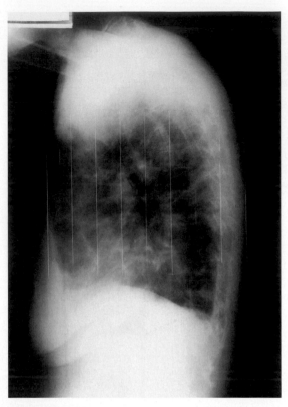

FIGURE 32-4 Guide shoe marks left by an improperly serviced turnaround assembly. (Courtesy Judy Williams.)

Direction of film transport

FIGURE 32-5 Pi line artifacts due to lack of processor cleaning. (Courtesy Rita Robinson.)

TABLE 32-2	Common Processing Artifacts
Appearance on Radiographic Film	**Cause**
Guide-shoe marks	Improper position or springing of guide shoes in turn-around assembly
Pi lines	Dirt or chemical stains on rollers
Sharp increase or decrease in OD	Dirty or warped rollers, which can leave sludge deposits on film
Uniform dull, gray fog	Improper or inadequate processing chemistry
Dichroic stain or "curtain effect"	Improper squeezing of processing chemicals from film
Small circular patterns of increased OD	Pressure caused by irregular or dirty rollers
Yellow-brown drops on film	Oxidized developer
Milky appearance	Unreplenished floor
Greasy appearance	Inadequate washing
Brittle appearance	Improper dryer temperature or hardener in the fixer

Chemical Fog

Chemical fog looks like light or radiation fog and is usually a uniform dull gray. Improper or inadequate processing chemistry can result in a special type of chemical fog called a **dichroic stain.** Dichroic means two colors. The dichroic stain appears as a curtain effect on the radiograph (Figure 32-6). Dichroic stain is a term generally applied to all chemical stains.

Chemical stains on a radiograph can appear yellow, green, blue, or purple. In slow processors, the chemistry may not be properly squeezed from the film and it either runs down the leading edge of the film or runs up the trailing edge. Both are called a **curtain effect.**

Wet-Pressure Sensitization

Wet-pressure sensitization is a common artifact produced in the developer tank (Figure 32-7). Irregular or dirty rollers cause pressure during development and produce small circular patterns of increased OD.

Processing artifacts in DR are different from those with screen-film because the method of producing the visible image is electronic rather than chemical. Image-

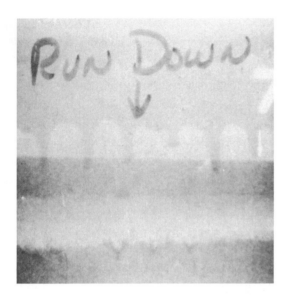

FIGURE 32-6 Excess chemistry runs down the leading edge of the film creating a "curtain" effect. (Courtesy William McKinney.)

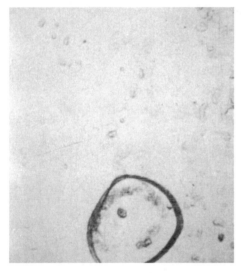

FIGURE 32-7 Wet-pressure sensitization caused by a dirty processor. (Courtesy William McKinney.)

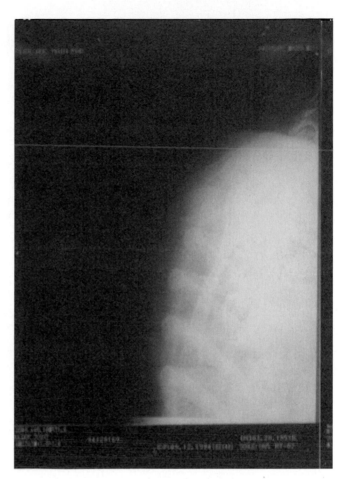

FIGURE 32-8 Failure of electronic processing can cause uninterpretable images in DR. (Courtesy Charles Willis.)

processing error can produce bizarre artifacts in DR. Interference with electronic components involved in processing DR images also occurs (Figure 32-8).

HANDLING AND STORAGE ARTIFACTS

A number of artifacts are caused by improper film storage conditions. Image fog can result if the temperature or the humidity is too high or if the film bin is not adequately shielded from radiation. Pressure marks can occur if film is stacked too high. Table 32-3 summarizes the storage artifacts discussed here.

 Proper facility design helps reduce handling and storage artifacts.

Light or Radiation Fog

White-light leaks in the darkroom or within the cassette cause streak-like artifacts of increased OD. If the safelight has an improper filter, if the safelight is too bright, or if the safelight is too close to the film-processing tray, the image will be fogged. Films left in the x-ray examination room during an exposure can become fogged by radiation. Radiation fog and safelight fog look alike.

Kink Marks

Characteristic artifacts can be caused by improper handling or storage either before or after processing. Rough handling before processing can cause scratches and kink marks, such as those shown in Figure 32-9. Although the kink mark may appear as a fingernail mark, it is not. It is caused by the kinking or abrupt bending of film. Both usually appear as increased OD.

TABLE 32-3	Common Handling and Storage Artifacts
Appearance on Radiographic Film	**Cause**
Fog	The temperature or humidity is too high
	The film bin is inadequately shielded from radiation
	The safelight is too bright, is too close to the processing tray, or has an improper filter
	The film has been left in the x-ray room during other exposures
Pressure or kink marks	The film is improperly or roughly handled
	The film is stacked too high in storage (the weight causes marks)
Streaks of increased OD	The darkroom or cassette has white-light leaks
Crown, tree, and smudge static	The temperature or humidity is too low
Yellow-brown stains	Thiosulfate is left on the film because of inadequate washing

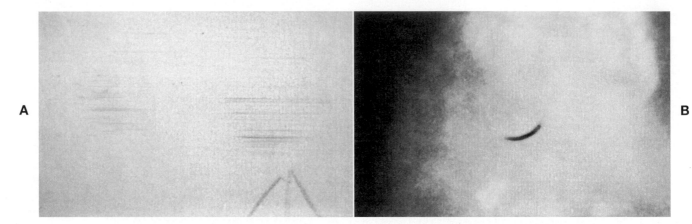

FIGURE 32-9 Preprocessing pressure artifacts can appear as scratches caused by heavy finger pressure on the feed tray and as "fingernail" marks caused by kinking of the film. **A,** scratches. **B,** "fingernail" marks. (Courtesy William McKinney.)

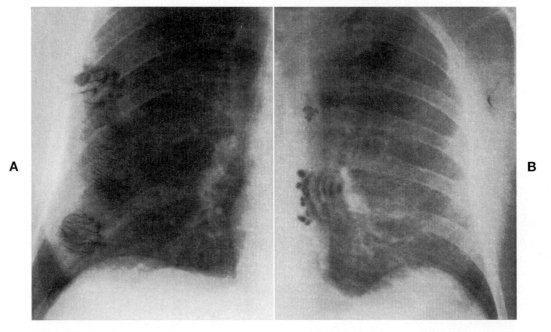

FIGURE 32-10 A, tree static. **B,** smudge static. These are the two most common types of static artifacts. (Courtesy Joel Gray.)

Static

Static is probably the most obvious artifact. It is caused by the buildup of electrons in the emulsion and is most noticeable during the winter or during periods of extremely low humidity. Three distinct patterns of static are crown, tree, and smudge. Tree static and smudge static are illustrated in Figure 32-10.

Handling and storage artifacts that occur in DR also differ from screen-film artifacts. Debris on the image receptor or in the optical path of CR, discoloration of the image receptor or fluorescent screens, fogging of the receptor during storage, "ghost images" from incomplete erasure, and "dead" detector elements can be considered handling and storage artifacts in DR (Figure 32-11).

Hypo Retention

The yellow-brown stain slowly appearing on a radiograph following a long storage time indicates a problem with hypo retention from the fixer. Not all of the residual thiosulfate from fixing was removed during washing, and silver sulfide slowly builds up and appears yellow in the stored radiograph.

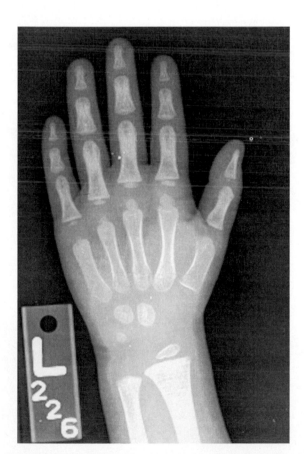

FIGURE 32-11 Debris on image receptor in DR can be confused with foreign bodies. (Courtesy Charles Willis.)

SUMMARY

An artifact is an undesirable OD that appears on the radiograph. Artifacts occur (1) during the radiographic exposure, (2) during the processing of the film, and (3) when the film is being handled and stored either before or after processing. Similar artifacts can occur in DR.

Exposure artifacts are a result of examination technique. They include patient motion, positioning errors, wrong screen-film combinations, double exposures, and improper grid positioning.

Processing artifacts are mostly pressure blemished on the film emulsion caused by the roller transport system in the processor. They include sludge from dirty rollers, chemical fog, roller marks, and wet-pressure sensitization.

CHALLENGE QUESTIONS

1. Define or otherwise identify:
   a. Exposure artifact
   b. Guide shoe
   c. Pick-off
   d. Pressure mark
   e. Kink mark
   f. Hypo retention
   g. Safelight
   h. Curtain effect
   i. Pi line
   j. Processing artifact
2. Why must records be kept when the QC technologist see artifacts?
3. Describe artifact.
4. List the three periods in diagnostic imaging in which artifacts tend to occur.
5. Give three examples of exposure artifacts.
6. How would a radiographer correct a blurred radiograph if it was due to patient motion?
7. What is the principal reason for double exposures?
8. Name three types of processing artifacts.
9. What is a dichroic stain?
10. How do guide-shoe marks occur?
11. Explain what 3.1416 inches has to do with pi lines.
12. Describe the cause of wet-pressure sensitization marks.
13. Explain three ways fog can occur on a radiograph.
14. What is the cause of a static artifact on the processed radiograph?
15. List the three kinds of static artifact patterns.
16. Why is it important for radiographers to be alert to film artifacts?
17. How can one best avoid processor artifacts?
18. What causes grid cutoff artifacts?
19. How do pressure-type artifacts appear?
20. What type of artifact does hypo retention cause?

PART V

PREGNANT?

or you think you might be...

tell your doctor
before getting
an x-ray or
prescription

RADIATION PROTECTION

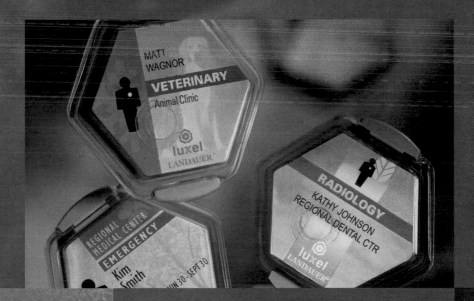

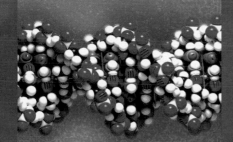

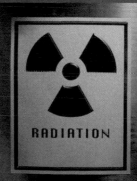

RADIATION

33

Human Biology

OBJECTIVES

At the completion of this chapter, the student should be able to do the following:

1. Discuss the cell theory of human biology
2. List and describe the molecular composition of the human body
3. Explain the parts and function of the human cell
4. Describe the processes of mitosis and meiosis
5. Evaluate the radiosensitivity of tissues and organs

OUTLINE

T IS KNOWN beyond a shadow of a doubt that x-rays are harmful. If sufficiently intense, x-rays can cause skin burns, cancer, leukemia, and other harmful effects. What is not known for certain is the degree of effect, if any, following diagnostic levels of x-radiation.

The benefits derived from diagnostic applications of x-rays are enormous. It is the job of the radiologic technologist, the radiologist, and the medical physicist to produce high-quality x-ray images with minimal radiation exposure. This approach results in the highest benefit with the lowest risk to patients and radiation workers. This is the practice of *ALARA*—"as low as reasonably achievable."

This chapter examines the concepts of human biology and discusses the known radiosensitivity of tissues, organs, and cells.

HUMAN RADIATION RESPONSE

The effect of x-rays on humans is the result of interactions at the atomic level (see Chapter 12). These atomic interactions take the form of ionization or excitation of orbital electrons and result in the deposition of energy in tissue. The deposited energy can result in a molecular change, the consequences of which can be measurable if the molecule involved is critical. Figure 33-1 summarizes the sequence of events between radiation exposure and latent whole-body injury.

When an atom is ionized, its chemical binding properties change. If the atom is a constituent of a large molecule, the ionization may result in breakage of the molecule or relocation of the atom within the molecule. The abnormal molecule may in time function improperly or cease to function, which can result in serious impairment or death of the cell.

 At each stage in the sequence, it is possible to repair radiation damage and recover.

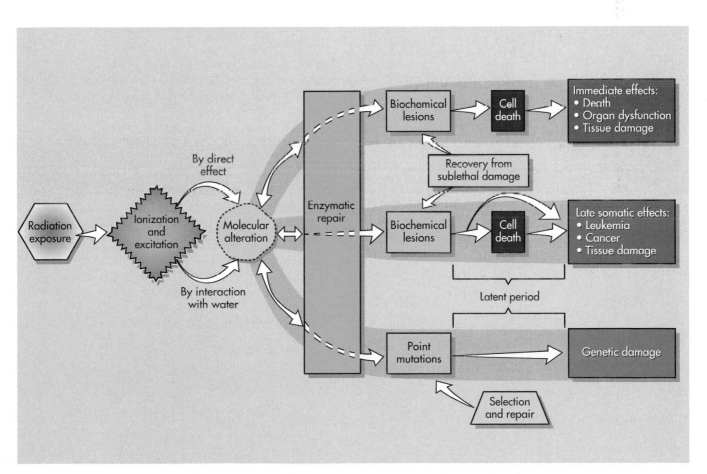

FIGURE 33-1 The sequence of events following radiation exposure of humans can lead to several radiation responses. At nearly every step, mechanisms for recovery and repair are available.

This process is reversible. Ionized atoms can become neutral again by attracting a free electron. Molecules can be mended by repair-enzymes. Cell and tissues can regenerate and recover from the radiation injury.

If the radiation response occurs within minutes or days after the radiation exposure, it is classified as an **early effect of radiation.** On the other hand, if the human injury is not observed for months or years, it is called a **late effect of radiation.**

A general classification scheme of the possible early and late human responses to radiation is shown in Box 33-1. In addition, many other radiation responses have been experimentally observed in animals. Most of the human responses have been observed following rather large radiation doses. But we are cautious and assume that even small doses are harmful.

Table 33-1 lists some of the human population groups in which many of these radiation responses have been observed.

 Radiobiology is the study of the effects of ionizing radiation on biologic tissue.

The ultimate goal of radiobiologic research is the accurate description of the effects of radiation on humans so that radiation can be used more safely in diagnosis and more effectively in therapy. Most radiobiologic research is designed to develop dose-response relationships so that the effect of planned doses can be predicted and the response to accidental exposure managed.

COMPOSITION OF THE BODY

At its most basic level, the human body is composed of atoms; radiation interacts at the atomic level. The atomic composition of the body determines the character and degree of the radiation interaction. The molecular and tissue composition defines the nature of the radiation response. Box 33-2 summarizes the atomic composition of the body and shows that over 85% of the body is hydrogen and oxygen.

Cell Theory

Radiation interaction at the atomic level results in molecular change, and this in turn can produce a cell deficient in normal growth and metabolism. Robert Hooke,

---

BOX 33-1 Human Responses to Ionizing Radiation

EARLY EFFECTS OF RADIATION ON HUMANS
1. Acute radiation syndrome
   a. Hematologic syndrome
   b. Gastrointestinal syndrome
   c. Central nervous system syndrome
2. Local tissue damage
   a. Skin
   b. Gonads
   c. Extremities
3. Hematologic depression
4. Cytogenetic damage

LATE EFFECTS OF RADIATION ON HUMANS
1. Leukemia
2. Other malignant disease
   a. Bone cancer
   b. Lung cancer
   c. Thyroid cancer
   d. Breast cancer
3. Local tissue damage
   a. Skin
   b. Gonads
   c. Eyes
4. Shortening of life span
5. Genetic damage
   a. Cytogenetic damage
   b. Doubling dose
   c. Genetically significant dose

EFFECTS OF FETAL IRRADIATION
1. Prenatal death
2. Neonatal death
3. Congenital malformation
4. Childhood malignancy
5. Diminished growth and development

TABLE 33-1	Human Populations in Which Radiation Effects Have Been Observed
Population	**Effect**
American radiologists	Leukemia, reduced life span
Atomic bomb survivors	Malignant disease
Radiation accident victims	Acute lethality
Marshall Islanders	Thyroid cancer
Uranium miners	Lung cancer
Radium watch-dial painters	Bone cancer
Patients treated with ^{131}I	Thyroid cancer
Children treated for enlarged thymus	Thyroid cancer
Patients with ankylosing spondylitis	Leukemia
Patients who underwent Thorotrast studies	Liver cancer
Irradiation in utero	Childhood malignancy
Volunteer convicts	Fertility impairment
Cyclotron workers	Cataracts

the English schoolmaster, first named the **cell** as the biologic building block in 1665. Shortly thereafter, in 1673, Anton van Leeuwenhoek accurately described a living cell based on his microscopic observations.

It was more than 100 years later, however, in 1838, that Schneider and Schwann showed conclusively that all plants and animals contain cells as their basic functional units. This is the **cell theory.**

The 1953 Watson and Crick description of the molecular structure of deoxyribonucleic acid (DNA) as the genetic substance of the cell was a major accomplishment. Precise mapping of the 30,000 human genes, which was completed in the year 2000, promises exceptional solutions to the detection and management of human disease.

Molecular Composition

There are five principal types of molecules in the body (Box 33-3). Four of these molecules—proteins, lipids (fats), carbohydrates (sugars and starches) and nucleic acids—are macromolecules.

 Macromolecules are very large molecules, sometimes consisting of hundreds of thousands of atoms.

Proteins, lipids, and carbohydrates are the principal classes of **organic molecules.** An organic molecule is life-supporting and contains carbon. One of the rarest molecules, a nucleic acid concentrated in the nucleus of a cell (DNA), is considered to be the most critical and radiosensitive target molecule.

Water is the most abundant molecule in the body and is the simplest. Water, however, plays a particularly important role in delivering energy to the target molecule, thereby contributing to radiation effects. In addition to water and the macromolecules, some trace elements and inorganic salts are essential to proper metabolism.

Water. The most abundant molecular constituent of the body is water. It consists of two atoms of hydrogen and one atom of oxygen (H_2O) and constitutes approximately 80% of human substance. Humans are basically made of structured water.

The water molecules exist both in the free-state and in the bound state, that is, bound to other molecules. They provide some form and shape, assist in maintaining body temperature, and enter into some biochemical reactions.

During vigorous exercise, body water is lost through perspiration to stabilize temperature and respiration. Water loss must be replaced to maintain **homeostasis,** which is the concept of the relative constancy of the internal environment of the human body.

Water and carbon dioxide are end products in the **catabolism** (breaking down into smaller units) of macromolecules. **Anabolism,** the production of large molecules from small, and catabolism are collectively called **metabolism.** Some athletes use anabolic steroids to build muscle mass, but harmful side effects may occur.

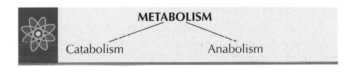
METABOLISM
Catabolism   Anabolism

Proteins. Approximately 15% of the molecular composition of the body is protein. Proteins are long-chain macromolecules that consist of a linear sequence of **amino acids** connected by **peptide bonds.** Twenty-two amino acids are used in **protein synthesis,** the metabolic production of proteins. The linear sequence, or arrangement, of these amino acids determines the precise function of the protein molecule.

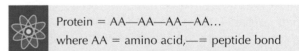
Protein = AA—AA—AA—AA...
where AA = amino acid,—= peptide bond

Figure 33-2 shows the general chemical form of a protein molecule. The generalized formula for a protein is $C_nH_nO_nN_nT_n$, where the subscript "n" refers to the number of atoms of each element in the molecule; T represents trace elements. In general, 50% of the mass of a protein molecule is carbon, 20% oxygen, 17% nitrogen, 7% hydrogen, and 6% other elements.

BOX 33-2   Atomic Composition of the Body

60.0% hydrogen
25.7% oxygen
10.7% carbon
 2.4% nitrogen
 0.2% calcium
 0.1% phosphorus
 0.1% sulfur
 0.8% trace elements

BOX 33-3   Molecular Composition of the Body

80% water
15% protein
 2% lipids
 1% carbohydrates
 1% nucleic acid
 1% other

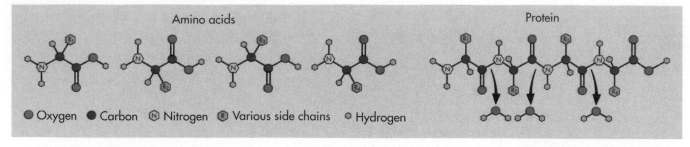

FIGURE 33-2 Proteins consist of amino acids linked by peptide bonds. The creation of the peptide bond requires the removal of a molecule of water.

Proteins have a variety of uses in the body. They provide structure and support. Muscles are very high in protein content. Proteins also function as enzymes, hormones, and antibodies.

Enzymes are molecules that are necessary in small quantities to allow a biochemical reaction to continue, even though they do not directly enter into the reaction.

Hormones are molecules that exercise regulatory control over some body functions, such as growth and development. Hormones are produced and secreted by the **endocrine glands**—the pituitary, adrenal, thyroid, parathyroid, pancreas, and gonads.

Antibodies constitute a primary defense mechanism of the body against infection and disease. The molecular configuration of an antibody may be precise and designed for attacking a particular type of invasive or infectious agent, the **antigen.**

Lipids. Lipids are organic macromolecules composed solely of carbon, hydrogen, and oxygen. They have the general formula $C_nH_nO_n$. Structurally, lipids have the form shown in Figure 33-3, and it is this structure that distinguishes them from carbohydrates. In general, lipids are composed of two kinds of smaller molecules, **glycerol** and **fatty acid.** Each lipid molecule is composed of one molecule of glycerol and three molecules of fatty acid.

Lipids are present in all tissues of the body and are the structural components of cell membranes. Lipids often are concentrated just under the skin and serve as a thermal insulator from the environment. Polar bears, for instance, have a particularly thick layer of subcutaneous fat (blubber) as a means of protection from the cold.

Lipids also serve as fuel for the body by providing energy stores. It is more difficult, however, to extract energy from lipids than from the other major fuel source, carbohydrates; this relationship, of course, is associated with one of the major dilemmas in modern nutrition—obesity.

Carbohydrates. Carbohydrates, like lipids, are composed solely of carbon, hydrogen, and oxygen, but their structure is different (Figure 33-4). This structural difference determines the contribution of the carbohydrate molecule to body biochemistry. The ratio of the

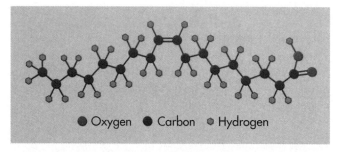

FIGURE 33-3 The structural configuration of a lipid is represented by a molecule of oleic acid: $CH_2(CH_2)7CH = CH(CH_2)_7COOH$.

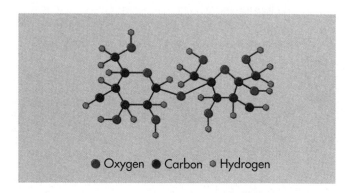

FIGURE 33-4 Carbohydrates are structurally different from lipids, even though their composition is similar. This is a molecule of sucrose, or ordinary table sugar: $(C_{12}H_{22}O_{11})$.

number of hydrogen atoms to oxygen atoms in a carbohydrate molecule is 2:1 (as in water), and a large fraction of this molecule consists of these atoms. Consequently, carbohydrates were first considered to be watered, or **hydrated,** carbons; hence their name.

Carbohydrates are also called **saccharides. Monosaccharides** and **disaccharides** are sugars. The chemical formula for glucose, a simple sugar, is $C_6H_{12}O_6$. These molecules are relatively small. **Polysaccharides** are large and include plant **starches** and animal **glycogen.** The chemical formula for a polysaccharide is $(C_6H_{10}O_5)_n$,

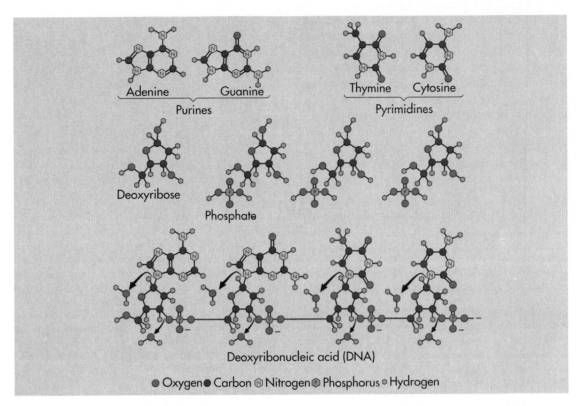

FIGURE 33-5 DNA is the control center for life. A single molecule consists of a backbone of alternating sugar (deoxyribose) and phosphate molecules. One of the four organic bases is attached to each sugar molecule.

where "n" is the number of simple sugar molecules in the macromolecule.

 The chief function of carbohydrates in the body is to provide fuel for cell metabolism.

Some carbohydrates are incorporated into the structure of cells and tissues to provide shape and stability. The human polysaccharide, glycogen, is stored in the tissues of the body and used as fuel only when quantities of the simple sugar, glucose, are inadequate.

Glucose is the ultimate molecule that fuels the body. Lipids can be catabolized into glucose for energy, but only with great difficulty. Polysaccharides are much more readily transformed into glucose. This explains why a chocolate bar, which is high in glucose, can provide a quick burst of energy for an athlete.

Nucleic Acids. Two principal nucleic acids are important to human metabolism: **DNA** and **ribonucleic acid (RNA)**. Located principally in the nucleus of the cell, DNA serves as the command or control molecule for cell function. The DNA contains all the hereditary information representing a cell and, of course, if the cell is a **germ cell,** all the hereditary information of the whole individual.

Located principally in the cytoplasm, RNA is also found in the nucleus. There are two types: messenger RNA (mRNA) and transfer RNA (tRNA). They are distinguished according to their biochemical functions. These molecules are involved in the growth and development of the cell through a number of biochemical pathways, notably protein synthesis.

The nucleic acids are very large and extremely complex macromolecules. Figure 33-5 shows the structural composition of DNA and how the component molecules are joined. DNA consists of a backbone composed of alternating segments of deoxyribose (a sugar) and phosphate. For each deoxyribose-phosphate conjugate formed, a molecule of water is removed.

 DNA is the radiation-sensitive target molecule.

Attached to each deoxyribose molecule is one of four different nitrogen-containing or nitrogenous organic bases: **adenine, guanine, thymine,** or **cytosine.** Adenine and guanine are **purines**; thymine and cytosine are **pyrimidines.**

The base-sugar-phosphate combination is called a **nucleotide,** and the nucleotides are strung together in one long-chain macromolecule. Human DNA exists as two of these long chains attached together in ladder fashion (Figure 33-6). The side rails of the ladder are the alternating sugar-phosphate molecules, and the rungs of the ladder consist of bases joined together by hydrogen bonds.

To complete the picture, the ladder is twisted about an imaginary axis like a spring. This produces a molecule with the **double-helix** configuration (Figure 33-7). The sequence of base bonding is limited to adenines bonded to thymines and cytosines bonded to guanines.

 Only adenine-thyroid and cytosine-guanine base-bonding is possible in DNA.

Structurally, RNA resembles DNA. In RNA, the sugar component is ribose rather than deoxyribose, and uracil replaces thymine as a base component. In contrast, RNA forms a single spiral, not a double helix.

The Human Cell

The principal molecular components of the human body are made of intricate cellular structures. The distribution of structures throughout the cell is reminiscent of the way the parts of an automobile are assembled. This assembly ensures proper growth, development, and function of the cell. Figure 33-8 is a cutaway view of a human cell with its principal structures labeled.

The two major structures of the cell are the **nucleus** and the **cytoplasm.** The principal molecular component of the nucleus is DNA, the genetic material of the cell. The nucleus also contains some RNA, protein, and water.

Most of the RNA is contained in a rounded structure, the **nucleolus.** The nucleolus is often attached to the nuclear membrane, a double-walled structure that at some locations is connected to the endoplasmic reticulum. The nature of this connection controls the passage of molecules, particularly RNA, from nucleus to cytoplasm.

The cytoplasm makes up the bulk of the cell and contains great quantities of all the molecular components

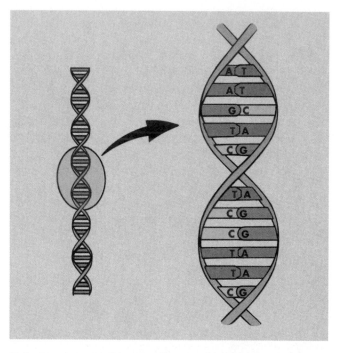

FIGURE 33-7 The DNA ladder is twisted about an imaginary axis to form a double helix.

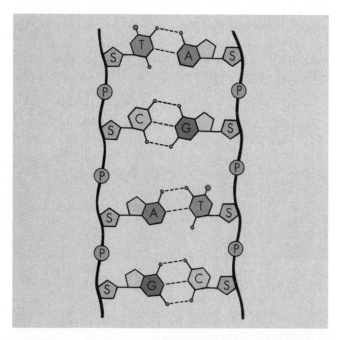

FIGURE 33-6 DNA consists of two long chains of alternating sugar and phosphate molecules fashioned like the side rails of a ladder with pairs of bases as rungs.

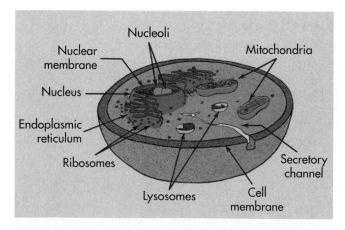

FIGURE 33-8 Schematic view of a human cell showing the principal structural components.

except DNA. A number of intracellular structures are found in the cytoplasm. The **endoplasmic reticulum** is a channel or series of channels that allows the nucleus to communicate with the cytoplasm.

The large bean-shaped structures are **mitochondria.** Macromolecules are digested in the mitochondria to produce energy for the cell. The mitochondria are therefore called the engine of the cell.

The small dot-like structures are **ribosomes.** Ribosomes are the site of protein synthesis and therefore are essential to normal cellular function. Ribosomes are scattered throughout the cytoplasm or the endoplasmic reticulum.

The small pea-like sacs are **lysosomes.** The lysosomes contain enzymes capable of digesting cellular fragments and sometimes the cell itself. Lysosomes help control intracellular contaminants.

All these structures, including the cell itself, are surrounded by membranes. These membranes consist principally of lipid-protein complexes that selectively allow small molecules and water to diffuse from one side to the other. These cellular membranes, of course, also provide structure and form for the cell and its components.

When the critical macromolecular cellular components are irradiated by themselves, a dose of approximately 1 Mrad (10 kGy_t) is required to produce a measurable change in any physical characteristic of the molecule.

When a macromolecule is incorporated into the apparatus of a living cell, only a few rads are necessary to produce a measurable biologic response. The lethal dose in some single-cell organisms, such as bacteria, is measured in kilorads, whereas human cells can be killed with a dose of less than 100 rad (1 Gy_t).

A number of experiments have shown that the nucleus is much more sensitive to the effects of radiation than the cytoplasm. Such experiments are conducted with either precise microbeams of electrons that can be focused and directed to a particular cell part or through the incorporation of the radioactive isotopes ³H and ¹⁴C into cellular molecules that localize exclusively to the cytoplasm or the nucleus.

Cell Function. Every human cell has a specific function in supporting the total body. Some differences are obvious, as with nerve cells, blood cells, and muscle cells. The similarities are also somewhat obvious.

In addition to its specialized function, each cell to some extent absorbs all molecular nutrients through the cell membrane and uses these nutrients in energy production and molecular synthesis. If this molecular synthesis is damaged by radiation exposure, the cell may malfunction and die.

Protein synthesis is a good example of a critical cellular function necessary for survival (Figure 33-9).

DNA, located in the nucleus, contains a molecular code that identifies which proteins the cell will make.

This code is determined by the sequence of base pairs (adenine-thymine and cytosine-guanine). A series of three base pairs, called a **codon,** identifies one of the 22 human amino acids available for protein synthesis.

This genetic message is transferred in the nucleus to a molecule of mRNA. The mRNA leaves the nucleus by way of the endoplasmic reticulum and makes its way to a ribosome, where the genetic message is transferred to yet another RNA molecule (tRNA).

The tRNA searches the cytoplasm for the amino acids for which it is coded. It attaches to the amino acid and carries it to the ribosome, where it is joined with other amino acids in sequence by peptide bonds to form the required protein molecule.

Interference with any phase of this procedure for protein synthesis could result in damage to the cell. Radiation interaction with the molecule having primary control over protein synthesis, DNA, is more effective in producing a response than radiation interaction with other molecules involved in protein synthesis.

Cell Proliferation. Although many thousands of rad are necessary to produce physically measurable disruption of macromolecules in vitro, single ionizing events at a particularly sensitive site of a critical target molecule are thought to be capable of disrupting cell proliferation.

 Cell proliferation is the act of a single cell or group of cells reproducing and multiplying in number.

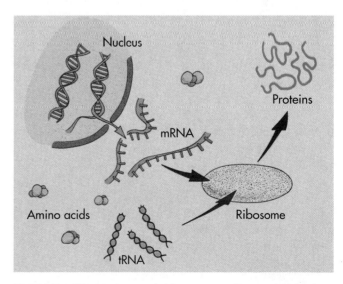

FIGURE 33-9 Protein synthesis is a complex process and involves many different molecules and cellular structures.

The human body has two general types of cells: **somatic cells** and **genetic cells.** The genetic cells are the oogonium of the female and the spermatogonium of the male. All other cells of the body are somatic cells. When somatic cells proliferate or divide, they undergo **mitosis.** Genetic cells undergo **meiosis.**

Mitosis. The cell biologist and the geneticist view the cell cycle differently (Figure 33-10). Each cycle includes the various states of cell growth, development, and division. The geneticist considers only two phases of the cell cycle: **mitosis (M)** and **interphase.**

Mitosis, the division phase, is characterized by four subphases: **prophase, metaphase, anaphase,** and **telophase.** The portion of the cell cycle between mitotic events is called interphase. Interphase is the period of growth of the cell between divisions.

The cell biologist usually identifies four phases of the cell cycle: M, G_1, S, and G_2. These phases of the cell cycle are characterized by the structure of the chromosomes, which contain the genetic material DNA. The **gap** in cell growth between M and S is G_1. G_1 is the pre-DNA synthesis phase.

The DNA synthesis phase is S. During this period, each DNA molecule is replicated into two identical daughter DNA molecules.

During S phase, the chromosome is transformed from a structure with two chromatids attached to a centromere to a structure with four chromatids attached to a centromere (Figure 33-11). The result is two pairs of homologous chromatids, that is, chromatids having precisely the same DNA content and structure.

The G_2 phase is the post-DNA synthesis gap of cell growth.

During interphase, the chromosomes are not visible; however, during mitosis, the DNA slowly takes the form of the chromosomes as seen microscopically. Figure 33-12 schematically depicts the process of mitosis.

During **prophase,** the nucleus swells and the DNA becomes more prominent and begins to take structural form. At **metaphase,** the chromosomes appear and are lined up along the equator of the nucleus. It is during metaphase that mitosis can be stopped and chromosomes can be studied carefully under the microscope.

 Radiation-induced chromosome damage is analyzed during metaphase.

Anaphase is characterized by each chromosome splitting at the centromere so that a centromere and two chro-

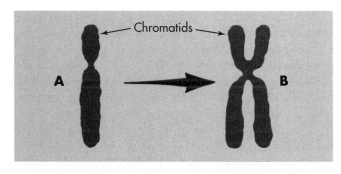

FIGURE 33-11 During the synthesis portion of interphase, the chromosomes replicate from a two-chromatid structure (**A**) to a four-chromatid structure (**B**).

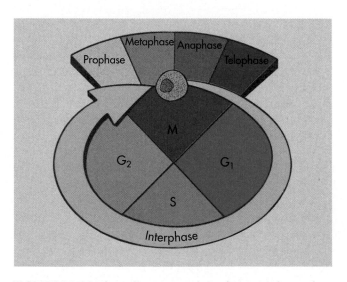

FIGURE 33-10 The cell's progress through one cycle involves several phases.

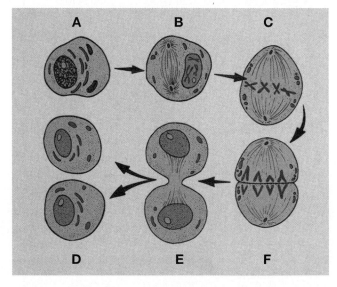

FIGURE 33-12 Mitosis is the phase of the cell cycle during which the chromosomes become visible, divide, and migrate to daughter cells. **A,** Interphase. **B,** Prophase. **C,** Metaphase. **D,** Anaphase. **E,** Telophase. **F,** Interphase.

matids are connected by a fiber to the poles of the nucleus. These poles are called **spindles** and the fibers are called **spindle fibers.** The number of chromatids per centromere has been reduced by half, and these newly formed chromosomes migrate slowly toward the spindle.

The final segment of mitosis, **telophase,** is characterized by the disappearance of the structural chromosomes into a mass of DNA and the closing off of the nuclear membrane like a dumbbell into two nuclei. At the same time the cytoplasm is divided into two equal parts, each accompanying one of the new nuclei.

Cell division is now complete. The two daughter cells appear precisely as the parent and contain exactly the same genetic material.

Meiosis. Genetic material can change during the division process of genetic cells, which is called **meiosis.** The genetic cells begin with the same number of chromosomes as somatic cells, 23 pairs (46 chromosomes). But for a genetic cell to be capable of marriage with another genetic cell, its complement of chromosomes must be reduced by half to 23 so that, following conception and the union of two genetic cells, the daughter cells will contain 46 chromosomes (Figure 33-13).

> Meiosis is the process whereby genetic cells undergo reduction division.

The genetic cell begins meiosis with 46 chromosomes, appearing as a somatic cell having completed the G_2 phase. The cell then progresses through the phases of mitosis into two daughter cells, each containing 46 chromosomes of two chromatids each. The names of the subphases are the same for both meiosis and mitosis.

Each of the daughter cells of this first division now progresses through a second division in which all the cellular material is divided, including the chromosomes. However, the second division is not accompanied by an S phase, and therefore there is no replication of DNA and consequently no duplication of the chromosomes.

The resulting granddaughter cells contain only 23 chromosomes each.

Each parent has undergone two division processes, resulting in four daughter cells. During the second division, some chromosomal material is exchanged among chromatids by a process called **crossing over.** Crossing over results in changes in genetic constitution and changes in inheritable traits.

Tissues and Organs

During the development and maturation of a human from the two united genetic cells, a number of different types of cells evolve. Collections of cells of similar structure and function form **tissues.** Box 33-4 is a breakdown of the composition of the body according to its tissue constituents.

These tissues in turn are precisely bound together to form **organs.** The tissues and the organs of the body serve as discrete units with specific functional responsibilities. Some tissues and organs combine into an overall integrated organization known as an **organ system.**

The principal organ systems of the body are the nervous system, the digestive system, the endocrine system, and the reproductive system. The effects of radiation that appear at the whole-body level result from damage to these organ systems, which in turn are a result of radiation injury to the cells of that system.

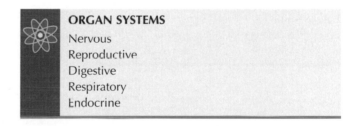
ORGAN SYSTEMS
Nervous
Reproductive
Digestive
Respiratory
Endocrine

The cells of a tissue system are identified by their rate of proliferation and their stage of development. Immature cells are called **undifferentiated cells, precursor cells,** or

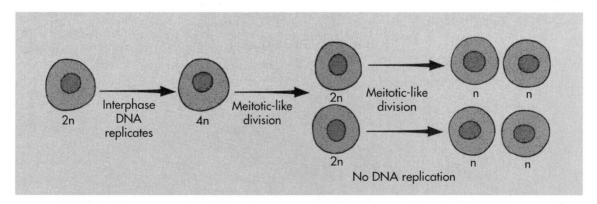

FIGURE 33-13 Meiosis is the process of reduction division, and it occurs only in reproductive cells. *n,* Number of similar chromosomes.

stem cells. As a cell matures through growth and proliferation, it can pass through various stages of differentiation into a fully functional and mature cell.

 Stem cells are more sensitive to radiation than mature cells.

The sensitivity of the cell to radiation is determined somewhat by its state of maturity and its functional role. Table 33-2 lists a number of different types of cells in the body according to their degree of radiosensitivity.

The tissues and organs of the body consist of both stem cells and mature cells. There are several types of tissue, which can be classified according to structural or functional features. These features influence the tissue's degree of radiosensitivity.

Epithelium is the covering tissue, and it lines all exposed surfaces of the body, both exterior and interior. Epithelium covers the skin, the blood vessels, the abdominal and chest cavities, and the gastrointestinal tract.

Connective and **supporting tissues** are high in protein and are composed principally of fibers that are usually highly elastic. Connective tissue binds tissues and organs together. Bone ligaments and cartilage are examples of connective tissue.

Muscle is a special type of tissue that can contract. It is found throughout the body and also is high in protein content.

Nervous tissue consists of specialized cells called **neurons** that have long, thin extensions from the cell to distant parts of the body. Nervous tissue is the avenue through which electrical impulses are transmitted throughout the body for control and response.

BOX 33-4 Tissue Composition of the Body

TISSUE	ABUNDANCE
Muscle	43%
Fat	14%
Organs	12%
Skeleton	10%
Blood	8%
Subcutaneous tissue	6%
Bone marrow	4%
Skin	3%

TABLE 33-2 Response to Radiation is Related to Cell Type

Radiosensitivity	Cell Type
High	Lymphocytes
	Spermatogonia
	Erythroblasts
	Intestinal crypt cells
Intermediate	Endothelial cells
	Osteoblasts
	Spermatids
	Fibroblasts
Low	Muscle cells
	Nerve cells

TABLE 33-3 Relative Radiosensitivity of Tissues and Organs Based on Clinical Radiation Oncology

Level of Radiosensitivity*	Tissue or Organ	Effects
High: 200–1000 rad (2–10 Gy$_t$)	Lymphoid tissue	Atrophy
	Bone marrow	Hypoplasia
	Gonads	Atrophy
Intermediate: 1000–1500 rad (10–50 Gy$_t$)	Skin	Erythema
	Gastrointestinal tract	Ulcer
	Cornea	Cataract
	Growing bone	Growth arrest
	Kidney	Nephrosclerosis
	Liver	Ascites
	Thyroid	Atrophy
Low: >5000 rad (>50 Gy$_t$)	Muscle	Fibrosis
	Brain	Necrosis
	Spinal	Transection

*The minimum dose delivered at the rate of approximately 200 rad/day (2 Gy$_t$/day) that will produce a response.

When these various types of tissue are combined to form an organ, they are identified according to two parts of the organ. The **parenchymal** part contains tissues that represent that particular organ, whereas the **stromal** part is composed of connective tissue and vasculature that provide structure to the organ.

The early effects of high-dose radiation result in observable organ damage. The various organs of the body exhibit a wide range of sensitivity to radiation. This radiosensitivity is determined by the function of the organ in the body, the rate at which cells mature in the organ, and the inherent radiosensitivity of the cell type.

A precise knowledge of these various organ radiosensitivities is unnecessary; however, knowledge of the general levels of radiosensitivity is helpful in understanding the effects of whole-body radiation exposure, particularly the acute radiation syndrome (Table 33-3).

SUMMARY

After radiation exposure, the human body responds in predictable ways. Radiobiology is the study of the effects of ionizing radiation on humans in order to refine knowledge of the expected response.

If a response occurs within minutes or days of exposure, it is called an early effect of radiation. If the injury is not observable for months or years, it is called a late effect of radiation exposure.

The cell is the basic functional unit of all plants and animals. At the molecular level, the human body is composed of mostly water, protein, lipid, carbohydrate, and nucleic acid. The two important nucleic acids in human metabolism are DNA and RNA.

DNA contains all the hereditary information in the cell. If the cell is a genetic cell, the DNA contains the hereditary information of the whole individual. DNA is a macromolecule made up of two long chains of base-sugar-phosphate combinations twisted into a double helix.

Major cellular function consists of protein synthesis and cell division. Mitosis is the growth, development, and division of cells. Meiosis is the term for the division of genetic cells.

Cells of similar structure bind together to form tissue. Tissue binds together to form organs. An overall integrated organization of tissue and organs is called an organ system.

The principal organ systems of the body are the nervous, digestive, endocrine, and reproductive systems.

The radiosensitivity of various tissue and organ systems varies widely. Reproductive cells are highly radiosensitive, whereas nerve cells are less radiosensitive.

CHALLENGE QUESTIONS

1. Define or otherwise identify:
   a. ALARA
   b. Cell theory
   c. Anabolism
   d. Carbohydrate
   e. M, G_1, S, G_2
   f. Epithelium
   g. Cytoplasm
   h. Enzyme
   i. Organic molecule
   j. Late effect of radiation
2. At what structural level do x-rays interact with humans to produce a radiation response?
3. How does ionizing radiation affect an atom within a large molecule?
4. List five human groups in which radiation effects have been observed.
5. What are the radiation effects on the populations mentioned in question 4?
6. What is the most abundant atom and the most abundant molecule in the body?
7. Name five possible effects of irradiation in vitro.
8. Why are humans basically a structured aqueous suspension?
9. What is the meaning of homeostasis?
10. How do proteins function in the human body?
11. What do carbohydrates do for us?
12. DNA is the abbreviation for what molecule?
13. Which molecule is considered the genetic material of the cell?
14. What is the function of the endoplasmic reticulum?
15. What is the approximate dose of radiation required to produce a measurable physical change in a macromolecule?
16. List the stages of cell division in a somatic cell.
17. List the stages of cell reduction division in a genetic cell.
18. What cell type is the most radiosensitive?
19. What type of tissue is the least radiosensitive?
20. List three early radiation effects and three late radiation effects in humans.

CHAPTER 34

Fundamental Principles of Radiobiology

OBJECTIVES

At the completion of this chapter, the student should be able to do the following:

1. State the law of Bergonie and Tribondeau
2. Describe the physical factors affecting radiation response
3. Describe the biologic factors affecting radiation response
4. Explain radiation dose-response relationships
5. Describe five types of radiation dose-response relationships

OUTLINE

SOME TISSUES are more sensitive than others to radiation exposure. Such tissues usually respond more rapidly and to lower doses of radiation.

Reproductive cells are more sensitive than nerve cells. This and other radiobiologic concepts were detailed in 1906 by two French scientists.

Physical factors and biologic factors affect the radiobiologic response of tissue. Most radiobiologic study arises from interest in radiation oncology. However, radiologic technologists must understand the effects of low-dose radiation exposure.

The study of radiobiology principally aims at establishing radiation dose-response relationships. A dose-response relationship is a mathematical and graphical function that relates radiation dose to the observed response.

soft tissue. It is another method of expressing **radiation quality** and determining the value of the **radiation weighting factor (W_R)** used in radiation protection (see Chapter 38). LET is expressed in units of kiloelectron volts of energy transferred per micrometer of track length in soft tissue (keV/μm).

The LET of diagnostic x-rays is approximately 3 keV/μm.

The ability of ionizing radiation to produce a biologic response increases as the LET of radiation increases. When LET is high, ionizations occur frequently, increasing the probability of interaction with the target molecule.

Relative Biologic Effectiveness

As the LET of radiation increases, the ability to produce biologic damage also increases. This relative effect is quantitatively described by the relative biologic effectiveness (RBE).

RELATIVE BIOLOGIC EFFECTIVENESS

$$RBE = \frac{\text{Dose of standard radiation necessary to produce a given effect}}{\text{Dose of test radiation necessary to produce the same effect}}$$

The standard radiation, by convention, is orthovoltage x-radiation in the range of 200 to 250 kVp. This type of x-ray beam was used for many years in radiation oncology and in essentially all early radiobiology research.

Diagnostic x-rays have an RBE of 1. Radiations with lower LET than diagnostic x-rays have an RBE less than 1, whereas radiations with higher LET have a higher RBE.

The RBE of diagnostic x-rays is 1.

LAW OF BERGONIE AND TRIBONDEAU

In 1906, two French scientists, Bergonie and Tribondeau, theorized and observed that radiosensitivity was a function of the metabolic state of the tissue being irradiated. This has come to be known as the law of Bergonie and Tribondeau and has been verified many times. Basically, the law states that the radiosensitivity of living tissue varies with maturation and metabolism (Box 34-1).

This law is principally interesting as a historical note in the development of radiobiology. It has found some application in radiation oncology. In diagnostic imaging, the law serves to remind us that the fetus is considerably more sensitive to radiation exposure than the child or the mature adult.

PHYSICAL FACTORS AFFECTING RADIOSENSITIVITY

When one irradiates tissue, the response of the tissue is determined principally by the amount of energy deposited per unit mass—the dose in rad (Gy$_t$). Even under controlled experimental conditions, however, when equal doses are delivered to equal specimens, the response may not be the same because of other modifying factors. A number of physical factors affect the degree of radiation response.

Linear Energy Transfer

Linear energy transfer (LET) is a measure of the rate at which energy is transferred from ionizing radiation to

Figure 34-1 shows the relationship between RBE and LET and identifies some of the more common types of radiation. Table 34-1 lists the approximate LET and RBE of various types of ionizing radiation.

Question: When mice are irradiated with 250 kVp x-rays, death occurs at 650 rad (6.5 Gy$_t$). If similar mice are irradiated with fast neutrons, death occurs at only 210 rad (2.1 Gy$_t$). What is the RBE for the fast neutrons?

Answer: RBE $= \dfrac{650 \text{ rad}}{210 \text{ rad}}$

$= 3.1$

TABLE 34-1	The LET and RBE of Various Radiations	
Type of Radiation	LET (keV/μm)	RBE
25 MV x-rays	0.2	0.8
^{60}Co rays	0.3	0.9
1 MeV electrons	0.3	0.9
Diagnostic x-rays	3.0	1.0
10 MeV protons	4.0	5.0
Fast neutrons	50.0	10
5 MeV alpha particles	100.0	20
Heavy nuclei	1000.0	30

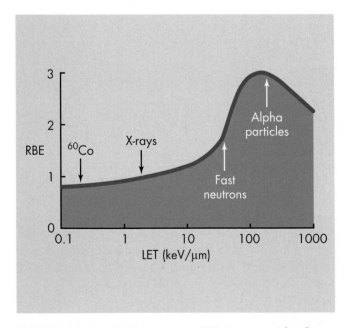

FIGURE 34-1 As LET increases, RBE increases also but a maximum value is reached followed by a lower RBE due to overkill.

Protraction and Fractionation

If a dose of radiation is delivered over a long period of time rather than quickly, the effect of that dose is lessened. Stated differently, if the time of irradiation is lengthened, a higher dose is required to produce the same effect. This lengthening of time can be accomplished in two ways.

If the dose is delivered continuously but at a lower dose rate, it is said to be **protracted**. Six hundred rad (6 Gy$_t$) delivered in 3 min (200 rad/min [2 Gy$_t$/min]) is lethal for a mouse. However, when 600 rad is delivered at the rate of 1 rad/hr (10 mGy$_t$/hr) for a total time of 600 hr, the mouse will survive.

 Dose protraction and fractionation cause less effect, allowing time for intracellular repair and tissue recovery.

If the 600 rad dose is delivered at the same dose rate, 200 rad/min, but in 12 equal fractions of 50 rad (500 mGy$_t$), each separated by 24 hr, the mouse will survive. In this situation the dose is said to be **fractionated**.

Dose fractionation has less effect because cells undergo repair and recovery between doses. Dose fractionation is used routinely in radiation oncology.

BIOLOGIC FACTORS AFFECTING RADIOSENSITIVITY

In addition to these physical factors, a number of biologic conditions alter the radiation response of tissue. Some of these factors have to do with the inherent state of the tissue, such as age and metabolic rate. Other factors are related to artificially introduced modifiers of the biologic system.

Oxygen Effect

Tissue is more sensitive to radiation when irradiated in the oxygenated, or aerobic, state than when irradiated under anoxic (without oxygen) or hypoxic (low-oxygen) conditions. This characteristic of tissue is called the oxygen effect and is described numerically by the **oxygen enhancement ratio (OER)**.

 OXYGEN ENHANCEMENT RATIO

OER = Dose necessary under anoxic conditions to produce a given effect

_____

Dose necessary under aerobic conditions to produce the same effect

Generally, tissue irradiation is conducted under conditions of full oxygenation. Hyperbaric (high-pressure) oxygen has been used in radiation oncology in an attempt to increase the radiosensitivity of nodular, avascular tumors, which are less radiosensitive than tumors with an adequate blood supply.

 Diagnostic x-ray imaging is performed under conditions of full oxygenation.

Question: When experimental mouse mammary carcinomas are clamped and irradiated under hypoxic conditions, the tumor control dose is 10,600 rad (106 Gy_t). When the tumors are not clamped and are irradiated under aerobic conditions, the tumor control dose is 4050 rad (40.5 Gy_t). What is the OER for this system?

Answer: $OER = \dfrac{10,600}{4050}$

$= 2.6$

The OER is LET-dependent (Figure 34-2). The OER is highest for low-LET radiation, having a maximum value of approximately 3, decreasing to approximately 1 for high-LET radiation.

Age

The age of a biologic structure affects its radiosensitivity. The response of humans is characteristic of this age-related radiosensitivity (Figure 34-3). Humans are most sensitive before birth.

Following birth, sensitivity decreases until maturity, at which time we are most resistant to radiation effects.

In old age, humans again become somewhat more radiosensitive.

Recovery

In vitro experiments show that human cells can recover from radiation damage. If the radiation dose is not sufficient to kill the cell before its next division (**interphase death**), then given sufficient time, the cell will recover from the **sublethal radiation damage** it has sustained.

 Interphase death occurs when the cell dies before replicating.

This intracellular recovery is due to a **repair** mechanism inherent in the biochemistry of the cell. Some types of cells have greater capacity for repair of sublethal damage than others. At the whole-body level, this recovery from radiation damage is assisted through **repopulation** by the surviving cells.

If a tissue or organ receives a sufficient radiation dose, it responds by shrinking. This is called **atrophy** and occurs because some cells die, disintegrate, and are carried away as waste products.

If a sufficient number of cells sustain only sublethal damage and survive, they may proliferate and repopulate the irradiated tissue or organ.

 The combined processes of intracellular repair and repopulation contribute to recovery from radiation damage.

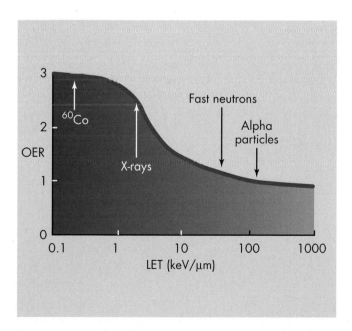

FIGURE 34-2 The OER is high for low LET radiation and decreases in value as the LET increases.

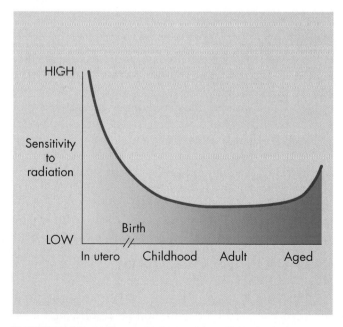

FIGURE 34-3 Radiosensitivity varies with age. Experiments with animals have shown that the very young and the very old are more sensitive to radiation.

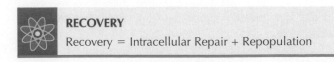

RECOVERY

Recovery = Intracellular Repair + Repopulation

Chemical Agents

Some chemicals can modify the radiation response of cells, tissues, and organs. For the chemical agents to be effective, they must be present at the time of irradiation. Post-irradiation application does not usually alter the degree of radiation response.

Radiosensitizers. Agents that enhance the effect of radiation are called **sensitizing agents.** Some examples are halogenated pyrimidines, methotrexate, actinomycin D, hydroxyurea, and vitamin K.

The halogenated pyrimidines become incorporated into the DNA of the cell and amplify radiation effects on that molecule. All the radiosensitizers have an effectiveness ratio of approximately 2; that is, if 90% of a cell culture is killed by 200 rad (2 Gy_t), then in the presence of a sensitizing agent, only 100 rad (1 Gy_t) is required for the same percentage of lethality.

Radioprotectors. The radioprotective compounds include molecules containing a sulfhydryl group (sulfur and hydrogen bound together), such as cysteine and cysteamine. Hundreds of others have been tested and found effective by a factor of approximately 2. For example, if 600 rad (6 Gy_t) is a lethal dose to a mouse, then in the presence of a radioprotective agent 1200 rad (12 Gy_t) would be required to produce lethality.

Radioprotective agents have not found human application because, to be effective, they must be administered at toxic levels. The protective agent can be worse than the radiation!

Hormesis

A growing body of radiobiologic evidence suggests that a little bit of radiation is good for you. Studies have shown that animals receiving low radiation doses live longer than controls. The prevailing explanation is that a little radiation stimulates hormonal and immune responses to other toxic environmental agents.

There are many nonradiation examples of hormesis. In large quantities fluoride is deadly. In small quantities it is a known tooth preservative.

Regardless of radiation hormesis, we continue to practice ALARA ("as low as reasonably achievable") vigorously as a known safe approach to radiation safety.

RADIATION DOSE-RESPONSE RELATIONSHIPS

Radiobiology is a relatively new science. Although some scientists were working with animals to observe the effects of radiation a few years after the discovery of x-rays, these studies were not experimentally sound, nor were their results applied. With the advent of the atomic age in the 1940s, however, interest in radiobiology increased enormously.

The object of nearly all radiobiologic research is the establishment of radiation dose-response relationships. A radiation dose-response relationship is a mathematical relationship between various radiation dose levels and the magnitude of the observed response.

Radiation dose-response relationships have two important applications in radiology. First, these experimentally determined relationships are used to design therapeutic treatment routines for patients with cancer.

Radiobiologic studies have also been designed to provide information on the effects of low-dose irradiation. These studies and the dose-response relationships obtained are the basis for our radiation control activities and are particularly significant to diagnostic radiology.

Every radiation dose-response relationship has two characteristics. It is either linear or nonlinear, and it is either threshold or nonthreshold. These characteristics can be described mathematically or graphically. This discussion avoids the math.

Linear Dose-Response Relationships

Figure 34-4 shows examples of the linear dose-response relationship, which is so-called because the response is directly proportional to the dose. When the radiation dose is doubled, the response to radiation is likewise doubled.

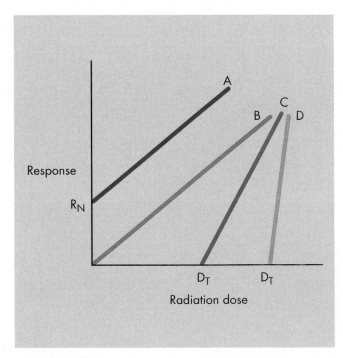

FIGURE 34-4 Linear dose-response relationships *A* and *B* are nonthreshold types; *C* and *D* are threshold types. R_N is the normal incidence or response with no radiation exposure.

Dose-response relationships *A* and *B* intersect the dose axis at zero or below (see Figure 34-4). These relationships are therefore the **linear, nonthreshold type.** In a nonthreshold dose-response relationship, any dose, regardless of its size, is expected to produce a response.

At zero dose, relationship *A* exhibits a measurable response, R_N. The level R_N is called the **natural** response level and indicates that even without radiation exposure that type of response, such as cancer, occurs.

> Radiation-induced cancer, leukemia, and genetic effects follow a linear-nonthreshold dose-response relationship.

Dose-response relationships *C* and *D* are identified as **linear, threshold** because they intercept the dose axis at some value greater than zero. The threshold dose for *C* and *D* is D_T.

At radiation doses below D_T, no response is expected. Relationship *D* has a steeper slope than *C*; therefore, above the threshold dose, any increment of dose produces a larger response if that response follows relationship *D* rather than *C*.

Nonlinear Dose-Response Relationships

All other radiation dose-response relationships are nonlinear (Figure 34-5). Curves *A* and *B* are **nonlinear, nonthreshold.** Curve *A* shows that a large response results from very little radiation dose. At high dose levels the radiation is not so efficient because an incremental dose at high levels results in less relative damage than the same incremental dose at low levels.

The dose-response relationship represented by curve *B* is just the opposite. Incremental doses in the low-dose range result in very little response. At high doses, however, the same increment of dose produces a much larger response.

Curve *C* is a **nonlinear, threshold** relationship. At doses below D_T no response is measured. As the dose is increased above D_T, it becomes increasingly effective per increment of dose until it reaches the dose corresponding to the inflection point of the curve.

The inflection point occurs when the curve stops bending up and begins bending down. Above this level, incremental doses become less effective. Relationship *C* is sometimes called an **S-type,** or **sigmoid-type,** radiation dose-response relationship.

> Skin effects resulting from high-dose fluoroscopy follow a sigmoid-type dose-response relationship.

We shall refer to these general types of radiation dose-response relationships in discussing the type and degree of human radiation injury. Diagnostic radiology is almost exclusively concerned with the late effects of radiation exposure and therefore with linear, nonthreshold dose-response relationships. For completeness, however, Chapter 36 briefly discusses early radiation damage.

Constructing a Dose-Response Relationship

Determining the radiation dose-response relationship for a whole-body response is tricky. It is very difficult to determine the degree of response, even that of early effects, because the number of experimental animals that can be used is usually small. It is nearly impossible to measure low-dose, late effects—the area of greatest interest to diagnostic imaging.

Therefore, we resort to irradiating a limited number of animals to very large doses of radiation in hopes of observing a statistically significant response. Figure 34-6 shows the results of such an experiment, in which four groups of animals were irradiated to a different dose. The observations on each group results in an ordered pair of data: a dose and the associated biologic response.

The error bars in each ordered pair indicate the confidence associated with each data point. The error bars on the dose measurements are very narrow; we can measure radiation dose very accurately. The error bars on the response, however, are very wide because of biologic variability and the limited number of observations at each dose.

The principal interest in diagnostic imaging is to estimate the response at very low radiation doses. Since this cannot be done directly, we **extrapolate** the

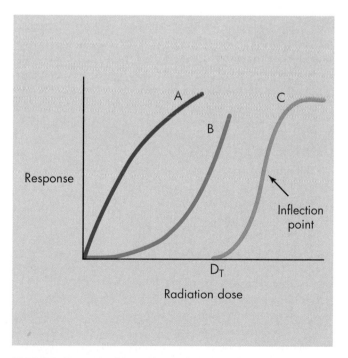

FIGURE 34-5 Nonlinear dose-response relationships can assume several shapes. Curves *A* and *B* are nonthreshold. Curve *C* is threshold. D_T, Threshold dose.

dose-response relationship from the high-dose, known region into the low-dose, unknown region.

This extrapolation invariably results in a **linear, non-threshold** dose-response relationship. Such an extrapolation, however, may not be correct because of the many qualifying conditions on the experiment.

The radiation dose-response relationship demonstrating radiation hormesis appears as in Figure 34-7 At

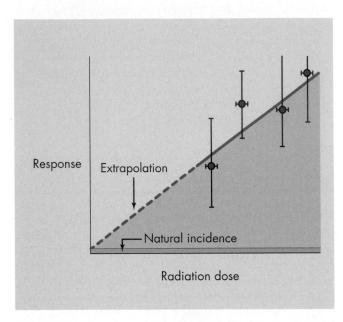

FIGURE 34-6 A dose-response relationship is produced by extrapolating high-dose experimental data to low doses.

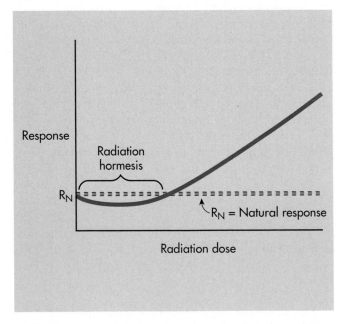

FIGURE 34-7 The dose response relationship for radiation hormesis.

very low doses, the irradiated subjects experience less response than the controls. The existence of radiation hormesis is highly controversial in radiation science. Regardless of its existence, no human radiation responses have been observed following doses less than 10 rad (100 mGy).

SUMMARY

In 1906, two French scientists first theorized that radiosensitivity was a function of the metabolic state of tissue being irradiated. Their theories are known as the Law of Bergonie and Tribondeau and state the following: (1) stem cells are radiosensitive, mature cells are less so, (2) young tissue is more radiosensitive than older tissue, (3) high metabolic activity is radiosensitive, low metabolic rate is radioresistant, and (4) increases in proliferation and growth rates of cells makes them more radiosensitive.

Physical and biologic factors affect tissue radiosensitivity. The physical factors are the LET, RBE, fractionation (dose delivered over a long time), and protraction.

The biologic factors affecting radiosensitivity are the oxygen effect, the age-related effect, and the recovery effect.

Some chemicals can modify the response of cells. They are called radiosensitizers and radioprotectors.

Radiobiology research concentrates on radiation dose-response relationships. In linear dose-response relationships, the response is directly proportional to the dose. In nonlinear dose-response relationships, varied doses produce varied responses.

The threshold dose is the level below which there is no response. The nonthreshold dose-response relationship means that any dose is expected to produce a response. For establishing radiation protection guidelines for diagnostic imaging, the linear, nonthreshold dose-response model is used.

CHALLENGE QUESTIONS

1. Define or otherwise identify:
    a. Linear energy transfer
    b. Standard radiation
    c. Oxygen enhancement ratio
    d. Repopulation
    e. Extrapolation
    f. Threshold dose
    g. Interphase death
    h. Dose protraction
    i. Radiation weighting factor
    j. Tribondeau
2. Write the formula for relative biologic effectiveness.
3. Give an example of fractionated radiation.
4. When is high pressure (hyperbaric) oxygen used in radiation oncology?

5. Write the formula for oxygen enhancement ratio.
6. How does age affect the radiosensitivity of tissue?
7. When a radiobiology experiment is conducted in vitro, what does that mean?
8. Name three agents that enhance the effect of radiation.
9. Name three radioprotective agents.
10. Are radioprotective agents used for human application?
11. Explain the meaning of a radiation dose-response relationship.
12. What occurs in a nonlinear radiation dose-response relationship?
13. Explain why the linear, nonthreshold dose-response relationship is used as model for diagnostic imaging radiation protection guides.
14. State two of the corollaries to the law of Bergonie and Tribondeau.

15. Approximately 800 rad of 220 kVp x-rays is necessary to produce death in the armadillo. Cobalt-60 gamma rays have a lower LET than 220 kVp x-rays; therefore, 940 rad is required for armadillo lethality. What is the RBE of ^{60}CO compared with 220 kVp?
16. Under fully oxygenated conditions, 90% of human cells in culture will be killed by 150 rad x-rays. If the cells are made anoxic, the dose required for 90% lethality is 400 rad. What is the OER?
17. What are the units of LET?
18. Describe how RBE and LET are related.
19. Is occupational radiation exposure fractionated, protracted, or continuous?
20. Describe how OER and LET are related.

Molecular and Cellular Radiobiology

OBJECTIVES

At the completion of this chapter, the student should be able to do the following:

1. Discuss three effects of in vitro irradiation of macromolecules
2. Explain the effects of radiation on DNA
3. Identify the chemical reactions involved in the radiolysis of water
4. Describe the effects of in vivo irradiation
5. Describe the principles of target theory
6. Discuss the kinetics of cell survival following irradiation

OUTLINE

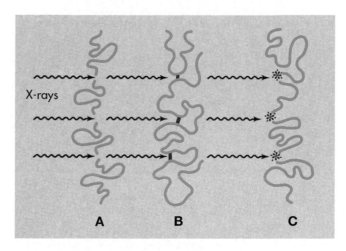

FIGURE 35-1 The results of irradiation of macro-molecules. **A**, Main-chain scission. **B**, Cross-linking. **C**, Point lesions.

VEN THOUGH the initial interaction between radiation and tissue occurs at the electron level, observable human radiation injury results from change at the molecular level. The occurrence of molecular lesions is categorized into effects on macromolecules and effects on water. This chapter discusses irradiation of macromolecules and the radiolysis of water.

Because the human body is an aqueous solution containing 80% water molecules, radiation interaction with water is the principal radiation interaction in the body. However, the ultimate damage is to the target molecule, DNA, which controls cellular metabolism and reproduction.

The effect of irradiation of macromolecules is quite different from that of irradiation of water. When macromolecules are irradiated **in vitro,** that is, outside the body or outside the cell, a considerable radiation dose is required to produce a measurable effect. Irradiation **in vivo,** that is, in the living cell, demonstrates that macromolecules are considerably more radiosensitive in their natural state.

 In vitro is irradiation outside of the cell or body. *In vivo* is irradiation in the body.

IRRADIATION OF MACROMOLECULES

A **solution** is a suspension of particles or molecules in a **fluid** such as water. A mixture of fluids such as water and alcohol is also a solution. When macromolecules are irradiated in solution in vitro, three major effects occur: main-chain scission, cross-linking, and point lesions (Figure 35-1).

Main-Chain Scission

Main-chain scission is the breakage of the backbone of the long-chain macromolecule. The result is the reduction of a long, single molecule into many smaller molecules, each of which may still be macromolecular.

Main-chain scission reduces not only the size of the macromolecule but also the **viscosity** of the solution. A viscous solution is one that is very thick and slow to flow, such as cold maple syrup. Tap water, on the other hand, has low viscosity. Measurements of viscosity determine the degree of main-chain scission.

Cross-Linking

Some macromolecules have small, spur-like side structures extending off the main chain. Others produce these spurs as a consequence of irradiation.

These side structures can behave as though they had a sticky substance on the end, and they attach to a neighboring macromolecule or to another segment of the same molecule. This process is called **cross-linking.** Radiation-induced molecular cross-linking increases the viscosity of a macromolecular solution.

Point Lesions

Radiation interaction with macromolecules also can result in disruption of single chemical bonds, producing **point lesions.** Such point lesions are not detectable but they can result in a minor modification of the molecule, which can in turn cause it to malfunction in the cell.

 At low radiation doses, point lesions are considered to be the cellular radiation damage resulting in the late radiation effects observed at the whole-body level.

Laboratory experiments have shown that all these types of radiation effects on macromolecules are reversible through intracellular repair and recovery.

Macromolecular Synthesis

Modern molecular biology has developed a generalized scheme for the function of a normal human cell. Molecular nutrients are brought to the cell and diffused through the cell membrane, where they are broken down (**catabolism**) into smaller molecules with an accompanying release of energy.

503

This energy is used in several ways but one of the more important ways is in the construction or **synthesis** of macromolecules from smaller molecules (**anabolism**). The synthesis of proteins and nucleic acids is critical to the survival of the cell and to its reproduction.

 Metabolism is catabolism (the reduction of nutrient molecules for energy) and anabolism (the production of large molecules for form and function).

Chapter 33 describes the scheme of protein synthesis and its dependence on nucleic acids. Proteins are manufactured by **translation** of the genetic code from tRNA, which had been **transferred** from mRNA. The information carried by the mRNA was in turn **transcribed** from the DNA. This chain of events is shown schematically in Figure 35-2.

Radiation damage to any of these macromolecules may result in cell death or late effects. Proteins are continuously synthesized throughout the cell cycle and occur in much more abundance than nucleic acids. Furthermore, multiple copies of specific protein molecules are always present in the cell. Consequently, proteins are less radiosensitive than nucleic acids.

Similarly, multiple copies of both types of RNA molecules are present in the cell, though they are less abundant than protein molecules. On the other hand, the DNA molecule, with its unique assembly of bases, is not so abundant.

 DNA is the most radiosensitive molecule.

DNA is synthesized somewhat differently from proteins. During the G_1 portion of interphase, the deoxyribose, phosphate, and base molecules accumulate in the nucleus. These molecules combine to form one large molecule that, during the S portion of interphase, is attached to an existing single chain of DNA (Figure 35-3). During G_1, the molecular DNA is in the familiar double-helix form.

 In G_1, there is half as much DNA as in G_2.

As the cell moves into S phase, the ladder begins to open up in the middle of each rung, much like a zipper. Now the DNA consists of only a single chain and there is no pairing of bases.

This state does not exist long, however, because the combined base-sugar-phosphate molecule attaches to the single-strand DNA sequence as determined by the permitted base pairing. Consequently, where there was one double-helix DNA molecule, there now are two similar molecules, each a duplicate of the original. The parent DNA is said to be replicated into two duplicate DNA daughter molecules.

Radiation Effects on DNA

DNA is the most important molecule in the human body because it contains the genetic information for each cell. Each cell has a nucleus containing DNA complexed with other molecules in the form of chromosomes. The chromosomes therefore control the growth and development of the cell, which in turn determine the characteristics of the individual (Figure 35-4).

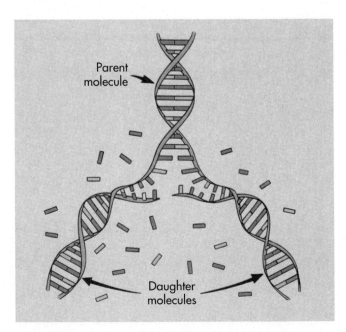

FIGURE 35-3 During S phase, the DNA separates like a zipper and two daughter DNA molecules are formed, each alike and each a replicate of the parent molecule.

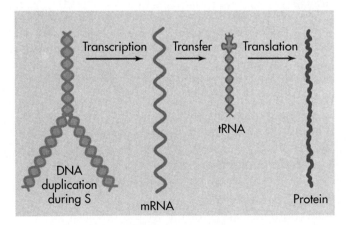

FIGURE 35-2 The genetic code of DNA is transcribed by mRNA and transferred to tRNA, which translates it into a protein.

If radiation damage to the DNA is severe enough, visible chromosome aberrations may be detected. Figure 35-5 is a representation of a normal chromosome and several distinct types of chromosome aberrations. Radiation-induced **chromosome aberrations,** or **cytogenetic damage,** are discussed more completely in Chapter 36.

The DNA molecule can be damaged without the production of a visible chromosome aberration. Although such damage is reversible, it can lead to cell death. If enough cells of the same type respond similarly, then a particular tissue or organ can be destroyed.

Damage to the DNA can also result in abnormal metabolic activity. The uncontrolled rapid proliferation of cells is the principal characteristic of radiation-induced malignant disease. If the damage to the DNA occurs in a germ cell, then it is possible that the response to the radiation exposure will not be observed until the following generation or even later.

The chromosome contains miles of DNA; therefore, when a visible aberration does appear, it signifies a considerable amount of radiation damage. Unobserved damage to the DNA can also produce responses at the cellular and whole-body level. The types of damage that can occur in the DNA molecule are as follows:

RADIATION RESPONSE OF DNA
1. Main-chain scission with only one side rail severed
2. Main-chain scission with both side rails severed
3. Main-chain scission and subsequent cross-linking
4. Rung breakage causing a separation of bases
5. A change in or loss of a base

The gross structural radiation response of DNA is diagrammed schematically in Figure 35-6. Although each of these effects results in a structural change in the DNA molecule, they are all reversible. In some of these types of damage the sequence of bases can be altered, and therefore the triplet code of codons may not remain intact. This represents a genetic mutation at the molecular level.

The fifth type of damage, the change or loss of a base, also destroys the triplet code and may not be reversible. This type of radiation damage is a molecular lesion of the DNA.

These molecular lesions are called **point mutations** and can be of either minor or major importance to the cell. One critical consequence of such point mutations is the transfer of the incorrect genetic code to one of the two daughter cells. This sequence of events is shown in Figure 35-7.

The three principal observable effects resulting from irradiation of DNA are cell death, malignant disease, and genetic damage. The latter two effects **at the molecular level** apparently conform to the **linear, nonthreshold** dose response relationship.

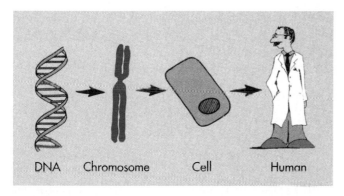

FIGURE 35-4 DNA is the target molecule for radiation damage. It forms chromosomes and controls cell and human growth and development.

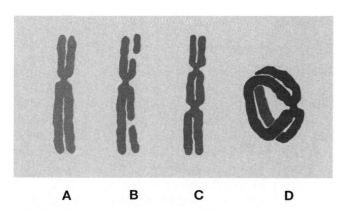

FIGURE 35-5 Normal and radiation damaged human chromosomes. **A,** Normal. **B,** Terminal deletion. **C,** Dicentric formation. **D,** Ring formation.

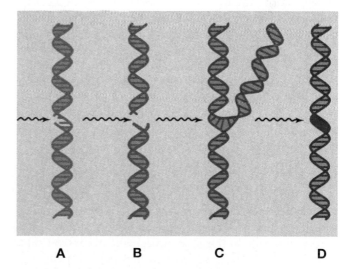

FIGURE 35-6 Types of damage that can occur in DNA. **A,** One side rail severed. **B,** Both side rails severed. **C,** Cross-linking. **D,** Rung breakage.

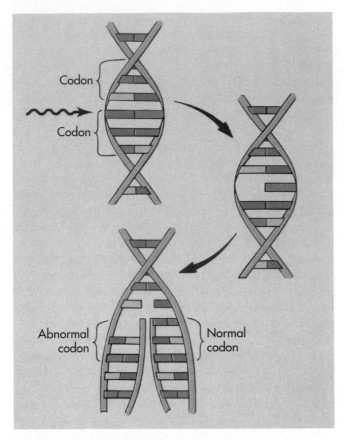

FIGURE 35-7 A point mutation results in the change or loss of a base, which creates an abnormal gene. This is therefore a genetic mutation that is passed to one of the daughter cells.

RADIOLYSIS OF WATER

Because the human body is an aqueous solution containing approximately 80% water molecules, irradiation of water represents the principal radiation interaction in the body. When water is irradiated, it dissociates into other molecular products; this action is called the **radiolysis of water** (Figure 35-8).

When an atom of water (H_2O) is irradiated, it is ionized and dissociates into two ions—an ion pair as shown by the following:

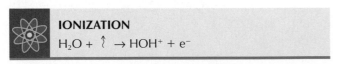

IONIZATION

$$H_2O + \text{\textasciitilde} \rightarrow HOH^+ + e^-$$

Following this initial ionization, a number of reactions can happen. First, the ion pair may rejoin into a stable water molecule. In this case, no damage occurs. Second, if these ions do not rejoin, it is then possible for the negative ion (the electron) to attach to another water molecule by the following reaction and produce yet a third type of ion.

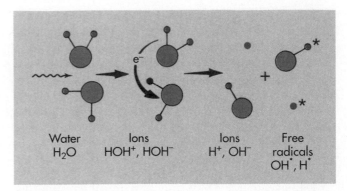

FIGURE 35-8 The radiolysis of water results in the formation of ions and free radicals.

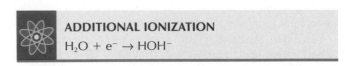

ADDITIONAL IONIZATION

$$H_2O + e^- \rightarrow HOH^-$$

The HOH^+ and HOH^- ions are relatively unstable and can dissociate into still smaller molecules as follows:

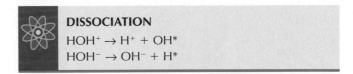

DISSOCIATION

$$HOH^+ \rightarrow H^+ + OH^*$$
$$HOH^- \rightarrow OH^- + H^*$$

The final result of the radiolysis of water is the formation of an ion pair, H^+ and OH^- and two free radicals, H^* and OH^*. The ions can recombine, and therefore no biologic damage would occur.

These types of ions are not unusual. Many molecules in aqueous solution exist in a loosely ionized state because of their structure. Salt ($NaCl$), for instance, easily dissociates into Na^+ and Cl^- ions. Even in the absence of radiation, water can dissociate into H^+ and OH^- ions.

 A free radical is an uncharged molecule containing a single unpaired electron in the outer shell.

The free radicals are another story. Free radicals are highly reactive. Free radicals are unstable and therefore exist with a lifetime of less than 1 ms. During that time, however, they are capable of diffusion through the cell and interaction at a distant site. Free radicals contain excess energy that can be transferred to other molecules to disrupt bonds and produce point lesions at some distance from the initial ionizing event.

The H^* and OH^* molecules are not the only free radicals that are produced during the radiolysis of water. The OH^* free radical can join with a similar molecule and form hydrogen peroxide.

HYDROGEN PEROXIDE

$OH^* + OH^* \rightarrow H_2O_2$

Hydrogen peroxide is poisonous to the cell and therefore acts as a toxic agent.

The H* free radical can interact with molecular oxygen to form the hydroperoxyl radical as follows:

HYDROPEROXYL FORMATION

$H^* + O_2 \rightarrow HO^*_2$

The hydroperoxyl radical, along with hydrogen peroxide, is considered to be the principal damaging product following the radiolysis of water. Hydrogen peroxide can also be formed by interaction of two hydroperoxyl radicals as follows:

HYDROGEN PEROXIDE FORMATION

$HO^*_2 + HO^*_2 \rightarrow H_2O_2 + O_2$

Some organic molecules, symbolized as RH, can become reactive free radicals as follows:

ORGANIC FREE RADICAL FORMATION

$RH + \uparrow \rightarrow RH^* \rightarrow H^* + R^*$

When oxygen is present, yet another species of free radical is possible as follows:

ORGANIC FREE RADICAL FORMATION

$R^* + O_2 \rightarrow RO^*_2$

Free radicals are energetic molecules because of their unique structure. This excess energy can be transferred to DNA and result in bond breaks.

DIRECT AND INDIRECT EFFECT

When biologic material is irradiated in vivo, the harmful effects of irradiation occur because of damage to a particularly sensitive molecule, such as DNA. Evidence for the direct effect of radiation comes from in vitro experiments wherein various molecules can be irradiated in solution. The effect is produced by ionization of the target molecule.

If the initial ionizing event occurs on the target molecule, the effect of radiation is direct.

On the other hand, if the initial ionizing event occurs on a distant, noncritical molecule, which then transfers the

energy of ionization to the target molecule, **indirect effect** has occurred. Free radicals, with their excess energy of reaction, are the intermediate molecules. They migrate to the target molecule and transfer their energy, which results in damage to that target molecule.

The principal effect of radiation on humans is indirect.

It is not possible to identify whether a given interaction with the target molecule resulted from direct or indirect effect. However, because the human body is 80% water and less than 1% DNA, we conclude that essentially all of the effects of irradiation in vivo result from indirect effect. When oxygen is present, as in living tissue, the indirect effects are amplified because of the additional types of free radicals that are formed.

Target Theory

The cell contains many species of molecules, most of which exist in overabundance. Radiation damage to such molecules probably would not result in noticeable injury to the cell because similar molecules would be available to continue to support the cell.

On the other hand, some molecules in the cell are considered to be particularly necessary for normal cell function. These molecules are not abundant; in fact, there may be only one such molecule. Radiation damage to such a molecule could affect the cell severely because there would be no similar molecules available as substitutes.

This concept of a sensitive key molecule is the basis for the **target theory**. According to target theory, for a cell to die after radiation exposure, its target molecule must be inactivated (Figure 35-9).

DNA is the target molecule.

The key molecular target is the DNA. Originally, target theory was used to represent cell lethality. It can be used equally well, however, to describe nonlethal radiation-induced cell abnormalities.

In target theory, the target is considered to be an area of the cell occupied by the target molecule or by a sensitive site on the target molecule. This area changes position with time because of intracellular molecular movement.

The interaction between radiation and cellular components is random; therefore, when an interaction does occur with a target, it occurs randomly. There is no favoritism of radiation to the target molecule. Its sensitivity to radiation occurs simply because of its vital function in the cell.

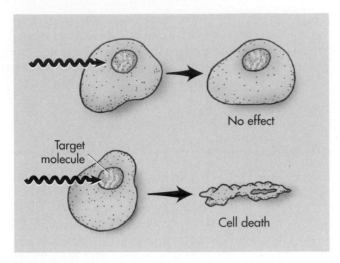

FIGURE 35-9 According to target theory, cell death will occur only if the target molecule is inactivated. DNA, the target molecule, is located in the cell nucleus.

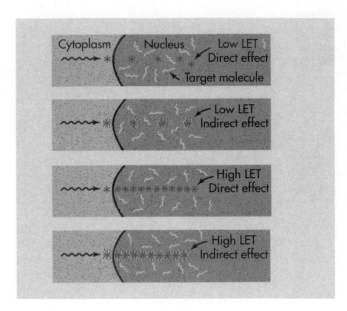

FIGURE 35-10 In the presence of oxygen, the indirect effect is amplified and the volume of action for low LET radiation is enlarged. The effective volume of action for high LET radiation remains unchanged, since maximum injury will have been inflicted by direct effect.

When radiation does interact with the target, a **hit** is said to have occurred. Radiation interaction with molecules other than the target molecule can also result in a hit. It is not possible to distinguish between a direct and an indirect hit.

 Hits occur through both direct and indirect effect.

When a hit occurs through indirect effect, the size of the target appears considerably larger because of the mobility of the free radicals. This increased target size contributes to the importance of the indirect effect of radiation.

Figure 35-10 illustrates some of the consequences of using target theory to explain the relationships among linear energy transfer (LET), the oxygen effect (OER), and direct versus indirect effect. With low-LET radiation, in the absence of oxygen, the probability of a hit on the target molecule is low because of the relatively large distances between ionizing events.

If oxygen is present, free radicals are formed and the volume of effectiveness surrounding each ionization is enlarged. Consequently, the probability of a hit is increased.

When high-LET radiation is used, the distance between ionizations is so close that the probability of a hit by direct effect is high. When oxygen is added to the system and high-LET radiation used, the added sphere of influence for each ionizing event, although somewhat larger, does not result in additional hits. The maximum number of hits has already been produced by direct effect with the high-LET radiation.

CELL-SURVIVAL KINETICS

Early radiation experiments at the cell level were conducted with simple cells, such as bacteria. It was not until the middle 1950s that laboratory techniques were developed to allow the growth and manipulation of human cells in vitro. Now cells can be grown in tubes, flasks, Petri dishes, or nearly any type of laboratory container.

One technique for measuring the lethal effects of radiation on cells is shown in Figure 35-11. If normal cells are planted individually in a Petri dish and incubated for 10 to 14 days, they divide many times and produce a visible **colony** consisting of many cells. This is cell **cloning.**

Following irradiation of such single cells, some do not survive and therefore fewer colonies are formed. A higher radiation dose leads to fewer colonies being formed.

 The lethal effects of radiation are determined by observing cell survival, not cell death.

Using a mathematical extension of target theory, two models of cell survival result. The **single-target, single-hit** model applies to biologic targets, such as enzymes, viruses, and simple cells like bacteria. The **multitarget, single-hit** model applies to more complicated biologic systems, such as human cells.

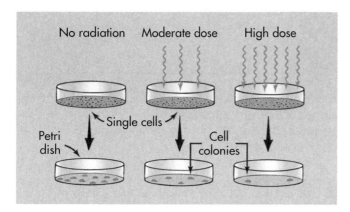

FIGURE 35-11 When single cells are planted in a Petri dish, they grow into visible colonies. Fewer colonies will develop if the cells are irradiated.

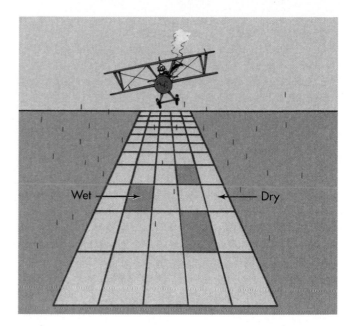

FIGURE 35-12 When rain falls on a dry pavement consisting of a large number of squares, the number of squares that remains dry decreases exponentially as the number of raindrops increases.

The following discussion concerns the equation of these models. The mathematics of these models is relatively unimportant but is given here for the interested student.

Single-Target, Single-Hit Model

Consider for a moment the situation illustrated in Figure 35-12. It is raining on a large concrete runway containing 100 squares. A square is considered wet when one or more raindrops have fallen on it.

When the first drop falls on the pavement, 1 of the 100 squares becomes wet. When the second drop falls, it will probably fall on a dry square and not the one already wet. Consequently, 2 out of 100 squares will be wet.

When the third raindrop falls, there will probably be 3 wet and 97 dry squares. As the number of raindrops increases, however, it becomes more probable that a given square will be hit by 2 or more drops.

Because the raindrops are falling **randomly**, the probability that a square will become wet is governed by a statistical law called the **Poisson distribution**. According to this law, when the number of raindrops is equal to the number of squares (100 in this case), 63% of the squares will be wet and 37% of the squares will be dry. If the raindrops had fallen **uniformly**, all 100 squares would become wet with 100 raindrops.

Radiation interacts randomly with matter.

Obviously, many of the 63 squares in this example have been hit twice or more. When the number of raindrops equals twice the number of squares, then 0.37×0.37, or 14, squares will be dry. Following 300 raindrops, only 5 squares will remain dry.

Examine a graph of the number of dry squares as a function of the number of raindrops (Figure 35-13). If the number of squares exposed to the rain were large or unknown, the scale on the right, expressed in percent, would be used.

The wet-squares analogy can be extended to the irradiation of a large number of biologic specimens—for example, 1000 bacteria. The bacteria presumably contain a single sensitive site, or **target**, that must be inactivated for the cell to die. As the 1000 bacteria are irradiated with increasing increments of dose, more are killed (Figure 35-14).

Just as with the wet squares, however, as the dose increases, some cells will suffer two or more hits. All hits per target in excess of one represent wasted radiation dose because the bacteria had already been killed by the first hit.

A hit is not simply an ionizing event, but rather an ionization that inactivates the target molecule.

When the radiation dose reaches a level sufficient to kill 63% of the cells (37% survival), it is called D_{37}. Following a dose equal to $2 \times D_{37}$, 14% of the cells would survive, and so on. D_{37} is a measure of the radiosensitivity of the cell. A low D_{37} represents a highly radiosensitive cell, and a high D_{37} represents radioresistance.

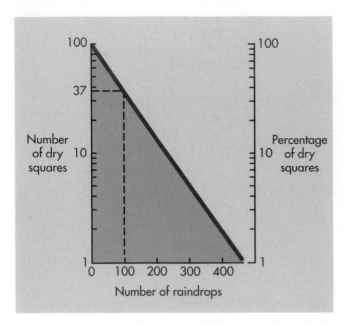

FIGURE 35-13 When the number of dry squares is plotted on semilogarithmic paper as a function of the number of raindrops, a straight line results because after a few drops some squares will be hit more than once.

 If there were no wasted hits (uniform interaction), D_{37} is the dose that would be sufficient to kill 100% of the cells.

The equation that describes the dose-response relationship represented by the graph in Figure 35-14 is the **single-target, single-hit** model of radiation-induced lethality as follows:

 **SINGLE-TARGET, SINGLE-HIT MODEL**

$$S = N/N_0 = e^{-D/D_{37}}$$

where S is the surviving fraction, N is the number of cells surviving a dose D, N_0 is the initial number of cells, and D_{37} is a constant dose related to the cell radiosensitivity.

Multitarget, Single-Hit Model

Returning to the wet-squares analogy, suppose that each pavement square were divided into two equal parts (Figure 35-15). By definition, each half must now be hit with a raindrop for the square to be considered wet. The first few raindrops will probably hit only one half

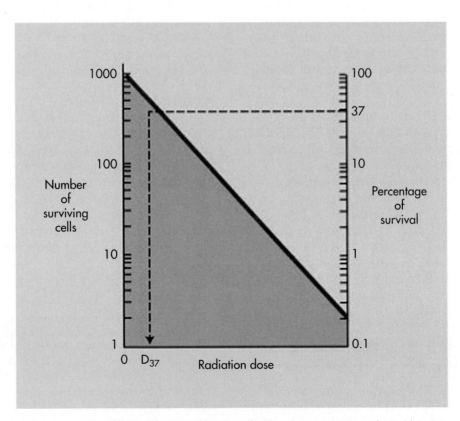

FIGURE 35-14 After the irradiation of 1000 cells, the dose-response relationship is exponential. The D_{37} is that dose that results in 37% survival.

of any given square, and therefore, following a very, light rain, no squares may be wet.

Many raindrops must fall before any single square suffers a hit in both halves so that it can be considered wet. This represents a **threshold because,** according to our definition, a number of raindrops can fall and all squares will remain dry.

As the number of raindrops increases, eventually some squares will have both halves hit and therefore be considered wet. This portion of the curve is represented by region A in Figure 35-16.

When a large number of raindrops has fallen, region C will be reached where every square will be at least half wet. When this occurs, each additional raindrop will produce a wet square. In region C the relation between number of raindrops and wet squares is that described by the single-target, single-hit model. The intermediate region B is the region of accumulation of hits.

Complex biologic specimens such as human cells are thought to have more than a single critical target. Suppose that the human cell has two targets, each of which has to be inactivated for the cell to die. This would be analogous to the square having two halves, each of which had to be hit by rain for it to be considered wet. Figure 35-17 is a graph of single-cell survival for human cells having two targets.

At very low radiation doses cell survival is nearly 100%. As the radiation dose increases, fewer cells survive because more sustain a hit in both target molecules.

At a high radiation dose, all cells that survive have one target hit. Therefore, at still all higher doses, the

dose-response relationship would appear as the single-target, single-hit model.

The model of cell survival just described is the multi-target, single-hit model as follows:

MULTITARGET, SINGLE-HIT MODEL

$S = N/N_0 = 1 - (1 - e^{-D/D_0})^n$

where S is the surviving fraction, N is the number of cells surviving a dose D, N_0 is the initial number of cells, D_0 is the dose necessary to reduce survival to 37% in the straight-line portion of the graph, and n is the *extrapolation number.*

The D_0 is called the **mean lethal dose** and is a constant related to the radiosensitivity of the cell. It is equal to D_{37} in the linear portion of the graph and therefore represents the dose that would result in one hit per target in the straight-line portion of the graph if no radiation were wasted.

A large D_0 indicates radioresistant cells, and a small D_0 is characteristic of radiosensitive cells.

The **extrapolation number** is also called the **target number.** When this type of experiment was first conducted with human cells, the observed extrapolation number was 2. That result agreed with the hypothesis that similar regions on two homologous chromosomes (an identical pair) had to

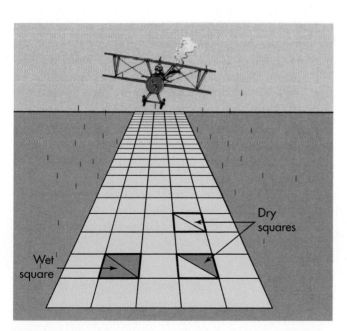

FIGURE 35-15 If each pavement square has two equal parts, each part must be hit for the square to be considered wet.

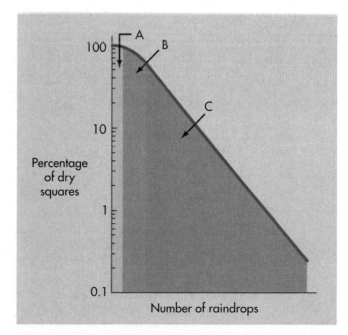

FIGURE 35-16 When a square contains two equal parts, both of which have to be hit to be considered wet, three regions of the dry square vs raindrops relationship can be identified.

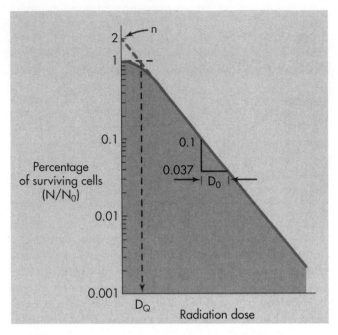

FIGURE 35-17 The multitarget, single-hit model of cell survival is characteristic of human cells containing two targets.

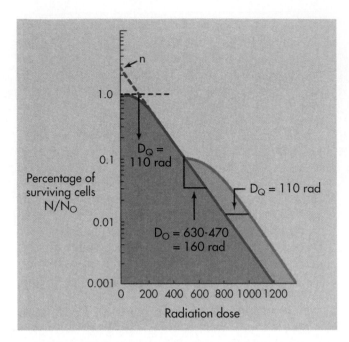

FIGURE 35-18 Split-dose irradiation results in a second cell survival curve with the same characteristics of the first displaced along the dose axis by D_Q.

be inactivated to produce cell death. Because chromosomes come in pairs, the experimental results confirmed the hypothesis.

Subsequent experiments, however, have resulted in extrapolation numbers ranging from 2 to 12, and therefore the precise meaning of n is unknown.

The D_Q is called the **threshold dose.** It is a measure of the width of the shoulder of the multitarget, single-hit model and is related to the capacity of the cell to recover from sublethal damage. Table 35-1 lists reported values for D_0 and D_Q for various experimental cell lines.

 A large D_Q indicates that the cell can readily recover from sublethal damage.

Recovery

The shoulder of the graph of the multitarget, single-hit model shows that for mammalian cells some damage must be accumulated before the cell dies. This accumulated damage is called **sublethal damage.** The wider the shoulder, the more sublethal damage that can be sustained and the higher the value of D_Q.

Figure 35-18 demonstrates the results of a **split-dose irradiation** designed to describe the capacity of a cell to recover from sublethal damage. This illustration shows a rather typical human cell survival curve with $D_0 = 160$ rad (1.6 Gy$_t$), $D_Q = 110$ rad (1.1 Gy$_t$), and $n = 2$. If one takes those cells that survive any large

TABLE 35-1	Dose (D_Q) for Various Experimental Mammalian Cell Lines	
Cell Type	D_0 (rad)	D_Q (rad)
Mouse oocytes	91	62
Mouse skin	135	350
Human bone marrow	137	100
Human fibroblasts	150	160
Mouse spermatogonia	180	270
Chinese hamster ovary	200	210
Human lymphocytes	400	100

dose (for example, 470 rad [4.7 Gy$_t$]) and re-incubates them in a growth medium, they will grow into another large population.

This new population of cells can then be used to perform a second cell survival experiment. When the cells that survived the first dose are subsequently subjected to additional incremental radiation doses, a second dose-response curve is generated that has precisely the same shape as the first.

Following such a split, the extrapolation number is the same and the mean lethal dose is the same, and the second dose-response curve is separated along the dose axis from the first dose-response curve by D_Q. For full recovery to occur, the time between such split doses must be at least as long as the cell generation time.

Such experiments show that cells that survive an initial radiation insult exhibit precisely the same characteristics as nonirradiated cells; therefore, the surviving cells have fully recovered from the sublethal damage produced by the initial irradiation.

 D_Q is a measure of the capacity to accumulate sublethal and the ability to recover from sublethal damage.

Question: From Figure 35-18, estimate the overall surviving fraction for a cell receiving a split-dose of 400 rad followed by 400 rad (4 Gy$_t$).

Answer: At a dose of 400 rad, approximately 0.15 of the cells survive. Therefore, at a split-dose of 400 rad and 400 rad, the surviving fraction should equal $0.15 \times 0.15 = 0.023$. The total dose is 800 rad (8 Gy$_t$), and the surviving fraction on the split-dose curve at 800 rad should equal 0.023, and it does. Had the 800 rad been delivered at one time, the surviving fraction would have been 0.012, as shown by the single-dose curve of Figure 35-18.

Cell-Cycle Effects

When human cells replicate by mitosis, the average time from one mitosis to another is called the **cell-cycle time** or the **generation time**. Most human cells that are in a state of normal proliferation have generation times of 10 to 20 hr.

Some specialized cells have generation times extending to hundreds of hours, and some cells, such as neurons (nerve cells), do not normally replicate. Longer generation times primarily result from a lengthening of the G$_1$ phase of the cell cycle.

 G$_1$ is the most time-variable of cell phases.

There are ways to take a randomly growing population of cells that are uniformly distributed in position throughout the cell cycle and **synchronize** them. A population of synchronized cells can then be subdivided into smaller populations and irradiated sequentially as they pass through the phases of the cell cycle.

Figure 35-19 represents results obtained from human fibroblasts. The fraction of cells surviving a given dose can vary by a factor of 10 from the most sensitive to the most resistant phase of the cell cycle.

This pattern of change in radiosensitivity as a function of phase in the cell cycle is the **age-response function**, which varies among cells. Cells in mitosis are al-

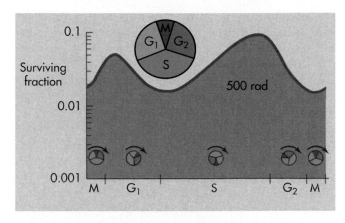

FIGURE 35-19 The age-response of human fibroblasts following irradiation, shows a minimum survival during the M phase and maximum survival during late S phase. Such cells are most radiosensitive during mitosis and most radioresistant during the late S phase.

ways most sensitive. The fraction of surviving cells is lowest in this phase. The next most sensitive phase of the cell cycle occurs at the G$_1$-S transition. The most resistant portion of the cell cycle is the late S phase.

 Human cells are most radiosensitive in M, most radioresistant in late S.

LET, RBE, and OER

Mammalian cell survival experiments have been used extensively to measure the effects of various types of radiation and to determine the magnitude of various dose-modifying factors, such as oxygen. Because the mean lethal dose, D_0, is related to radiosensitivity, the ratio of D_0 for one condition of irradiation compared with another is a measure of the effectiveness of the dose modifier, whether it is physical or biologic.

If the same cell type is irradiated by two different radiations under identical conditions, results may appear as in Figure 35-20. At the very high LET (as with alpha particles and neutrons), the cell-survival kinetics follow the single-target, single-hit model. With low-LET radiation (x-rays), the multitarget, single-hit model applies.

The mean lethal dose following low-LET irradiation is always greater than that following high-LET irradiation. If the low-LET D_0 represents x-rays, then the ratio of one D_0 to another equals the relative biologic effectiveness (RBE) for the high-LET radiation as follows:

 RELATIVE BIOLOGIC EFFECTIVENESS

$$RBE = \frac{D_0 \ (\text{x-radiation}) \ \text{to produce an effect}}{D_0 \ (\text{test radiation}) \ \text{to produce the same effect}}$$

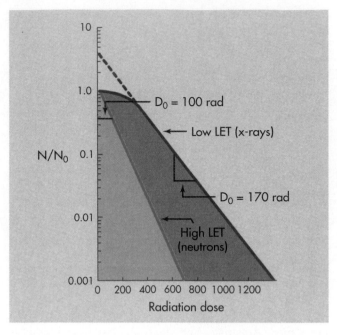

FIGURE 35-20 Representative cell survival curves following exposure to 200 kVp x-rays and 14 MeV neutrons.

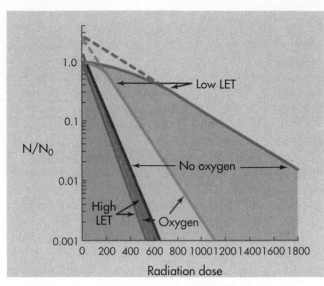

FIGURE 35-21 Cell survival cures for human cells irradiated in the presence and absence of oxygen with high and low LET radiation.

Question: Figure 35-20 shows the radiation dose-response relationship of human fibroblasts exposed to x-rays and to 14 MeV neutrons. The D_0 following x-radiation is 170 rad (1.7 Gy_t); the D_0 for neutron irradiation is 100 rad (1 Gy_t). What is the RBE of 14 MeV neutrons relative to x-rays?

Answer: $RBE = \dfrac{170 \text{ rad}}{100 \text{ rad}}$

$$= 1.7$$

 Irradiation of mammalian cells with high-LET radiation follows the single-target, single-hit model.

The most completely studied dose modifier is oxygen. The presence of oxygen maximizes the effect of low-LET radiation. When hypoxic or anoxic cells are exposed, a considerably higher dose is required to produce a given effect.

With high-LET radiation, there is little difference between the response of oxygenated cells and anoxic cells. Figure 35-21 shows typical cell-survival curves for each of these combinations of LET and oxygen.

Such experiments are designed to measure the magnitude of the oxygen effect. The OER determined from single-cell survival experiments is defined as follows:

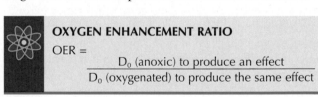

OXYGEN ENHANCEMENT RATIO

$$OER = \frac{D_0 \text{ (anoxic) to produce an effect}}{D_0 \text{ (oxygenated) to produce the same effect}}$$

Question: With reference to Figure 35-21, what is the estimated OER for human cells exposed to low-LET radiation and to high-LET radiation?

Answer: Low LET, no oxygen D_0 = 340 rad
Low LET, oxygen D_0 = 140 rad

$$OER = \frac{340 \text{ rad}}{140 \text{ rad}} = 2.4$$

High LET, no oxygen, D_0 = 90 rad
High LET, oxygen, D_0 = 70 rad

$$OER = \frac{90 \text{ rad}}{70 \text{ rad}} = 1.3$$

The interrelationships among LET, RBE, and OER are complex. However, it is LET that determines the magnitude of RBE and OER.

SUMMARY

When macromolecules are irradiated in vitro, three major effects occur: (1) main-chain scission, (2) cross-linking, and (3) disruption of single chemical bonds in a macromolecule, causing point lesions. All three types of damage are reversible through intercellular repair and recovery.

DNA, with its unique assembly of bases, is not abundant in the cell. As a result, DNA is the most radiosensitive of all macromolecules. Chromosome aberrations or abnormal metabolic activity can result from DNA damage. DNA irradiation has three observable effects: cell death, malignant disease, and genetic damage.

Because the human body is 80% water, irradiation of water is the principal interaction in the body. Water dissociates into free radicals that are highly reactive and can diffuse through the cell to cause damage at some distance.

The initial ionizing event is said to be a direct effect if the interaction occurs with a DNA molecule. If the ionizing event occurs with water and transfers that energy to DNA, the event is said to be an indirect effect.

The concept of a sensitive key molecule in a cell is the basis for the target theory. For a cell to die after radiation exposure, the target molecule, DNA, must be inactivated.

Radiation exposure results in two models of cell survival. The single-target, single-hit model applies to simple cells such as bacteria. The multitarget, single-hit model implies a dose threshold. However, at higher doses, the relationship becomes a single-hit, single-target model. Experiments in cell recovery show that cells can recover from sublethal radiation damage.

CHALLENGE QUESTIONS

1. Define or otherwise identify:
   a. In vitro
   b. Cytogenetic damage
   c. Point mutation
   d. Free radical
   e. Target theory
   f. D_{37}
   g. Mean lethal dose
   h. Radiation hit
   i. Extrapolation number
   j. D_Q

2. List the effects of irradiation of macromolecules in solution in vitro.
3. How is solution viscosity used to determine the degree of radiation macromolecular damage?
4. What is the difference between catabolism and anabolism?
5. In what phase of the cell cycle does the DNA ladder open up in the middle of each rung and consist of only a single chain?
6. Name the three principal observable effects of DNA irradiation.
7. Differentiate between transcription, transfer, and translation when applied to molecular genetics.
8. Draw a diagram illustrating the point mutations of DNA that transfer the incorrect genetic code to one of the two daughter cells.
9. Write the formula for the radiolysis of water in which the atom of water is ionized and dissociates into two ions.
10. What happens to radiation-induced free radicals within the cell?
11. What is the target theory of radiobiology.
12. Does radiation interact with tissue uniformly or randomly?
13. Draw cell survival curves to show the difference between irradiation with low-LET and high-LET radiation.
14. What is the difference between in vitro and in vivo?
15. Complete the following chemical equations:
    H_2O + Radiation → ?
    HOH^+ (dissociation) → ?
    HOH^- (dissociation) → ?
16. The D_{37} of a cellular species that follows the single-target, single-hit model is 150 rad. What percentage of cells will survive 450 rad?
17. What is the RBE of alpha radiation if the D_0 is 40 rad, compared with 180 rad for x-rays?
18. What is the difference between direct effect and indirect effect?
19. How does the radiosensitivity of human cells vary with stages of the cell cycle?
20. Draw cell-survival curves to show the difference between low-LET irradiation of aerobic cells and anoxic cells.

Early Effects of Radiation

OBJECTIVES

At the completion of this chapter, the student should be able to do the following:

1. Describe the three acute radiation syndromes
2. Identify the two stages leading to acute radiation lethality
3. Define $LD_{50/60}$
4. Discuss local tissue damage following high-dose irradiation
5. Review the cytogenetic effects following radiation exposure

OUTLINE

DURING THE 1920s and the 1930s, it would not have been unusual for a radiologic technologist to visit the hematology laboratory once a week for a routine blood examination. Before the introduction of personnel radiation monitors, periodic blood examination was the only way to monitor x-ray workers.

There was great concern over the danger of occupational radiation exposure. Today's occupational radiation exposures are quite low. Still, the radiologic technologist must understand the early effects of high radiation dose.

This chapter explores such early effects from the most severe (death) to the most worrisome today (skin effects). The chapter also reviews hematologic and cytogenetic effects.

To produce a radiation response in humans within a few days to months, the dose must be substantial. Such a response is called **early effect** of radiation exposure. A dose of this magnitude is rare in diagnostic radiology.

These early effects have been studied extensively with laboratory animals, and there are even some data from observations of humans. This chapter considers only the more important effects as identified in Table 36-1, along with the minimum radiation dose necessary to produce each.

Early radiation responses are called **deterministic.** Deterministic radiation responses are those that exhibit increasing severity with increasing radiation dose. Furthermore, there is usually a dose threshold.

ACUTE RADIATION LETHALITY

Death, of course, is the most devastating human response to radiation exposure. No cases of death following diagnostic x-ray exposure have been recorded, although some early x-ray pioneers died from the late effects of x-ray exposure. In each of these cases, however, the total radiation dose was extremely high by today's standards.

Acute radiation-induced human lethality is of only academic interest in diagnostic radiology. Diagnostic x-ray beams are neither intense enough nor large enough to cause death.

Diagnostic x-ray beams always result in partial-body exposure, which is less harmful than whole-body exposure.

Some accidental exposures of persons in the nuclear weapons and nuclear energy fields have resulted in immediate death, but the number of such accidents has been small considering the length and activity of the atomic age. The unfortunate incident at Chernobyl in April 1986 is the one notable exception.

Thirty people at Chernobyl experienced the acute radiation syndrome and died. A number of minor late effects have been observed. No one died or was even seriously exposed in the March 1979 incident at the nuclear power reactor at Three Mile Island, Pennsylvania. Employment in the nuclear power industry is a safe occupation.

The sequence of events following high-level radiation exposure leading to death within days or weeks is called the **acute radiation syndrome.** There are, in fact, three separate syndromes that are dose-related and that follow a rather distinct course of clinical responses.

These syndromes are **hematologic death, gastrointestinal (GI) death,** and **central nervous system (CNS) death.** The clinical signs and symptoms of each are outlined in Table 36-2. CNS death requires radiation doses in excess of 5000 rad (50 Gy$_t$) and results in death within hours. Hematologic death and GI death follow lower exposures and require a longer time for death to occur.

In addition to the three lethal syndromes, two other periods are associated with acute radiation lethality. The **prodromal period** consists of acute clinical symptoms that occur within hours of exposure and continue for up to a day or two. Following the prodromal period, there may be a **latent period,** during which time the subject is free of visible effects.

Prodromal Period

At radiation doses above approximately 100 rad delivered to the total body, the signs and symptoms of radiation sickness may appear within a matter of minutes to hours. The symptoms of this early radiation sickness most often take the form of nausea, vomiting, diarrhea, and a reduction in the white cells of the peripheral blood (leukopenia).

This immediate response of radiation sickness is the prodromal period.

The prodromal period may last from a few hours to a couple of days. The severity of the symptoms is dose-related; at doses in excess of 1000 rad (10 Gy$_t$), the symptoms can be violent. At still higher doses, the duration of the prodromal syndrome becomes shorter, until it is difficult to separate the prodromal syndrome from the period of manifest illness.

Latent Period

After the period of initial radiation sickness, there is a period of apparent well-being called the latent period. The latent period extends from hours or less (at doses in excess of 5000 rad) to weeks (at doses from 100 to 500 rad).

 The latent period is the time after exposure during which there is no sign of radiation sickness.

The latent period is sometimes mistakenly thought to indicate an early recovery from a moderate radiation dose. It may be different, however, giving no indication of the extensive radiation response yet to follow.

Manifest Illness

The dose necessary to produce a given syndrome and the mean survival time are the principal quantitative measures of human radiation lethality (see Table 36-2). Although ranges of dose and resulting mean survival times are given, there is rarely a precise difference in the

dose and time-related sequence of events associated with each syndrome. At very high radiation doses, the latent period disappears altogether. At very low radiation doses, there may be no prodromal period.

Hematologic Syndrome. Radiation doses in the range of approximately 200 to 1000 rad produce the hematologic syndrome. The subject initially experiences mild symptoms of the prodromal syndrome, which appear in a matter of a few hours and may persist for several days.

The latent period that follows can extend as long as 4 weeks and is characterized by a general feeling of wellness. There are no obvious signs of illness, although the number of cells in the peripheral blood declines during this time.

 The hematologic syndrome is characterized by a reduction in white cells, red cells, and platelets.

The period of **manifest illness** is characterized by possible vomiting, mild diarrhea, malaise, lethargy, and fever. Each of the types of blood cells follows rather characteristic patterns of cell depletion. If the dose is not lethal, recovery begins in 2 to 4 weeks, but it may take as long as 6 months for full recovery.

If the radiation injury is severe enough, the reduction in blood cells continues unchecked until the body's defense against infection is nil. Just before death, hemorrhage and dehydration may be pronounced. Death occurs because of generalized infection, electrolyte imbalance, and dehydration.

Gastrointestinal (GI) Syndrome. Radiation doses of approximately 1000 to 5000 rad (10 to 50 Gy_t) result in the **GI syndrome**. The prodromal symptoms of vomiting and diarrhea occur within hours of exposure and persist for hours to as long as a day. A latent period of 3 to 5 days follows, during which time no symptoms are present.

The manifest illness period begins with a second wave of nausea and vomiting, followed by diarrhea. The victim experiences a loss of appetite (anorexia) and may become lethargic.

TABLE 36-1	Principal Early Effects of Radiation Exposure on Humans and the Approximate Threshold Dose

Effect	Anatomic Site	Threshold Dose
Death	Whole-body	200 rad / 2 Gy_t
Hematologic depression	Whole-body	25 rad / 0.25 Gy_t
Skin erythema	Small field	200 rad / 2 Gy_t
Epilation	Small field	300 rad / 3 Gy_t
Chromosome aberration	Whole-body	5 rad / 50 mGy_t
Gonadal dysfunction	Local tissue	10 rad / 0.1 mGy_t

TABLE 36-2	Summary of Acute Radiation Lethality		
Period	Approximate Dose (rad)	Mean Survival Time (Days)	Clinical Signs and Symptoms
Prodromal	>100	—	Nausea, vomiting, diarrhea
Latent	100–10,000	—	None
Hematologic	200–1000	10–60	Nausea, vomiting, diarrhea, anemia, leukopenia, hemorrhage, fever, infection
Gastrointestinal	1000–5000	4–10	Same as hematologic *plus* electrolyte imbalance, lethargy, fatigue, shock
Central nervous system	>5000	0–3	Same as gastrointestinal *plus* ataxia, edema, vasculitis, meningitis

The diarrhea persists and becomes more severe, leading to loose and then watery and bloody stools. Supportive therapy cannot prevent the rapid progression of symptoms that ultimately leads to death within 4 to 10 days of exposure.

 GI death occurs principally because of severe damage to the cells lining the intestines.

Intestinal cells are normally in a rapid state of proliferation and are continuously being replaced by new cells. The turnover time for this cell renewal system in a normal person is 3 to 5 days.

Radiation exposure kills the most sensitive cells—stem cells—and this controls the length of time until death. When the intestinal lining is completely denuded of functional cells, fluids pass uncontrollably across the intestinal membrane, electrolyte balance is destroyed, and conditions promote infection.

At doses consistent with the GI syndrome, measurable and even severe hematologic changes occur. It takes longer time for the cell renewal system of the blood to develop mature cells from the stem cell population; therefore, there is not enough time for maximum hematologic effects to occur.

Central Nervous System (CNS) Syndrome. Following a radiation dose in excess of approximately 5000 rad (50 Gy$_t$), a series of signs and symptoms occur that lead to death within a matter of hours to days. First, severe nausea and vomiting begins, usually within a few minutes of exposure.

During this initial onset, the victim may become extremely nervous and confused, complain of a burning sensation in the skin, lose vision, and even lose consciousness within the first hour. This may be followed by a latent period lasting up to 12 hours, during which time the earlier symptoms subside or disappear.

After the latent period is the period of manifest illness, during which time the symptoms of the prodromal stage return, but more severely. The person becomes disoriented, loses muscle coordination; has difficulty breathing; may go into convulsive seizures; experiences loss of equilibrium, ataxia, and lethargy; lapses into a coma; and dies.

Regardless of the medical attention given the patient, the symptoms of manifest illness appear rather suddenly and always with extreme severity. At radiation doses high enough to produce CNS effects, the outcome is always death within a few days of exposure.

 The ultimate cause of death in CNS syndrome is an elevated fluid content of the brain.

The CNS syndrome is characterized by increased intracranial pressure, inflammatory changes in the blood vessels of the brain (vasculitis), and inflammation of the meninges (meningitis).

At doses sufficient to produce CNS damage, damage to all other organs of the body is equally severe. The classic radiation-induced changes in the GI tract and the hematologic system cannot occur because there is insufficient time between exposure and death for them to appear.

LD$_{50/60}$

If experimental animals are irradiated with varying doses of radiation, for example, 100 to 1000 rad (1 to 10 Gy$_t$), the plot of the percentage dying as a function of radiation dose would appear as in Figure 36-1. This figure illustrates the radiation dose-response relationship for acute human lethality.

 The LD$_{50/60}$ is the dose of radiation to the whole-body that causes 50% of the irradiated subjects to die within 60 days.

At the lower dose of approximately 100 rad (1 Gy$_t$), no one is expected to die. Above approximately 600 rad (6 Gy$_t$), all those irradiated die unless vigorous medical support is available. Above 1000 rad (10 Gy$_t$), even vigorous medical support does not prevent death.

 Acute radiation lethality follows a nonlinear, threshold dose-response relationship.

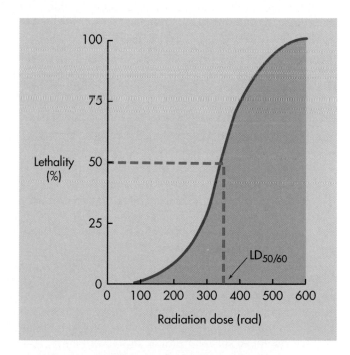

FIGURE 36-1 Radiation-induced death in humans follows a nonlinear, threshold dose-response relationship.

TABLE 36-3	Approximate LD$_{50/60}$ for Various Species after Whole-body Radiation Exposure	
Species	**LD$_{50/60}$ (rad)**	
Pig	250	
Dog	275	
Human	350	
Guinea pig	425	
Monkey	475	
Opossum	510	
Mouse	620	
Goldfish	700	
Hamster	700	
Rat	710	
Rabbit	725	
Gerbil	1050	
Turtle	1500	
Armadillo	2000	
Newt	3000	
Cockroach	10,000	

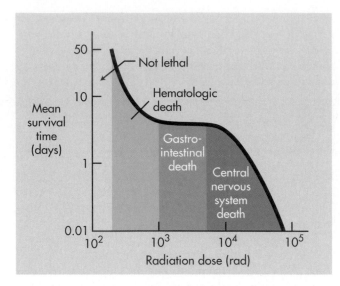

FIGURE 36-2 Mean survival time after radiation exposure shows three distinct regions. If death is due to hematologic or CNS effects, the mean survival time will vary with dose. If GI effects cause death, it occurs in approximately 4 days.

If death is to occur, it usually happens within 60 days of exposure. Acute radiation lethality is measured quantitatively by the LD$_{50/60}$, which is approximately 350 rad (3.5 Gy$_t$) for humans. With clinical support, humans can tolerate much higher doses; the maximum is reported to be 850 rad (8.5 Gy$_t$). Table 36-3 lists values of LD$_{50/60}$ for various species.

Sometimes additional measures of acute lethality are identified. LD$_{10/60}$ and LD$_{90/60}$ indicate a dose resulting in 10% lethality or 90% lethality within 60 days, respectively. LD$_{50/30}$ is the lethal dose to 50% of subjects when the observed survival time is shortened to 30 days. Normally, this is not much different from the LD$_{50/60}$.

Question: From Figure 36-1, estimate the radiation dose that will produce 25% lethality in humans within 60 days.

Answer: First, draw a horizontal line from the 25% level on the y-axis until it intersects the S curve. Now, drop a vertical line from this point to the x-axis. This intersection with the x-axis occurs at the LD$_{25/60}$, which is approximately 250 rad (2.5 Gy$_t$).

Mean Survival Time

As the whole-body radiation dose increases, the average time between exposure and death decreases. This time is known as the **mean survival time**. A graph of radiation dose versus mean survival time is shown in Figure 36-2. This graph has three distinct regions associated with the three radiation syndromes.

As the radiation dose increases from 200 to 1000 rad (2 to 10 Gy$_t$), the mean survival time decreases from approximately 60 to 4 days, and this region is consistent with death resulting from the hematologic syndrome. Mean survival time is dose-dependent with the hematologic syndrome.

In the dose range associated with the GI syndrome, however, the mean survival time remains relatively constant, at 4 days. With larger doses, those associated with the CNS syndrome, the mean survival time is again dose-dependent, varying from approximately 3 days to a matter of hours.

LOCAL TISSUE DAMAGE

When only part of the body is irradiated, compared with whole-body irradiation, a higher dose is required to produce a response. Every organ and tissue of the body can be affected by partial-body irradiation. The effect is cell death, resulting in a shrinkage of the organ or tissue. This can lead to total lack of function for that organ or tissue, or it can be followed by recovery.

 Atrophy is the shrinkage of an organ or tissue due to cell death.

There are many examples of local tissue damage immediately after radiation exposure. In fact, if the dose is high enough, any local tissue will respond. The manner in which local tissues respond depends on their intrinsic radiosensitivity and the kinetics of cell proliferation and maturation. Examples of local tissues that can be affected immediately are skin, gonads, and bone marrow.

Effects on Skin

The tissue with which we have most experience is the skin. Normal skin consists of three layers: an outer layer (the epidermis), an intermediate layer of connective tissue (the dermis), and a subcutaneous layer of fat and connective tissue.

The skin has additional accessory structures, such as hair follicles, sweat glands, and sensory receptors (Figure 36-3). All the cell layers and the accessory structures participate in the response to radiation exposure.

The skin, like the lining of the intestine, represents a continuing cell renewal system, only at a much slower rate than that experienced by intestinal cells. Almost 50% of the cells lining the intestine are replaced every day, whereas the skin cells are replaced at the rate of only approximately 2% per day.

The outer skin layer, the epidermis, consists of several layers of cells, the lowest layer being the **basal cells**. The basal cells are the **stem cells** that mature as they migrate to the surface of the epidermis. Once these cells arrive on the surface as mature cells, they are slowly lost and have to be replaced by new cells from the basal layer.

 Damage to basal cells results in the earliest manifestation of radiation injury to the skin.

In earlier times, the tolerance of the patient's skin determined the limitations of radiation oncology with **orthovoltage x-rays** (200 to 300 kVp x-rays). The object of x-ray therapy is to deposit energy in the tumor while sparing the surrounding normal tissue.

Because the x-rays must pass through the skin to reach the tumor, the skin was necessarily subjected to higher radiation doses than the tumor. The resultant skin damage was **erythema** (a sunburn-like reddening of the skin), followed by **desquamation** (ulceration and denudation of the skin), which often required interruption of the therapy.

After a single dose of 300 to 1000 rad (3 to 10 Gy$_t$), an initial mild erythema may occur within the first or second day. This first wave of erythema then subsides, only to be followed by a second wave that reaches maximum intensity in about 2 weeks.

At higher doses, this second wave of erythema is followed by a moist desquamation, which in turn may lead to a dry desquamation. Moist desquamation is known as **clinical tolerance** for radiation therapy.

During radiation therapy, the skin is exposed in a fractionated scheme, usually approximately 200 rad/day (2 Gy$_t$/d), 5 days a week. To assist the radiation on-

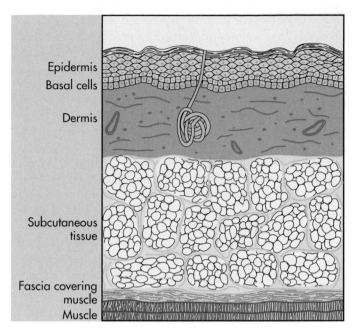

FIGURE 36-3 A sectional view of the anatomic structures of the skin. The basal cell layer is most radiosensitive.

cologist in planning patient treatments, isoeffect curves have been generated that accurately project the dose necessary to produce skin erythema or clinical tolerance after a prescribed treatment routine (Figure 36-4). Contemporary radiation oncology uses high-energy x-radiation from linear accelerators, which spares the skin from radiation damage.

Erythema was perhaps the first observed biologic response to radiation exposure. Many of the early x-ray pioneers, including Roentgen, suffered skin burns induced by x-rays. One of the hazards to the patient during the early years of radiology was x-ray–induced erythema.

During those years, x-ray tube potentials were so low that it was usually necessary to position the tube very close to the patient's skin; exposures of 10 to 30 min were often required. Often the patient would return several days later suffering from an x-ray burn.

These skin effects follow a nonlinear, threshold dose-response relationship similar to that described for radiation-induced lethality. Small doses of x-radiation do not cause erythema. Extremely high doses of x-radiation cause erythema in all persons so irradiated.

Whether intermediate radiation doses produce erythema depends on the individual's radiosensitivity, the dose rate, and the size of the irradiated skin field. Analysis of persons irradiated therapeutically with superficial x-rays has shown that the **skin erythema dose** required to affect 50% of those irradiated (**SED$_{50}$**), is about 500 rad (5 Gy$_t$).

Before the definition of the roentgen and the development of accurate radiation-measuring apparatus, the skin was observed and its response to radiation used in formulating radiation protection practices. The unit used was the SED$_{50}$, and permissible radiation exposures were specified in fractions of SED$_{50}$.

Another response of the skin to radiation exposure is **epilation** or loss of hair. For many years soft x-rays (10 to 20 kVp), called **grenz rays,** were used as the treatment of choice for skin diseases, such as tinea capitis (ringworm).

Tinea capitis of the scalp, not uncommon in children, was successfully treated by grenz radiation; unfortunately, the patient's hair would fall out for weeks or even months. Sometimes, an unnecessarily high dose of grenz rays resulted in permanent epilation.

High-dose fluoroscopy has focused more attention on the response of the skin to x-rays. The longer fluoroscopy times required for cardiovascular and interventional procedures, coupled with allowed exposure rates exceeding 20 R/min, is of great concern. Injuries to patients have been reported, and steps are being taken to establish better control over such exposures. Table 36-4 summarizes the potential effects of high-dose fluoroscopy.

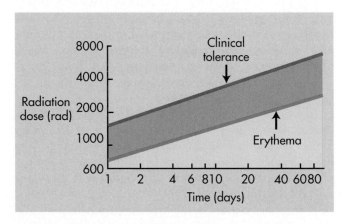

FIGURE 36-4 These isoeffect curves show the relationship between the number of daily fractions and the total radiation dose that will produce erythema or moist desquamation. As the fractionation of the dose increases, so does the total dose required.

Effects on Gonads

The human gonads are critically important target organs. As an example of local tissue effects, they are particularly sensitive to radiation. Responses to doses as low as 10 rad have been observed. Because these organs produce the germ cells that control fertility and heredity, their response to radiation has been studied extensively.

Much of what is known in the area of both the type of radiation response and dose-response relationships have been derived from numerous animal experiments. Some significant data are also available from human populations. Radiotherapy patients, radiation accident victims, and volunteer convicts have all provided data to allow a rather complete description of the gonadal response to radiation.

The cells of the testes (the male gonads) and the ovaries (the female gonads) respond differently to radiation because of differences in progression from the stem cell phase to the mature cell. Figure 36-5 illustrates this progression, indicating the most radiosensitive phase of cell maturation.

 Ovaries and testes produce oogonia and spermatogonia, which mature into ovum and sperm, respectively.

Germ cells are produced by both ovaries and testes, but they develop from the stem cell phase to the mature cell phase at different rates and at different times. This process of development is called **gametogenesis.**

The stem cells of the ovaries are the **oogonia,** and they multiply in number only before birth, during fetal life. The oogonia reach a maximum number of several million and then begin to decline because of spontaneous degeneration.

During late fetal life, many **primordial follicles** grow to encapsulate the oogonia, which become **oocytes.** These follicle-containing oocytes remain in a suspended state of growth until puberty. By the time of prepuberty, the number of oocytes has been reduced to only several hundred thousand.

TABLE 36-4	Potential Radiation Responses of Skin from High-Dose Fluoroscopy	
Potential Radiation Response	**Threshold Dose**	**Approximate Time of Onset**
Early transient erythema	200 rad / 2 Gy$_t$	Hours
Main erythema	600 rad / 6 Gy$_t$	10 d
Temporary epilation	300 rad / 3 Gy$_t$	3 wk
Permanent epilation	700 rad / 7 Gy$_t$	3 wk
Moist desquamation	1800 rad / 18 Gy$_t$	4 wk

Commencing at puberty, the follicles rupture with regularity, ejecting a mature germ cell, the **ovum.** Only 400 to 500 such ova are available for fertilization (number of years of menstruation times 13 per year).

The germ cells of the testes are continually being produced from stem cells progressively through a number of stages to maturity, and like the ovaries, the testes provide a sustaining cell-renewal system.

The male stem cell is the **spermatogonia,** which matures into the **spermatocyte.** The spermatocyte in turn multiplies and develops into a **spermatid,** which finally differentiates into the functionally mature germ cell, the **spermatozoa** or **sperm.** The maturation process from stem cell to spermatozoa requires 3 to 5 weeks.

Ovaries. Irradiation of the ovaries early in life reduces their size (atrophy) by germ cell death. After puberty, such irradiation also causes suppression and delay of menstruation.

 The most radiosensitive cell during female germ cell development is the oocyte in the mature follicle.

Radiation effects on the ovaries depend somewhat on age. At fetal life and early childhood, the ovaries are especially radiosensitive. They decline in sensitivity, reaching a minimum in the age range of 20 to 30 years, and then increase continually with age.

Doses as low as 10 rad (100 mGy$_t$) in the mature female may delay or suppress menstruation. A dose of approximately 200 rad (2 Gy$_t$) produces temporary infertility; approximately 500 rad (5 Gy$_t$) to the ovaries produces permanent sterility.

In addition to the destruction of fertility, irradiation of the ovaries of experimental animals has been shown to produce genetic mutations. Even moderate doses, such as 25 to 50 rad (250 to 500 mGy$_t$), have been associated with measurable increases in genetic mutations. Evidence also indicates that oocytes surviving such a modest dose can repair some genetic damage as they mature into ova.

Testes. The testes, like the ovaries, atrophy after high doses of radiation. Much data on testicular damage have been gathered from observations of volunteer convicts and patients treated for carcinoma in one testis while the other was shielded. Many investigators have recorded normal births to such patients whose remaining functioning testis received a radiation dose between 50 and 300 rad (0.5 and 3 Gy$_t$).

The spermatogonial stem cells are the most sensitive phase in the gametogenesis of the spermatozoa. After irradiation of the testes, the maturing cells, spermatocytes, and spermatids are relatively radioresistant and continue to mature. Consequently, there is no significant reduction in spermatozoa until several weeks after exposure; therefore, fertility continues during this time, during which the irradiated spermatogonia would have developed into mature spermatozoa had they survived.

Radiation doses as low as 10 rad (100 mGy$_t$) can reduce the number of spermatozoa (Table 36-5) in a manner reminiscent of the radiation response of the ovaries. With increasing dose, the depletion of spermatozoa becomes greater and extends over a longer period.

Two hundred rad (2 Gy$_t$) produces temporary infertility, which commences approximately 2 mo following irradiation and persists for up to 12 mo. Five hundred rad (5 Gy$_t$) to the testes produces permanent sterility. Even following doses sufficient to produce permanent sterility, the male normally retains his ability to engage in sexual intercourse.

Male gametogenesis is a self-renewing system; some evidence suggests that the most hazardous mutations are the genetic ones induced in surviving postspermatogonial cells. Consequently, after testicular irradiation of doses exceeding approximately 10 rad (100 mGy$_t$), the male should refrain from procreation for 2 to 4 mo until all cells that were in the spermatogonial and

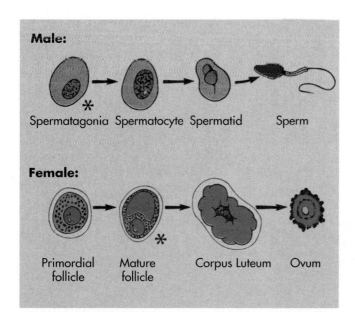

FIGURE 36-5 Progression of germ cells from the stem cell phase to the mature cell. Asterisk indicates the most radiosensitive cell.

TABLE 36-5	Response of Ovaries and Testes to Radiation	
Approximate Dose	**Response**
10 rad / 0.1 Gy$_t$	Minimal detectable
200 rad / 2 Gy$_t$	Temporary infertility
500 rad / 5 Gy$_t$	Sterility

postspermatogonial stages at the time of irradiation have matured and disappeared.

This reduces but probably does not eliminate any increase in genetic mutations because of the persistence of the stem cell. Evidence from animal experiments suggests that genetic mutations undergo some repair even when the stem cell is irradiated.

HEMATOLOGIC EFFECTS

If you were a radiologic technologist in practice during the 1920s and the 1930s, you might have visited the hematology laboratory once a week for a routine blood examination. Before the introduction of personnel radiation monitors, periodic blood examination was the only monitoring performed on x-ray and radium workers. The examination included total cell counts and a white cell (leukocyte) differential count.

Most institutions had a radiation safety regulation such that, if the leukocytes were depressed by greater than 25% of normal level, the employee was either given time off or assigned to nonradiation activities until the count returned to normal.

 Under no circumstances is a periodic blood examination recommended as a feature of any current radiation protection program.

What was not entirely understood at that time was that the minimum whole-body dose necessary to produce a measurable hematologic depression was approximately 25 rad (250 mGy$_t$). These workers were being heavily irradiated by today's standards.

Hemopoietic System

The hemopoietic system consists of bone marrow, circulating blood, and lymphoid tissue. Lymphoid tissues are the lymph nodes, spleen, and thymus. With this system, the principal effect of radiation is a depressed number of blood cells in the peripheral circulation. Time- and dose-related effects on the various types of circulating blood cells are determined by the normal growth and maturation of these cells.

All cells of the hemopoietic system apparently develop from a single type of stem cell (Figure 36-6). This stem cell is called a **pluripotential stem cell** because it can develop into several different types of mature cells.

Although the spleen and thymus manufacture one type of leukocyte (the lymphocyte), most circulating blood cells, including lymphocytes, are manufactured in the bone marrow. In a child, the bone marrow is rather uniformly distributed throughout the skeleton. In an adult, the active bone marrow responsible for producing circulating cells is restricted to flat bones, such as the ribs, sternum, and skull, and the ends of long bones.

From the single pluripotential stem cell, a number of cell types are produced. Principally these are the **lymphocytes** (those involved in the immune response), the **granulocytes** (scavenger type of cells used to fight bacteria), **thrombocytes** (also called platelets and involved in

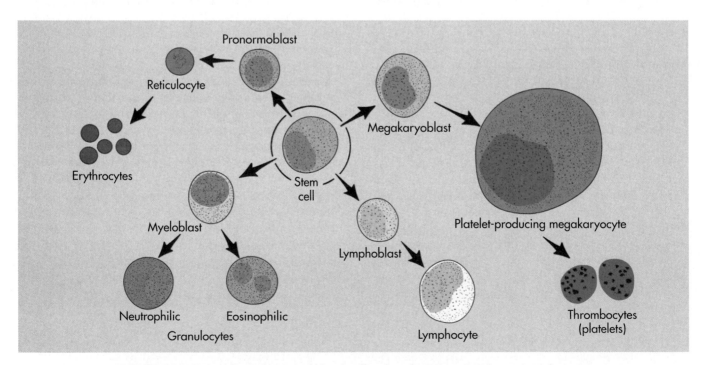

FIGURE 36-6 Four principal types of blood cells – lymphocytes, granulocytes, erythrocytes, and thrombocytes – develop and mature from a single pluripotential stem cell.

the clotting of blood to prevent hemorrhage), and **erythrocytes** (red blood cells that are the transportation agents for oxygen). These cell lines develop at different rates in the bone marrow and are released to the peripheral blood as mature cells.

While in the bone marrow, the cells proliferate in number, differentiate in function, and mature. The developing granulocytes and erythrocytes spend about 8 to 10 days in the bone marrow. Thrombocytes have a lifetime of approximately 5 days in the bone marrow.

Lymphocytes are produced over varying times and have varying lifetimes in the peripheral blood. Some are thought to have lives measured in terms of hours and others in terms of years. In the peripheral blood, the granulocytes have a lifetime of only a couple of days. Thrombocytes have a lifetime of approximately 1 week and erythrocytes a lifetime of nearly 4 months.

The hemopoietic system, therefore, is another example of a cell renewal system. Normal cell growth and development determine the effect of radiation on this system.

Hemopoietic Cell Survival

The principal response of the hemopoietic system to radiation exposure is a decrease in the number of all types of blood cells in the circulating peripheral blood. Lethal injury to the stem cells causes the depletion of these mature circulating cells.

Figure 36-7 shows the radiation response of three circulating cell types. Examples are given for low, moderate, and high radiation doses showing that the degree of cell depletion increases with increasing dose. These fig-

ures are the results of observations on experimental animals, radiotherapy patients, and the few radiation accident victims.

Following exposure, the first cells to become affected are the lymphocytes. These cells are reduced in number (**lymphopenia**) within minutes or hours following exposure, and they are very slow to recover. Because the response is so immediate, the radiation effect is apparently a direct one on the lymphocytes themselves rather than on the stem cells.

The lymphocytes and the spermatogonia are the most radiosensitive cells in the body.

Granulocytes experience a rapid rise in number (granulocytosis), followed first by a rapid decrease and then a slower decrease in number (granulocytopenia). If the radiation dose is moderate, then an abortive rise in granulocyte count may occur 15 to 20 days following irradiation. Minimum granulocyte levels are reached approximately 30 days following irradiation. Recovery, if it is to occur, takes approximately 2 months.

The depletion of platelets (thrombocytopenia) following irradiation develops more slowly, again because of the longer time required for the more sensitive precursor cells to reach maturity. Thrombocytes reach a minimum in about 30 days and recover in approximately 2 months, similar to the response kinetics of granulocytes.

The erythrocytes are less sensitive than the other blood cells, apparently because of their very long life-

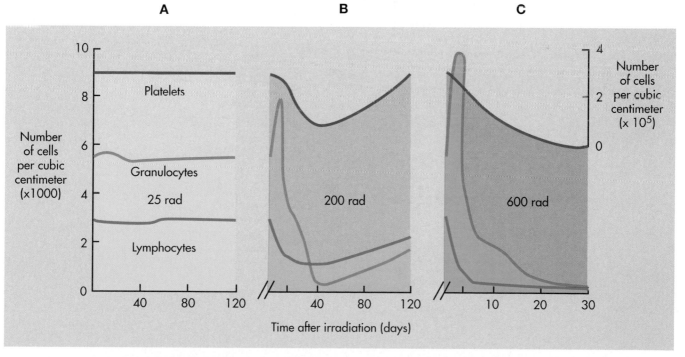

FIGURE 36-7 These graphs show the radiation response of the major circulating blood cells. **A,** 25 rad. **B,** 200 rad. **C,** 600 rad.

time in the peripheral blood. Injury of these cells is not apparent for a matter of weeks. Total recovery may take 6 months to a year.

CYTOGENETIC EFFECTS

A technique developed in the early 1950s contributed enormously to human genetic analysis and radiation genetics. The technique calls for a culture of human cells to be prepared and treated so that the chromosomes of each cell can be easily observed and studied. This has resulted in many observations on radiation-induced chromosome damage.

 Cytogenetics is the study of the genetics of cells, particularly cell chromosomes.

The photomicrograph shown in Figure 36-8 shows the chromosomes of a human cancer cell following radiation therapy. The many chromosome aberrations represent a high degree of damage.

Radiation cytogenetic studies have shown that nearly every type of chromosome aberration can be radiation-induced and that some aberrations may be specific to radiation. The rate of induction of chromosome aberrations is related in a complex way to the radiation dose and differs among the various types of aberrations.

 Radiation-induced chromosome aberrations follow a nonthreshold dose-response relationship.

Attempts to measure chromosome aberrations in patients following diagnostic x-ray examination have been largely unsuccessful. However, some studies involving high-dose fluoroscopy have shown radiation-induced chromosome aberrations soon after the examination.

Without question, high doses of radiation cause chromosome aberrations. Low doses no doubt also do so, but it is technically difficult to observe aberrations at doses that are less than approximately 5 rad (50 mGy$_t$). An even more difficult task is identifying the link between radiation-induced chromosome aberrations and latent illness or disease.

When the body is irradiated, all cells can suffer cytogenetic damage. Such damage is classified here as an early response to radiation because, if the cell survives, the damage manifests during the next mitosis following the radiation exposure.

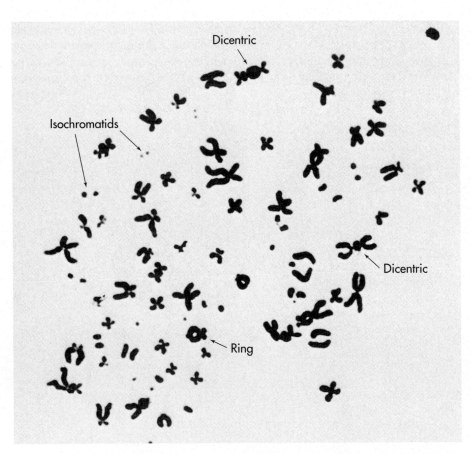

FIGURE 36-8 Chromosome damage in an irradiated human cancer cell. (Courtesy Neil Wald.)

Human peripheral lymphocytes are most often used for cytogenetic analysis, and these lymphocytes do not move into mitosis until stimulated in vitro by an appropriate laboratory technique.

Cytogenetic damage to the stem cells is sustained immediately but may not be manifested for the considerable time required for that stem cell to reach maturity as a circulating lymphocyte.

Although chromosome damage occurs at the time of irradiation, it can be months and even years before the damage is measured. For this reason, chromosome abnormalities in their circulating lymphocytes persist in some workers who were irradiated in industrial accidents 20 years ago.

Normal Karyotype

The human chromosome consists of many long strings of DNA mixed with a protein and folded back on itself many times. See Figure 33-11, which shows a normal chromosome as it would appear in the G_1 phase of the cell cycle, when only two chromatids are present, and in the G_2 phase of the cell cycle following DNA replication. The chromosome structure of four chromatids represented for the G_2 phase is that which is visualized in the metaphase portion of mitosis.

For certain types of cytogenetic analyses of the chromosomes, photographs are taken and enlarged so that each chromosome can be cut out like a paper doll and paired with its sister into a chromosome map, which is called a **karyotype** (Figure 36-9).

Each cell has 22 pairs of autosomes and a pair of sex chromosomes, the X chromosome from the female and the Y chromosome from the male.

Structural radiation damage to individual chromosomes can be visualized without constructing a karyotype. These are the single- and double-hit chromosome aberrations. Reciprocal translocations require a karyotype for detection. Point genetic mutations are undetectable even with karyotype construction.

Single-Hit Chromosome Aberrations

When radiation interacts with chromosomes, the interaction can occur through direct or indirect effect. In either mode, these interactions result in a **hit**. The hit, however, is somewhat different from the hit described previously in radiation interaction with DNA.

The DNA hit results in an invisible disruption of the molecular structure of the DNA. A chromosome hit, on the other hand, produces a visible derangement of the chromosome. Because the chromosomes contain DNA, this indicates that such a hit has disrupted many molecular bonds and severed many chains of DNA.

A chromosome hit represents severe damage to the DNA.

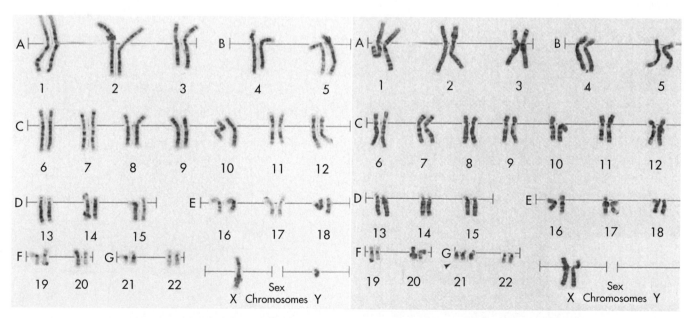

FIGURE 36-9 A photomicrograph of the human cell nucleus at metaphase shows each chromosome distinctly. The karyotype is made by cutting and pasting each chromosome like paper dolls and aligning them largest to smallest. The left karyotype is male, the right female. (Courtesy Carolyn Caskey Goodner.)

Single-hit effects produced by radiation during the G_1 phase of the cell cycle are shown in Figure 36-10. The breakage of a chromatid is called **chromatid deletion.** During S phase, both the remaining chromosome and the deletion are replicated.

The chromosome aberration visualized at metaphase consists of a chromosome with material missing from the ends of two sister chromatids and two acentric (without a centromere) fragments. These fragments are called **isochromatids.**

Chromosome aberrations can also be produced by single-hit events during the G_2 phase of the cell cycle (see Figure 36-10). The probability that ionizing radiation will pass through sister chromatids to produce isochromatids is low. Usually the radiation produces a chromatid deletion in only one arm of the chromosome. The result is a chromosome with an arm that is obviously missing genetic material and a chromatid fragment.

Multi-Hit Chromosome Aberrations

A single chromosome can sustain more than one hit. Multi-hit aberrations are not uncommon (Figure 36-11).

In the G_1 phase of the cell cycle, ring chromosomes are produced if the two hits occur on the same chromosome. Dicentrics are produced when adjacent chromosomes each suffer one hit and recombine. The mechanism for the joining of chromatids depends on a condition called **stickiness** that is radiation-induced and appears at the site of the severed chromosome.

Similar aberrations can be produced in the G_2 phase of the cell cycle; however, such aberrations again require that (1) either the same chromosome be hit two or more times or (2) adjacent chromosomes be hit and joined together. However, these are rare.

Reciprocal Translocations. The multi-hit chromosome aberrations previously described represent rather severe damage to the cell. At mitosis, the acentric fragments are either lost or attracted to only one of the daughter cells because they are unattached to a spindle fiber. Consequently, one or both of the daughter cells can be missing considerable genetic material.

Reciprocal translocations are multi-hit chromosome aberrations that require karyotypic analysis for detection (Figure 36-12). Radiation-induced reciprocal translocations result in no loss of genetic material, simply a rearrangement of the genes. Consequently, all or nearly all genetic codes are available; they simply may be organized in an incorrect sequence.

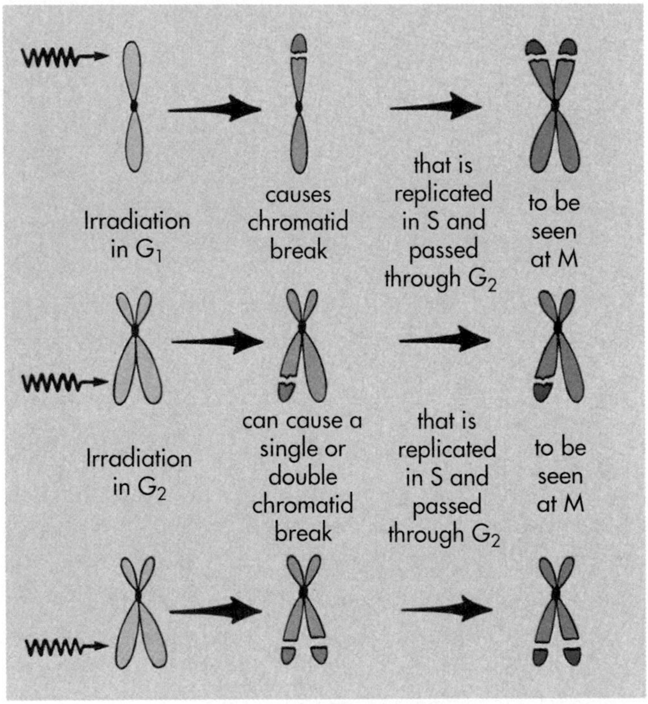

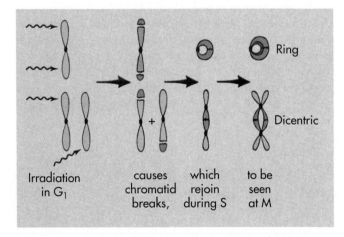

FIGURE 36-11 Multi-hit chromosome aberrations after irradiation in G_1 result in ring and dicentic chromosomes in addition to chromatid fragments. Similar aberrations can be produced by irradiation during G_2 but they are rarer.

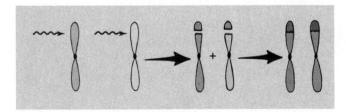

FIGURE 36-12 Radiation-induced reciprocal translocations are multi-hit chromosome aberrations that require karyotypic analysis for detection.

FIGURE 36-10 Single-hit chromosome aberrations after irradiation in G_1 and G_2. The aberrations are visualized and recorded during the M phase.

Kinetics of Chromosome Aberration

At very low doses of radiation, only single-hit aberrations occur. When the radiation dose exceeds approximately 100 rad (1 Gy$_t$), the frequency of multi-hit aberrations increases more rapidly.

The general dose-response relationship for production of single- and multi-hit aberrations is shown in Figure 36-13. Single-hit aberrations are produced with a **linear, nonthreshold** dose-response relationship. Multi-hit aberrations are produced following a **nonlinear, nonthreshold** relationship. A number of investigators have experimentally determined these relationships.

RADIATION DOSE-RESPONSE RELATIONSHIPS FOR CYTOGENETIC DAMAGE

Single-Hit: $Y = a + bD$

Multi-Hit: $Y = a + bD + cD^2$

where Y is the number of single- or multi-hit chromosome aberrations, a is the naturally occurring frequency of chromosome aberrations, and b and c are radiation dose (D) coefficients of damage for single- and multi-hit aberrations, respectively

Some laboratories use cytogenetic analysis as a biologic radiation dosimeter. The multi-hit aberrations are considered to be the most significant in terms of latent human damage. If the radiation dose is unknown yet not life-threatening, the approximate chromosome aberration frequency is two single-hit aberrations per rad per 1000 cells and one multi-hit aberration per 10 rad per 1000 cells.

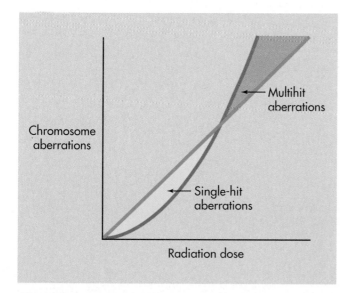

FIGURE 36-13 Dose-response relationships for single-hit aberrations is linear, nonthreshold, whereas that for multi-hit aberrations is nonlinear, nonthreshold.

SUMMARY

After exposure to a high radiation dose, humans can experience a response within a few days to a few weeks. This immediate response is called an early effect of radiation exposure. Such early effects are usually deterministic—the severity of response is dose-related and there is no dose threshold.

The sequence of events following high-dose radiation exposure leading to death within days or weeks is called the acute radiation syndrome, which includes the hematologic syndrome, GI syndrome, and CNS syndrome. The syndromes are dose-related.

LD$_{50/60}$ is the dose of radiation to the whole body in which 50% of the subjects will die within 60 days. For humans, this dose is estimated at 350 rad. As radiation dose increases, the time between exposure and death decreases.

When only part of the body is irradiated, higher doses are tolerated. Examples of local tissue damage are effects on the skin, gonads, and bone marrow. The first manifestation of radiation injury to the skin is damage to the basal cells. Resulting skin damage is erythema, desquamation, or epilation.

Radiation of the male testes can result in a reduction of spermatozoa. A dose of 200 rad produces temporary infertility. A dose of 500 rad to the testes produces permanent sterility. In the male as in the female, the stem cell is the most radiosensitive phase.

The hemopoietic system consists of bone marrow, circulating blood, and lymphoid tissue. The principal effect of radiation on this system is fewer blood cells in the peripheral circulation. Radiation exposure decreases the number of all precursor cells, which reduces the number of mature cells in the circulating blood. Lymphocytes and spermatogonia are considered the most radiosensitive cells in the body.

The study of chromosome damage from radiation exposure is called cytogenetics. Chromosome damage takes on the following different forms: (1) chromatid deletion, (2) dicentric chromosome aberration, and (3) reciprocal translocations.

CHALLENGE QUESTIONS

1. Define or otherwise identify:
   a. GI death
   b. Latent period
   c. LD$_{50/30}$
   d. Erythema
   e. Clinical tolerance
   f. Primordial follicle
   g. Erythrocyte
   h. Karyotype
   i. Epilation
   j. Multi-hit aberration

2. What is the minimum dose that results in reddening of the skin?

3. Explain the prodromal syndrome.

4. The clinical signs and symptoms of the manifest illness stage of acute radiation lethality are classified into what three groups?

5. During which stage of the acute radiation syndrome is recovery stimulated?

6. What dose of radiation results in the gastrointestinal syndrome?

7. Why does death occur with the GI syndrome?

8. Identify the cause of death from the CNS syndrome.

9. Describe the stages of gametogenesis in the female. Identify the most radiosensitive phases.

10. What cells arise from pluripotential stem cells?

11. Discuss the maturation of basal cells in the epidermis.

12. What two cells are the most radiosensitive cells in the human body?

13. Describe the changes in mean survival time with increasing dose.

14. What are the approximate values of $LD_{50/60}$ and SED_{50} in humans?

15. What are the four principal blood cell lines and the function of each?

16. Diagram the mechanism for the production of a reciprocal translocation.

17. List the clinical signs and symptoms of the hematologic syndrome.

18. What mature cells form from the pluripotential stem cell?

19. If the normal incidence of singe hit-type chromosome aberrations is 0.15 per 100 cells and the dose coefficient is 0.0094, how many such aberrations would be expected following a dose of 38 rad?

20. If the normal incidence of multi-hit chromosome aberrations is 0.082 and the dose coefficient is 0.0047, how many dicentrics per 100 cells would be expected following a whole-body dose of 16 rad?

Late Effects of Radiation

OBJECTIVES

At the completion of this chapter, the student should be able to do the following:

1. Define late effects of radiation exposure
2. Identify the radiation dose needed to produce late effects
3. Discuss the results of epidemiologic studies of persons exposed to radiation
4. List the local tissue effects of low-dose radiation to various types of organs
5. Explain the estimates of radiation risk
6. Analyze radiation-induced leukemia and cancer
7. Review the risks of low dose radiation to fertility and pregnancy

OUTLINE

ARLY EFFECTS of radiation exposure are produced by high radiation doses. Late effects of radiation exposure are the result of low doses delivered over a long time period.

The radiation exposures experienced by personnel in diagnostic imaging are low dose and low linear energy transfer (LET). In addition, the exposures in diagnostic imaging are delivered intermittently over long periods.

The principal late effects of low-dose radiation over long periods are radiation-induced malignancy and genetic effects. Life span shortening and effects on local tissues have also been reported as late effects, but these are not considered significant. Radiation protection guides are based on the suspected or observed late effects of radiation and on an assumed linear, nonthreshold dose–response relationship.

This chapter reviews these late effects and introduces the subject of risk estimation. Radiation effects during pregnancy are of considerable importance in diagnostic x-ray imaging, and such effects are discussed here.

The radiation exposures that we experience in diagnostic radiology are low and of low LET, and are chronic in nature because they are delivered intermittently over long periods of time. Therefore, late radiation effects are of particular importance.

The principal late effects are radiation-induced malignancy and genetic effect. Most late effects are also known as **stochastic** effects. Stochastic effects of radiation exposure exhibit an increasing incidence of response—not severity—with increasing dose. There is no dose threshold for a stochastic response.

> Our radiation protection guides are based on the late effects of radiation and on linear, nonthreshold dose–response relationships.

Studies of large numbers of people exposed to a toxic substance require considerable statistical analyses. Such studies are called **epidemiologic studies** and they are required when the number of persons affected is small.

Epidemiologic studies of people exposed to radiation are difficult because (1) the dose is usually not known

TABLE 37-1	Minimum Population Sample Required to Show That the Given Radiation Dose Significantly Elevated the Incidence of Leukemia
Dose	**Required Sample Size (No. of People)**
5 rad (0.05 Gy$_t$)	6,000,000
10 rad (0.1 Gy$_t$)	1,600,000
15 rad (0.15 Gy$_t$)	750,000
20 rad (0.2 Gy$_t$)	500,000
50 rad (0.5 Gy$_t$)	100,000

but presumed to be low, and (2) the frequency of response is very low. Consequently, the results of radiation epidemiologic studies do not carry the statistical accuracy that observations of early radiation effects do.

Table 37-1 illustrates the difficulty of the problem. It shows the minimum number of persons that must be observed as a function of radiation dose definitely to link an increase in the incidence of leukemia with the radiation dose in question.

LOCAL TISSUE EFFECTS
Skin

In addition to the early effects of erythema and desquamation and late-developing carcinoma, chronic irradiation of the skin can result in severe nonmalignant changes. Early radiologists who performed fluoroscopic examinations without protective gloves developed a very callused, discolored, and weathered appearance to the skin of their hands and forearms. In addition, the skin would be very tight and brittle and sometimes severely crack or flake.

This late effect was observed many years ago in radiologists and is called **radiodermatitis**. The dose necessary to produce such an effect is very high. No such effects occur in the current practice of radiology.

Chromosomes

Irradiation of blood-forming organs can produce hematologic depression as an early response or leukemia as a late response. Chromosome damage in the circulating lymphocytes can be produced as both an early and a late response.

The types and frequency of chromosome aberrations have been described previously; however, even a low dose of radiation can produce chromosome aberrations that may not be apparent until many years after the radiation exposure. For example, individuals irradiated accidentally with rather high radiation doses continue to show chromosome abnormalities in their peripheral lymphocytes for as long as 20 years.

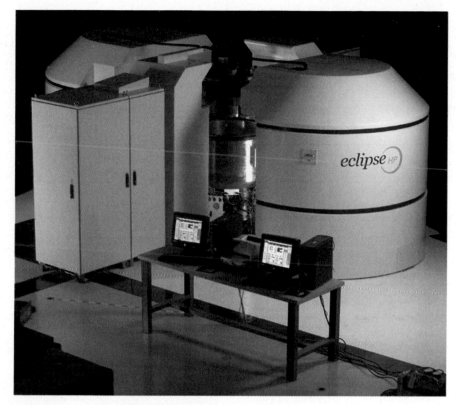

FIGURE 37-1 Cyclotron used to produce radionuclides for nuclear medicine. (Courtesy CTI, Molecular Imaging, Inc.)

This late effect presumably occurs because of radiation damage to the lymphocytic stem cells. These cells may not be stimulated into replication and maturation for many years.

Cataracts

In 1932, E. O. Lawrence of the University of California developed the first **cyclotron**, a 5-inch-diameter machine capable of accelerating charged particles to very high energies. These charged particles are used as "bullets" that are shot at the nuclei of target atoms in the study of nuclear structure. By 1940, every university physics department of any worth had built its own cyclotron and was engaged in what has become high-energy physics.

The modern cyclotron is used principally to produce radionuclides for use in nuclear medicine (Figure 37-1), especially fluorine-18 for positron emission tomography (PET). The largest particle accelerators in the world are located at Argonne National Laboratory in the United States and at CERN in Switzerland. These accelerators are used to discover the ultimate fine structure of matter and to describe exactly what happened at the moment of the creation of the universe.

Early cyclotrons were located in one room and a beam of high-energy particles was extracted through a tube and steered and focused by electromagnets onto the target material in the adjacent room. At that time,

sophisticated electronic equipment was not available for controlling this high-energy beam.

The cyclotron physicists used a tool of the radiologist, the fluorescent screen, to aid in locating the high-energy beam. Unfortunately, in so doing, these physicists would receive high radiation doses to the lens of the eye because they had to look directly into the beam.

In 1949, the first paper reporting cataracts in cyclotron physicists appeared. By 1960, several hundred such cases of radiation-induced cataracts had been reported. This was particularly tragic because there were few high-energy physicists.

 Radiation-induced cataracts occur on the posterior pole of the lens.

On the basis of these observations and animal experimentation, several conclusions can be drawn regarding radiation-induced cataracts. The radiosensitivity of the lens of the eye is age dependent. The older the individual, the greater the radiation effect and the shorter the latent period. Latent periods varying from 5 to 30 years have been observed in humans, and the average latent period is approximately 15 years. High-LET radiation, such as neutron and proton radiation, has a high relative biologic effectiveness (RBE) for the production of cataracts.

The dose–response relationship for radiation-induced cataracts is nonlinear, threshold.

If the lens dose is high enough, in excess of approximately 1000 rad (10 Gy$_t$), cataracts develop in nearly 100% of those who are irradiated. The precise level of the threshold dose is difficult to assess.

Most investigators would suggest that the threshold after an acute x-ray exposure is approximately 200 rad (2 Gy$_t$). The threshold after fractionated exposure, such as that we receive in radiology, is probably in excess of 1000 rad (10 Gy$_t$).

Occupational exposures to the lens of the eye are too low to require protective lens shields for radiologic technologists. It is nearly impossible for a medical radiation worker to reach the threshold dose.

Radiation administered to patients undergoing head and neck examination by either fluoroscopy or computed tomography can be significant. In computed tomography, the lens dose can be 5 rad per slice. In this situation, however, usually no more than one or two slices intersect the lens. In either case, protective lens shields are not normally required. However, in computed tomography it is common to modify the examination to reduce the dose to the eyes.

LIFE SPAN SHORTENING

There have been many experiments conducted with animals after both acute and chronic exposure that show that irradiated animals die young. Figure 37-2 is redrawn from several such representative experiments and shows that the relationship between life span shortening and dose is apparently linear, nonthreshold. When all the animal data are considered collectively, it is difficult to attempt a meaningful extrapolation to humans.

 At worst, humans can expect a reduced life span of approximately 10 days for every rad.

The data presented in Table 37-2 were compiled by Cohen of the University of Pittsburgh and extrapolated from various statistical sources of mortality. The expected loss of life in days is given as a function of occupation, disease, or other condition.

As one can see, the most grievous risk is being male rather than female. Whereas the average life shortening caused by occupational accidents is 74 days, that for radiation workers is only 12 days.

 Radiologic technology is a safe occupation.

Radiation-induced life span shortening is nonspecific— that is, there are no characteristic diseases associated

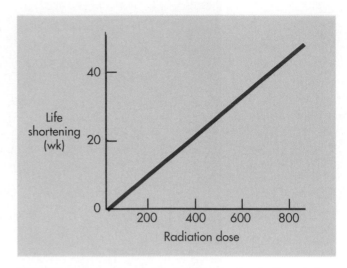

FIGURE 37-2 In chronically irradiated animals, the relationship between extent of life shortening and dose appears linear, nonthreshold. This graph shows the representative results of several such experiments with mice.

TABLE 37-2	Risk of Life Span Shortening as a Consequence of Occupation, Disease, or Various Other Conditions
Risky Condition	**Expected Days of Life Lost**
Being male rather than female	2800
Heart disease	2100
Being unmarried	2000
One pack of cigarettes a day	1600
Working as a coal miner	1100
Cancer	980
30 pounds overweight	900
Stroke	520
All accidents	435
Service in Vietnam	400
Motor vehicle accidents	200
Average occupational accidents	74
Speed limit increase from 55 to 65 mph	40
Radiation worker	12
Airplane crashes	1

with it and it does not include late malignant effects. It is simply accelerated premature aging and death.

One investigator has evaluated the death records of radiologic technologists who operated field x-ray equipment during World War II. These imaging systems were poorly designed and inadequately shielded so that the technologists received higher-than-normal exposures. Seven thousand such technologists have been studied, and no radiation effects have been observed.

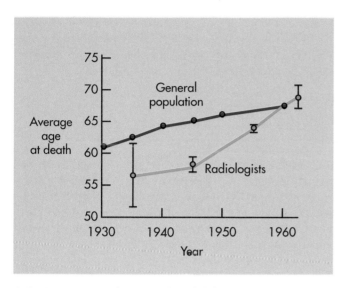

FIGURE 37-3 Radiation-induced life span shortening is shown for American radiologists. The age at death in the radiologists was less than that of the general population, but this difference has disappeared.

TABLE 37-3	Death Statistics for Three Groups of Physicians	
Died During	**Median Age at Death**	**Age-Adjusted Deaths per 1000**
1935 to 1944		
RSNA	71.4	18.4
ACP	73.4	15.4
AAOO	76.2	13.0
1945 to 1954		
RSNA	72.0	16.4
ACP	74.8	13.7
AAOO	76.0	11.9
1955 to 1958		
RSNA	73.5	13.6
ACP	76.0	11.4
AAOO	76.4	10.6

ACP, American College of Physicians; *AAOO*, American Academy of Ophthalmology and Otolaryngology; *RSNA*, Radiological Society of North America.

An investigation of health effects from radiation exposure of American radiologic technologists is currently underway. This is a mail survey covering many work-related conditions of approximately 150,000 subjects, which will take many years to complete. Early reports show no effects.

Observations on human populations have not been totally convincing. No life span shortening has been observed in the atomic bomb survivors, and some received rather substantial radiation doses. Life span shortening in radium watch-dial painters, x-ray patients, and other human radiation-exposed populations has not been reported.

American radiologists are one population that has been fairly extensively studied, and early radiologists appeared to have reduced life span. Such a study has many shortcomings, not the least of which is its retrospective nature. Figure 37-3 shows the results obtained when the age at death for radiologists was compared with the age at death for the general population. Radiologists dying in the early 1930s were approximately 5 years younger than the average age at death of the general population. However, this difference in age at death had shrunk to zero by 1965.

A more thorough study used two other physician groups as controls rather than the general population. Table 37-3 summarizes the results of this investigation. The physician groups observed in this study were members of the Radiological Society of North America (RSNA) as the high-risk group and members of the American Academy of Ophthalmology and Otolaryngology (AAOO) as the low-risk group. Members of the American College of Physicians (ACP) represented an intermediate-risk group.

A comparison of the median age at death and age-adjusted death rates for these physician specialties demonstrates a significant difference in age at death during the early years of radiology.

RISK ESTIMATES

The early effects of high-dose radiation exposure are usually easy to observe and measure. The late effects are also easy to observe, but it is nearly impossible to associate a particular late response with a previous radiation exposure.

Consequently, precise dose–response relationships are often not possible to formulate, and we therefore resort to **risk estimates**. There are three types of risk estimates—relative, excess, and absolute risk—and they each represent different statements of risk and have different dimensions.

Relative Risk

If one observes a large population for late radiation effects without having any precise knowledge of the radiation dose to which they were exposed, then the concept of **relative risk** is used. The relative risk is computed by comparing the number of persons in the exposed population showing a given late effect with the number who show the same late effect in an unexposed population.

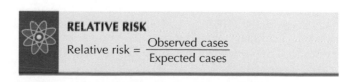

RELATIVE RISK

$$\text{Relative risk} = \frac{\text{Observed cases}}{\text{Expected cases}}$$

A relative risk of 1.0 indicates no risk at all. A relative risk of 1.5 indicates that the frequency of a late response is 50% higher in the irradiated population compared with the nonirradiated population.

Relative risk for radiation-induced late effects of particular importance observed in human populations are in the range of 1 to 2.

Occasionally, an investigation results in the identification of a relative risk of less than 1. This would indicate that the exposed population receives some protective benefit, which is consistent with the theory of radiation hormesis. However, the usual interpretation of such studies is that the results are not statistically significant, either because of the small number of observations or because of inadequate identification of irradiated and control populations.

> The theory of radiation hormesis suggests that very low radiation doses are beneficial.

There is some evidence to support the principle of **radiation hormesis**. Radiation hormesis suggest that low levels of radiation, less than approximately 10 rad (100 mGy$_t$), are good for you! Such low doses may provide a protective effect by stimulating molecular repair and immunologic response mechanisms. Nevertheless, radiation hormesis remains a theory at this time, and until it is proven, we will continue to practice ALARA—as low as reasonably achievable.

An example of a reported dose–response relationship indicating radiation hormesis was shown in Figure 34-7. The low-dose region where the relative risk is less than 1 is the hormetic region. The crossover at a relative risk of 1 is usually in the 5- to 20-rad (50- to 200-mGy$_t$) range.

Question: In a study of radiation-induced leukemia after diagnostic levels of radiation, 227 cases were observed in 100,000 persons so irradiated. The normal incidence of leukemia in the United States is 150 cases per 100,000. Based on these data, what is the relative risk of radiation-induced leukemia?

Answer: $\text{Relative risk} = \dfrac{\text{Observed cases}}{\text{Expected cases}}$

$$\dfrac{227}{100,000} \div \dfrac{150}{100,000} = \dfrac{0.00227}{0.00150} = 1.51$$

Excess Risk

Often, when an investigation of human radiation response indicates the induction of some late effect, the magnitude of the effect is reflected by the excess cases induced. Leukemia, for instance, is known to occur spontaneously in nonirradiated populations. If the leukemia incidence in an irradiated population exceeds that which is expected, then the difference between the observed number of cases and the expected number would be excess risk.

EXCESS RISK
Excess risk = Observed cases − Expected cases

The excess cases in this instance are assumed to be radiation induced. To determine the number of excess cases, one must be able to measure the observed number of cases in the irradiated population and compare them with the number that would have been expected on the basis of known population levels.

Question: Twenty-three cases of skin cancer were observed in a population of 1000 radiologists. The incidence in the general population is 0.5/100,000. How many excess skin cancers were produced in the population of radiologists?

Answer: Excess cases = Observed cases − Expected cases

$$= \dfrac{23}{1000} - \dfrac{0.5}{100,000}$$

$$= \dfrac{23}{1000} - \dfrac{0.005}{1000}$$

$$\simeq 23$$

Because none would be expected, all 23 cases represent radiation risk.

Absolute Risk

If at least two different dose levels are known, then it may be possible to determine an absolute risk factor. Unlike the relative risk, which is a dimensionless ratio, the absolute risk has units of number of cases/10⁶ persons/ rad/yr. Absolute risk of radiation-induced malignant disease is approximately 10 cases/10⁶ persons/rad/yr. This value is a considerable simplification of the results of many studies.

To determine the absolute radiation risk, one must assume a linear dose–response relationship. If the dose–response relationship is assumed to be nonthreshold, then only one dose level is required. The value of the absolute radiation risk is equal to the slope of the dose–response relationship (Figure 37-4). The error bars on each data point indicate the precision of the observation of response.

Question: The absolute risk for radiation-induced breast cancer is approximately 6 cases/10⁶ persons/rad/yr for a 20-year at-risk period. If 100,000 women receive 100 mrad during

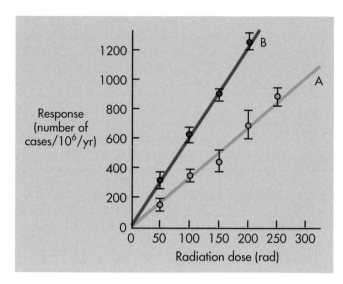

FIGURE 37-4 Slope of the linear, nonthreshold dose–response relationship is equal to the absolute risk. *A* and *B* show absolute risks of 3.4 and 6.2 cases per 10^6 persons/rad/year, respectively.

TABLE 37-4	Summary of the Incidence of Leukemia in Atomic Bomb Survivors		
	Hiroshima	**Nagasaki**	**Total**
Total number of survivors in study	74,356	25,037	99,393
Observed cases of leukemia	102	42	144
Expected cases of leukemia	39	13	52

mammography, how many cancers would be expected to be induced?

Answer: (6 cases/106 persons/rad/yr) (10^5 persons) (0.1 rad) (20 years) = 1.2 cases

Question: There are approximately 300,000 American radiologic technologists and they receive an annual effective dose of 10 mrem. What is the expected number of annual deaths because of this occupational exposure?

Answer: (10 cases/10^6 persons/rad/yr) (0.3 × 10^6) (0.01 rad) = (10 cases) (0.003) = 0.03 cases/yr

The reader should realize that death from malignant disease occurs in approximately 20% of the population.

RADIATION-INDUCED MALIGNANCY

All the late effects, including radiation-induced malignancy, have been observed in experimental animals, and from these animal experiments dose–response relationships have been developed. At the human level, these late effects have been observed, but often there are insufficient data precisely to identify the dose–response relationship. Consequently, some of the conclusions drawn regarding human responses are based in part on animal data.

Leukemia

When one considers radiation-induced leukemia in laboratory animals, there is no question that this response is real and that the incidence increases with increasing

radiation dose. The form of the dose–response relationship is apparently linear and nonthreshold. A number of human population groups have exhibited an elevated incidence of leukemia after radiation exposure: atomic bomb survivors, American radiologists, radiotherapy patients, and children irradiated in utero, to name a few.

Atomic Bomb Survivors. Probably the greatest wealth of information that we have on radiation-induced leukemia in humans results from observations of the survivors of the atomic bombings of Hiroshima and Nagasaki. At the time of the bombing, approximately 300,000 people lived in those two cities. Nearly 100,000 were killed from the blast and early effects of radiation. Another 100,000 people received significant doses of radiation and survived. The remainder were unaffected because their radiation dose was less than 10 rad (100 mGy$_t$).

After World War II, scientists of the Atomic Bomb Casualty Commission (**ABCC**), now known as the Radiation Effects Research Foundation (**RERF**), attempted to determine the radiation dose received by each of the atomic bomb survivors in both cities. They estimated the dose to each survivor by considering not only distance from the explosion but also terrain, type of bomb, type of building construction if the survivor was inside, and other factors that might influence dose.

A summary of the data obtained by these investigations is given in Table 37-4, and the data analysis is shown graphically in Figure 37-5. After the high doses delivered by the bombs, the leukemia incidence is as much as 100 times that in the nonirradiated population. Even though there are large error bars at each dose increment, the response appears linear, nonthreshold.

If, however, one expands the data in the low-dose region (e.g., below 200 rad), one could conclude that a threshold exists in the neighborhood of 50 rad. Nevertheless, neither this information nor other available information is interpreted to support a threshold response.

 Radiation-induced leukemia follows a linear, nonthreshold dose–response relationship.

Figure 37-6 demonstrates the temporal distribution of the onset of leukemia in the atomic bomb survivors for the 40 years after the bombings. The data are presented as cases per 100,000 and include for comparison the leukemia rate in the population at large and in the nonexposed populations of the bombed cities. There was a rather rapid rise in leukemia incidence that reached a plateau after approximately 5 years. The incidence declined slowly for approximately 20 years, when it reached the natural level experienced by the nonexposed.

 Radiation-induced leukemia is considered to have a latent period of 4 to 7 years and an at-risk period of approximately 20 years.

The at-risk period is that time after irradiation during which one might expect the radiation effect to occur. The at-risk period for radiation-induced cancer is lifetime.

The data from the atomic bomb survivors show without a doubt that the radiation exposure to those survivors caused the later development of leukemia. It is interesting, however, to reflect on some additional aspects of these events.

Of the 300,000 total resident population, 335 persons are estimated to have survived doses in excess of 600 rad. The leukemia risk estimates are based on only 144 cases in the total exposed population. Acute leukemia and chronic myelocytic leukemia were observed most often in the atomic bomb survivors.

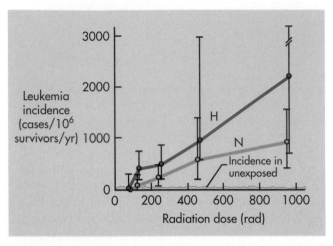

FIGURE 37-5 Data from the atomic bomb survivors of Hiroshima (H) and Nagasaki (N) suggest a linear, nonthreshold dose–response relationship.

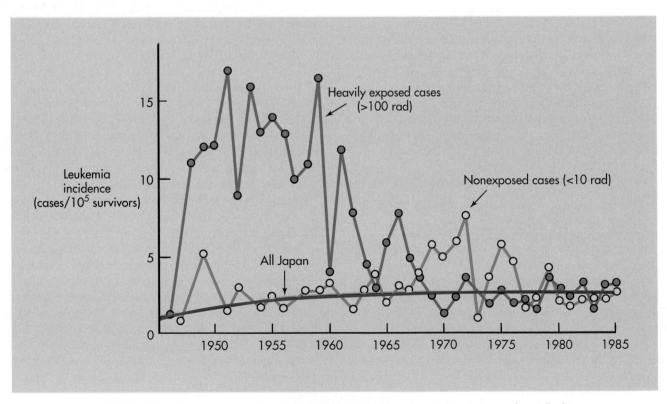

FIGURE 37-6 The incidence of leukemia in the atomic bomb survivors increased rapidly for the first few years, then declined to natural incidence by approximately 1975.

Chronic lymphocytic leukemia is rare, and therefore, not considered to be a form of radiation-induced leukemia.

Taken to the final analysis, the data from the atomic bomb survivors pointed to an absolute risk of 1.5 cases/10⁶ persons/rad/yr. The overall relative risk based on the total number of observed leukemia deaths (144) versus the number of expected leukemia deaths (52) is approximately 3:1.

Radiologists. By the second decade of radiology, reports of pernicious anemia and leukemia in radiologists began to appear. In the early 1940s, several investigators had reviewed the incidence of leukemia in American radiologists and found it alarmingly high. These early radiologists functioned without the benefit of modern radiation protection devices and procedures, and many served as both radiation oncologists and diagnostic radiologists.

It has been estimated that some of these early radiologists received doses exceeding 100 rad/yr (1 Gy,/yr). Currently, American radiologists do not exhibit an elevated incidence of leukemia compared with other physician specialists.

A rather exhaustive study of mortality in radiologists in Great Britain covering the period from the turn of the century to 1960 did not show such an elevated risk of leukemia. The reasons for such a different experience between American and British radiologists are unknown. Some suggest that it is because radiation therapy procedures in Great Britain have always been attended by medical physicists, who presumably were conscious of radiation safety.

Studies of radiation-induced leukemia in American radiologic technologists consistently show no evidence of any radiation effect.

Ankylosing Spondylitis Patients. In the 1940s and 1950s, particularly in Great Britain, it was common practice to treat patients with ankylosing spondylitis with radiation. Ankylosing spondylitis is an arthritis-like condition of the vertebral column.

Such patients cannot walk upright or move except with great difficulty. For relief, they would be given fairly high doses of radiation to the spinal column, and the treatment was quite successful. Patients who previously had to walk hunched over were able to stand erect.

Radiation therapy was a permanent cure and remained the treatment of choice for approximately 20 years, until it was discovered that some who had been cured by radiation were dying from leukemia. The graphic results on the observations of these patients are shown in Figure 37-7.

During the period from 1935 to 1955, 14,554 male patients were treated at 81 different radiation therapy centers in Great Britain. Review of the treatment records showed the dose to the bone marrow of the spinal column ranged from 100 to 4000 rad (1 to 40 Gy).

Fifty-two cases of leukemia occurred in this population. When this incidence of leukemia is compared with that of the general population, the relative risk is 10:1.

The absolute risk can be obtained from these data by determining the slope of the best-fit line through the data points (Figure 37-8). Such an analysis gives a result of approximately 0.8 cases/10⁶ persons/rad/yr. If 95%

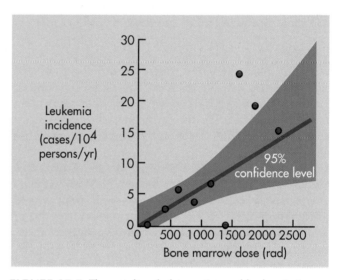

FIGURE 37-7 The results of observations of leukemia in patients with ankylosing spondylitis treated with x-ray therapy suggest a linear, nonthreshold dose–response relationship.

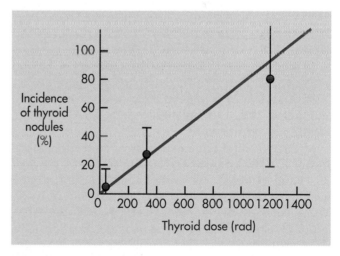

FIGURE 37-8 Radiation-induced preneoplastic thyroid nodularity in three groups of persons whose thyroid glands were irradiated in childhood follows a linear, nonthreshold dose–response relationship.

confidence limits are placed on the data, one could not rule out the possibility of a threshold dose at approximately 300 rad.

Leukemia in Other Populations. There have been a number of studies designed to link leukemia incidence with environmental radiation. Natural background radiation levels increase in general with altitude and with latitude, but the range of levels observed is not sufficient to demonstrate a causal relationship with leukemia.

Other population groups that have provided evidence, both positive and negative, regarding the leukemia-inducing action of radiation are radium watch-dial painters, children receiving superficial x-ray treatment, and some additional adult radiation therapy groups.

Cancer

What has been discussed regarding radiation-induced leukemia also can be reported for radiation-induced cancer. We do not have quite as much human data concerning cancer as for leukemia. Nevertheless, it can be said without question that radiation can cause cancer.

The relative risks and absolute risks are shown to be similar to those reported for leukemia. Many types of cancer have been implicated as radiation induced, and a discussion of the more important ones is in order.

It is not possible to link any case of cancer to a previous radiation exposure, regardless of its magnitude, because cancer is so common. Approximately 20% of all deaths are caused by cancer; therefore, any radiation-induced cancers are obscured. Leukemia, on the other hand, is a relatively rare disease, which makes analysis of radiation-induced leukemia easier.

Thyroid Cancer. Thyroid cancer has developed in three groups of patients whose thyroid glands were irradiated in childhood. The first two groups, called the Ann Arbor series and the Rochester series, consist of individuals who, in the 1940s and early 1950s, were treated shortly after birth for thymic enlargement. The thymus is a gland lying just below the thyroid gland that can enlarge shortly after birth in response to infection.

At these facilities, radiation was often the treatment of choice. After a dose of up to 500 rad (5 Gy$_t$), the thymus gland would shrink so that all enlargement disappeared. No further problems were evident until up to 20 years later, when thyroid nodules and thyroid cancer began to develop in some of these patients.

Another group included 21 children who were natives of the Rongelap Atoll in 1954; they were subjected to high levels of fallout during a hydrogen bomb test. The winds shifted during the test, carrying the fallout over an adjacent inhabited island rather than one that had been evacuated. These children received radiation doses to the thyroid gland from both external exposure and internal ingestion of approximately 1200 rad (12 Gy$_t$).

If one computes the incidence of thyroid nodularity, considered **preneoplastic**, in these three groups and plots this incidence as a function of estimated dose, the result is that shown in Figure 37-8. Admittedly, the error bars on both the dose data and the incidence levels are large. Still, the implication of a linear, nonthreshold dose–response relationship is clear.

Data are just now becoming available on the nearly 100,000 persons exposed to radiation from the 1989 Chernobyl incident. No excess leukemia or cancer has been observed in this population. There is a small increase in thyroid nodularity.

Bone Cancer. Two population groups have contributed an enormous amount of data showing that radiation can cause bone cancer. The first group consists of the radium watch-dial painters.

In the 1920s and 1930s, there were various small laboratories whose employees, mostly female, worked at benches painting watch dials with paint laden with radium sulfate. To prepare a fine point on the paintbrushes, the employees would touch the tip of the brush to the tongue. In this manner, substantial quantities of radium were ingested.

Radium salts were used because the emitted radiation, principally alpha and beta particles, would continuously excite the luminous compounds so the watch dial would glow in the dark. Current technology uses harmlessly low levels of tritium (^{3}H) and promethium (^{147}Pm) for this purpose.

When ingested, the radium would behave metabolically like calcium and deposit in bone. Because of radium's long half-life (1620 years) and alpha emission, these employees received radiation doses up to 50,000 rad (500 Gy$_t$) to bone.

Seventy-two bone cancers in approximately 800 persons have been observed during a follow-up period in excess of 50 years. Analysis of these data has disclosed an overall relative risk of 122:1. The absolute risk is equal to 0.11 cases/10^6 persons/rad/yr.

Another population in whom excess bone cancer developed is patients treated with radium salts for a variety of diseases, from arthritis to tuberculosis. Such treatments were common practice in many parts of the world until about 1950.

Skin Cancer. Skin cancer usually begins with the development of a radiodermatitis. Significant data have been developed from several reports of skin cancer induced in radiation therapy recipients treated with orthovoltage (200 to 300 kVp) or superficial x-rays (50 to 150 kVp).

Radiation-induced skin cancer follows a threshold dose–response relationship.

From these data, we conclude that the latent period is approximately 5 to 10 years, but we do not have enough data to assign absolute risk values. When the dose delivered to the skin was in the range of 500 to 2000 rad (5 to 20 Gy_t), the relative risk of developing skin cancer was 4:1. If the dose was 4000 to 6000 rad (40 to 60 Gy_t) or 6000 to 10,000 rad (60 to 100 Gy_t), the relative risks were 14:1 and 27:1, respectively.

Breast Cancer. In Chapter 22, some of the radiographic techniques used in mammography were discussed. The radiation dose to mammography patients is considered in a later chapter. Here, we discuss the risk of radiation-induced breast cancer.

A continuing controversy exists regarding the risk of radiation-induced breast cancer, with implications for breast cancer detection by x-ray mammography. Concern over such risk first surfaced in the mid-1960s after reports were published of breast cancer developing in patients with tuberculosis.

Tuberculosis was for many years treated by isolation in a sanitarium. During the patient's stay, one mode of therapy was to induce a pneumothorax in the affected lung, and this was done under non–image-intensified fluoroscopy. Many patients received multiple treatments and up to several hundred fluoroscopic examinations.

Precise dose determinations are not possible, but levels of several hundred rad would have been common. In some of these patient populations, the relative risk for radiation-induced breast cancer was shown to be as high as 10:1.

One such population exhibited no excess risk. This finding, however, was explained as a consequence of the fluoroscopic technique. In the positive studies, the patient faced away from the radiologist, toward the fluoroscopic x-ray tube, during exposure. In the study that reported negative findings, the patients were imaged facing the radiologist so that the radiation beam entered posteriorly. The breast tissue was exposed only to the low-intensity beam exiting the patient.

Additional studies have produced results suggesting radiation-induced breast cancer developed in patients treated with x-rays for acute postpartum mastitis. The dose to these patients ranged from 75 to 1000 rad (0.75 to 10 Gy_t). The relative risk factor in this population was approximately 3:1.

Radiation-induced breast cancer has also been observed in the atomic bomb survivors. Through 1980, observations on nearly 12,000 women who received radiation doses to the breasts of 10 rad or more showed a relative risk of 4:1.

In some of these studies, only one breast was irradiated. In nearly every such case, breast cancer developed only in the irradiated breast. These patients have now been followed for up to 25 years. On the basis of all available data regarding radiation-induced breast cancer, the best estimate for absolute risk is 6 cases/10^6 persons/rad/yr.

Lung Cancer. Early in the 20th century, it was observed that approximately 50% of the workers in the Bohemian pitchblende mines of Germany died of lung cancer. Lung cancer incidence in the general population was negligible by comparison. The dusty mine environment was considered to be the cause of this lung cancer. Now it is known that radiation exposure from radon in the mines contributed to the incidence of lung cancer in these miners.

Observations of the American uranium miners active in the Colorado plateau in the 1950s and 1960s have also shown elevated levels of lung cancer. The peak of this activity occurred in the early 1960s, when there were approximately 5000 miners active in nearly 500 underground mines and 150 open-pit mines. Most of the mines were worked by less than 10 men; therefore, for such a small operation, one could expect a lack of proper ventilation.

The radiation exposure in these mines occurred because of the high concentration of uranium ore. Uranium, which is radioactive with a very long half-life of 10^9 years, decays through a series of radioactive nuclides by successive alpha and beta emissions, each accompanied by gamma radiation.

One of the decay products of uranium is **radon** (^{222}Rn). This radionuclide is a gas that emanates through the rock to produce a high concentration in air. When breathed, the radon can be deposited in the lung, where it undergoes additional successive series of decay to a stable isotope of lead.

During these subsequent decay actions, several alpha particles are released, resulting in a rather high local dose. Also, alpha particles are high-LET radiation, and therefore have a high RBE.

To date, more than 4000 uranium miners have been observed and they have received estimated doses to lung tissue as high as 3000 rad (30 Gy_t); on this basis, the relative risk was approximately 8:1. Interestingly, smoking uranium miners have a relative risk of approximately 20:1.

The available data indicate a dose–response relationship that is linear, nonthreshold with an absolute risk of 1.3 cases/10^6 persons/rad/yr.

Liver Cancer. Thorium dioxide (ThO_2) in a colloidal suspension known as **Thorotrast** was widely used in diagnostic radiology between 1925 and 1945 as a contrast agent for angiography. Thorotrast was approximately 25% ThO_2 by weight and it contained several radioactive isotopes of thorium and its decay products. Radiation that was emitted produced a dose in the ratio of approximately 100:10:1 of alpha, beta, and gamma radiation, respectively.

The use of Thorotrast has been shown to be responsible for several types of carcinoma after a latent period of approximately 15 to 20 years. After extravascular injection, it is carcinogenic at the site of the injection. After intravascular injection, ThO_2 particles are deposited in phagocytic cells of the reticuloendothelial system and are concentrated in the liver and spleen. Its half-life and high alpha radiation dose has resulted in many cases of cancer in these organs.

TOTAL RISK OF MALIGNANCY

On the basis of many of these observations on human population groups after exposure to low-level radiation, and considering all the risk estimates taken collectively for leukemia and cancer, a number of simplified conclusions can be made. The overall absolute risk for induction of malignancy is approximately 8 cases/10,000-rad (8×10^{-2} Sv^{-1}), with the at-risk period extending for 20 to 25 years after exposure. Lethality from radiation-induced malignant disease is projected at 50%. Therefore, approximately 400 deaths from radiation-induced malignancy can be expected after an exposure of 1 rad to 10,000 persons. The risk of death from radiation-induced malignant disease is 4/10,000-rad (4×10^{-2} Sv^{-1}).

Three Mile Island

To make these values somewhat more meaningful, we can consider the celebrated Three Mile Island incident in 1979. There were approximately 2,000,000 people residing within an 80-km (50-mile) radius of Three Mile Island, on the Susquehanna River in Pennsylvania.

On the basis of population statistics, one would expect to observe approximately 330,000 cancer deaths in these persons. During the total period of the radiation incident, the average dose to persons living within a 160-km (100-mile) radius was 1.5 mrad (15 μGy_t); to those within the 80-km (50-mile) radius, it was 8 mrad (80 μGy_t).

Applying 8 mrad as an upper limit, one can predict that the Three Mile Island incident will result in no more than one additional malignant death as a result of this population radiation exposure. Clearly, this response is not detectable in the face of approximately 400,000 natural cancer deaths in that population.

PREDICTED RADIATION-INDUCED DEATHS AT THREE MILE ISLAND

2×10^6 people $\times$ 4 deaths/10^4 people-rad $\times$ 0.0015 rad = 1.2 deaths

TABLE 37-5	BEIR Committee Estimated Excess Mortality From Malignant Disease in 100,000 People	
	Male	**Female**
Normal expectation	20,560	16,680
Excess cases		
Single exposure to 10 rad (100 mGy$_t$)	770	810
Continuous exposure to 1 rad/yr (10 mGy$_t$/yr)	2880	3070
Continuous exposure to 100 mrad/yr (1 mGy$_t$/yr)	520	600

BEIR Committee

The Committee on the Biologic Effects of Ionizing Radiation (BEIR), an arm of the National Academy of Sciences, has reviewed the data on late effects of low-dose, low-LET radiation. Their 1990 report showed the results summarized in Table 37-5, and they are considered authoritative.

The BEIR committee examined three situations. First, they estimated the excess mortality from malignant disease after a one-time accidental exposure to 10 rad; such a situation is highly unlikely in radiology. Second, they considered the response to a dose of 1 rad/yr for life; this situation is possible in diagnostic radiology but is certainly rare. Finally, they considered excess radiation-induced cancer mortality after a continuous dose of 100 mrad/yr. This is still considerably higher than the experience of most radiologic technologists, but can serve as a good upper limit of occupational radiation risk.

Assuming a linear, nonthreshold dose–response relationship, these analyses showed an additional 800 cases of malignant disease death in a population of 100,000 after 10 rad and an additional 550 deaths after 100 mrad/yr. These cases are in addition to the normal incidence of cancer death, which is approximately 19,000 per 100,000 persons.

 The BEIR Committee has further stated that because of the uncertainty in their analysis, less than 1 rad/yr may not be harmful.

The BEIR Committee has also analyzed the available human data with regard to the age at exposure, with a limited time of expression of effects, and whether the response was **absolute** or **relative**. This requires additional definitions of these terms. If one is irradiated at an early age and the response is limited in time, the radiation-induced excess malignant disease appears as a bulge on

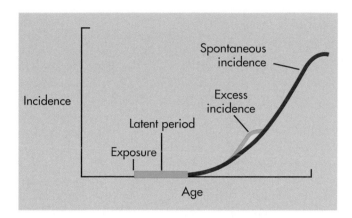

FIGURE 37-9 Exposure at an early age can result in an excess bulge of cancer after a latent period.

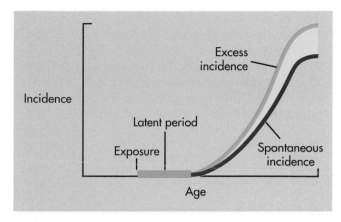

FIGURE 37-11 The relative risk model predicts that the excess radiation-induced cancer risk is proportional to the natural incidence.

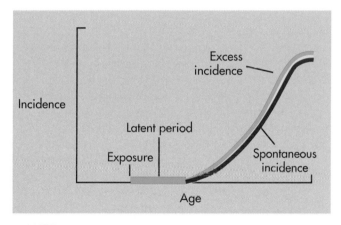

FIGURE 37-10 The absolute risk model predicts that the excess radiation-induced cancer risk is constant for life.

TABLE 37-6	Average Annual Risk of Death From Various Causes	
Cause	**Your Chance of Dying This Year**
All causes (all ages)	1 in 100
20 cigarettes per day	1 in 280
Heart disease	1 in 300
Cancer	1 in 520
All causes (25-year-old)	1 in 700
Stroke	1 in 1200
Motor vehicle accident	1 in 4000
Drowning	1 in 30,000
Alcohol (light drinker)	1 in 50,000
Air travel	1 in 100,000
Radiation, 100 mrad	1 in 100,000
Texas Gulf Coast hurricane	1 in 4,500,000
Being a rodeo cowboy	1 in 6,200,000

the age–response relationship (Figure 37-9). Childhood leukemia is a good example.

An **absolute age–response relationship** is shown in Figure 37-10. Here, the increased incidence of cancer is a constant number of cases after a minimal latent period. Most subscribe to a **relative age–response relationship**, where the increased incidence of cancer is proportional to the natural incidence (Figure 37-11).

Perhaps the best way to present these radiation risk data is to compare them with other known causes of death. As one might imagine, there are volumes of tables that analyze risk. This information is presented in simplified form in Table 37-6.

Note that in these common situations, risk from radiation exposure is near the bottom of the list. Our actual occupational risk is even less because we use protective apparel during fluoroscopy, and the radiation risk estimate assumes whole-body exposure.

RADIATION AND PREGNANCY

Since the first medical applications of x-rays, there has been concern and apprehension regarding the effects of radiation before, during, and after pregnancy. Before pregnancy, the concern is interrupted fertility. During pregnancy, concern is directed to possible congenital effects in newborns. The postpregnancy concerns are related to the suspected genetic effects. All these effects have been demonstrated in animals and some have been observed in humans.

Effects on Fertility

The early effect of high-level radiation on the interruption of fertility in both men and women is discussed in Chapter 36. There is ample evidence to show that such an effect does exist and is dose related. The effects of low-dose, long-term irradiation on fertility, however, are less well defined.

Animal data in this area are lacking. Those that are available indicate that, even when radiation is delivered at the rate of 100 rad per year, there is no noticeable depression in fertility.

 Low-dose, chronic irradiation does not impair fertility.

There have been two national surveys of American radiologists, one reported in 1927 and the other in 1955. In each case, a finding of depressed fertility and increased congenital abnormalities in the offspring of radiologists was reported. Both studies have been questioned because of their experimental methods. The conclusions reported are not generally accepted.

The health effects analysis of 150,000 American radiologic technologists mentioned earlier has indicated no effect on fertility. The number of births during a 12-year sampling period equaled the number expected.

Irradiation in Utero

Irradiation in utero concerns the following two types of exposures: that of the radiation worker and that of the patient. The recommended techniques and radiation control procedures associated with these exposed persons are considered fully in Chapter 40. Here, we consider the biologic effects of such irradiation.

Substantial animal data are available to describe fairly completely the effects of relatively high doses of radiation delivered during various periods of gestation. Because the embryo is a rapidly developing cell system, it is particularly sensitive to radiation. With age, the embryo (and then the fetus) becomes less sensitive to the effects of radiation, and this pattern continues into adulthood.

After maturity, radiosensitivity increases with age. Figure 37-12 is a summary of the observed $LD_{50/60}$ in mice exposed at various times, showing this aggregated radiosensitivity. Such findings are of particular concern because a diagnostic x-ray exposure often occurs when pregnancy is unknown.

 All observations point to the first trimester during pregnancy as the most radiosensitive period.

The effects of radiation in utero are time related and dose related. They include prenatal death, neonatal death, congenital abnormalities, malignancy induction, general impairment of growth, genetic effects, and mental retardation. Figure 37-13 is redrawn from studies designed to observe the effects of a 200-rad (2-Gy_t) dose

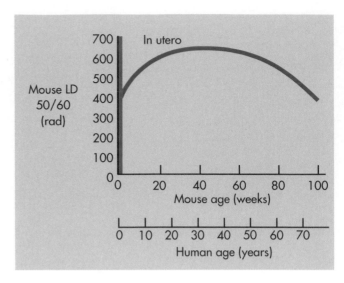

FIGURE 37-12 $LD_{50/60}$ of mice in relation to age at time of irradiation.

delivered at various stages in utero in mice. The scale along the x-axis indicates the approximate comparable time in humans.

Within **2 weeks** of fertilization, the most pronounced effect of a high radiation dose is prenatal death, which is manifested as a spontaneous abortion. Observations in radiation therapy patients have confirmed this effect, but only after very high doses.

On the basis of animal experimentation, it would appear that this response is very rare. Our best estimate is that a 10-rad (100-mGy_t) dose during the first 2 weeks will induce perhaps a 0.1% rate of spontaneous abortion. This is in addition to the 25% to 50% normal incidence of spontaneous abortions.

Fortunately, this response is of the all-or-none variety: Either there is a radiation-induced abortion, or the pregnancy will carry to term with no ill effect.

 The first 2 weeks of pregnancy may be of least concern because the response is all-or-nothing.

During the period of **major organogenesis,** from the 2nd through the 10th week, two effects may occur. Early in this period, skeletal and organ abnormalities can be induced. As major organogenesis continues, congenital abnormalities of the central nervous system may be observed if the pregnancy is carried to term.

If the radiation-induced congenital abnormalities are severe enough, the result will be neonatal death. After a dose of 200 rad (2 Gy_t) to the mouse, nearly 100% of the fetuses suffered significant abnormalities. In 80%, it was sufficient to cause neonatal death.

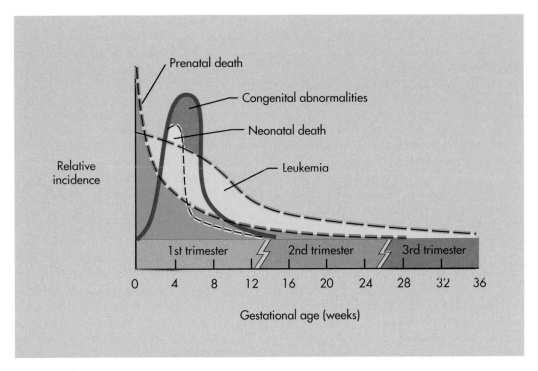

FIGURE 37-13 After 200 rad delivered at various times in utero, a number of effects can be observed.

Such effects are rare after diagnostic levels of exposure and are essentially undetectable after radiation doses of less than 10 rad (100 mGy$_t$). A dose of 10 rad (100 mGy$_t$) during organogenesis is expected to increase the incidence of congenital abnormalities by 1% above the natural incidence. To complicate matters, there is approximately a 5% incidence of naturally occurring congenital abnormalities in the unexposed population.

Irradiation in utero at the human level has been associated with childhood malignancy by a number of investigators. Perhaps the most complete study of this effect was conducted by Alice Stewart and co-workers in a project known as the Oxford Survey, a study of childhood malignancy in England, Scotland, and Wales.

Nearly every such case of childhood malignancy in these countries since 1946 has been investigated. Each case was first identified and then investigated by interview with the mother, review of the hospital charts, and review of the physician records.

Each "case" of childhood malignancy was matched with a "control" for age, sex, place of birth, socioeconomic status, and other demographic factors. The control subject was a child who matched with the "case" in all respects except the control did not have cancer or leukemia. The Oxford Survey is being continued at this time and has now considered more than 10,000 cases and a like number of matched control subjects.

Although the Oxford Survey has reviewed all malignancies, it is the findings of radiation-induced leukemia

TABLE 37-7	Relative Risk of Childhood Leukemia After Irradiation In Utero by Trimester
Time of X-Ray Examination	**Relative Risk**
First trimester	8.3
Second trimester	1.5
Third trimester	1.4
Total	**1.5**

that have been of particular importance. Table 37-7 shows the results of this survey in terms of relative risk.

 The relative risk of childhood leukemia after irradiation in utero is 1.5.

A relative risk of 1.5 for the development of childhood leukemia after irradiation in utero is significant. This indicates an increase of 50% over the nonirradiated rate. The number of cases involved, however, is small.

The incidence of childhood leukemia in the population at large is approximately 9 cases per 100,000 live births. According to the Oxford Survey, if all 100,000 had been irradiated in utero, perhaps 14 cases of leukemia would have resulted. Although these findings have been substantiated in several American populations, there is no consensus among radiobiologists that this effect after such low doses is indeed real.

There are other effects after irradiation in utero that have been studied rather fully in animals and have been observed in some human populations. An unexpected finding in offspring of the atomic bomb survivors is mental retardation. Children of exposed mothers have performed poorly in IQ tests and have demonstrated poor scholastic performance compared with unexposed Japanese children.

These differences are marginal, yet significant. When assessed by test scores, measurable mental retardation is apparent in approximately 6% of all children. A 10-rad dose in utero is expected to increase this incidence by an additional 0.5%.

Radiation exposure in utero does retard the growth and development of the newborn. Irradiation in utero, principally during the period of major organogenesis, has been associated with microcephaly (small head) and, as discussed, mental retardation.

The human data bearing on these effects are obtained from patients irradiated medically, the atomic bomb survivors, and the residents of the Marshall Islands who were exposed to radioactive fallout in 1954 during weapons testing. For instance, the heavily irradiated children at Hiroshima are, on the average, 2.25 cm (0.9 in) shorter, 3 kg (6.6 lb) lighter, and 1.1 cm (0.4 in) smaller in head circumference than members of the nonirradiated control groups.

These effects, as well as mental retardation, have been observed principally in those receiving doses in excess of 100 rad (1 Gy_t) in utero. The lack of appropriate and sensitive tests of mental function makes it impossible to draw similar conclusions at doses below 100 rad (1 Gy_t).

A summary of the effects of irradiation in utero is given in Table 37-8. There are four responses of concern to radiology: spontaneous abortion, congenital abnormalities, mental retardation, and childhood malignancy.

Spontaneous abortion causes the least concern of the four because it is an all-or none effect. Congenital abnormalities, mental retardation, and childhood malignancy are of real concern, but it should be recognized that the probability of such a response after a fetal dose of 10 rad (100 mGy_t) is nil. Furthermore, 10 rad (100 mGy_t) to the fetus is very rarely experienced in radiology.

The form of the dose–response relationship for each of these effects is unknown. However, several appear to be linear and nonthreshold when based on doses greater than 100 rad (1 Gy_t). When large experimental animal populations were acutely exposed, the minimum reported dose for observing such effects as statistically significant was approximately 10 rad (100 mGy_t).

No evidence in either humans or animals indicates that the levels of radiation exposure currently experienced occupationally and medically are responsible for any such effects on growth and development.

Although our efforts for protecting the unborn from the harmful effects of radiation are principally directed at diagnostic x-ray exposures, we must also be aware of similar hazards from radioisotope examinations. For example, radioiodine is known to concentrate principally in the thyroid gland. After administration of radioactive iodine, the dose to thyroid tissue will be several orders of magnitude higher than the whole-body dose because of this organ concentration effect.

The thyroid gland begins to function at approximately 10 weeks of gestation, and because radioiodine readily crosses the placental barrier from the mother's blood to the fetal circulation, radioiodine should be administered during pregnancy only in trace doses and before the 10 week gestation period. At any time thereafter, the hazard of such an administration increases.

Genetic Effects

Unfortunately, our weakest area of knowledge in radiation biology is the area of radiation genetics. Essentially all the data indicating that radiation causes genetic effects have come from large-scale experiments with either flies or mice.

 We do not have any data suggesting radiation-induced genetic effects in humans.

TABLE 37-8	Summary of Effects After 10 Rad In Utero		
Time of Exposure	**Type of Response**	**Natural Occurrence**	**Radiation Response**
0–2 wk	Spontaneous abortion	25%	0.1%
2–10 wk	Congenital abnormalities	5%	1%
2–15 wk	Mental retardation	6%	0.5%
0–9 mo	Malignant disease	8/10,000	12/10,000
0–9 mo	Impaired growth and development	1%	Nil
0–9 mo	Genetic mutation	10%	Nil

Observations of the atomic bomb survivors have shown no radiation-induced genetic effects, and descendants of survivors are now into the third generation. Other human populations have likewise provided only negative results. Consequently, in the absence of accurate human data, there is no choice but to rely on information from experimental laboratory studies.

In 1927, the Nobel prize–winning geneticist H. J. Muller from the University of Texas reported the results of his irradiation of *Drosophila*, the fruit fly. He irradiated mature flies before procreation and then measured the frequency of lethal mutations in the offspring. The radiation doses used were thousands of rad, but, as the data of Figure 37-14 show, the dose–response relationship for radiation-induced genetic damage is unmistakably linear, nonthreshold.

From Muller's studies, other conclusions were drawn. Radiation does not alter the quality of mutations but rather increases the frequency of those mutations that are observed spontaneously. Muller's data showed no dose rate or dose fractionation effects. Hence, he concluded that such mutations were single-hit phenomena.

It was principally on the basis of Muller's work that the National Council on Radiation Protection in 1932 lowered the recommended dose limit and acknowledged officially for the first time the existence of nonthreshold radiation effects. Since then, all radiation protection guides have assumed a linear, nonthreshold dose–response relationship and have been based on the suspected genetic, as well as somatic, effects of radiation.

The only other experimental work of any significance is that of Russell. Beginning in 1946, he began to irradiate a large mouse colony with radiation dose rates that varied from 0.001 to 90 rad/min (0.01 to 900 mGy$_t$/min), with total doses up to 1000 rad (10 Gy$_t$). These studies are continuing and observations have now been made on over 8 million mice! The experiment requires the observation of seven specific genes that control readily recognizable characteristics, such as ear shape, coat color, and eye color.

Russell's data show that a dose rate effect does exist, which would indicate that the mouse has the capacity to repair genetic damage. He has confirmed the linear, nonthreshold form of the dose–response relationship and has not detected any types of mutations that did not occur naturally.

The average mutation rate per unit dose in the mouse is approximately 15 times that observed in the fruit fly. Whether an increased sensitivity exists in humans relative to the mouse is unknown.

 The doubling dose is that dose of radiation that produces twice the frequency of genetic mutations as would have been observed without the radiation.

From these experimental studies the concept of the doubling dose has been developed. The doubling dose in humans is estimated to lie in the range between 50 and 250 rad (0.5 and 2.5 Gy$_t$).

So, what is the significance of all this in our daily practice? What is the significance to either patients or radiologic technologists? First, it can be said with certainty that the incidence of radiation-induced genetic mutations after the levels of exposure experienced in diagnostic radiology is essentially zero (Box 37-1).

BOX 37-1   Additional Conclusions Regarding Radiation Genetics

Radiation-induced mutations are usually harmful.

Any dose of radiation, however small, to a germ cell results in some genetic risk.

The frequency of radiation-induced mutations is directly proportional to dose, so that a linear extrapolation of data obtained at high doses provides a valid estimate of low-dose effects.

The effect depends on radiation protraction and fractionation.

For most prereproductive life, the woman is less sensitive to the genetic effects of radiation than the man.

Most radiation-induced mutations are *recessive*. These require that the mutant genes be present in both the male and the female to produce the trait. Consequently, such mutations may not be expressed for many generations.

The frequency of radiation-induced genetic mutations is extremely low. It is approximately 10^{-7} mutation/rad/gene.

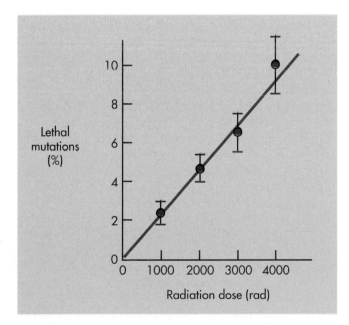

FIGURE 37-14 Irradiation of flies by H. J. Muller showed the genetic effects to be linear, nonthreshold. Note that the doses were exceedingly high.

Under nearly all such diagnostic exposures, no action is required; however, should a high radiation dose be experienced (e.g., in excess of 10 rad), some protective action may be required. The prefertilized egg, in its various stages, exhibits a constant sensitivity to radiation; however, it also demonstrates some capacity for repair of genetic damage. If repair occurs, it is rapid, and therefore a delay in procreation of only a few days may be appropriate. In the male, on the other hand, it might be prudent to refrain from procreation for a period of 60 days to allow cells that were in a resistant stage of development at the time of exposure to mature to functioning spermatids.

SUMMARY

The late effects of radiation exposure occur a long time after exposure. Late effects can develop from high-dose, short-term exposure, but the concern in diagnostic imaging is low-dose exposures over time.

Many epidemiologic studies have reported positive results; however, there are problems: (1) The exact dose is usually not known, and (2) the frequency of observable response is low. Most late effects are stochastic—the incidence of response is dose related and there is no dose threshold.

Local tissues can be affected by low-dose radiation. The late effects appear as nonmalignant changes in the skin. The skin shows a weathered, callused, and discolored appearance. Chromosome damage in circulating lymphocytes and cataracts in the lens of the eye have been observed as late effects of radiation exposure.

Because dose–response relationships are not precise when observing late effects of radiation exposure, risk estimates are used to estimate radiation response in a population. Relative risk is calculated when the population's radiation dose is not known. Relative risk is computed by comparing the number of persons in the exposed population with late effects to the number in an unexposed population in whom the same condition developed. Excess risk determines the magnitude of the late effect as the difference between cases and control subjects.

The effects of low-dose, long-term irradiation in utero can include the following: prenatal death, neonatal death, congenital abnormalities, malignancy, impairment of growth, genetic effects, and mental retardation. However, these abnormalities are based on doses greater than 100 rad, with the minimum reported doses in animal experiments at approximately 10 rad. There is no evidence at either the human or animal level to indicate that the levels of radiation exposure currently experienced occupationally or medically are responsible for any such effects on fetal growth or development.

CHALLENGE QUESTIONS

1. Define or otherwise identify:
   a. Epidemiology
   b. In utero
   c. ABCC-RERF
   d. Thorotrast
   e. Major organogenesis
   f. The Oxford Survey
   g. H. J. Muller
   h. Doubling dose
   i. Radon (^{222}Rn)
   j. Radium watch-dial painters
2. What population experienced radiation-induced cataracts?
3. What is the risk of life span shortening for radiation workers?
4. What is the significance of the change in death statistics of American radiologists from the 1935 to 1944 time period to the 1955 to 1958 time period?
5. There are approximately 300,000 radiologic technologists in the United States and their annual exposure is 50 mrem (0.5 mSv). Assuming a 40-year working period, how many are likely to die from their occupational radiation exposure?
6. What is the absolute risk when three cases of radiation-induced leukemia develop per year in 100,000 persons after an average dose of 2 rad?
7. When should excess risk be used as the preferable risk index?
8. Twenty million people in Scandinavia were exposed to an average 0.7 mrad as a result of Chernobyl. Assuming an absolute risk of 10 cases/10^6/rad/yr over a 30-year period, how many malignancies will be induced?
9. What is the suspected reason why British radiologists did not have an elevated risk of leukemia compared with American radiologists?
10. Discuss the experience of radiation-induced leukemia in ankylosing spondylitis patients.
11. Why was the thymus gland irradiated in the Ann Arbor and Rochester series? What were the late effects of the thymus irradiation?
12. Discuss the way bone cancer developed in watch-dial painters in the 1920s and 1930s.
13. Explain the risk of radon gas to uranium miners.
14. During the period of the Three Mile Island incident, what was the average dose to persons living within a 100-mile radius of the nuclear plant?
15. What are the effects on fertility from low-dose, long-term irradiation?
16. Is it true that most radiation-induced mutations are recessive?

17. In a population of 30,367 irradiated persons, 13 cases of leukemia developed; in a control population of 86,672 persons, 31 cases of leukemia developed. What was the relative risk?
18. What is the absolute risk if 32 cases of leukemia develop per year in 100,000 persons after an average dose of 2 rad?
19. How many cases of radiation-induced leukemia are suspected to have occurred in the atomic bomb survivors?
20. What is the difference between relative risk and excess risk?

CHAPTER 38

Health Physics

OBJECTIVES

At the completion of this chapter, the student should be able to do the following:

1. Define health physics
2. List the cardinal principles of radiation protection and discuss the ALARA concept
3. Explain the meaning of NCRP and the concept of dose limits
4. Name the recommended dose limits for radiation workers and the public
5. Discuss the radiosensitivity of the stages of pregnancy
6. Describe the recommended management procedures for pregnant radiation workers and for the pregnant patient

OUTLINE

Cardinal Principles of Radiation Protection
    Minimize Time
    Maximize Distance
    Maximize Shielding
Dose Limits
    Whole-Body Dose Limits
    Dose Limits for Tissues and Organs
    Public Exposure
    Educational Considerations
X-Rays and Pregnancy
    Radiobiologic Considerations
    Pregnant Technologist
    Management Principles
    Pregnant Patient

MMEDIATELY AFTER their discovery, x-rays were applied to the healing arts. It was recognized within months, however, that radiation could cause harmful effects.

The first American fatality from radiation exposure was Thomas Edison's assistant, Clarence Dally. Since then, a great deal of effort has been devoted to developing equipment, techniques, and procedures to control radiation levels and reduce unnecessary radiation exposure to radiation workers and the public.

The cardinal principles for radiation protection are simplified rules to provide safety in radiation areas for occupational workers. In 1931, the first dose-limiting recommendations were made. Today, the National Council on Radiation Protection and Measurements (NCRP) continuously reviews the recommended dose limits.

Providing radiation protection for workers and public is the practice of health physics. Health physicists design equipment, calculate and construct barriers, and develop administrative protocols to maintain radiation exposures as low as reasonably achievable (ALARA). That is the substance of this chapter.

The term *health physics* was coined during the early days of the Manhattan Project, the secret wartime effort to develop the atomic bomb. The group of physicists and physicians responsible for the radiation safety of persons involved in the production of atomic bombs were the first health physicists. Thus, the health physicist is a radiation scientist concerned with the research, teaching, or operational aspects of radiation safety.

Health physics is concerned with providing occupational radiation protection and minimizing radiation dose to the public.

CARDINAL PRINCIPLES OF RADIATION PROTECTION

All health physics activity in radiology is designed to minimize radiation exposure of patients and personnel. Three cardinal principles of radiation protection developed for nuclear activities—**time, distance,** and **shielding**—find

---

equally useful application in diagnostic radiology. By observing these cardinal principles, radiation exposure can be minimized (Box 38-1).

Minimize Time

The dose to an individual is directly related to the duration of exposure. If the time during which one is exposed to radiation is doubled, the exposure will be doubled, as follows:

TIME

Exposure = Exposure rate × Exposure time

Question: A radiation worker is exposed to 230 mR/hr (2.3 mGy$_a$/hr) from a radiation source. If the worker remains at that position for 36 minutes, what will be the total occupational exposure?

Answer: Occupational exposure $= 230\,\text{mR/hr}\,\dfrac{36\,\text{min}}{60\,\text{min/hr}}$

$= 138\,\text{mR}$

Question: The parent of a patient is asked to remain next to the patient during fluoroscopy, where the radiation exposure level is 600 mR/hr (6 mGy$_a$/hr). If the allowable daily exposure is 50 mR, how long may the parent remain? (Figure 38-1)

Answer: Time = Exposure ÷ Exposure rate
= 50 mR ÷ 600 mR/hr
= $\frac{1}{12}$ hour
= 8 minutes

During radiography, the time of exposure is kept to a minimum to reduce motion blur. During fluoroscopy, the time of exposure should also be kept to a minimum to reduce patient and personnel exposure. This is an area of radiation protection not directly controlled by the radiologic technologist.

Radiologists are trained to depress the fluoroscopic foot switch in an alternating fashion, sequencing **on-off**

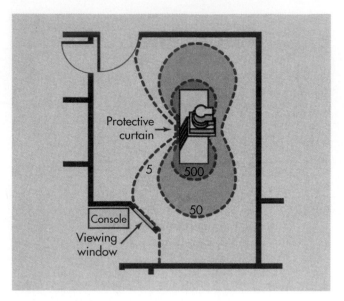

FIGURE 38-1 Typical isoexposure contours during fluoroscopic examination (mR/hr).

rather than continuous **on** during the course of the examination. A repeated up-and-down motion on the fluoroscopic foot switch permits a high-quality examination to be made with a considerably reduced exposure to the patient. The use of pulsed progressive fluoroscopy can reduce patient dose by a factor of 0.1 or less.

The **5-minute reset timer** on all fluoroscopes reminds the radiologist that a considerable fluoroscopic time has elapsed. The timer records the amount of x-ray beam on-time. Most fluoroscopic examinations take less than 5 minutes. Only during difficult interventional radiology procedures should it be necessary to exceed 5 minutes of exposure time.

Question: A fluoroscope emits 4.2 R/min (42 mGy$_a$/min) at the tabletop for every milliampere of operation (4.2 R/mAmin). What is the patient exposure in a barium enema examination that is conducted at 1.8 mA and requires 2.5 minutes of fluoroscopic time?

Answer: Patient exposure $= \left(\dfrac{4.2\,\text{R}}{\text{mAmin}} \right)(1.8\,\text{mA})(2.5\,\text{min})$

$= 18.9\,\text{R}$

Maximize Distance

As the distance between the source of radiation and a person increases, the radiation exposure decreases rapidly. The decrease in exposure is calculated using the inverse square law, discussed in Chapter 5.

 If the distance from the source exceeds five times the source diameter, it can be treated as a point source.

Most radiation sources are point sources. The x-ray tube target, for example, is a point source of radiation. The scattered radiation generated in a patient appears, however, to come not from a point source but rather from an extended area source. As a rule of thumb, even an extended source can be considered a point source at sufficient distance.

 DISTANCE
Assume a point source and apply the inverse square law.

Question: An x-ray tube has an output intensity of 2.6 mR/mAs at 100-cm source-to-image receptor distance (SID) when operated at 70 kVp. What would be the radiation exposure 350 cm from the target?

Answer: $\dfrac{I_1}{I_2} = \dfrac{d_2{}^2}{d_1{}^2}$

$I_1 = I_2 \dfrac{d_2{}^2}{d_1{}^2}$

$= (2.6\,\text{mR/mAs}) \left(\dfrac{100\,\text{cm}}{350\,\text{cm}} \right)^2$

$= (2.6\,\text{mR/mAs})(0.082)$

$= 0.21\,\text{mR/mAs}$

In radiography, the distance from radiation source to patient is usually fixed by the type of examination, and the radiologic technologist is positioned behind a protective barrier.

During fluoroscopy, the radiologic technologist can exercise good radiation protection procedures. Figure 38-1 shows the approximate radiation exposure levels at waist height during a fluoroscopic examination. The lines on the plot plan are called **isoexposure lines** and represent positions of equal radiation exposure in the fluoroscopy room. At the normal position for a radiologist or a radiologic technologist, the exposure rate at this position is approximately 300 mR/hr (3 mGy$_a$/hr).

 During fluoroscopy, the radiologic technologist should remain as far from the patient as practicable.

During portions of the examination, when it is not necessary for the radiologic technologist to remain close to the patient, the technologist should step back. Two steps back, the exposure rate is only approximately 5 mR/hr (50 µGy$_a$/hr). This reduction in exposure does not follow the inverse square law because during fluoroscopy, the patient is an extended source of radiation because of scattered x-rays generated within the body.

Question: What is the approximate occupational exposure of a radiologic technologist at a position where the exposure rate is 300 mR/hr, and farther back where the exposure rate is 20 mR/hr during a fluoroscopic examination lasting 4 minutes, 15 seconds?

Answer: Occupational exposure equals
First position: (300 mR/hr)(4.25 min)
                                  (1 hr/60 min) = 21.25 mR
Second position: (20 mR/hr)(4.25 min)
                                  (1 hr/60 min) = 1.4 mR

Maximize Shielding

Positioning shielding between the radiation source and exposed persons greatly reduces the level of radiation exposure. Shielding used in diagnostic radiology usually consists of lead, although conventional building materials are also used. The amount that a protective barrier reduces radiation intensity can be estimated if the half-value layer (HVL) or the 10th-value layer (TVL) of the barrier material is known. The HVL is defined and discussed in Chapter 12. The TVL is similarly defined as follows:

One TVL is the thickness of absorber that reduces the radiation intensity to one-tenth its original value.

Table 38-1 shows approximate HVLs and TVLs for lead and concrete for diagnostic x-ray beams between 40 and 150 kVp.

SHIELDING
1 TVL = 3.3 HVL

Question: When operated at 80 kVp, an x-ray imaging system emits 3.6 mR/mAs at an SID of 100 cm. How much shielding (concrete or lead) would be required to reduce the intensity to less than 0.25 mR/mAs?

Answer: The amount of shielding in the first or second column of the following data will reduce the beam intensity to the value in the third column. The last row is the answer.

Pb (mm)	Concrete (in)	Beam intensity (mR/mAs)
0	0	3.60
0.19	0.42	1.80
0.38	0.84	0.60
0.57	1.26	0.45
0.76	1.68	0.23

Question: An x-ray imaging system is used strictly for chest radiography at 125 kVp. The useful beam is always pointed to a wall containing 0.8 mm Pb shielding. How much additional shielding will be required if the workload doubles?

Answer: When the workload doubles, so will the exposure on the other side of the wall. From Table 38-1, it is seen that one HVL, or 0.27 mm Pb, will be necessary to reduce that exposure to its original level.

Another example of the application of shielding in radiology is the use of protective apparel. Protective aprons usually contain 0.5 mm Pb. This is approximately equivalent to 2 HVLs, which should reduce occupational exposure to 25%. Actual measurements show that such protective aprons reduce exposure to approximately 10% because scattered x-rays are often incident on the apron at an oblique angle.

Usually, applications of the cardinal principles of radiation protection involve a consideration of all three. The typical problem involves a known radiation level at a given distance from the source.

The level of exposure at any other distance, behind any shielding, for any length of time can be calculated. The order in which these calculations are made makes no difference.

Question: The operating kVp of a radiographic imaging system rarely exceeds 100 kVp. The

TABLE 38-1	Approximate Half-value and Tenth-value Layers of Lead and Concrete at Various Tube Potentials			
	HVL		**TVL**	
Tube Potential	**Lead (mm)**	**Concrete (in)**	**Lead (mm)**	**Concrete (in)**
40 kVp	0.03	0.13	0.06	0.40
60 kVp	0.11	0.25	0.34	0.87
80 kVp	0.19	0.42	0.64	1.4
100 kVp	0.24	0.60	0.80	2.0
125 kVp	0.27	0.76	0.90	2.5
150 kVp	0.28	0.86	0.95	2.8

HVL, Half-value layer; *TVL*, tenth-value layer.

output intensity is 4.6 mR/mAs at 100-cm SID. The distance to a desk on the other side of the wall to which the x-ray beam is directed is 200 cm. The wall contains 0.96 mm Pb, and 300 mAs is anticipated daily. If the exposure is to be restricted to 2 mR/wk, how long each day may the desk be occupied?

Answer: Daily x-ray output at 100 cm =
$$(4.6 \text{ mR/mAs})(300 \text{ mAs}) = 1380 \text{ mR}$$
Daily output at 200 cm =
$$(1380)(100/200)^2 = 345 \text{ mR}$$
Daily output behind 0.96 mm Pb or 4 HVLs = 22 mR
$$= 110 \text{ mR/wk}$$
$$\text{Time allowed} = \frac{2mR}{110 \text{ mR/wk}} = 0.018 \text{ week}$$
$$= 43 \text{ minutes}$$

However, this analysis does not take into account the x-ray beam attenuation by the patient, which is approximately 2 TVLs or 0.01. Therefore,

Daily output behind 0.96 mm Pb and the patient = $(110 \text{ mR})(0.01) = 1.1 \text{ mR}$

$$\text{Time allowed} = \frac{2 \text{ mR}}{1.1 \text{ mR/wk}} =$$
$$1.8 \text{ wk (unlimited)}$$

Question: Suppose an analysis shows that if an administrator remains at his or her desk for more than 24 minutes each week, the occupational dose limit will be exceeded. How much additional protective lead would be required?

Answer: Full occupancy is 40 hr × 60 min/hr =
$$2400 \text{ min}$$
$$\frac{2400 \text{ min}}{24 \text{ min}} = 100$$

That is, 2 TVLs or an additional 1.6 mm Pb.

Figure 38-2 illustrates the use of these cardinal principles of radiation protection during a typical clinical situation.

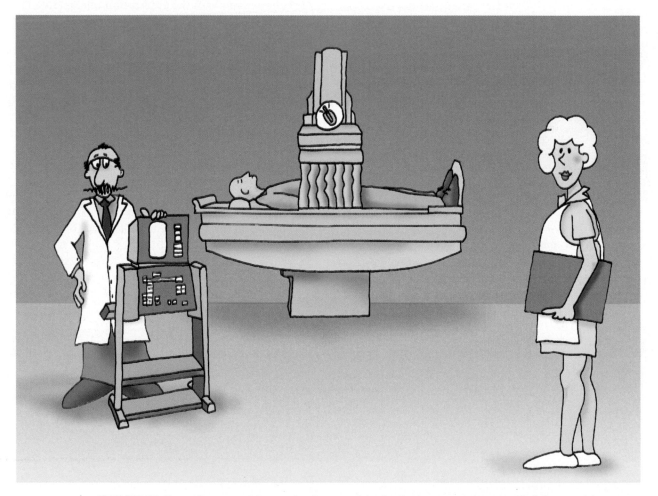

FIGURE 38-2 Application of the cardinal principles of radiation protection in radiology.

DOSE LIMITS

A continuing effort of health physicists has been the description and identification of occupational dose limits. For many years, a **maximum permissible dose (MPD)** was specified. The MPD was the dose of radiation that would be expected to produce no significant radiation effects.

At radiation doses below the MPD, no responses should occur. At the level of the MPD, the risk is not zero, but it is small—lower than the risk associated with other occupations and reasonable in light of the benefits derived. The concept of MPD is now obsolete and has been replaced by dose limits (DL).

Whole-Body Dose Limits

The National Council on Radiation Protection (NCRP) has assessed risk based on data from the reports of the National Academy of Sciences (Biologic Effects of Ionizing Radiation [BEIR] Committee) and the National Safety Council (Table 38-2) to establish DLs. State and federal government agencies routinely adopt these recommended dose limits as law. Current DLs are prescribed for various organs as well as the whole body, and for various working conditions. If one received the DL each year, the lifetime risk will not exceed 10^{-4} yr^{-1}.

 DLs imply that if received annually, the risk of death would be less than 1 in 10,000.

The value 10^{-4} yr^{-1} is the approximate risk of death to those working in safe industries. The DLs recommended by the NCRP ensure that radiation workers have the same risk as those in safe industries.

Question: Suppose all 300,000 American radiologic technologists receive the DL (5000 mrem) this year. How many would be expected to die prematurely?

Answer: $(300,000)(10^{-4}) = 30$

But of course, they actually receive approximately 50 mrem/yr; therefore, the expected mortality is as follows:

$$30 \left(\frac{50}{5000} \right) = 0.3; \text{ less than 1!}$$

Particular care is taken to make certain that no **radiation worker** receives a radiation dose in excess of the DL. The DL is specified only for occupational exposure. It should not be confused with medical x-ray exposure received as a patient. Although patient dose should be kept low, there is no patient DL.

The first DL, 50,000 mrem/wk (500 mSv/wk), was recommended in 1902. The current DL is 100 mrem/wk (1 mSv/wk). Through the years there has been a downward revision of the DL. The history of these continuing recommendations is given in Table 38-3 and is shown graphically in Figure 38-3.

In the early years of radiology, the DL consisted of a single value considered the safe working level for whole-body exposure. It was based primarily on the known acute response to radiation exposure and presumed that a **threshold dose** existed.

Today the DL is specified not only for whole-body exposure but also for partial-body exposure, organ exposure, and exposure of the general population, again excluding medical exposure as a patient and exposure from natural sources (Table 38-4).

These DLs included in Table 38-4 were first published by the NCRP in 1987 and further refined in 1993. They replace the previous MPDs, which had been in effect since 1959.

These DLs have been adopted by state and federal regulatory agencies and are now the law of the United States. Notice that SI units are preferred.

The basic annual DL is 50 mSv/yr (5000 mrem/yr). The DL for the lens of the eye is 150 mSv/yr (15 rem/yr), and that for other organs is 500 mSv/yr (50 rem/yr).

The cumulative whole-body DL is 10 mSv (1000 mrem) times one's age in years. The DL during pregnancy is 5 mSv (500 mrem), but once pregnancy is declared, the monthly exposure shall not exceed 0.5 mSv (50 mrem).

 Current DLs are based on a *linear, nonthreshold dose–response relationship;* they are considered to be an acceptable level of occupational radiation exposure.

In practice, at least in diagnostic radiology, it is seldom necessary to exceed even 1/10 the appropriate DL.

TABLE 38-2	Fatal Accident Rates in Various Industries
Industry	**Rate (× 10^{-4} yr^{-1})**
Trade	0.4
Manufacture	0.4
Service	0.4
Government	0.9
Radiation workers	0.9
All groups	0.9
Transport	2.2
Public utilities	2.2
Construction	3.1
Mining	4.3
Agriculture	4.4

However, because the basis for the DL assumes a linear, nonthreshold dose–response relationship, **all unnecessary** radiation exposure should be avoided.

Occupational exposure is described as *dose equivalent* in units of milliseivert (millirem). DLs are specified as *effective dose (E)*. This scheme has been adopted to afford more precision in radiation protection practices.

The effective dose (E) concept accounts for different types of radiation because of their varying relative biologic effectiveness. Effective dose also considers the relative radiosensitivity of various tissues and organs.

These are particularly important considerations when a protective apron is worn. Wearing a protective apron reduces radiation dose to many tissues and organs to near zero. Therefore, effective dose is much less than that recorded by a collar-positioned radiation monitor.

EFFECTIVE DOSE

Effective dose (E) = Radiation weighting factor (W_r) × Tissue weighting factor (W_t) × Absorbed dose

Adoption of this scheme is progressing. For our purposes, effective dose (E) is the quantity of importance. It is expressed in mSv (mrem) and is the basis for our DLs.

As seen in Table 38-5, the radiation weighting factor (W_r) is equal to 1 for the types of radiation we use in medicine. The value of W_r for other types of radiation depends on the LET of that radiation.

The tissue weighting factor (W_t) accounts for the relative radiosensitivity of various tissues and organs. Tissues with a higher value of W_t are more radiosensitive. These are shown in Table 38-6.

TABLE 38-3	Historical Review of Dose Limits for Occupational Exposure		
Year	Recommendation	Approximate Daily Dose Limit (mrem)	Source
1902	Dose limited by fogging of a photographic plate after 7-minute contact exposure	10,000	Rollins
1915	Lead shielding of tube needed (no numeric exposure levels given)		British Roentgen Society
1921	General methods to reduce exposure		British X-ray and Radium Protection Committee
1925	"It is entirely safe if an operator does not receive every thirty days a dose exceeding 1/100 of an erythema dose."	200	Mutscheller
1925	10% of a SED per year	200	Sievert
1926	One SED per 90,000 working hours	40	Dutch Board of Health
1928	0.000028 of a SED per day	175	Barclay and Cox
1928	0.001 of a SED per month 5 R per day permissible for the hands	150	Kaye
1931	Limit exposure to 0.2 R per day	200	Advisory Committee on X-ray and Radium Protection of the United States
1932	0.001 of a SED per month	30	Failla
1934	5 R per day permissible for the hands	5000	Advisory Committee on X-ray and Radium Protection of the United States
1936	0.1 R per day	100	Advisory Committee on X-ray and Radium Protection of the United States
1941	0.02 R per day	20	Taylor
1943	200 mR per day is acceptable	200	Patterson
1959	5 rem per year, 5 (N-18) rem accumulated	20	National Council on Radiation Protection and Measurements
1987	50 mSv per year, 10 × N mSv cumulative	20	National Council on Radiation Protection and Measurements
1991	20 mSv per year	8	International Commission on Radiation Protection

SED, Skin erythema dose.

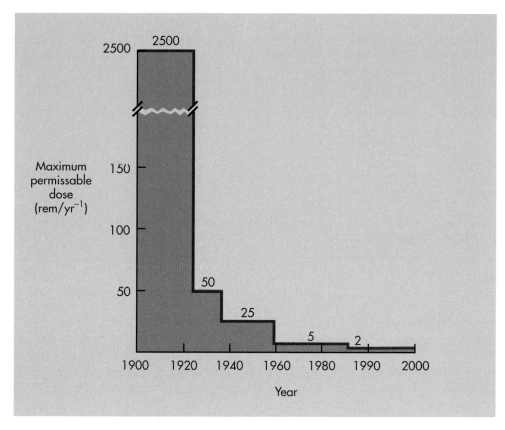

FIGURE 38-3 Dose limits over the past century.

TABLE 30-4	Dose Limits Recommended by the National Council on Radiation Protection and Measurements

A. Occupational exposures
  1. Effective dose
    a. Annual: 50 mSv (5000 mrem)
    b. Cumulative: 10 mSv × age (1000 mrem × age)

  2. Equivalent annual dose for tissues and organs
    a. Lens of eye   150 mSv (15 rem)
    b. Thyroid, skin, hands, and feet   500 mSv (50 rem)
B. Public exposures (annual)
  1. Effective dose, frequent exposure   1 mSv (100 mrem)
  2. Equivalent dose for tissues and organs
    a. Lens of eye   15 mSv (1500 mrem)
    b. Skin, hands, and feet   50 mSv (5000 mrem)
C. Education and training exposures (annual)
  1. Effective dose   1 mSv (100 mrem)
  2. Equivalent dose for tissues and organs
    a. Lens of eye   15 mSv (1500 mrem)
    b. Skin, hands, and feet   50 mSv (5000 mrem)
D. Embryo–fetus exposures
  1. Total equivalent dose   5 mSv (500 mrem)
  2. Equivalent dose in 1 month   0.5 mSv (50 mrem)
E. Negligible individual dose (annual)   0.01 mSv (10 mrem)

TABLE 38-5	Weighting Factors for Various Types of Radiation
Type of Energy Range	**Radiation Weighting Factor (W_r)**
X- and gamma rays, electrons	1
Neutrons, energy	
< 10 keV	5
10 keV to 100 keV	10
>100 keV to 2 MeV	20
> 2 MeV to 20 MeV	10
>20 MeV	5
Protons	2
Alpha particles	20

TABLE 38-6	Weighting Factors for Various Tissues
Tissue	**Tissue Weighting Factor (W_t)**
Gonad	0.20
Active bone marrow	0.12
Colon	0.12
Lung	0.12
Stomach	0.12
Bladder	0.05
Breast	0.05
Esophagus	0.05
Liver	0.05
Thyroid	0.05
Bone surface	0.01
Skin	0.01

Practical implementation of these DLs and weighting factors does not change our previous approach. The DL is sufficiently high that it rarely, if ever, is exceeded in diagnostic radiology.

With a collar-positioned radiation monitor, a change in procedure is necessary to estimate effective dose (E). Because essentially all of our radiation exposure occurs during fluoroscopy and the trunk is shielded by a lead apron, the response of the monitor overestimates the effective dose (E).

A conversion factor of 0.3 should be applied to the collar monitor–reported value to estimate effective dose (E). If a protective apron is not worn (e.g., a radiographer who does no fluoroscopy), then the monitor response may be considered the effective dose.

Dose Limits for Tissues and Organs

The whole-body DL of 50 mSv/yr (5000 mrem/yr) is an effective dose, which takes into account the weighted average to various tissues and organs. In addition, the NCRP identifies several specific tissues and organs with specific recommended dose limits.

Skin. Some organs of the body have a higher DL than the whole-body DL. The DL for the skin is 500 mSv/yr (50 rem/yr).

This limit is not normally of concern in diagnostic radiology because it applies to nonpenetrating radiation such as alpha and beta radiation and very soft x-rays. Radiologic technologists exclusively engaged in mammography or nuclear medicine are highly unlikely to sustain radiation exposures to the skin in excess of 10 mSv/yr (1000 mrem/yr).

Extremities. Radiologists often have their hands near the primary fluoroscopic radiation beam, and therefore extremity exposure may be of concern. The DL for the extremities is the same as that for the skin, 500 mSv/yr (50 rem/yr).

These radiation levels are quite high and under normal circumstances should not even be approached. For certain occupational groups, such as interventional radiologists and nuclear medicine technologists, extremity personnel monitors should be provided. Such devices are worn on the wrist or the finger.

Public Exposure

Individuals in the general population are limited to 5 mSv/yr (500 mrem/yr) if the exposure is infrequent. If the exposure is frequent, such as hospital workers who may regularly visit x-ray rooms, the DL is 1 mSv/yr (100 mrem/yr).

 The DL established for nonoccupationally exposed persons is 1/10 of that for the radiation worker.

This 1 mSv/yr is the DL that medical physicists use when computing the thickness of protective barriers. If a barrier separates an x-ray examining room from an area occupied by the general public, then the shielding is designed so that the annual exposure of an individual in the adjacent area cannot exceed 1 mSv/yr (100 mrem/yr).

If the adjacent area is occupied by radiation workers, then the shielding must be sufficient to maintain an annual exposure level less than 10 mSv/yr (1000 mrem/yr). This approach to shielding derives from the 10 mSv × N cumulative DL.

Radiation exposure of the general public or individuals in the population is rarely measured because it is not necessary. Most radiology personnel do not receive even this level of exposure.

Educational Considerations

There are several special situations associated with the whole-body occupational DL. Students younger than 18 years of age may not receive more than 1 mSv/yr (100 mrem/yr) during the course of their educational activities. This is included in and not in addition to the 1 mSv (100 mrem) permitted each year as a nonoccupational exposure.

Consequently, student radiologic technologists younger than 18 years of age may be engaged in x-ray imaging, but their exposure must be monitored and must remain below 1 mSv/yr (100 mrem/yr). Because of this, it is general practice not to accept underaged persons into schools of radiologic technology unless their 18th birthday is within sight.

In keeping with **ALARA,** even more changes in the DL are on the way. The International Commission on Radiological Protection (ICRP) issued a number of recommendations, including an annual whole-body DL of 20 mSv (2000 mrem). Such a reduction is currently under consideration in the United States.

X-RAYS AND PREGNANCY

Two situations in diagnostic radiology require particular care and action. Both are associated with pregnancy. Their importance is obvious from both a physical and an emotional standpoint.

Radiobiologic Considerations

The severity of the potential response to radiation exposure in utero is both time related and dose related, as discussed in Chapter 37. Unquestionably, the period most sensitive to radiation exposure occurs before birth. Furthermore, the fetus is more sensitive early in pregnancy than late in pregnancy. As a general rule, the higher the radiation dose, the more severe will be the radiation response.

Time Dependence. A grave misconception is that the most critical time for irradiation is during the first 2 weeks, when it is most unlikely that the expectant mother knows of her condition. In fact, this is the time during pregnancy when such irradiation is least hazardous.

The most likely biologic response to irradiation during the first 2 weeks of pregnancy is resorption of the embryo, and therefore no pregnancy. No other response is likely.

There is no concern over the possibility of the induction of congenital abnormalities during the first 2 weeks of pregnancy. Such a response has not been demonstrated in experimental animals or humans after any level of radiation dose.

The time from approximately the 2nd week to the 10th week of pregnancy is called the period of **major organogenesis.** During this time, the major organ systems of the fetus are developing. If the radiation dose is sufficient, congenital abnormalities may result.

Early in organogenesis, the most likely congenital abnormalities are associated with skeletal deformities. Later in this period, neurologic deficiencies are more likely to occur.

During the second and third trimesters of pregnancy, the responses previously noted are unlikely. The results of numerous investigations strongly suggest that if a response occurs after diagnostic irradiation during the latter two trimesters, the principal response would be the appearance of malignant disease during childhood.

These responses to irradiation during pregnancy require a very high radiation dose before there is significant risk of occurrence. No such responses would occur at less than 25 rad (250 mGy).

Such dose levels are highly unlikely, yet possible with patients who receive multiple x-ray examinations of the abdomen or pelvis. They are essentially impossible with radiologic technologists because their occupational exposures are so low. There are no other significant responses after irradiation in utero.

Dose Dependence. As one might imagine, virtually no information is available at the human level to construct dose–response relationships for irradiation in utero. There is, however, a large body of data from animal irradiation, particularly rats and mice, from which such relationships can be estimated. The statements that follow, although attributed to human exposure, represent estimates based on extrapolation from animal studies.

After an in utero radiation dose of 200 rad (2 Gy), it is nearly certain that each of the effects noted previously will occur. The likelihood is small, however, that an exposure of this magnitude would be experienced in diagnostic radiology.

Spontaneous abortion after irradiation during the first 2 weeks of pregnancy is unlikely at radiation doses less than 25 rad (250 mGy). The precise nature of the dose–response relationship is unknown, but a reasonable estimate of risk suggests that 0.1% of all conceptions would be resorbed after a dose of 10 rad (100 mGy).

The response at lower doses would be proportionately lower. Keep in mind, however, that the incidence of spontaneous abortion in the absence of radiation exposure is estimated to be in the 25% to 50% range.

In the absence of radiation exposure, approximately 5% of all live births exhibit a manifest congenital abnormality. A 1% increase in congenital abnormalities is estimated to follow a 10-rad (100-mGy) fetal dose, with a proportionately lower increase at lower doses.

The induction of a childhood malignancy after irradiation in utero is difficult to assess. Risk estimates are even lower than those reported for spontaneous abortion and congenital abnormalities. Our best approach to assessing risk of childhood malignancy is to use a relative risk estimate.

During the first trimester, the relative risk of radiation-induced childhood malignancy is in the range of 5 to 10; it drops to approximately 1.4 during the third trimester. The overall relative risk is accepted to be 1.5, a 50% increase over the naturally occurring incidence.

Pregnant Technologist

When a radiologic technologist becomes pregnant, she should notify her supervisor. The pregnancy then becomes **declared** and the DL becomes 0.5 mSv/mo (50 mrem/mo). The supervisor should then review her previous radiation exposure history because this aids in deciding what protective actions are necessary.

The DL for the fetus is 5 mSv (500 mrem) for the period of pregnancy, a dose level that most radiologic technologists will not reach regardless of pregnancy. Although some may receive doses that exceed 5 mSv/yr (500 mrem/yr), most receive less than 1 mSv/yr (100 mrem/yr).

This is usually indicated with the personnel monitoring device positioned at the collar above the protective apron. The exposure at the waist under the protective apron does not normally exceed 10% of these values, and therefore, under normal conditions, specific protective action is not necessary.

Most lead protective aprons are 0.5 mm lead equivalent. These provide approximately 90% attenuation at 75 kVp, which is sufficient. One millimeter lead equivalent protective aprons are available, but such thickness is not necessary, particularly in view of the additional weight of the apron. Back problems during pregnancy constitute a greater hazard than radiation exposure.

The length of the apron need not extend below the knees, but wraparound aprons are preferred during pregnancy. If necessary, a special effort should be made to provide an apron of proper size because of its weight.

 The pregnant radiologic technologist should be provided with a second personnel monitoring device.

An additional radiation monitor should be positioned under the protective apron at waist level. The exposure reported on this second monitor should be maintained on a separate record and identified as exposure to the fetus.

Do not allow the monitors to be switched and the record confused. Try color-coding—red for the collar badge (red neck!) and yellow for the waist badge (yellow belly!). Additional or thicker lead aprons are not normally necessary (Figure 38-4).

Experience with the use of such an additional monitor shows consistently that exposures to the fetus are insignificant. Suppose, for instance, that a pregnant radiologic technologist wearing a single radiation monitor at collar level receives 10 mSv (1000 mrem) during the 9-month period. The dose at waist level under a protec-

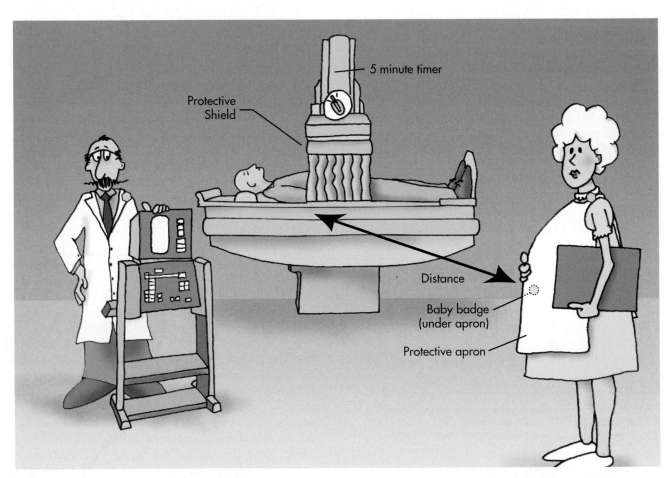

FIGURE 38-4 During fluoroscopy when pregnant, a second "baby monitor" should be positioned under the protective apron.

tive apron would be less than 10% of the collar dose, or 1 mSv (100 mrem).

Attenuation by the maternal tissues overlying the fetus reduces the dose to the fetus to approximately 30% of the abdominal skin dose, or 300 μSv (30 mrem). Consequently, when normal protective measures are taken, it is nearly impossible for a radiologic technologist to even approach the fetal DL of 5 mSv (500 mrem).

Management Principles

It should be clear that the probability of a harmful effect after any occupational radiation exposure received in diagnostic imaging is highly unlikely. A biologic response is very rarely expected and has not been observed in radiologic personnel for the past 50 years or so.

Nevertheless, it is essential for the director of radiology to incorporate three steps into the radiation protection program: new employee training, periodic in-service training, and counseling during pregnancy.

New Employee Training. The initial step for any administrative protocol dealing with pregnant employees involves orientation and training. During these orientation discussions, all female employees should be instructed as to their responsibility regarding pregnancy and radiation.

Each radiologic technologist should be provided with a copy of the facility radiation protection manual and other appropriate materials. This material might include a one-page summary of doses, responses, and proper radiation control working habits (Table 38-7).

The new employee should then read and sign a form (Figure 38-5) indicating that she has been instructed in this area of radiation protection. An important point to be made by signing this document is that the employee will voluntarily notify her supervisor when she is pregnant or suspects she is pregnant.

In-Service Training. Every well-run radiology service maintains a regular schedule of in-service training. Usually, this training is conducted at monthly intervals, but sometimes more often. At least twice each year such training should be devoted to radiation protection, and a portion of these sessions should be directed at the potentially pregnant employee.

The material to be covered in such sessions is outlined in Table 38-7. Although it is good to review doses and responses, it is probably more appropriate to emphasize radiation control procedures. These, of course, affect the radiation safety of all radiologic technologists, not just the pregnant technologist.

A review of personnel monitoring records is particularly important. A helpful procedure is to post the most recent radiation monitoring report for all to see. The year-end report should be initialed by each radiologic technologist, and the director of radiology should be sure that the technologists understand the nature and magnitude of their annual exposure.

Through such training, radiologic personnel will realize that their occupational exposure is minimal, usually less than 10% of the DL.

EMPHASIZE

The effective RDL is 50 mSv/yr (5000 mrem/yr)

Environmental background radiation is approximately 1 mSv/yr (100 mrem/yr)

Occupational exposures are closer to the latter than the former

Counseling During Pregnancy. The director of radiology takes the next action when the radiologic technologist declares her pregnancy. First, the director

TABLE 38-7	Pregnancy in Diagnostic Radiology
Human responses to low-level x-ray exposure	
Life span shortening	10 days/rad
Cataracts	None below 200 rad
Leukemia	10 cases/10^6/rad/yr
Cancer	2 cases/10^4/rad
Genetic effects	Doubling dose = 50 rad
Death from all causes	2 deaths/10^4/rad
Effects of irradiation in utero	
0–14 days	Spontaneous abortion: 25% natural incidence; 0.1% increase/10 rad
2–10 weeks	Congenital abnormalities: 5% natural incidence; 1% increase/10 rad
2nd–3rd trimester	Cell depletion: no effect at < 50 rad
	Latent malignancy: 4:10,000 natural incidence; 6:10,000/rad
0–9 months	Genetic effects: 10% natural incidence; 5×10^{-7} mutations/rad
Protective measures for the pregnant radiologic technologist	
Two occupational radiation monitors	
Dose limit: 5 mSv/9 mo, 0.5 mSv/mo	

> ### New Employee Notification
>
> This is to certify that _____ , a new employee of this radiologic facility, has received instructions regarding mutual responsibilities should she become pregnant during this employment.
>
> In addition to personal counseling by _____ , she has been given to read several documents dealing with pregnancy in diagnostic radiology. Furthermore, the additional reading material that follows is available in the departmental office:
>
> 1. *Review of NCRP radiation dose limit for embryo and fetus in occupationally-exposed women,* NCRP Report No 53, Washington, DC, 1977, National Council on Radiation Protection and Measures.
> 2. *Medical radiation exposure of pregnant and potentially pregnant women,* NCRP Report No 54, Washington, DC, 1977, National Council on Radiation Protection and Measures.
> 3. Wagner, LK et al: *Exposure of the pregnant patient to diagnostic radiation,* Philadelphia, 1985, JB Lippincott.
> 4. *The effects on populations of exposure to low levels of ionizing radiation,* Washington, DC, 1990, National Academy of Sciences.
>
> I understand that should I become pregnant and I decide to declare my pregnancy, it is my responsibility to inform my supervisor of my condition so that additional protective measures can be taken.
>
> _____   _____
> Supervisor   Employee
>
>
> _____
> Date

FIGURE 38-5 Form for new employee notification.

should counsel the employee, including a review of her radiation exposure history and any future modifications to her schedule that are appropriate.

 Under no circumstance should termination or involuntary leave of absence occur as a consequence of pregnancy.

In all likelihood, a review of the employee's previous radiation exposure history will show a low exposure profile. Those who wear the radiation monitor positioned at the collar, as recommended, and who are heavily involved in fluoroscopy, may receive an exposure greater than 5 mSv/yr (500 mrem/yr). Such employees, however, are protected by lead aprons so that exposure to the trunk of the body would not normally exceed 500 µSv (50 mrem per year).

This review of occupational radiation exposure is the appropriate time to emphasize that the DL during pregnancy is 5 mSv (500 mrem) and 0.5 mSv/mo (50 mrem/mo). Furthermore, it should be shown that this DL refers to the fetus and not to the radiologic technologist. The level of 5 mSv (500 mrem) to the fetus during gestation is considered an absolutely safe radiation exposure level.

In view of this discussion, the director of radiology should point out to the radiologic technologist that an alteration in her work schedule is not normally required.

For radiologic technologists involved in radiation oncology, nuclear medicine, or ultrasonography, a similar consultation and level of modification as previously discussed is appropriate. In radiation oncology, the pregnant technologist may continue her normal workload but should be advised not to participate in brachytherapy applications.

In nuclear medicine, the pregnant technologist should handle only small quantities of radioactive material. She should not elute radioisotope generators or inject millicurie quantities of radioactive material.

Ultrasound technologists are not normally classified as radiation workers. A sizable portion of ultrasound patients, however, are nuclear medicine patients, and therefore become a potential source of exposure to the

Acknowledgment of Radiation Risk During Pregnancy

I, _____ , do acknowledge that I have received counseling from _____ regarding my employment responsibilities during my pregnancy.

It is clear to me that there is a vanishingly small probability that my employment will in any way adversely affect my pregnancy. The reading material listed below has been made available to me to demonstrate that the additional risk during my pregnancy is much less than that for most occupational groups. I further understand that, although I may be assigned to low-exposure duties and provided with a second radiation monitor, these are simply added precautions and do not in any way convey that any assignment in this department is especially hazardous during pregnancy.

1. *Review of NCRP radiation dose limit for embryo and fetus in occupational-exposed women*, NCRP Report No 53, Washington, DC, 1977, National Council on Radiation Protection and Measures.
2. *Medical radiation exposure of pregnant and potentially pregnant women*, NCRP Report No 54, Washington, DC, 1977, National Council on Radiation Protection and Measures.
3. Wagner, LK et al: *Exposure of the pregnant patient to diagnostic radiation*, Philadelphia, 1985, JB Lippincott.
4. *The effects of populations of exposure to low levels of ionizing radiation*, Washington, DC, 1990, National Academy of Sciences.

_____
Supervisor

_____
Employee

_____
Date

FIGURE 38-6 Form for acknowledgment of radiation risk during pregnancy.

ultrasonographer. This is a remote risk because the quantity of radioactivity used is so low. It may be advisable during the pregnancy to provide the ultrasonographer with a radiation monitor.

Finally, the pregnant technologist should be required to read and sign a form (Figure 38-6) attesting to the fact that she has been given proper attention and that she understands that the level of risk associated with her employment is much less than that experienced by nearly all occupational groups.

The Pregnant Patient

Safeguards against accidental irradiation early in pregnancy present complex administrative problems. This situation is particularly critical during the first 2 months of pregnancy, when such a condition may not be suspected and when the fetus is particularly sensitive to radiation exposure. After 2 months, the risk of irradiating an unknown pregnancy becomes small because the patient is usually aware of her condition.

If the state of pregnancy is known, then under some circumstances the radiologic examination should not be conducted. One should never knowingly examine a pregnant patient with x-rays unless a documented decision to do so has been made. When such an examination does proceed, it should be conducted with all of the previously discussed techniques for minimizing patient dose.

When a pregnant patient must be examined, the examination should be done with precisely collimated beams and carefully positioned protective shields. The use of high kVp technique is most appropriate in such situations. The administrative protocols that can be used to ensure that we do not irradiate pregnant patients vary from complex (elective booking) to simple (posting).

Elective Booking. The most direct way to ensure against the irradiation of an unsuspected pregnancy is to institute **elective booking**. This requires that the clinician, radiologist, or radiologic technologist determine the time of the patient's previous menstrual cycle. X-ray examinations in which the fetus is not in or near the primary beam may be allowed, but they should be accompanied by pelvic shielding.

Ideally, the referring physician should be responsible for determining the menstrual cycle and for withholding the examination request if there is any question about

---

X-Ray Consent for Women of Childbearing Age

X-ray examinations of abdomen and pelvis exposing the uterus to radiation are:

Abdomen (KUB)	Colon (barium enema)	Pyelograms (IVP and retrograde)
Stomach (UGI)	Gallbladder	Cystograms
Small Intestine (SI)	Hips, sacrum, coccyx	Lumbar spine and pelvis
All nuclear medicine studies		

The 10 days after onset of menstural period are generally considered safe for x-ray examinations.

Onset of last menstural period   Date _____   Date today _____

I am pregnant	Yes _____	No _____	Don't know _____
I have had a hysterectomy	Yes _____	No _____	Don't know _____
I use an IUD	Yes _____	No _____	Don't know _____

I recognize that if I am pregnant and have radiation to the abdomen, there is a possibility of injury to the fetus. However, I understand that the likelihood of such injury is slight and that my physician feels that the information to be gained from this examination is important to my health. I therefore wish to have this x-ray examination performed now.

_____
Name of examination

_____
Signature of patient

_____
Witness

FIGURE 38-7 X-ray consent for women of childbearing age.

---

its necessity. This may require a radiologist-sponsored educational program that can be easily conducted at regularly scheduled medical staff meetings.

Patient Questionnaire. An alternative procedure is to have the patient herself indicate her menstrual cycle. In many radiology departments, the patient must complete an information form before examination.

These forms often include questions such as "Are you or could you be pregnant?" and "What was the date of your last menstrual period?" Figure 38-7 is an example of such a simple, yet effective questionnaire for protecting against irradiation of a pregnant patient.

Posting. If neither elective booking nor the request form seems appropriate to a radiology service, an equally successful method is to post signs of caution in the radiology waiting room. Such signs could read "Are you pregnant or could you be? If so, inform the radiologic technologist," or "Warning—special precautions are necessary if you are pregnant," or "Caution—if there is any possibility that you are pregnant, it is very important that you inform the radiologic technologist before you have an x-ray examination."

Figure 38-8 is a helpful poster available from the National Center for Devices and Radiological Health. Such posting satisfies our responsibility to the patient and to the health care facility.

It has been estimated that fewer than 1% of all women referred for x-ray examination are potentially pregnant. If a pregnant patient escapes detection and is irradiated, however, what is the subsequent responsibility of the radiology service to the patient, and what should be done?

The first step is to estimate the fetal dose. The medical physicist should be consulted immediately and requested to estimate the fetal dose. If a preliminary review of the examination techniques used (e.g., type of examination, kVp, and mAs) determines that the dose may have exceeded 1 rad (10 mGy$_t$), a more complete dosimetric evaluation should be conducted.

Table 38-8 presents representative radiation levels for many examinations. With a knowledge of the types of examinations performed and the techniques and apparatus used, the medical physicist can accurately determine the fetal dose. Test objects and dosimetry mate-

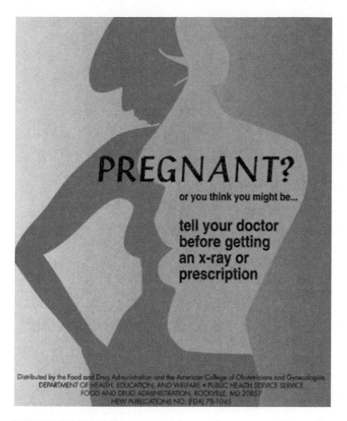

FIGURE 38-8 Wall posters with warnings concerning radiation and pregnancy are available from the National Center for Devices and Radiological Health. (Courtesy National Center for Devices and Radiological Health.)

Examination	Entrance Skin Exposure (mR)	Fetal Dose (mrad)
Skull (lateral)	70	0
Cervical spine (AP)	110	0
Shoulder	90	0
Chest (PA)	10	0
Thoracic spine (AP)	180	1
Cholecystogram (PA)	150	1
Lumbosacral spine (AP)*	250	80
Abdomen or KUB (AP)*	220	70
Intravenous pyelogram (IVP)*	210	60
Hip*	220	50
Wrist or foot	5	0

TABLE 38-8   Representative Entrance Exposures and Fetal Doses for Frequently Performed Radiographic Examinations with a 400-Speed Image Receptor

AP, Anteroposterior; *IVP*, intravenous pyelogram; *KUB*, kidneys, ureters, bladder; *PA*, posteroanterior.
*Gonadal shields should be used if possible.

rials are available to ensure that this determination can be made with confidence.

Once the fetal dose is known, the referring physician and radiologist should determine the stage of gestation at which the x-ray exposure occurred. With this information, there are only two alternatives: Allow the patient to continue to term or terminate the pregnancy.

Recommendation for abortion after diagnostic x-ray exposure is rarely indicated. Because the natural incidence of congenital anomalies is approximately 5%, no such effects can reasonably be considered a consequence of diagnostic x-ray doses. Manifest damage to the newborn is unlikely at fetal doses below 25 rad (250 mGy$_t$), although some suggest that lower doses may cause mental developmental abnormalities.

In view of the available evidence, a reasonable approach is to apply a 10- to 25-rad rule. Below 10 rad (100 mGy$_t$), a therapeutic abortion is not indicated unless there are additional risk factors involved. Above 25 rad (250 mGy$_t$), the risk of latent injury may justify a therapeutic abortion.

Between 10 and 25 rad, the precise time of irradiation, the emotional state of the patient, the effect an additional child would have on the family, and other social and economic factors must be carefully considered.

Fortunately, experience with such situations has shown that fetal doses have been consistently low. The fetal dose rarely exceeds 5 rad (50 mGy$_t$) after a series of x-ray examinations.

SUMMARY

Health physics is concerned with the research, teaching, and operational aspects of radiation exposure. The three cardinal principles developed for radiation workers are as follows: Minimize time of radiation exposure, maximize the distance from the radiation source, and include shielding to reduce radiation exposure. ALARA (as low as reasonably achievable) defines the principal concept of radiation protection.

DLs are prescribed by the NCRP for various organs, the whole body, and various working conditions so that the lifetime risk of each year's occupational exposure does not exceed 10^{-4} per year.

The NCRP recommends a cumulative whole-body DL of 10 mSv times one's age in years. The DL during pregnancy is 5 mSv. In diagnostic imaging, however, it is seldom necessary to exceed 1/10 the appropriate DL.

Occupational radiation exposure is measured in milliseiverts (millirems), and the description of such exposure is effective dose (E). Effective dose accounts for type of radiation and the relative radiosensitivity of tissues and organs.

The radiobiology of pregnancy requires particular attention to the pregnant radiologic technologist and the pregnant patient. The pregnant radiologic technologist should be provided with a second radiation monitoring device to be worn under the protective apron at waist level. Posting the waiting room and examination room with education signs meets our responsibility to the pregnant patient.

CHALLENGE QUESTIONS

1. Define or otherwise identify:
   a. Health physics
   b. TVL
   c. NCRP
   d. Effective dose
   e. ALARA
   f. Tissue weighting factor (W_r)
   g. Fetal DL
   h. Extremity monitor
   i. Major organogenesis
   j. Elective booking
2. Write the equation for the radiation dose as a function of time of exposure.
3. What is the function of the 5-minute reset timer on a fluoroscopy imaging system?
4. A fluoroscope emits 3.5 R/mA-minute at the table top for every mA of operation. What is the approximate patient entrance skin exposure (ESE) after a 3.2-minute fluoroscopic examination of 1.5 mA?
5. What are the three cardinal principles of radiation protection?
6. What does the value 10^{-4} yr^{-1} mean in regard to the NCRP recommended dose limits?
7. How do some radiation occupational groups such as nuclear medicine technologists monitor their extremity doses?
8. What is the whole-body occupational DL for radiography students younger than 18 years of age?
9. What is the embryo's response to irradiation above 25 rad during the first 2 weeks after conception?
10. During the fetal period of major organogenesis, what radiation responses are possible?
11. State the management protocol for the pregnant radiologic technologist.
12. What information regarding radiation protection should be covered in regularly scheduled in-service training classes?
13. What procedure should be followed if a patient is examined and subsequently discovers that she is pregnant?
14. The output intensity of a radiographic unit is 4.2 mR/mAs. What is the total output after a 200-ms exposure at 300 mA?
15. What is the approximate patient skin dose after a 3.2-minute fluoroscopic examination of 1.5 mA?
16. List five procedures that could result in a measurable fetal dose.
17. How can the three cardinal principles of radiation protection be best applied in diagnostic radiology?
18. What exposure will a radiologic technologist receive when exposed for 10 minutes at 4 m from a source with intensity of 100 mR/hr at 1 m while wearing a protective apron equivalent to 2 HVLs?
19. What wartime effort coined the term *health physicist*?
20. The collar-positioned monitor of a fluoroscopist records 0.9 mSv (90 mrem) during a month. This represents approximately what effective dose (E)?

Designing for Radiation Protection

OBJECTIVES

At the completion of this chapter, the student should be able to do the following:

1. Name the leakage radiation limit for x-ray tubes
2. List nine radiation protection features of a radiographic imaging system
3. List nine radiation protection features of a fluoroscopic imaging system
4. Discuss the design of primary and secondary radiation barriers
5. Describe the three types of radiation dosimeters used in diagnostic imaging

OUTLINE

The SID indicator must be accurate to within 2% of the indicated SID.

NUMBER OF features of modern x-ray imaging systems designed to improve radiographic quality were discussed in previous chapters. Many of these features are also designed to reduce patient dose during x-ray examinations. For instance, proper beam collimation contributes to improved image contrast and is also effective in reducing patient dose.

More than 100 individual radiation protection devices and accessories are associated with modern x-ray imaging systems. Some are characteristic of either radiographic or fluoroscopic imaging systems and some are mandated by federal regulation for all diagnostic x-ray imaging systems. A description of the devices required for all diagnostic x-ray imaging systems follows.

RADIOGRAPHIC PROTECTION FEATURES

Many radiation protection devices and accessories are associated with modern x-ray imaging systems. Two that are appropriate for all diagnostic x-ray imaging systems relate to the protective housing of the x-ray tube and to the control panel.

Protective X-Ray Tube Housing. Every x-ray tube must be contained within a protective housing that reduces leakage radiation during use.

Leakage radiation must be less than 100 mR/hr (1 mGy$_a$/hr) at a distance of 1 m from the protective housing.

Control Panel. The control panel must indicate the conditions of exposure and positively indicate when the x-ray tube is energized. These requirements are usually satisfied with kVp and mA indicators. Sometimes visible or audible signals indicate when the x-ray beam is energized.

X-ray beam-on must be positively and clearly indicated to the operator.

Source-to-Image Receptor Distance Indicator

A source-to-image receptor distance (SID) indicator must be provided. It can be as simple as a tape measure attached to the tube housing, or as advanced as lasers.

Collimation

Light-localized, variable-aperture rectangular collimators should be provided. Cones and diaphragms may replace the collimator for special examinations. The attenuation of the useful beam by the collimator shutters must be equivalent to that attenuated by the protective housing.

The x-ray beam and light beam must coincide to within 2% of the SID.

Question: Most radiographs are taken at an SID of 100 cm. How much difference is allowed between the projection of the light field and the x-ray beam at the image receptor?

Answer: 2% of 100 cm = 2 cm

Positive-Beam Limitation

Automatic, light-localized, variable-aperture collimators were required on all but special x-ray imaging systems manufactured in the United States between 1974 and 1994. These positive-beam-limiting (PBL) devices are no longer required but continue to be a part of most new radiographic imaging systems. They must be adjusted so that with any film size in use and at all standard SIDs the collimator shutters automatically provide an x-ray beam equal to the image receptor.

The PBL must be accurate to within 2% of the SID.

Beam Alignment

In addition to proper collimation, each radiographic tube should be provided with a mechanism to ensure proper alignment of the x-ray beam and the image receptor. It does no good to align the light field and the x-ray beam if the image receptor is not also aligned.

Filtration

All general-purpose diagnostic x-ray beams must have a total filtration (inherent plus added) of at least 2.5 mm Al when operated above 70 kVp. Radiographic tubes operated between 50 and 70 kVp must have at least 1.5 mm Al. Below 50 kVp, a minimum of 0.5 mm Al total filtration is required. X-ray tubes designed for mammography usually have 30 μm Mo or 60 μm Rh filtration.

As was discussed in Chapter 31, it is not normally possible physically to examine and measure the thickness of each component of total filtration. An accurate measurement of half-value layer (HVL) is sufficient. If the HVL is equal to or greater than the value given in Table 31-3 at the various kVps, total filtration is adequate.

Question: The following data are obtained on a three-phase radiographic imaging system operating at 70 kVp, 100 mA, 100 ms. Is the filtration adequate?

Added filtration (mm Al)	0	0.5	1.0	1.5	2.0	3.0	4.0	5.0
Exposure (mR)	87	74	65	56	49	39	31	25

Answer: A plot of these data indicates an HVL of 2.5 mm Al. Table 31-3 shows that at 70 kVp, an HVL of 2.2 mm Al or greater is sufficient. The filtration is adequate.

Reproducibility

For any given radiographic technique, the output radiation intensity should be constant from one exposure to another. This is checked by making repeated exposures at the same technique and observing the average variation in radiation intensity.

 The variation in x-ray exposure should not exceed 5%.

Linearity

When adjacent mA stations are used, for example, 100 mA and 200 mA, and exposure time is adjusted for constant mAs, the output radiation intensity should remain constant. When the exposure time remains constant, causing the mAs to increase in proportion to the increase in mA, radiation intensity should be proportional to mAs.

 The maximum acceptable variation in linearity is 10% from one mA station to an adjacent mA station.

This takes any inaccuracy in the exposure timer out of the analysis. The radiation intensity is expressed in units of mR/mAs (mGy_a/mAs).

Operator Shield

It must not be possible to expose an image receptor while the radiologic technologist stands outside a fixed protective barrier, usually the console booth. The exposure control should be fixed to the operating console and not to a long cord. The radiologic technologist may be in the examination room during exposure, but only if protective apparel is worn.

Mobile X-Ray Imaging System

A protective lead apron should be assigned to each mobile x-ray imaging system. The exposure switch of such an imaging system must allow the operator to remain at least 2 m from the x-ray tube during exposure. Of course, the useful beam must be directed away from the radiologic technologist while positioned at this minimum distance.

FLUOROSCOPIC PROTECTION FEATURES

The features of fluoroscopic imaging systems that follow are primarily intended to reduce patient and personnel exposure.

Source-to-Skin Distance

One would think that increasing the distance between any x-ray tube and the patient would result in reduced patient dose because of the increased distance. This is true, but to maintain the exposure to the image intensifier, the mA needs to be increased to compensate for the increased distance. Because of the divergence of the x-ray beam, the entrance skin exposure (ESE) is less for the required exit exposure as the source-to-skin distance (SSD) is increased.

 The SSD must be not less than 38 cm on stationary fluoroscopes and not less than 30 cm on mobile fluoroscopes.

Review Figure 39-1, where a 20-cm abdomen is 5 HVLs thick. If the fluoroscopic x-ray tube is moved from 40 cm SSD to 20 cm SSD, there is a great increase in ESE. The exposure required at the image intensifier is 1 mR.

The ESEs will be 2.25 mR and 4.0 mR, respectively, solely because of the divergence of the x-ray beam—the inverse square law. Add the x-ray attenuation of 5 HVLs for each geometry, and the respective ESEs become 72 mR and 128 mR.

Primary Protective Barrier

The image intensifier assembly serves as a primary protective barrier and must be 2 mm Pb equivalent. It must be coupled with the x-ray tube and interlocked so that the fluoroscopic x-ray tube cannot be energized when the image intensifier is in the parked position.

Filtration

The total filtration of the fluoroscopic x-ray beam must be at least 2.5 mm Al equivalent. The tabletop, patient cradle, or other material positioned between the x-ray tube and the tabletop are included as part of the total filtration. When the filtration is unknown, the HVL should be measured. The minimum HVL reported in Table 31-3 must be met so that adequate filtration can be assumed.

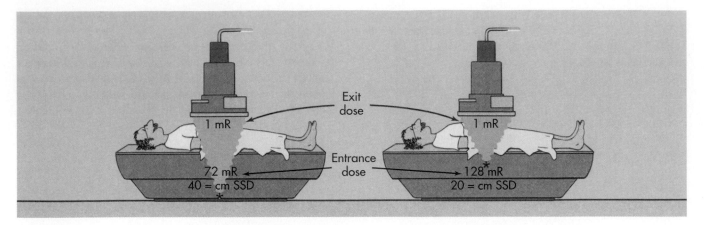

FIGURE 39-1 Patient entrance skin exposure (ESE) is higher when the fluoroscopic x-ray tube is too close to the tabletop.

Collimation

The fluoroscopic x-ray beam collimators must be adjusted so that an unexposed border is visible on the image monitor when the input phosphor of the image intensifier is positioned 35 cm above the tabletop and the collimators are fully open. For automatic collimating devices, such an unexposed border should be visible at all heights above the tabletop. The collimator shutters should track with height above the tabletop.

Exposure Control

The fluoroscopic exposure control should be of the dead-man type; that is, if the operator should drop dead, the exposure would be terminated—unless, of course, he or she falls on the switch! The conventional foot pedal or pressure switch on the image intensifier tower satisfies this condition.

Bucky Slot Cover

During fluoroscopy, the Bucky tray is moved to the end of the examining table, leaving an opening in the side of the table approximately 5 cm wide at gonadal level. This opening should automatically be covered with at least 0.25 mm Pb equivalent.

Protective Curtain

A protective curtain or panel of at least 0.25 mm Pb equivalent should be positioned between the fluoroscopist and the patient. Figure 39-2 shows the typical isoexposure distribution for a fluoroscope. Without the curtain and Bucky slot cover, the exposure of radiology personnel is many times higher.

Cumulative Timer

A cumulative timer that produces an audible signal when the fluoroscopic time has exceeded 5 minutes must be provided. This device is designed to make sure

the radiologist is aware of the relative beam-on time during each procedure. The assisting radiologic technologist should record total fluoroscopy beam-on time for each examination.

Dose Area Product

The intensity of the x-ray beam at the tabletop of a fluoroscope should not exceed 2.1 R/min (21 mGy$_a$/min) for each mA of operation at 80 kVp. If there is no optional high-level control, the intensity must not exceed 10 R/min (100 mGy$_a$/min) during fluoroscopy. If an optional *high-level control* is provided, the maximum tabletop intensity allowed is *20 R/min (200 mGy$_a$/min)*. There is no limit on x-ray intensity when the image is recorded, as in cineradiography or videography.

The overall carcinogenic risk to a patient depends on radiation dose and the volume of tissue exposed. Dose refers to the energy deposited locally and is the quantity that best reflects the potential for injury to that tissue. It does not depend on the area exposed.

Dose area product (DAP) is a quantity that reflects not only dose but also the volume of tissue irradiated, and therefore may be a better indicator of risk than dose. DAP is expressed in R-cm^2 (cGy-cm^2).

DAP increases with increasing field size even if the dose remains unchanged. Smaller field size results in lower DAP, and thus less risk because a smaller amount of tissue is exposed.

DAP may be used to monitor radiation output from radiographic and fluoroscopic imaging systems. DAP meters are becoming more common on x-ray imaging systems. Typically, the device is placed near the x-ray source beyond the collimator and before the beam enters the patient. To obtain a measure of the risk for injury to the skin where the beam enters the patient, dose can be derived by dividing the DAP measurement by the area of the beam at the skin. Using DAP to monitor radiation

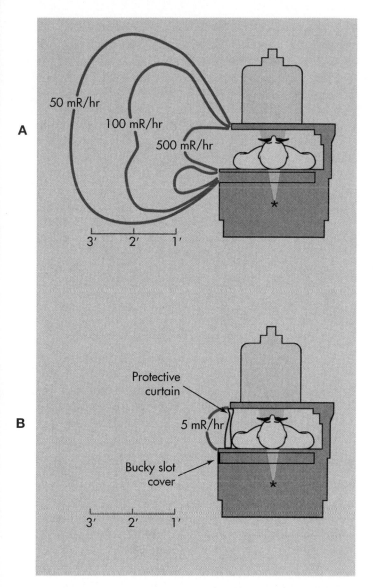

FIGURE 39-2 **A,** Isoexposure profile for an unshielded fluoroscope demonstrates need for protective curtains and Bucky slot covers. **B,** Exposure profile with these protective devices.

usage is a good way to implement radiation management procedures and keep patient exposures low.

DESIGN OF PROTECTIVE BARRIERS

In designing a radiology department or an individual x-ray examination room, it is not sufficient to consider only general architectural characteristics. Great attention must be given to the location of the x-ray imaging system in the examination room.

The use of adjoining rooms is also of great importance when designing for radiation safety. It is often necessary to insert protective barriers, usually sheets of lead, in the walls of x-ray examination rooms. If the radiology facility is located on an upper floor, then it may be necessary to shield the floor as well.

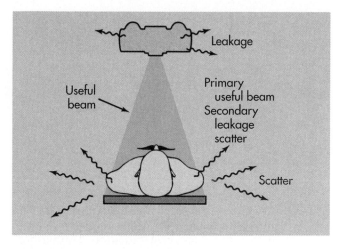

FIGURE 39-3 Three types of radiation—the useful beam, leakage radiation, and scatter radiation—must be considered in designing the protective barriers of an x-ray room.

A great number of factors are considered when designing a protective barrier. This discussion touches only on the fundamentals and some basic definitions. Whenever new x-ray facilities are being designed or old ones renovated, a medical physicist must be consulted for assistance in designing proper radiation shielding.

Type of Radiation

For the purpose of protective barrier design, three types of radiation are considered (Figure 39-3). Primary radiation is the most intense, and therefore the most hazardous and the most difficult to shield.

When a chest board is positioned on a given wall, it is sometimes necessary to provide shielding directly behind the chest board in addition to that specified for the rest of the wall. Any wall to which the useful beam can be directed is designated a **primary protective barrier.**

 Primary radiation is the useful beam.

Lead bonded to sheet rock or wood paneling is most often used as a primary protective barrier. Such lead shielding is available in various thicknesses and it is specified for architects and contractors in units of pounds per square foot (lb/ft²).

Concrete, concrete block, or brick may be used instead of lead. As a rule of thumb, 4 inches of masonry is equivalent to 1/16 inch of lead. Table 39-1 shows available lead thicknesses and equivalent thicknesses of concrete.

There are two types of secondary radiation: **scatter radiation** and **leakage radiation.** Scatter radiation results when the useful beam intercepts any object, causing

TABLE 39-1	Lead and Concrete Equivalents for Primary Protective Barriers				
LEAD			**CONCRETE**		
(mm)	(in)	(lb/ft²)	(cm)	(in)	
0.4	1/64	1	2.4	1 3/8	
0.8	1/32	2	4.8	1 7/8	
1.2	3/64	3	7.2	2 7/8	
1.6	1/16	4	9.6	3 3/4	

TABLE 39-2	Equivalent Material Thicknesses for Secondary Barriers				
	SUBSTITUTES				
Computed Lead Required	Steel (mm)	Glass (mm)	Gypsum (mm)	Wood (mm)	
0.1	0.5	1.2	2.8	19	
0.2	1.2	2.5	5.9	33	
0.3	1.8	3.7	8.8	44	
0.4	2.5	4.8	12	53	

some x-rays to be scattered. For the purpose of protective shielding calculations, the scattering object can be considered as a new source of radiation. During both radiography and fluoroscopy, the patient is the single most important scattering object.

 The intensity of scatter radiation 1 m from the patient is approximately 0.1% of the intensity of the useful beam at the patient.

Question: The patient ESE is 410 mR (4.1 mGy$_a$) for a kidney, ureter, and bladder (KUB) examination. What will be the approximate radiation exposure 1 m from the patient? At 3 m from the patient?

Answer: At 1 m: 410 mR × 0.1% = 410 mR × 0.001

$$= 0.41 \text{ mR} = 410 \ \mu\text{R}$$

At 3 m: $= 0.41 \text{ mR} = (1/3)^2$
$= 0.41 \text{ mR} (1/9)$
$= 0.036 \text{ mR} = 36 \ \mu\text{R}$

Leakage radiation is that radiation emitted from the x-ray tube housing in all directions other than that of the useful beam. If the x-ray tube housing is properly designed, the leakage radiation will never exceed the regulatory limit of 100 mR/hr (1 mGy$_a$/hr) at 1 m. Although in practice, leakage radiation levels are much less than this limit, 100 mR/hr at 1 m is used for barrier calculations.

Barriers designed to shield areas from secondary radiation are called **secondary protective barriers.** Secondary protective barriers are always less thick than primary protective barriers.

Often, lead is not required for secondary protective barriers because the computation usually results in less than 0.4 mm Pb. In such cases, conventional gypsum board, glass, or lead acrylic is adequate.

Many walls that are secondary protective barriers can be adequately protected with four thicknesses of 5/8-inch gypsum board. Operating console barriers are secondary protective barriers—the useful beam is never directed at the operating console booth. Four thicknesses of gypsum

board and ½-inch plate glass may be all that is necessary. Sometimes glass walls ½ to 1 inch thick can be used for control booth barriers. Table 39-2 gives equivalent thicknesses for secondary protective barrier materials.

Question: What percentage of the recommended dose limit (100 mrem/wk) will be incident on a control booth barrier located 3 m from the x-ray tube and patient? Assume the x-ray output is 3 mR/mAs and that the weekly beam-on time is 5 minutes at an average 100 mA, a generous assumption.

Answer: *From scatter radiation, the barrier will receive:*
Total primary beam = 3 mR/mAs × 10 mA × 5 min × 60 s/min
= 90,000 mR
Scatter radiation = 90,000 mR × 1/1000 × $(1/3)^2$
= 10 mR
From leakage radiation, the barrier will receive:
Leakage radiation at 1 m = 100 mR/hr × 5/60 hr = 8.3 mR
Leakage radiation = 8.3 mR $(1/3)^2$
= 0.9 mR
Total secondary radiation = 10 mR + 0.9 mR
= 10.9 mR or 11% of the recommended dose limit

This analysis is representative of the clinical environment. The estimated exposure is to the control booth barrier, not to the radiologic technologist. The composition of the barrier and the additional distance will reduce technologist exposure even more. This is the reason that personnel radiation exposure during radiography is very low.

 Radiologic technologists receive most of their occupational radiation exposure during fluoroscopy.

Factors Affecting Barrier Thickness

Many factors must be taken into consideration when calculating the required protective barrier thickness. A thorough discussion of these factors is beyond the scope of this book; however, a definition of each is useful for understanding the problems involved.

Distance. The thickness of a barrier naturally depends on the distance between the source of radiation and the barrier. The distance is that to the adjacent occupied area, not to the inside of the wall of the x-ray room.

A wall along which an x-ray imaging system is positioned probably requires more shielding than the other walls of the room. In such case, the leakage radiation may be more hazardous than the scatter radiation or even the useful beam. It may be desirable to position the x-ray imaging system in the middle of the room because then no single wall is subjected to especially intense radiation exposure.

Occupancy. The use of the area being protected is of principal importance. If the area were a rarely occupied closet or storeroom, the required shielding would be less than if it were an office or laboratory occupied 40 hours per week.

This concept reflects the **time of occupancy factor (T)**. Table 39-3 reports the occupancy levels of various areas as suggested by the National Council on Radiation Protection and Measurements (NCRP).

Control. An area occupied primarily by radiology personnel and patients is called a **controlled area**. The design limits for a controlled area are based on the proportionate weekly exposure, and therefore require that the barrier reduce the exposure to a worker in the area to less than 100 mrem (1 mSv/wk).

Design limits for a controlled area are based on the annual recommended dose limit of 5000 mrem/yr (50 mSv/yr).

An **uncontrolled area** can be occupied by anyone, and therefore the maximum exposure rate allowed is based on the recommended dose limit for the public of 100 mrem/yr (1 mSv/yr). This is equivalent to 2 mrem/wk (20 μSv/wk), which is the design limit for an uncontrolled area. Furthermore, the protective barrier should ensure that no individual will receive more than 2.5 mrem (25 μSv) in any one hour.

Workload. The shielding required for an x-ray examination room depends on the level of radiation activity in that room. The greater the number of examinations performed each week, the thicker the shielding required.

This characteristic is called **workload (W)** and has units of milliampere-minutes per week (mAmin/wk). A busy, general-purpose x-ray room may have a workload

TABLE 39-3	Levels of Occupancy of Areas That May be Adjacent to X-Ray Rooms, as Suggested by the NCRP
Occupancy	**Area**
Full	Work areas (e.g., offices, laboratories, shops, wards, nurses' stations), living quarters, children's play areas, occupied space in nearby buildings
Frequent	Corridors, restrooms, patient rooms
Occasional	Waiting rooms, stairways, unattended elevators, janitors' closets, outside area

of 500 mAmin/wk. Rooms in private offices have workloads of less than 100 mAmin/wk.

Question: The plans for a community hospital call for two x-ray examination rooms. The estimated patient load for each room is 15 patients per day, and each patient will average 3 films taken at 80 kVp, 70 mAs. What is the projected workload of each room?

Answer: 15 patients/day × 5 days/wk =

$$75 \text{ patients/wk}$$
$$75 \text{ patients/wk} \times 3 \text{ films/pt} = 225 \text{ films/wk}$$
$$225 \text{ films/wk} \times 70 \text{ mAs/film} =$$
$$1,5750 \text{ mAs/wk}$$
$$15,750 \text{ mAs/wk} \times \frac{1 \text{ min}}{60 \text{ s}} = 262.5 \text{ mAmin/wk}$$

For combination radiographic/fluoroscopic imaging systems, usually only the radiographic workload need be considered for barrier calculations. When the fluoroscopic x-ray tube is energized, a primary protection barrier in the form of the fluoroscopic screen always intercepts the useful x-ray beam. Consequently, the primary barrier requirements are always much less for fluoroscopic x-ray beams than for radiographic x-ray beams.

Use Factor. The percentage of time during which the x-ray beam is on and directed toward a particular wall is called the **use factor (U)** for that wall. The NCRP recommends that walls be assigned a use factor of ¼ and the floor a use factor of 1.

Studies have shown these recommendations to be high, and therefore very conservative. Many medical physicists suggest that primary barriers in fact do not exist. All barriers are secondary because the useful beam is always intercepted by the patient and the image receptor.

If an x-ray room has a special design, other use factors may be assigned. A room designed strictly for chest

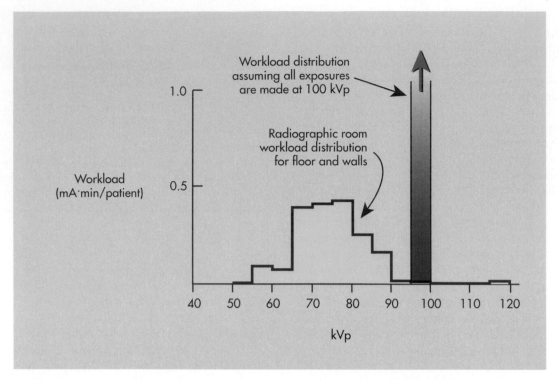

FIGURE 39-4 Workload distribution of clinical voltage.

radiography has one wall with a use factor of 1. All others have a use factor of zero for primary radiation, and thus would be considered secondary radiation barriers.

The ceiling is nearly always considered a secondary protective barrier. For a secondary barrier, leakage and scatter radiation are present 100% of the time that the x-ray tube is energized.

 The use factor for secondary barriers is always 1.

kVp. The final consideration in the design of an x-ray protective barrier is the penetrability of the x-ray beam. For protective barrier calculations, kVp is used as the measure of penetrability. Most modern x-ray imaging systems are designed to operate at up to 150 kVp. Most examinations, however, are conducted at an average of 75 kVp.

Usually, constant operation is assumed at a kVp greater than that actually used: 100 kVp for general radiography, 30 kVp for mammography. Therefore, it is more likely for the protective barrier to be too thick than too thin.

Alternatively, a workload distribution such as those shown in Figure 39-4 may be used. Workload distribution results in a more precise determination of required barrier thickness, but it is a considerably more difficult computation.

Measurements of radiation exposure outside the x-ray examination room always result in radiation levels far less than that anticipated by calculation. The total beam-on time is always less than that assumed. The average kVp is usually closer to 75 kVp than to 100 kVp.

The calculations do not account for the fact that the patient and image receptor always intercept the useful beam. Therefore, although the calculations are intended to result in a dose limit of 100 mrem/wk or 2 mrem/wk outside the x-ray room, rarely will the actual exposure exceed 1/10 of those dose limits. To confirm this for yourself, keep records for 1 week of kVp, mAs, and beam direction.

RADIATION DETECTION AND MEASUREMENT

Instruments are designed to detect radiation or to measure radiation, or to do both. Those designed for detection usually operate in the **pulse** or **rate** mode and are used to indicate the presence of radiation. In the pulse mode, the presence of radiation is indicated by a ticking, chirping, or beeping sound. In the rate mode, the instrument response is in mR/hr or R/hr.

Instruments designed to measure the intensity of radiation usually operate in the **integrate** mode. They accumulate the signal and respond with a total exposure (mR or R). Such application is called **dosimetry,** and the radiation measuring devices are called **dosimeters.**

TABLE 39-4	Radiation Detection and Measuring Device Characteristics and Uses
Device	**Characteristics—Uses**
Photographic emulsion	Limited range, sensitive, energy dependent—personnel monitoring, imaging
Ionization chamber	Wide range, accurate, portable—survey for radiation levels >1 mR/hr
Proportional counter	Laboratory instrument, accurate, sensitive—assay of small quantities of radionuclides
Geiger-Muller counter	Limited to <100 mR/hr, portable—survey for low radiation levels and radioactive contamination
Optically stimulated dosimetry	Wide range, accurate, sensitive—newest personnel monitoring device
Thermoluminescence dosimetry	Wide range, accurate, sensitive—personnel monitoring, stationary area monitoring
Scintillation detection	Limited range, very sensitive, stationary or portable instruments—photon spectroscopy, imaging

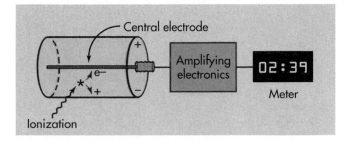

FIGURE 39-5 The ideal gas-filled detector consists of a cylinder of gas and a central collecting electrode. When a voltage is maintained between the central electrode and the wall of the chamber, electrons produced in ionization can be collected and measured.

era, an imaging device used in nuclear medicine, and it is also used in most computed tomography (CT) imaging systems.

Gas-Filled Detectors

Three types of gas-filled radiation detectors exist: ionization chambers, proportional counters, and Geiger-Muller detectors. Although they are different in response characteristics, each is based on the same principle of operation. As radiation passes through gas, it ionizes atoms of the gas. The electrons released in ionization are detected as an electrical signal proportional to the radiation intensity.

 The ionization of gas is the basis for gas-filled radiation detectors.

The earliest radiation detection device was the photographic emulsion, and it is still a primary means of radiation detection and measurement. However, other devices have been developed that have more favorable characteristics than the photographic emulsion for some applications. Table 39-4 lists most of the currently available radiation detection and measurement devices, along with some of their principal characteristics and uses.

It is apparent that film has two principal applications in diagnostic radiology: the making of a radiograph and the personnel radiation monitor (film badge). The photographic process was discussed in Chapters 13 and 14. Use of film as a radiation monitor is covered in Chapter 40.

Four other types of radiation detection devices are of particular importance in diagnostic radiology. The gas-filled radiation detector is used widely as a device to measure radiation intensity and to detect radioactive contamination. Thermoluminescence dosimetry (TLD) and optically stimulated dosimetry (OSL) are used for both patient and personnel radiation monitoring. Scintillation detection is the basis for the gamma cam-

Consider an ideal gas-filled detector as shown schematically in Figure 39-5. It consists of a cylinder filled with air or any of a number of other gases.

Along the central axis of the cylinder is positioned a rigid wire called the **central electrode.** If a voltage difference is impressed between the central electrode and the wall such that the wire is positive and the wall negative, then any electrons liberated in the chamber by ionization will be attracted to the central electrode.

These electrons form an electric signal, either as a pulse of electrons or as a continuous current. This electric signal is then amplified and measured. Its intensity is proportional to the radiation intensity that caused it.

In general, the larger the chamber, the more gas molecules there are available for ionization, and therefore the more sensitive the instrument. Similarly, if the chamber is pressurized, then more molecules are available for ionization and even higher sensitivity results.

 A high sensitivity means that an instrument can detect very low radiation intensities.

Sensitivity is not the same as **accuracy.** A high accuracy means that an instrument can detect and **precisely measure** the intensity of a radiation field. Instrument accuracy is controlled by the overall electronic design of the device.

Region of Recombination. If the voltage across the chamber of the ideal gas-filled detector is slowly increased from zero to a high level, the resulting electric signal in the presence of a fixed radiation level will increase in stages (Figure 39-6). In the first stage, when the voltage is very low, no electrons are attracted to the central electrode. The ion pairs produced in the chamber recombine. This is known as the **region of recombination,** shown as stage *R* in Figure 39-6.

Ion Chamber Region. As the chamber voltage is increased, a condition is reached where every electron released by ionization is attracted to the central electrode and collected. The voltage at which this occurs varies according to the design of the chamber, but for most conventional instruments it is in the range of 100 to 300 V.

This portion of the gas-filled detector performance curve is known as the **ionization region,** indicated by *I* in the Figure 39-6. Ion chambers are operated in this region.

A number of different types of ion chambers are used in radiology, the most familiar being the portable survey instrument (Figure 39-7). This instrument is used principally for area radiation surveys. It can measure a wide range of radiation intensities, from 1 mR/hr (10 μGy$_a$/hr) to several thousand R/hr (Gy$_a$/hr).

The ion chamber is the instrument of choice for measuring the radiation intensity in areas around a fluoroscope, around radionuclide generators and syringes, in the vicinity of patients containing therapeutic quantities of radioactive materials, and outside of protective barriers.

There are other, more accurate, ion chambers, which are used for the precise calibration of the output intensity of diagnostic x-ray imaging systems (Figure 39-8).

Another application of a precision ion chamber is the dose calibrator (Figure 39-9). These devices find daily use in nuclear medicine laboratories for the assay of radioactive material.

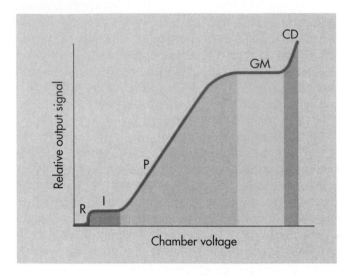

FIGURE 39-6 The amplitude of the signal from a gas-filled detector increases in stages as the voltage across the chamber is increased.

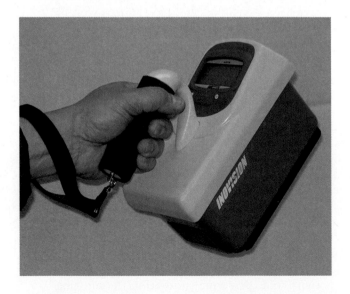

FIGURE 39-7 This portable ion chamber survey instrument is useful for radiation surveys when exposure levels are in excess of 1 mR/hr. (Courtesy Cardinal Health, Inc.)

Proportional Region. As the chamber voltage of the ideal gas-filled detector is increased still farther above the ionization region, electrons of the filling gas released by primary ionization are accelerated more rapidly to the central electrode. The faster these electrons travel, the higher the probability that they will cause additional ionization on their way to the central electrode. These additional ionizations result in additional electrons called **secondary electrons.**

These secondary electrons are also attracted to the central electrode and collected. The total number of electrons collected in this fashion increases with increasing chamber voltage. The result is a rather large electron pulse for each primary ionization. This stage of the voltage response curve is known as the **proportional region.**

Proportional counters are sensitive instruments that are used primarily as stationary laboratory instruments for the assay of small quantities of radioactivity. There are some portable survey instruments that operate in the proportional region, but these are usually used to detect only alpha and beta radiation.

One characteristic of proportional counters that makes them particularly useful is their ability to distinguish between alpha and beta radiation. Nevertheless, proportional counters find little applications in clinical radiology.

Geiger-Muller Region. The fourth region of the voltage response curve for the ideal gas-filled chamber is the **Geiger-Muller (G-M) region.** This is the region in which Geiger counters operate.

In the G-M region, the voltage across the ionization chamber is sufficiently high that, when a single ionizing event occurs, a cascade of secondary electrons is produced in a fashion similar to a very brief, yet violent, chain reaction. The effect is that nearly all the molecules of the gas are ionized, liberating a large number of electrons. This results in a large electron pulse.

When sequential ionizing events occur soon after one another, the detector may not be capable of responding to a second event if the filling gas has not been restored to its initial condition. Therefore, a **quenching agent** is added to the filling gas of the Geiger counter to enable the chamber to return to its original condition; subsequent ionizing events can then be detected. The minimum time between ionizations that can be detected is known as the **resolving time.**

Geiger counters are used for contamination control in nuclear medicine laboratories. As portable survey instruments, they are used to detect the presence of

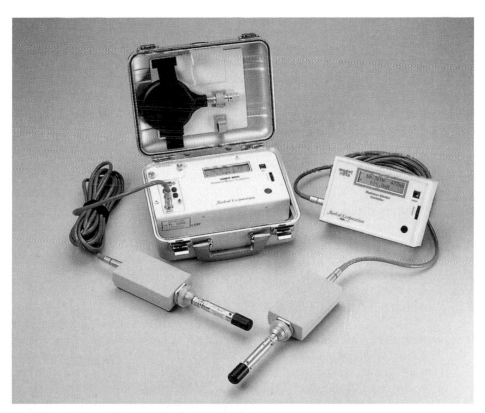

FIGURE 39-8 This ion chamber dosimeter is used for accurate measurement of diagnostic x-ray beams. (Courtesy Radcal Corp.)

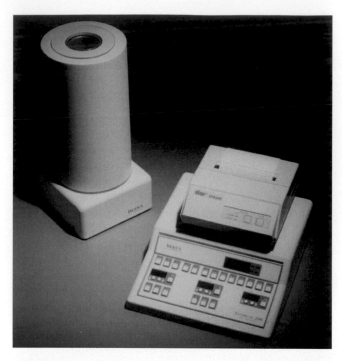

FIGURE 39-9 This configuration of an ion chamber is called a *dose calibrator*. It is used in nuclear medicine to measure accurately quantities of radioactive material. (Courtesy Biodex Medical Systems, Inc.)

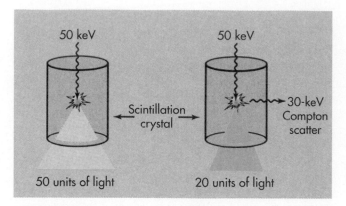

FIGURE 39-10 During scintillation, the intensity of light emitted is proportional to the amount of energy absorbed in the crystal.

radioactive contamination on work surfaces and laboratory apparatus.

They are not particularly useful as dosimeters because they are difficult to calibrate for varying conditions of radiation. Geiger counters are sensitive instruments capable of detecting and indicating single ionizing events. If equipped with an audio amplifier and speaker, one can even hear the crackle of individual ionizations.

The Geiger counter does not have a very wide range. Most instruments are limited to less than 100 mR/hr (1 mGy$_a$/hr).

Region of Continuous Charge. If the voltage across the gas-filled chamber is increased still further, a condition is reached whereby a single ionizing event completely discharges the chamber, as in operation in the G-M region. Because of the high voltage, however, electrons continue to be stripped from atoms of the filling gas, producing a continuous current or signal from the chamber.

In this condition of continuous discharge, the instrument is useless for the detection of radiation, and continued operation in this region results in damage. The region of continuous discharge is indicated as *CD* in Figure 39-5.

Scintillation Detectors

Scintillation detectors are used in several areas of radiologic science. The scintillation detector is the basis for the gamma camera in nuclear medicine and is used in the detector arrays of most CT imaging systems.

The Scintillation Process. Certain types of material scintillate when irradiated; that is, they emit a flash of light immediately in response to absorption of an x-ray. The amount of light emitted is proportional to the amount of energy absorbed by the material.

Consider, for example, the two x-ray interactions diagrammed in Figure 39-10. If a 50-keV x-ray interacts photoelectrically in the crystal, all the energy (50 keV) would reappear as light. If, however, that same x-ray interacts by a Compton scattering event in which only 20 keV of energy was absorbed, then a proportionately lower quantity of light would be emitted in the scintillation.

Only those materials with a particular crystalline structure scintillate. At the atomic level, the process involves the rearrangement of valence electrons into traps. The return of the electron from the trap to its normal position is immediate in scintillation and delayed in luminescence. This property was considered under an earlier discussion of luminescence (Chapter 15).

Types of Scintillation Phosphors. Many different types of liquids, gases, and solids can respond to ionizing radiation by scintillation. Scintillation detectors are most often used to indicate individual ionizing events and are incorporated into either fixed or portable radiation detection devices. They can be used to measure radiation either in the rate mode or integrate mode.

Nearly all the noble gases can be made to respond to radiation by scintillation. Such applications are rare, however, because the detection efficiency is very low and the probability of interaction therefore is small.

Liquid scintillation detectors are frequently used in the research laboratory to detect the low-energy beta emissions from carbon-14 (^{14}C) and tritium (^{3}H). Because they present a relatively harmless radiation hazard and are easily incorporated into biologic molecules, ^{14}C and ^{3}H are useful research radionuclides.

These radionuclides emit low-energy beta particles with no associated gamma rays. This makes them hard to detect. With liquid scintillation counting, however, the biologic molecules can be mixed with a liquid scintillation phosphor so that the beta emission interacts directly with the phosphor, causing a flash of light to be emitted. Liquid scintillation counters have nearly 100% detection efficiency for beta radiation.

By far the most widely used scintillation phosphors are the inorganic crystals—thallium-activated sodium iodide (NaI:Tl) or thallium-activated cesium iodide (CsI:Tl). The **activator atoms** of thallium are impurities grown into the crystal to control the spectrum of the light emitted and to enhance its intensity.

The NaI:Tl crystals are incorporated into gamma cameras; CsI:Tl is the phosphor incorporated into image-intensifier tubes as the input phosphor. Both types of crystals have been incorporated into CT imaging system detector arrays. However, many of today's CT imaging systems use cadmium tungstate ($CdWO_4$) or a ceramic as the scintillation detector.

The Scintillation Detector Assembly. Light produced during scintillation is emitted isotropically, that is, with equal intensity in all directions. Consequently, when used as radiation detectors, scintillation crystals are enclosed in aluminum with a polished inner surface in contact with the crystal. This allows the light flash to be reflected internally to the one face of a crystal that is not enclosed, called the **window.**

The aluminum containment is also necessary to seal the crystal hermetically. A **hermetic seal** is one that prevents the crystal from coming into contact with air or moisture. This is necessary because many scintillation crystals are **hygroscopic;** that is, they absorb moisture. When moisture is absorbed, the crystals swell and crack. Cracked crystals are not useful because the crack produces an interface that reflects and attenuates the scintillation.

Figure 39-11 shows the basic components of a single crystal–photomultiplier (PM) tube assembly representative of the type used in a portable survey instrument. The detector portion of the assembly is the NaI:Tl crystal contained in the aluminum hermetic seal. Coupled to the window of the crystal is a PM tube that converts the light flashes from the scintillator into an electric signal of pulses.

The PM tube is an electron vacuum tube that contains a number of elements. The tube consists of a **glass envelope,** which provides structural support for the internal elements and maintains the vacuum inside the tube.

The portion of the glass envelope that is coupled to the scintillation crystal is called the **window of the tube.** The crystal window and the PM tube window are sandwiched together with a silicone grease, which provides **optical coupling** so that the light emitted by the scintil-

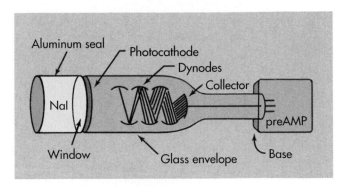

FIGURE 39-11 Scintillation detector assembly characteristics of the type used in a portable survey instrument.

lator is transmitted to the interior of the PM tube with minimum loss.

As the light passes from the crystal into the PM tube, it is incident on a thin metal coating called a **photocathode,** which consists of a compound of cesium, antimony, and bismuth. Electrons are emitted from the photocathode by a process called **photoemission** that is similar to thermionic emission in the filament of an x-ray tube, except that the stimulus is light rather than heat.

 A photocathode is a device that emits electrons when illuminated.

The flash of light from the scintillation crystal therefore is incident on the photocathode and electrons are released by photoemission. The number of electrons emitted is directly proportional to the intensity of the light.

These photoelectrons are accelerated to the first of a series of platelike elements called **dynodes.** Each dynode serves to amplify the electron pulse by **secondary electron emission.** For each electron incident on the dynode, several secondary electrons are emitted and directed to the next stage. Consequently, there is an electron gain for each dynode in the PM tube.

 The dynode gain is the ratio of secondary electrons to incident electrons.

The number of dynodes and the gain of each dynode determine the overall electron gain of the PM tube. Photomultiplier tube gain is the dynode gain raised to the power of the number of dynodes.

PHOTOMULTIPLIER TUBE GAIN

PM tube gain = g^n

where dynode gain is g, and n is equal to the number of dynodes.

Question: An eight-stage PM tube (eight dynodes) has a dynode gain of three (three electrons emitted for each incident electron). What is the PM tube gain?

Answer: PM tube gain = 3^8
= 6561

The last platelike element of the PM tube is called the collecting electrode or **collector.** The collector absorbs the electron pulse from the last dynode and conducts it to the **preamplifier.** The preamplifier provides an initial state of pulse amplification. It is attached to the **base** of the PM tube, a structure to provide support for the glass envelope and internal structures.

The overall result of scintillation detection is that a single photon interaction produces a burst of light; this in turn, produces photoelectron emission, which is then amplified to produce a relatively large electron pulse.

 The size of the electron pulse is proportional to the energy absorbed by the crystal from the incident photon.

It is this property of scintillation detection that promotes its use as an energy-sensitive device for **gamma spectrometry** using **pulse height analysis.** Through such application, unknown gamma emitters can be identified and more sensitive radioisotope imaging can be accomplished, by counting only those pulses having energy representing a total gamma ray absorption.

Scintillation detectors are sensitive devices for x-rays and gamma rays. They are capable of measuring radiation intensities as low as single-photon interactions. This property of scintillation detectors results in their use as portable radiation devices in much the same manner as Geiger counters.

A portable scintillation detector is more sensitive than a Geiger counter because it has much higher detection efficiency. For this application, the scintillation detector would be used to monitor the presence of contamination and perhaps low levels of radiation.

Thermoluminescence Dosimetry

Some materials glow when heated. This is the thermally stimulated emission of visible light, called *thermoluminescence.* In the early 1960s, Cameron and coworkers at the University of Wisconsin experimented with some thermoluminescent materials and were able to show that exposure to ionizing radiation caused some materials to glow particularly brightly when subsequently heated.

 TLD is the emission of light by a thermally stimulated crystal following irradiation.

This radiation-induced thermoluminescence has been developed into a sensitive and accurate method of radiation dosimetry for personnel radiation monitoring and for measuring patient dose during diagnostic and therapeutic radiation procedures. Personnel and patient radiation monitoring are discussed in Chapter 40; however, at this time it is important to know some of the basic principles of TLD (Figure 39-12).

After irradiation, the TLD phosphor is placed on a special dish or planchet for analysis in an instrument called a *TLD analyzer.* The temperature of the planchet can be carefully controlled. Directly viewing the planchet is a PM tube. The PM tube is the same type of light-sensitive and light-measuring vacuum tube described previously as a major component of scintillation detectors.

The PM tube–planchet assembly is in a chamber with a light-tight seal. The output signal from the PM tube is amplified and displayed.

The Glow Curve. As the temperature of the planchet is increased, the amount of light emitted by the TLD increases in an irregular manner. Figure 39-13 shows the light output from lithium fluoride (LiF) as the temperature increases. There are several prominent peaks in the graph, and each occurs because of a specific electron transition in the TL crystals.

Such a graph is known as a **glow curve,** and each TL material has a characteristic glow curve. Both the height of the highest temperature peak and the total area under the curve are directly proportional to the energy deposited in the TLD by ionizing radiation. The TLD analyzers are electronic instruments designed to measure the height of the glow curve or the area under the curve and relate this to exposure or dose through a conversion factor.

Types of Thermoluminescence Dosimetry Material. Many materials, including some body tissues, exhibit the property of radiation-induced thermoluminescence. Materials that are used for TLD, however, are somewhat

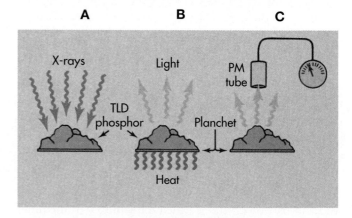

FIGURE 39-12 Thermoluminescence dosimetry is a multistep process. **A,** Exposure to ionizing radiation. **B,** Subsequent heating. **C,** Measurement of the intensity of the emitted light.

limited in number and are principally types of inorganic crystals. Lithium fluoride (LiF) is the most widely used TLD material. It has an atomic number of 8.2, and therefore has x-ray absorption properties similar to that of soft tissue.

LiF is relatively sensitive. It can measure doses as low as 5 mrad (50 μGy_t) with modest accuracy, and at doses exceeding 10 rad (100 mGy_t), its accuracy is better than $\pm 5\%$.

 Lithium fluoride is a nearly tissue-equivalent radiation dosimeter.

Calcium fluoride (CaF) activated with manganese (CaF$_2$:Mn) has a higher effective atomic number (Z = 16.3) than LiF, and this makes it considerably more sensitive to ionizing radiation. CaF$_2$:Mn can measure radiation doses of less than 1 mrad (10 μGy_t) with moderate accuracy. Other types of TLDs are available, and Table 39-5 lists some thermoluminescent phosphors and their principal characteristics and applications.

Properties of Thermoluminescence Dosimetry. A particular advantage of TLD is size. The TLD can be obtained in several solid crystal shapes and sizes. Rectangular rods measuring 1 × 1 × 6 mm and flat chips measuring 3 × 3 × 1 mm are the most popular sizes. The TLD can also be obtained in powder form, which allows for its irradiation in nearly any configuration. TLDs are also available with the phosphor matrixed with Teflon or plated onto a wire and sealed in glass.

The TLD is reusable. When irradiated, the energy absorbed by the TLD remains stored until released as visible light by heat during analysis. The heating restores the crystal to its original condition and makes it ready for another exposure.

The TLD responds proportionately to dose. If the dose is doubled, the TLD response also is doubled.

The TLD is rugged, and its small size makes it useful for monitoring dose in small areas, such as body cavities. The TLD does not respond to individual ionizing events, and therefore it cannot be used in a rate meter type of instrument. The TLD is suitable only for integral dose measurements, but it does not give immediate results. It must be analyzed after irradiation for dosimetry results.

Optically Stimulated Luminescence

An additional radiation dosimeter especially adapted for personnel monitoring was developed by Landauer in the late 1990s (Figure 39-14). The process is called *optically stimulated luminescence* (OSL) and uses aluminum oxide (Al$_2$O$_3$) as the radiation detector.

Irradiation of the Al$_2$O$_3$ stimulates some electrons into an excited state. During processing, laser light stimulates these electrons, causing them to return to their ground state with the emission of visible light. The intensity of the visible light emission is proportional to the radiation dose received by the Al$_2$O$_3$.

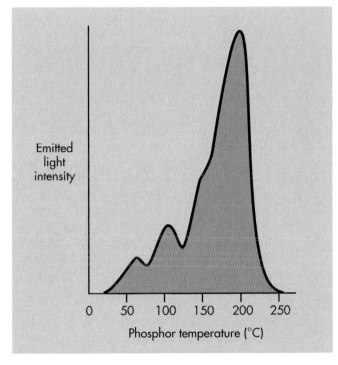

FIGURE 39-13 Thermoluminescence glow curve for LiF.

TABLE 39-5	Some Thermoluminescent Phosphors and Their Characteristics and Uses			
	Lithium Fluoride	**Lithium Borate**	**Calcium Fluoride**	**Calcium Sulfate**
Composition	LiF	Li$_2$B$_4$O$_7$:Mn	CaF$_2$:Mn	CaSO$_4$:Dy
Density × 10^3 (kg/m^3)	2.64	2.5	3.18	2.61
Effective atomic number	8.2	7.4	16.3	15.3
Temperature of main peak (°C)	195	200	260	220
Principal use	Patient and personnel dose	Research	Environmental monitoring	Environmental monitoring

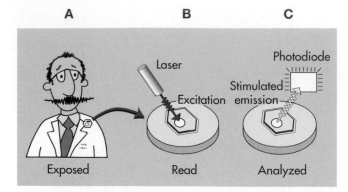

A **B** **C**

Laser

Photodiode

Excitation

Stimulated emission

Exposed   Read   Analyzed

FIGURE 39-14 Optically stimulated dosimetry is a multistep process. **A,** Exposure to ionizing radiation. **B,** Laser illumination. **C,** Measurement of the intensity of the stimulated light emission.

The OSL process is not unlike TLD. Both are based on stimulated luminescence. However, OSL has several advantages over TLD, especially as applied to occupational radiation monitoring.

With a minimum reportable dose of 1 mrad, OSL is more sensitive than TLD. OSL has a precision of ±1 mrad, which beats TLD. Other features of OSL include reanalysis for confirmation of dose, qualitative information about exposure conditions, wide dynamic range, and excellent long-term stability.

SUMMARY

There are many radiation protection devices, accessories, and protocols associated with modern x-ray imaging systems. This chapter discusses the radiation protection devices that are common to all radiographic and fluoroscopic imaging systems. Many of the devices are federally mandated; others are features added by manufacturers.

Leakage radiation emitted by the x-ray tube during exposure must be contained by a protective x-ray tube housing. The limit of leakage must be no more than 100 mR per hour at a distance of 1 m from the housing. The control panel must indicate exposure by either kVp and mA meters or visible and audible signals.

Great attention is given to the design of radiographic rooms, to the placement of x-ray imaging systems, and to the use of adjoining rooms. There are two types of protective barriers: primary barriers and secondary barriers. Primary barriers intercept the useful x-ray beam and require the most lead or concrete. Secondary barriers protect personnel from scatter and leakage radiation.

Dosimeters are instruments designed to detect and measure radiation. Other than photographic emulsion, there are four types of highly accurate devices for measuring radiation. The gas-filled detectors are the ionization chamber, the proportional counter, and the Geiger-Muller counter. The scintillation detector is a very sensitive device used in nuclear medicine. Two other radiation detection devices used especially for occupational radiation monitoring are thermoluminescence dosimetry and optically stimulated luminescence.

CHALLENGE QUESTIONS

1. Define or otherwise identify:
   a. TLD
   b. Use factor
   c. Diagnostic protective x-ray tube housing
   d. Glow curve
   e. Primary protective barrier
   f. X-ray linearity
   g. Secondary radiation
   h. Occupancy factor
   i. Geiger-Muller region
   j. Resolving time
2. What do audible and visible signals indicate on the radiographic control console?
3. List as many devices used for radiation protection on radiographic equipment as you can.
4. What is the result if the x-ray beam and the film are not properly aligned?
5. What filtration is used for mammography equipment operated below 30 kVp?
6. How are reproducibility and linearity different when measuring the intensity of the x-ray beam?
7. What characteristics of fluoroscopic equipment are designed for radiation protection?
8. How can filtration be measured if the amount of inherent and added filtration is unknown?
9. Name the three types of radiation exposure that are of concern when designing protective barriers.
10. List four factors that are taken into consideration when designing a barrier for a radiographic room.
11. What is the difference between a controlled area and an uncontrolled area?
12. What are the units of workload for an x-ray examination room?
13. Explain the use factor (U) as it relates to a protective barrier in an x-ray examination room.
14. Why is the use factor for secondary barriers always 1?
15. Name the three gas-filled dosimeters.
16. Discuss the properties of TLD that make it suitable for personnel monitoring.
17. Which modality of diagnostic imaging uses scintillation detection as a radiation detection process?
18. What are the two most widely used scintillation phosphors?
19. A photomultiplier has nine dynodes, each of which has a gain of 2.2. What is the overall tube gain?
20. Given the following conditions of operation, compute the weekly workload.
    20 patients per day
    3.2 films per patient
    80 mAs per view on average

CHAPTER 40

Radiation Protection Procedures

OBJECTIVES

At the completion of this chapter, the student should be able to do the following:

1. Discuss the units and concepts of occupational radiation exposure
2. Indicate three ways that patient dose can be reported
3. Describe the intensity and distribution of radiation dose in mammography and computed tomography
4. Discuss ways to reduce occupational radiation exposure
5. Explain occupational radiation monitors and where they should be positioned
6. Discuss personnel radiation monitoring reports
7. List the available thicknesses of protective apparel
8. Discuss ALARA principles applied to patient radiation safety
9. Identify screening x-ray examinations that are no longer routinely performed
10. Discuss factors affecting patient radiation dose
11. Explain when to use gonadal shields

OUTLINE

Occupational Radiation Exposure
Patient Dose
   Estimation of Patient Dose
   Patient Dose in Special Examinations
Reduction of Occupational Radiation Exposure
   Personnel Monitoring
   Personnel Monitoring Report
   Protective Apparel
   Position
   Patient Holding
Reduction of Unnecessary Patient Dose
   Unnecessary Examinations
   Repeat Examinations
   Radiographic Technique
   Image Receptor
   Patient Positioning
   Specific Area Shielding

ALL MEDICAL health physics activity is directed in some way to minimizing the radiation exposure of radiologic personnel and the radiation dose to patients during x-ray examination. Radiation exposure of radiologists and radiologic technologists is measured with occupational radiation monitors. Patient dose is usually estimated by conducting simulated x-ray examinations with human phantoms and test objects.

If radiation control procedures are adopted, occupational radiation exposure and patient dose can be kept acceptably low. Health physicists subscribe to **ALARA**—keep all radiation exposure **as low as reasonably achievable**. Radiologic technologists should follow this guide as well.

OCCUPATIONAL RADIATION EXPOSURE

Radiation dose is measured in units of rads (Gy_t). Radiation exposure is measured in roentgens (Gy_a). When the exposure is to radiologic technologists and radiologists, the proper unit is the rem (Sv).

The rem is the unit of effective dose and is used for radiation protection purposes. Although **exposure, dose,** and **effective dose** have precise and different meanings, they are often used interchangeably in radiology because they have approximately the same numeric value.

When properly used, exposure (R, Gy_a) refers to radiation intensity in air. Dose (rad, Gy_t) measures the radiation energy absorbed as a result of radiation exposure, and is used to identify irradiation of patients. Effective dose (rem, Sv) identifies the biologic effectiveness of the radiation energy absorbed. This unit is applied to occupationally exposed persons and to population exposure.

Although the recommended dose limit for radiologic personnel is 50 mSv/yr (5000 mrem/yr), experience has shown that considerably lower exposures than this are routine. The occupational radiation exposure of radiologic personnel engaged in general x-ray activity should not normally exceed 1 mSv/yr (100 mrem/yr).

Radiologists usually receive slightly higher exposures than radiologic technologists. This is because the radiologist receives most of his or her exposure during fluoroscopy and is usually closer to the radiation source, the patient, during such procedures. Table 40-1 reports the results of an analysis of the annual occupational radiation exposure of radiologic personnel. Clearly, the radiation exposures are low.

TABLE 40-1 Occupational Radiation Exposure of Radiologic Personnel

Exposure Category	Value
Average whole-body dose	0.7 mSv/yr
Those receiving less than the minimum detectable dose	53%
Those receiving <1 mSv/yr	88%
Those receiving >50 mSv/yr	0.05%

Fluoroscopy. Unquestionably, the highest occupational exposure of diagnostic x-ray personnel occurs during fluoroscopy and mobile radiography. During radiographic exposure, the radiologist is rarely present and the radiologic technologist is behind the console protective barrier.

When fixed protective barriers are not available, such as during mobile examination, the mobile x-ray imaging system is equipped with an exposure cord long enough to allow the technologist to leave the immediate examination area. The radiologic technologist should wear a protective apron for each such mobile examination.

During fluoroscopy, both radiologist and radiologic technologist are exposed to relatively high levels of radiation. Personnel exposure, however, is directly related to the x-ray beam-on time. With care, personnel exposures can be maintained ALARA.

Question: A barium enema examination requires 2.5 minutes of fluoroscopic x-ray beam time. If the radiographer is exposed to 250 mR/hr, what will be his or her occupational radiation exposure?

Answer: Exposure = exposure rate × time
= 250 mR/hr × 2.5 minutes
= 250 mR/hr × 0.0417 hour
= 10.4 mR

Remote fluoroscopy results in low personnel exposures because personnel are not in the x-ray examination room with the patient. Some fluoroscopes have the x-ray tube over the table and the image receptor under the table. This geometry offers some advantage to image quality, but personnel exposures are higher because the secondary radiation (scatter + leakage) levels are higher.

This condition should be kept in mind during mobile and C-arm fluoroscopy. It is best to position the x-ray tube under the patient during mobile and C-arm fluoroscopy (Figure 40-1).

Interventional Radiology. Personnel engaged in interventional radiology procedures often receive higher exposures than do those in general radiologic practice

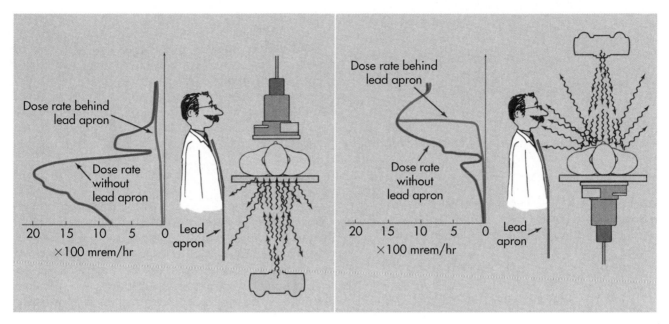

FIGURE 40-1 Scatter radiation during portable fluoroscopy is more intense with the x-ray tube over the patient. (Courtesy Stephen Balter.)

because of longer fluoroscopic x-ray beam-on time. The frequent absence of a protective curtain on the image intensifier tower and the extensive use of cineradiography also contribute to higher personnel exposure.

Extremity exposure during interventional radiology procedures may be significant. Even with protective gloves, exposure of the forearm can approach the recommended dose limit of 500 mSv/yr (50 rem/yr) if care is not taken. Without protective gloves, excessive hand exposures are possible.

 Extremity monitoring must be provided for interventional radiologists.

Mammography. Personnel exposures associated with mammography are low because the low kVp of operation results in less scatter radiation. Usually, a long exposure cord and a conventional wall or window wall are sufficient to provide adequate protection.

Rarely does a room used strictly for mammography require protective lead shielding. Dedicated mammography x-ray units have personnel protective barriers made of lead glass, lead acrylic, and even plate glass as an integral component. Usually, such barriers are totally adequate.

Computed Tomography. Personnel exposures in computed tomography (CT) facilities are low. Because the CT x-ray beam is finely collimated and only secondary radiation is present in the examination room, the radiation levels are low compared with those expe-

rienced in fluoroscopy. Figure 40-2 shows the isoexposure profiles for both the horizontal and vertical planes of a multislice spiral CT imaging system. These data are given as mR/360 degrees rotation and they show that personnel can be permitted to remain in the room during imaging. However, protective apparel should always be worn in such situations.

Question: It is necessary for a radiologic technologist to remain in the CT room at midtable position during a 20-scan examination. What would be the occupational exposure if no protective apron were worn?

Answer: From Figure 40-2, we may assume an exposure of 0.1 mR/scan.

Occupational exposure = 0.1 mR/scan ×
$$20 = 2 \text{ mR}$$

Of course, with a protective apron, the trunk of the body would receive essentially zero.

Surgery. Nursing personnel and others working in the operating room and in intensive care units are sometimes exposed to radiation from mobile x-ray imaging systems and C-arm fluoroscopes. Although these personnel are often anxious about such exposures, many studies have shown that their occupational exposure is near zero and certainly is no cause for concern. It usually is not necessary to provide occupational radiation monitors for such personnel.

Mobile Radiology. Occupational radiation monitors are not necessary during mobile radiography except for the radiologic technologist and anyone required to

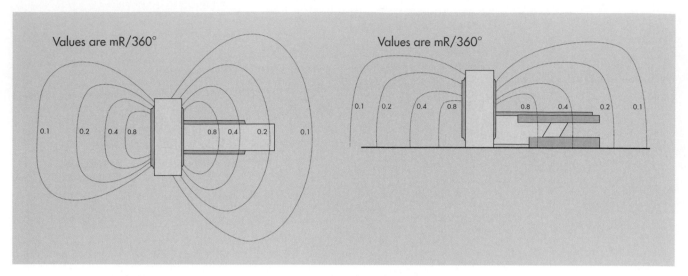

FIGURE 40-2 Isoexposure profiles (in mR/360 degrees) in both the horizontal and the vertical planes for multislice spiral computed tomography.

restrain or hold patients. Personnel who regularly operate or are in the immediate vicinity of a C-arm fluoroscope should wear an occupational radiation monitor in addition to protective apparel. During C-arm fluoroscopy, the x-ray beam may be on for a relatively long time and the beam can be pointed in virtually any direction.

It should **never** be necessary for radiologic personnel to exceed 50 mSv/yr (5000 mrem/yr). In smaller hospitals, emergency centers, and private clinics, occupational exposures rarely exceed 5 mSv/yr (500 mrem/yr). As Table 40-1 reported, average exposures in most facilities are less than 1 mSv/yr (100 mrem/yr).

PATIENT DOSE

The exposure of patients to medical x-rays is commanding increased attention in our society for two reasons.

First, the frequency of x-ray examination is increasing among all age groups, at a rate of approximately 10% per year in the United States. This rate of increase is exceeded in many other countries. This indicates that physicians are relying more and more on x-ray diagnosis to assist them in patient care, even taking into account the newer imaging modalities.

This is to be expected. X-ray diagnosis is considered much more accurate today than in the past. More rigorous training programs required of radiologists and radiologic technologists and improvements in diagnostic x-ray imaging systems allow for more difficult, but more substantive, x-ray examinations. Efficacy and diagnostic accuracy are much improved.

Second, there is increasing concern among public health officials and radiation scientists regarding the risk that is associated with medical x-ray exposure. Acute effects on superficial tissues after angiointerventional procedures are being reported with increasing frequency.

The possible late effects of diagnostic x-ray exposure are of concern, and therefore attention must be given to good radiation control practices. When a diagnosis can be obtained with lower radiation dose, it should be because of reduced risk. This is in keeping with **ALARA.**

Estimation of Patient Dose

Patient dose from diagnostic x-rays is usually reported in one of three ways. The exposure to the entrance surface or **entrance skin exposure (ESE)** is most often reported because it is easy to measure.

The **gonadal dose** is important because of the possible genetic responses to medical x-ray exposure. The dose to the gonads is not difficult to measure or estimate.

The dose to the **bone marrow** is important because bone marrow is the target organ believed responsible for radiation-induced leukemia. Bone marrow dose cannot be measured directly; it is estimated from ESE.

Table 40-2 presents some representative values of ESE and gonadal dose for various x-ray examinations. The mean marrow dose for each procedure is also presented. Note that these are only approximate values and should not be used to estimate patient dose at any facility.

In any given x-ray facility, actual doses delivered may be considerably different. Efficiency of x-ray production and image receptor speed are the most important variables.

These values do provide for relative dose comparisons among various radiologic examinations. Doses during fluoroscopy are too dependent on technique, equipment, and beam-on time to be easily estimated. Usually, such doses must be measured.

Entrance Skin Exposure. ESE is most often referred to as the *patient dose.* It is widely used because it is easy to measure and reasonably accurate estimates can be made in the absence of measurements.

TABLE 40-2	Representative Radiation Quantities From Various Diagnostic X-Ray Procedures			
Examination	Technique (kVp/mAs)	Entrance Skin Exposure (mR)	Mean Marrow Dose (mrad)	Gonad Dose (mrad)
Skull	76/50	200	10	< 1
Chest	110/3	10	2	< 1
Cervical spine	70/40	150	10	< 1
Lumbar spine	72/60	300	60	225
Abdomen	74/60	400	30	125
Pelvis	70/50	150	20	150
Extremity	60/5	50	2	< 1
CT (head)	125/300	3000	20	50
CT (pelvis)	124/400	4000	100	3000

CT, Computed tomography.

Thermoluminescence dosimeters (TLDs) are most often used. The size, sensitivity, and accuracy of TLDs make them very satisfactory patient radiation monitors.

A small grouping or pack of 3 to 10 TLDs can easily be taped to the patient's skin in the center of the x-ray field. Because the response of the TLD is proportional to exposure and dose, the TLD can be used to measure all levels experienced in diagnostic radiology. With proper laboratory technique, the results of such measurements are accurate to within 5%.

Two rather straightforward methods for estimating ESE are available in the absence of patient measurements. The first requires the use of a nomogram such as that shown in Figure 40-3. This figure contains a family of curves from which one can estimate the output intensity of a radiographic unit if the technique is known or assumed. The output intensity of different x-ray imaging systems varies widely, so the use of this nomogram method is good only to perhaps ±50%.

Using this nomogram first requires knowledge of the total filtration in the x-ray beam. This is usually available from the medical physics report, but if not, 3 mm Al is a good estimate. Next, identify the kVp and mAs of the intended examination.

Draw a vertical line rising from the value of total filtration until it intersects with the kVp of the examination. From this intersection, draw a horizontal line to the left until it intersects the mR/mAs axis. The resulting mR/mAs value is the approximate output intensity of the radiographic unit. Multiply this value times the examination mAs value to obtain the approximate patient exposure.

Question: With reference to Figure 40-3, estimate the ESE from a lateral skull film taken at 66 kVp, 150 mAs, with a radiographic unit having 2.5 mm Al total filtration.

Answer: Estimate the intersection between a vertical line rising from 2.5 mm Al and a horizontal

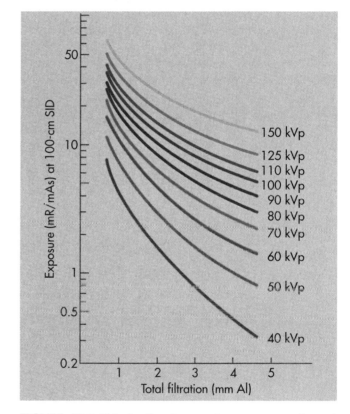

FIGURE 40-3 This family of curves is a nomogram for estimating output x-ray intensity from a single-phase radiographic unit. (Courtesy John R. Cameron.)

line through 66 kVp. Extend the horizontal line to the y-axis and read 3.8 mR/mAs.
3.8 mR/mAs × 150 = 570 mR

A better approach requires that a medical physicist construct a nomogram such as that shown in Figure 40-4 for each radiographic unit. A straight edge between any kVp and mAs value will cross the ESE scale at the correct mR value.

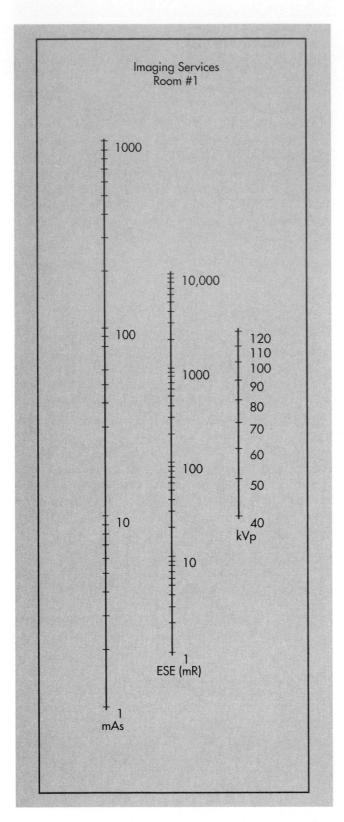

Imaging Services
Room #1

1000

10,000

100   120
                             110
          1000   100
                             90

                             80

                             70

                             60
          100
                             50

10   40
                             kVp

          10

                          1
          ESE (mR)

1
mAs

FIGURE 40-4 This type of nomogram is very accurate but must be fashioned individually for each radiographic unit. (Courtesy Michael D. Harpen.)

Question: Using the nomogram of Figure 40-4, what is the ESE when a radiographic exposure is made at 66 kVp, 150 mAs?

Answer: The line is drawn as shown and crosses the ESE scale at 1800 mR.

A third method for estimating ESE requires that one know the output intensity for at least one operating condition. During the annual or special radiation control survey and calibration of an x-ray facility, the medical physicist measures this output intensity, usually in units of mR/mAs at 80 cm, the approximate source-to-skin distance (SSD), or at 100 cm, the source-to-image receptor distance (SID). At 70 kVp, radiographic output intensity varies from approximately 2 to 10 mR/mAs at 80 cm SSD.

With this calibration value available, one would first make adjustment for a different SSD by applying the inverse square law.

Question: The output intensity of a radiographic unit is reported as 3.7 mR/mAs (37 (Gy_a/mAs)) at 100 cm SID. What is the intensity at 75 cm SSD?

Answer: At 75 cm SSD the intensity will be greater by $(100/75)^2 = (1.32)^2 = 1.78$
$$3.7 \text{ mR/mAs} \times 1.78 = 6.6 \text{ mR/mAs}$$

Having the ESE, one scales this according to the kVp and mAs of the examination. Output intensity varies according to the square of the ratio in the change in kVp. Refer to Chapter 11 to review this relationship.

Question: The output intensity at 70 kVp and 75 cm SSD is 6.6 mR/mAs (66 $\mu Gy_a/mAs$). What is the output intensity at 76 kVp?

Answer: At higher kVp, the output intensity is greater by the square of the ratio of the kVp.
$$(76/70)^2 = (1.09)^2 = 1.18$$
$$6.6 \text{ mR/mAs} \times 1.18 = 7.8 \text{ mR/mAs}$$

The final step in estimating ESE is to multiply the output intensity in mR/mAs by the examination mAs value because they are proportional.

Question: If the radiographic technique for an intravenous pyelogram calls for 80 mAs, what is the ESE when the output intensity is 7.8 mR/mAs (78 $\mu Gy_a/mAs$)?

Answer: 7.8 mR/mAs × 80 mAs = 624 mR

These steps can be combined into a single calculation as illustrated in the following example.

Question: The output intensity for a radiographic unit is 4.5 mR/mAs (4.5 $\mu Gy_a/mAs$) at 70 kVp and 80 cm. If a lateral skull film is taken at 66 kVp, 150 mAs, what will be the ESE at an 80-cm SSD? What would be the skin dose at a 90-cm SSD?

Answer: *At 80 cm SSD*

$$\text{Dose} = (4.5 \text{ mR/mAs})\left(\frac{66 \text{ kVp}}{70 \text{ kVp}}\right)^2 (150 \text{ mAs})$$

$$= 600 \text{ mR}$$

At 90 cm SSD

$$\text{Dose} = (600 \text{ mR})\left(\frac{80}{90}\right)^2$$

$$= 474 \text{ mR}$$

ESE in fluoroscopy is much more difficult to estimate because the x-ray field moves and sometimes varies in size. If the field were of one size and stationary, ESE would be directly related to exposure time.

 For the average fluoroscopic examination, one can assume an ESE of 3 R/min.

Question: A fluoroscopic procedure requires 2.5 min at 90 kVp, 2 mA. What is the approximate ESE?

Answer: ESE = (4 R/min)(2.5 min)
= 10 R

Mean Marrow Dose. The hematologic effects of radiation are rarely experienced in diagnostic radiology. It is appropriate, however, that we understand the mean marrow dose, which is one measure of patient dose during diagnostic procedures.

The mean marrow dose is the average radiation dose to the entire active bone marrow. For instance, if during a particular examination, 50% of the active bone marrow were in the primary beam and received an average dose of 25 mrad (250 μGy$_t$), the mean marrow dose would be 12.5 mrad (125 μGy$_t$).

Table 40-2 includes the approximate mean marrow dose in adults for various radiographic examinations. In children, these levels would in general be less because the radiographic techniques used are considerably less.

Table 40-3 shows the distribution of active bone marrow in the adult, and this gives some clue as to which diagnostic x-ray procedures involve exposure to large amounts of bone marrow.

In the United States, the mean marrow dose from diagnostic x-ray examinations averaged over the entire population is approximately 100 mrad/yr (1 mGy$_t$/yr). Such a dose never results in the hematologic responses described in Chapter 36. It is a dose concept, however, used to estimate, on a population basis, the risk of one late effect of radiation—leukemia.

TABLE 40-3	Distribution of Active Bone Marrow in Adults
Anatomic Site	**Percentage of Bone Marrow**
Head	10
Upper limb girdle	8
Sternum	3
Ribs	11
Cervical vertebrae	4
Thoracic vertebrae	13
Lumbar vertebrae	11
Sacrum	11
Lower limb girdle	29
Total	**100**

Genetically Significant Dose. Measurements and estimates of gonad dose are important because of the suspected genetic effects of radiation. Although the gonad dose from diagnostic x-rays is low for each individual, it may have some significance in terms of population effects.

 The genetically significant dose (GSD) is the gonad dose that, if received by every member of the population, would produce the total genetic effect on the population as the sum of the individual doses actually received.

The population gonad dose of importance is the **GSD**, the radiation dose to the population gene pool. Thus, it is a weighted-average gonad dose. It takes into account those persons who are irradiated and those who are not, and averages the results. The GSD can be estimated only through large-scale epidemiologic studies.

 GENETICALLY SIGNIFICANT DOSE

$$GSD = \frac{\Sigma DN_x P}{\Sigma N_T P}$$

Where Σ is the mathematical symbol meaning to sum or add values, D is the average gonad dose per examination, N_x is the number of persons receiving x-ray examinations, N_T is the total number of persons in the population, and P (progeny) is the expected future number of children per person.

For computational purposes, therefore, the GSD considers the age, sex, and expected number of children for each person examined with x-rays. It also acknowledges the various types of examinations and the gonadal dose per examination type.

Estimates of GSD have been conducted in many different countries (Table 40-4). The estimate reported by the U.S. Public Health Service is 20 mrad/yr (200 (Gy$_t$/yr). Thus, this is a genetic radiation burden over and above the existing natural background radiation level of approximately 100 mrad/yr (1 mGy$_t$/yr). The genetic effects of this total GSD, 120 mrad/y (1.2 mGy$_t$/yr), are not detectable.

Patient Dose in Special Examinations

Dose in Mammography. Because of the considerable application of x-rays for examination of the female breast and the concern for the induction of breast cancer by radiation, it is imperative that we have some understanding of the radiation doses involved in such examinations.

Screen-film and digital mammography currently are the only acceptable techniques. Direct-exposure film and xeromammography are no longer used.

An ESE of approximately 800 mR/view (8 mGy$_a$/view) is normal. Increasing the x-ray tube potential much beyond 26 kVp degrades the image unacceptably, and therefore further dose reduction by technique manipulation is unlikely. Faster films and screens, however, may make even lower-dose mammography possible.

Radiographic grids are used in most screen-film mammography examinations. Grid ratios of 4:1 and 5:1 are most popular. The contrast enhancement produced by using such grids is significant, but so is the increase in patient dose. Patient dose is increased by approximately two times with the use of such grids compared with nongrid technique.

The values stated for patient dose in mammography can be misleading. Because of the low x-ray energies used in mammography, the dose falls off very rapidly as the x-ray beam penetrates the breast. If the ESE for a craniocaudad view is 800 mR (8 mGy$_a$), the dose to the midline of the breast may be only 100 mrad (1.0 mGy$_t$).

Fortunately, it is known that the risk of an adverse biologic response from mammography is small. Certainly, it is nothing about which a patient should be concerned. Any possible response, however, is related to the average radiation dose to glandular tissue, and not the skin exposure. **Glandular dose (D$_g$)** varies in a complicated way with variations in x-ray beam quality and quantity.

 Glandular dose is approximately 15% of the ESE.

Specification of an ESE can also be misleading when one considers a two-view examination, such as that used for screening (Figure 40-5). Consider an examination consisting of craniocaudad and mediolateral oblique views. The craniocaudad and the mediolateral oblique views produce an ESE of 800 mR (8 mGy$_a$) each.

It would be incorrect to describe this total examination procedure as resulting in an ESE of 1.6 R (16 mGy$_a$). Skin exposures from different projections cannot be added. We must either specify the skin exposure for each view or attempt to estimate the total D$_g$.

The total D$_g$ can be estimated by approximating that the contribution from each view will be 15% of the ESE. Consequently, the total D$_g$ would be the sum of (0.15 × 800 = 120 mrad [1.2 mGy$_t$]) contribution from each of the craniocaudad and mediolateral oblique views. The total D$_g$ would, therefore be 240 mrad (2.4 mGy$_t$).

 Glandular dose should not exceed 100 mrad/view with contact mammography and 300 mrad/view with a grid.

From this discussion, it would seem that patient dose in mammography can be considerably reduced if the number of views is restricted. The axillary view should not be done routinely. For screening programs, no more than two views per breast are advisable.

Dose in Computed Tomography Imaging. An important consideration in CT imaging, as with any x-ray procedure, is not only the skin dose but also the distribution of dose to internal organs and tissues during imaging.

On the basis of skin dose, CT results in a somewhat higher dose than most other diagnostic x-ray procedures. The skin dose delivered by a series of contiguous CT slices is much higher than that delivered by a single radiographic view. A typical radiographic head or body examination, however, often involves several views. Furthermore, for many CT examinations, considerably less tissue volume is irradiated than in conventional radiography.

However, because of increasing use of spiral CT and multislice imaging, CT must often be considered a high-dose procedure. U.S. Public Health Service data suggest

TABLE 40-4	Estimated Genetically Significant Dose From Diagnostic X-Ray Examination
Population	**Genetically Significant Dose (mrad)**
Denmark	22
Great Britain	12
Japan	27
New Zealand	12
Sweden	72
United States	20

that 5% of all x-ray examinations are CT, yet CT accounts for 35% of total patient dose. The CT dose is approximately equal to the average fluoroscopic dose.

As was pointed out in Chapters 29 and 30, CT differs in many important ways from other x-ray examinations. A radiograph can be likened to a photograph taken with a flash—the patient is "floodlighted" with x-rays to expose the image receptor directly.

On the other hand, CT images the patient with a fine, collimated beam of x-rays. This difference in radiation delivery also means that the **dose distribution** from CT is different from that in radiographic procedures.

The CT dose is nearly uniform throughout the imaging volume for a head examination. CT at midline results in 50% of the ESE for body CT. Radiographic and fluoroscopic dose is high at the entrance surface and very low at the exit surface.

Part of the dose efficiency of CT arises because of the precise collimation of the x-ray beam. Scatter radiation increases patient dose and reduces radiographic contrast. Because CT uses narrow, well-collimated x-ray beams, scatter radiation is significantly reduced and contrast resolution significantly improved. Thus, a larger percentage of the x-rays contributes usefully to the image.

The precise collimation used in CT means that only a well-defined volume of tissue is irradiated for each image. The ideal x-ray beam for CT would have sharp boundaries. There would be no overlap between adjacent images. Thus, the dose delivered to a patient from a series of ideal contiguous CT images should be the same as that from a single slice.

Figure 40-6 illustrates, however, how this ideal situation cannot be attained in practice. The size of the focal spot of the x-ray tube blurs the sharp boundaries of the section. Also, the x-ray beam is not precisely parallel, and some spreading occurs as the beam crosses the image field.

If a series of adjacent images is performed with an automatically indexed patient couch, the couch movement must be precise. If the couch moves too much between images, some tissue will be missed. If it moves too little, some tissue in each image will be doubled-exposed.

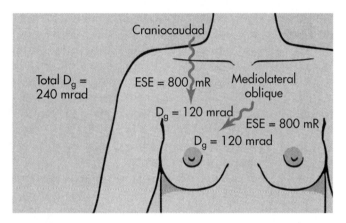

FIGURE 40-5 Two mammographic exposures result in a total glandular dose that is the sum of the individual glandular doses.

It is essential that CT collimators be periodically monitored for proper adjustment.

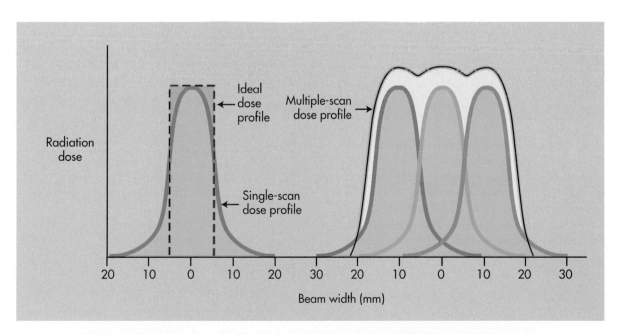

FIGURE 40-6 Patient dose distribution in multislice spiral computed tomography is complicated because the profile of the x-ray beam cannot be made sharp.

Finally, and perhaps most important, if the prepatient collimators are too wide, tissues near the interface of each image may receive twice the dose than they otherwise should. Thus, in practice, a series of adjacent images delivers a slightly higher dose than a single image because of the overlapping dose profiles.

Typical CT doses range from 3000 to 5000 mrad (30 to 50 mGy$_t$) during head imaging and 4000 to 6000 mrad (40 to 60 mGy$_t$), during body imaging. These values are only approximate and vary widely depending on the type of CT imaging system and the examination technique.

Because the CT x-ray beam is well collimated, the area of irradiation can be precisely controlled. Thus, radiosensitive organs such as the eyes can be selectively avoided.

Shields as protection from the primary x-ray beam in CT are of little use. Not only does the metal from these shields produce terrible artifacts in the image but also the rotational scheme of the x-ray source greatly reduces their effectiveness. The patient, however, can effectively be shielded from the low levels of scatter radiation as long as the direct x-ray beam does not intersect the shield.

Patient dose during spiral CT is somewhat more difficult to assess than the dose during conventional CT. At a pitch of 1.0:1, the patient dose is approximately the same. At a higher pitch, the dose is reduced compared with conventional CT. At a lower pitch, patient dose is increased.

As with any radiographic procedure, many factors influence patient dose. For CT imaging, a generalization is possible.

COMPUTED TOMOGRAPHY PATIENT DOSE

$$\text{Patient Dose} = k \, \frac{IE}{\sigma^2 w^3 h}$$

where k is a conversion factor, I is a beam intensity in mAs, E is average beam energy in keV (approximately 1/2 kVp), σ is a system noise, w is pixel size, and h is slice thickness.

Note that, as with radiography, patient dose is proportional to the x-ray beam intensity. It is also directly proportional to the average beam energy. Other factors are variables that are unique to CT imaging.

Sigma (σ) is noise. This is equivalent to quantum mottle in screen-film radiography and represents random statistical variations in the CT numbers. The w stands for the pixel size, one of the determinants of spatial resolution. The last factor, h, is the slice thickness.

A reduction in either the noise or slice thickness, while other factors remain constant, increases patient dose.

All other factors being equal, a low noise, high-resolution CT image results in higher patient dose. The challenge in CT, as indeed with all x-ray imaging, is not so much to deliver fantastically good resolution and low noise (because this could be achieved at the cost of very high patient dose) but to use the x-ray beam efficiently, producing the best possible image at a reasonable dose to the patient.

REDUCTION OF OCCUPATIONAL RADIATION EXPOSURE

The radiologic technologist can do much to minimize occupational radiation exposure. Most exposure control procedures do not require sophisticated equipment or especially rigorous training, but simply a conscientious attitude in the performance of assigned duties. Most equipment characteristics, technique changes, and administrative procedures designed to minimize patient dose also reduce occupational exposure.

In diagnostic radiology, at least 95% of the radiologic technologist's occupational radiation exposure come from fluoroscopy and mobile radiography. Attention to the cardinal principles of radiation protection (time, distance, and shielding) and ALARA are the most important aspects of occupational radiation control.

During fluoroscopy, the radiologist should minimize x-ray beam-on time. This can be done by careful technique, which includes intermittent activation of the fluoroscopic views rather than one long period of x-ray beam-on time. It is a common radiation protection practice to maintain a log of fluoroscopy time by recording the x-ray beam-on time using the 5-minute reset timer.

During fluoroscopy, the radiologic technologist should step back from the table when his or her immediate presence and assistance are not required. The radiologic technologist should also take maximum advantage of all protective shielding, including apron, curtain, and Bucky slot cover … and the **radiologist.**

Each mobile x-ray unit should have a protective apron assigned to it.

The radiologic technologist should wear a protective apron during all mobile examinations and maintain maximum distance from the source. The primary beam should never be pointed at the radiologic technologist or other nearby personnel.

The exposure cord on a portable x-ray unit must be at least 2 m long.

During radiography, the radiologic technologist is positioned behind a control booth barrier. These barriers are usually considered secondary barriers because they intercept only leakage and scatter radiation. Consequently, leaded glass and leaded gypsum board are often unnecessary for such barriers.

 The useful beam should never be directed toward the operating console.

Other work assignments in diagnostic imaging, such as scheduling, darkroom duties, and filing, result in essentially no occupational radiation exposure.

Occupational Radiation Monitoring

The level of occupational exposure to radiologists and radiologic technologists depends on the type and frequency of activity in which they are engaged. Determining the quantity of radiation they receive requires a program of occupational radiation monitoring. Occupational radiation monitoring refers to procedures instituted to estimate the amount of radiation received by individuals who work in a radiation environment.

 Occupational radiation monitoring is required when there is any likelihood that an individual will receive more than 1/10 of the recommended dose limit.

Most clinical diagnostic imaging personnel must be monitored; however, it usually is not necessary to monitor diagnostic radiology secretaries and file clerks. Furthermore, it usually is not necessary to monitor operating room personnel, except perhaps those routinely involved in cystoscopy and C-arm fluoroscopy.

 The occupational radiation monitor offers no protection against radiation exposure!

The occupational radiation monitor simply measures the quantity of radiation to which the monitor was exposed, and therefore is simply an indicator of the exposure of the wearer. There are basically three types of personnel monitors in use in diagnostic radiology: film badges, TLDs, and optically stimulated luminescence (OSL) dosimeters.

Regardless of the type of monitor, it is essential that it be obtained from a certified laboratory. In-house processing of radiation monitors should not be attempted.

Film Badges. Film badges came into general use during the 1940s and have been used widely in diagnostic radiology ever since. Film badges are specially designed devices in which a film similar to dental radiographic film is sandwiched between metal filters inside a plastic holder. Figure 40-7 is a view of several typical occupational radiation monitors.

The film incorporated into a film badge is special radiation dosimetry film that is particularly sensitive to x-rays. The optical density on the exposed and processed film is related to the exposure received by the film badge.

Carefully controlled calibration, processing, and analyzing conditions are necessary for the film badge to measure accurately occupational radiation exposure. Usually, exposures less than 10 mR (100 μGy_a) are not measured by film badge monitors, and the film badge vendor will report only that a minimum exposure (M) was received. When higher exposures are received, they can be accurately reported.

The metal filters, along with the window in the plastic film holder, allow estimation of the x-ray energy. The usual filters are made of aluminum and copper.

When the radiation exposure is a result of penetrating x-rays, the image of the filters on the processed film is faint and there may be no image at all of the window in the plastic holder. If the badge is exposed to soft x-rays, the filters are well imaged and the optical densities under the filters allow estimation of the x-ray energy.

Often the filters to the front of the film badge differ in shape from the filters to the back of the film badge. Radiation that had entered through the back of the film badge would normally indicate that the person wearing the badge received considerably higher exposure than indicated because the x-rays would have penetrated through the body before interacting with the film badge.

 Film badges must be worn with their proper side to the front.

Several advantages of film badge occupational radiation monitors continue to make them popular. They are inexpensive, easy to handle, easy to process, and reasonably accurate, and have been in use for several decades.

Film badge monitors also have disadvantages. They cannot be reused and because they incorporate film as the sensing device, they cannot be worn for more than 1 month because of possible fogging caused by temperature and humidity.

Film badge monitors should never be left in an enclosed car or other area where excessive temperatures may occur. The fogging produced by elevated temperature and humidity results in a falsely high evaluation of exposure.

Thermoluminescence Dosimeters. The sensitive material of the TLD monitor (Figure 40-8) is lithium fluoride (LiF) in crystalline form, either as a powder or more often as a small chip approximately 3 mm square and 1 mm thick. When exposed to x-rays, the TLD

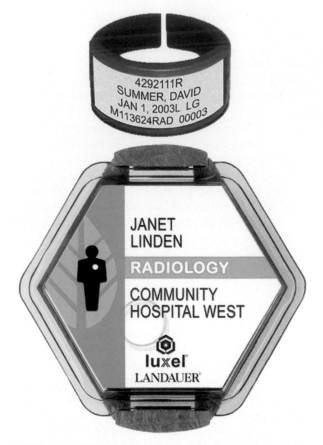

FIGURE 40-7 Some representative radiation monitors. Many have metal filters incorporated to help identify the type of radiation and its energy. (Courtesy Landauer, Inc.)

absorbs energy and stores it in the form of excited electrons in the crystalline lattice.

When heated, these excited electrons fall back to their normal orbital state with the emission of visible light. The intensity of visible light is measured with a photomultiplier tube and is proportional to the radiation dose received by the crystal. This sequence was described in Chapter 39.

The TLD occupational radiation monitor has several advantages over film. It is more sensitive and more accurate than a film badge monitor. Properly calibrated TLD monitors can measure exposure as low as 5 mR (50 μGy_a). The TLD monitor does not suffer from loss of information after exposure to excessive heat or humidity.

 TLDs can be worn for intervals up to 1 year.

The primary disadvantage of TLD personnel monitoring is cost. The price of a typical TLD monitoring ser-

vice is perhaps twice that of film badge monitoring. If the frequency of monitoring is quarterly, however, the cost is about the same.

Optically Stimulated Luminescence. OSL dosimeters (Figure 40-9) are worn and handled just as film badges and TLDs, and are approximately the same size. The OSL dosimeters have some advantages over all of the previous dosimeters.

Where to Wear the Occupational Radiation Monitor. Much discussion and research in health physics have gone into providing precise recommendations about where a radiologic technologist should wear the occupational radiation monitor. The official publications of the National Council on Radiation Protection and Measurements (NCRP) offer suggestions that have been adopted as regulations in most states.

Many radiologic technologists wear their personnel monitors in front at the waist or chest level because it is convenient to clip the badge over a belt or a shirt pocket. If the technologist is not involved in fluoroscopic procedures, these locations are acceptable.

If the radiologic technologist participates in fluoroscopy, then the occupational radiation monitor should be positioned on the collar above the protective apron.

The recommended dose limit of 5000 mrem/yr (50 mSv/yr) refers to the effective dose (E). It has been shown that during fluoroscopy, when a protective apron is worn, exposure to the collar region is approximately 20 times greater than that to the trunk of the body beneath the protective apron. So, if the occupational radiation monitor is worn beneath the protective apron, it will record a falsely low exposure and will not indicate what could be a hazardous exposure to unprotected body parts.

In some clinical situations—during pregnancy and for extremity monitoring—it may be advisable to wear more than one radiation monitor. The abdomen should be monitored during pregnancy. The extremities should be monitored during interventional procedures when the radiologist's hands are in close proximity to the useful beam. Nuclear medicine technologists should wear extremity monitors when handling millicurie quantities of radioactive material.

Occupational Radiation Monitoring Report

State and federal regulations require that the results of the occupational radiation monitoring program be recorded in a precise fashion and maintained for review. Annual, quarterly, monthly, or weekly monitoring periods are acceptable.

The occupational radiation monitoring report must contain a number of specific items of information (Fig-

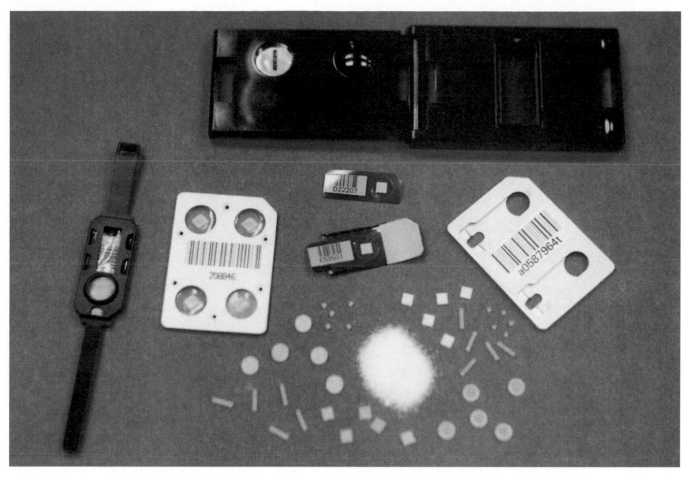

FIGURE 40-8 Thermoluminescence dosimeters are available as chips, disks, rods, and powder. They are used for area and environmental radiation monitoring and especially for occupational radiation monitoring. (Courtesy Bicron.)

ure 40-10). These various items are identified on the header of the columns.

The exposure data that must be included on the form are the current exposure and the cumulative annual exposure. Separate radiation monitors, such as extremity monitors or fetal monitors, are identified separately from the whole-body monitor.

Occasionally, if occupational exposure involves low energy radiation, dose to the skin might occur that is greater than the dose of penetrating radiation. In such cases, the skin dose is separately identified. There are areas on the report for neutron radiation exposure to accommodate nuclear reactor and particle accelerator workers.

When a radiologic technologist changes employment, the total radiation exposure history must be transferred to the records of the new employer. Consequently, when one leaves a job, one should automatically receive a report of the total radiation exposure history at that facility. Such a report should be given automatically; if it is not, it must be requested.

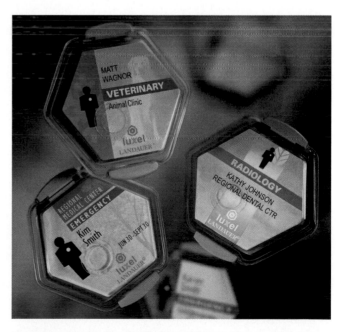

FIGURE 40-9 Optically stimulated luminescence dosimeters. (Courtesy Landauer, Inc.)

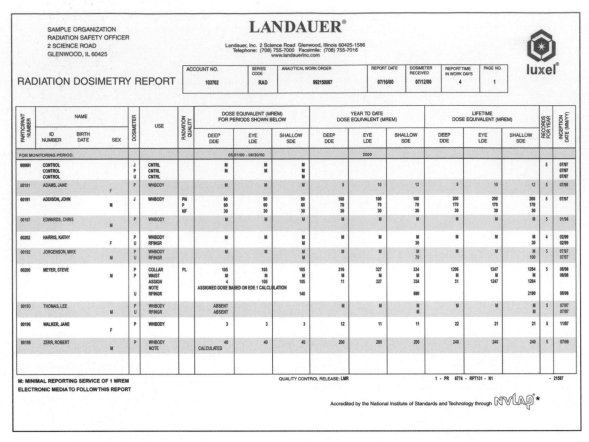

FIGURE 40-10 Occupational radiation monitoring report must include the items of information shown here. (Courtesy Landauer, Inc.)

When establishing an occupational radiation monitoring program, the supplier of the monitor should be informed of the type of radiation facility involved. That information influences the method of calibration of the monitors and the control monitors.

The control monitor should never be stored in or adjacent to a radiation area. It should be kept in a distant room or office. After processing, the response of the control monitor is subtracted from each individual monitor. That way, the report for each individual monitor represents only occupational radiation exposure.

> The control monitor measures the background exposure during transportation, handling, and storage.

All monitors should be returned to the supplier together and in a timely fashion so they can be processed together. Lost or inadvertently exposed monitors must be evaluated and an estimate of the true exposure should be made by the medical physicist.

Protective Apparel

The operating console is usually positioned behind fixed protective barriers during diagnostic radiographic procedures. During fluoroscopy or mobile radiography, radiologic personnel are in the examination room and near the x-ray source.

> Protective apparel must be worn during fluoroscopy and mobile radiology.

Protective gloves and aprons are available in many sizes and shapes. They are usually constructed of lead-impregnated vinyl. Some protective garments are impregnated with tin or other metals because other metals have some advantages over lead as a shielding material in the diagnostic x-ray energy range.

The normal thicknesses for protective apparel are 0.25, 0.5, and 1 mm of lead equivalent. The garments themselves are much thicker than these dimensions, but they provide shielding equivalent to that thickness of lead (Table 40-5). Protection of at least 0.25 mm Pb is required.

TABLE 40-5	Some Physical Characteristics of Protective Lead Aprons				
			PERCENTAGE X-RAY ATTENUATION		
Equivalent Thickness (mm Pb)		Weight (lb)	50 kVp	75 kVp	100 kVp
0.25		3–10	97	66	51
0.50		6–15	99.9	88	75
1.00		12–25	99.9	99	94

Maximum exposure reduction is obtained with the 1 mm lead equivalent garment, but an apron of this material can weigh as much as 10 kg (22 lb). The wearer could be exhausted by end of the fluoroscopy schedule just from having to carry the protective apron. The x-ray attenuation at 75 kVp for 0.25 mm lead equivalent and 1 mm lead equivalent is 66% and 99%, respectively.

 0.5 mm lead equivalent protective aprons are a workable compromise between unnecessary weight and desired protection.

Protective aprons for interventional radiology should be of the wrap-around type. During these procedures, there can be a lot of personnel movement and some, such as an anesthesiologist, may even have their back to the radiation source.

When not in use, protective apparel must be stored on properly designed racks. If they are continuously folded or heaped in the corner, cracks can develop. At least once a year, aprons and gloves should be fluoroscoped to be sure that no such cracks appear. If fluoroscopy is not available, high-kVp radiography (e.g., 120 kVp/10 mAs) may be used (see Figure 31-6).

Position

During fluoroscopy, all personnel should remain as far from the patient as possible, keeping the front of the apron facing the radiation source at all times. After loading spot films, the radiologic technologist should take a step or two backwards from the table when his or her presence is not required. The radiologist should use the dead man's foot switch sparingly. Naturally, when x-ray beam-on time is high, the radiation exposure to patient and personnel will be proportionately high.

Patient Holding

Many patients referred for x-ray examination are not physically able to support themselves. Examples are infants, the elderly, and the incapacitated. Mechanical restraining devices should be available for such patients. Otherwise, a relative or friend accompanying the pa-

tient should be asked to help. As a last resort, other hospital employees such as nurses and orderlies may be used **occasionally** to hold patients.

 Radiology staff should never hold patients.

When it is necessary to have another person hold the patient, protective apparel must be provided to that person. An apron and gloves are necessary, and the holder should be carefully positioned and instructed so that he or she is not exposed to the useful beam. Because the holder is often the mother of a child patient, be sure to ask if she could be pregnant.

REDUCTION OF UNNECESSARY PATIENT DOSE

The radiologic technologist has considerable control over many sources of unnecessary patient dose. Unnecessary patient dose is defined as any radiation dose that is not required for the patient's well-being or proper management and care.

Unnecessary Examinations

The radiologic technologist has practically no control over what some consider the largest source of unnecessary patient dose, that is, the unnecessary x-ray examination. This is almost exclusively the radiologist's or clinician's responsibility. Radiologic technologists can help by inquiring if the patient has had a previous x-ray examination. If so, perhaps those images should be obtained for review before continuing.

Unfortunately, this source of unnecessary patient dose presents a serious dilemma for the radiologist and the clinician. Many x-ray examinations are knowingly requested when the yield of helpful information may be extremely low or nonexistent. When such an examination is performed, the benefit to the patient in no way compensates for the radiation dose.

If the examination is not performed, however, the clinician and radiologist may be severely criticized if the patient's management results in failure. Even though the examination in question would have contributed little, if anything, to effective patient management, the radiologist may even be sued. In such situations, the radiologist is caught between the proverbial "rock and a hard place."

Routine x-ray examinations should not be performed when there is no precise medical indication. Substantial evidence shows that such examinations are of little benefit because they are not cost-effective and the disease detection rate is very low. Examples of such cases follow:

- **Mass screening for tuberculosis.** General screening has not been found effective. Better methods of tuberculosis testing are now available. Some x-ray screening in high-risk groups (e.g., medical and paramedical personnel), in service personnel posing a potential community hazard (e.g., food handlers or teachers), and in special occupational groups (e.g., miners and workers having contact with beryllium, asbestos, glass, or silica) may be appropriate.
- **Hospital admission.** Chest x-ray examinations for routine hospital admission when there is no clinical indication of chest disease should not be performed. Among patients who might be candidates for such examination are those admitted to the pulmonary service.
- **Preemployment physicals.** Chest and lower back x-ray examinations are not justified because the knowledge gained about previous injury or disease is nil.
- **Periodic health examinations.** Many physicians and health care organizations promote annual or biannual physical examinations. Certainly, when such an examination is conducted on an asymptomatic patient, it should not include x-ray examination, especially fluoroscopic examination.
- **Whole-body multislice spiral CT screening.** Some facilities now offer this procedure to the public for self-referral. Until there is evidence of a significant disease detection rate, this should not be done. The radiation dose is too high.

Repeat Examinations

One area of unnecessary radiation exposure that the radiologic technologist can influence is that of repeat examinations. The frequency of repeat examinations has been variously estimated to range as high as 10% of all examinations. In the typical busy hospital facility, the rate of repeat examinations does not normally exceed 5%. Examinations with the highest repeat rates are lumbar spine, thoracic spine, and abdomen.

Some repeat examinations are caused by equipment malfunctions. However, most are caused by radiologic technologist error. Studies of causes of repeat examinations have shown that improper positioning and poor radiographic technique resulting in an image too light or too dark are primarily responsible for repeats.

Motion and improper collimation are responsible for some repeats. Infrequent errors that also contribute to repeat examinations are dirty screens, use of improperly loaded cassettes, light leaks, chemical fog, artifacts caused by a dirty processor, wrong projection, improper patient preparation, grid errors, and multiple exposure.

Radiographic Technique

In general, the use of high-kVp technique results in reduced patient dose. Increasing the kVp is always associated with a reduction in mAs to obtain an acceptable radiographic optical density, and this in turn results in reduced patient dose.

This dose reduction occurs because the patient dose is linearly related to the mAs but is related to approximately the square of the kVp. An area of radiography where high-kVp technique is widely accepted is examination of the chest.

Question: A lateral skull radiograph is obtained at 64 kVp, 80 mAs and results in an ESE of 400 mR (4 mGy$_a$). If the tube potential is increased to 74 kVp (15% increase) and the mAs reduced by half to 40 mAs, the optical density will remain the same. What will be the new ESE?

Answer: $\text{Dose} = (400 \text{ mR}) \left(\dfrac{40 \text{ mAs}}{80 \text{ mAs}} \right) \left(\dfrac{74 \text{ kVp}}{64 \text{ kVp}} \right)^2$

$= (400 \text{ mR})(0.5)(1.34)$
$= 267 \text{ mR}$

Of course the radiologist must be the final judge of radiographic quality. Increasing kVp even slightly may result in images that have too low contrast for proper interpretation by the radiologist.

Proper collimation is essential to good radiographic technique. Positive beam limitation does not prevent the radiologic technologist from reducing the field size still further by collimation. By using collimation, not only is the patient dose reduced but the image quality is improved with enhanced contrast resolution because scatter radiation is also reduced.

Image Receptor

The image receptor should be selected first for the type of examination being performed, and second for the radiation dose necessary to produce a good-quality image. It should be kept in mind that it is screen speed rather than film speed that principally controls the patient dose.

The fastest-speed screen-film combination consistent with the nature of the examination should be used.

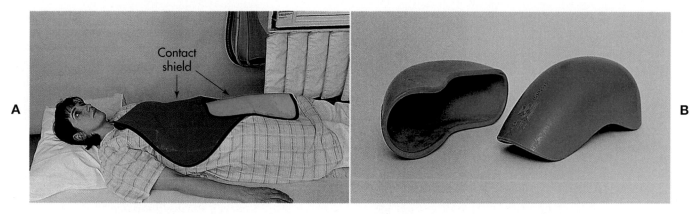

FIGURE 40-11 Examples of useful contact gonad shields, which can be a piece of vinyl-lead **(A)** or shaped **(B).**

Rare earth and other fast screens should be used when possible. The routine application of such screens in orthopedic, chest, and magnification radiography is appropriate. In some applications, the use of such fast systems may result in bothersome quantum mottle, but this again must be decided by the radiologist. Usually, 400-speed systems are now used for general radiography.

Patient Positioning

When examining the upper extremities or breast, especially with the patient in a seated position, care should be taken that the useful beam does not intercept the gonads. Position the patient lateral to the useful beam and provide a protective apron as a shield.

Specific Area Shielding

X-ray examinations result in a partial-body exposure, although most radiation protection guides and radiation response information are based on whole-body exposure. The partial-body nature of the x-ray examination is controlled by proper beam collimation and the use of specific area shielding.

Use of specific area shielding is indicated when a particularly sensitive tissue or organ is in or near the useful beam. The lens of the eye, the breasts, and the gonads are frequently shielded from the primary radiation beam. There are two types of specific area shielding devices: the **contact shield** and the **shadow shield.**

Lens shields are always of the contact type. The contact shielding device is positioned directly on the patient. Gonad shields, on the other hand, can be of either the contact or the shadow type.

Breast shields are contact shields recommended for use during scoliosis examinations. Such examinations often consist of an AP projection subjecting the juvenile breasts to primary beam x-irradiation. The PA projection, however, is equally satisfactory because

---

BOX 40-1 Gonad Shielding

Gonad shielding should be considered for all patients, especially children and those who are potentially reproductive. As an administrative procedure, this would include all patients younger than 40 years of age and perhaps even older men.

Gonad shielding should be used when the gonads lie in or near the useful beam.

Proper patient positioning and beam collimation should not be relaxed when gonad shields are in use.

Gonad shielding should be used only when it does not interfere with obtaining the required diagnostic information.

---

magnification is of little importance. The PA projection results in a breast dose of only approximately 1% of the AP projection.

Figure 40-11 shows some examples of contact gonad shields. When such contact shields are not purchased commercially, a properly cut piece of protective material is perfectly adequate. Shapes such as hearts, diamonds, triangles, and squares have been used effectively, especially for children.

An example of the shadow shield is shown in Figure 40-12. This type of shield is just as effective as the contact shield and is more acceptable for use with adult patients. The use of such devices, however, requires careful attention on the part of the radiologic technologist.

The shield must shadow the gonads without interfering with the desired anatomy. Improper positioning of the shadow shield can result in a repeat examination and increased patient dose. Shadow shields are particularly useful during surgery where sterile procedure is required. Box 40-1 lists the main points of gonadal shielding.

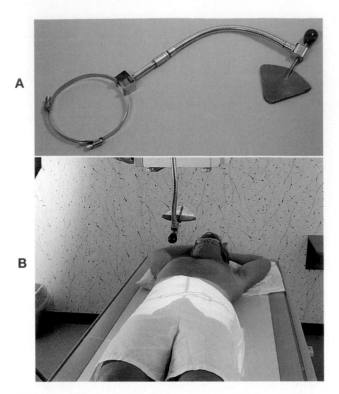

FIGURE 40-12 **A,** Shadow shield. **B,** Shadow shield suspended above the beam-defining system casts a shadow over the gonads. (Courtesy Nuclear Associates.)

SUMMARY

Although the dose limit for occupational workers is 50 mSv/yr, most radiologic personnel receive less than 0.5 mSv/yr. Radiologists may receive a higher dose if engaged in a heavy fluoroscopy schedule.

Patient dose from diagnostic x-rays is usually recorded in one of the following three ways: (1) ESE, (2) mean marrow dose, or (3) gonadal dose. TLDs are the monitor of choice for patient radiation dose. Knowing the output intensity of at least one x-ray technique and the SSD, the medical physicist can estimate the ESE for any patient examination. For fluoroscopic examinations, a good general assumption for the ESE is 4 R/min.

Because 95% of occupational exposure comes from fluoroscopy and mobile radiography, the radiologic technologist should follow these guidelines for reducing occupational exposure:
1. During mobile radiography, wear an apron, maintain maximum distance from the source, and never direct the primary beam toward others.
2. During fluoroscopy, step back from the table if not needed and use shielding, including an apron, curtain, Bucky slot cover, and the radiologist.

3. During radiography, stand behind the control booth and never direct the primary beam toward the control booth barrier.

Personnel monitoring is required when there is any likelihood that an individual will receive more than 1/10 the dose limit. The various personnel radiation monitors are (1) film badges, (2) TLDs, and (3) OSL dosimeters. Film badges are widely used because they are inexpensive and accurate, but they must be changed monthly. The OSL is very sensitive and accurate and may be worn for up to 1 year. For general use, the radiographer should wear the personnel monitor at waist or chest level; however, during fluoroscopy, the monitor is worn on the collar outside the protective apron.

Radiographers and occupational workers should never be used to hold patients during an exposure.

Use of specific area shielding is indicated when sensitive tissue or a sensitive organ is in or near the primary beam. Gonadal shielding should be considered for all patients of reproductive age and when the gonads are in or near the primary beam. Gonadal shielding should be used only when it does not interfere with the required diagnostic information.

CHALLENGE QUESTIONS

1. Define or otherwise identify:
   a. ALARA
   b. GSD
   c. Image receptor
   d. Shadow shield
   e. Mean marrow dose
   f. Personnel monitor
   g. The units of x-radiation output intensity
   h. Glandular dose
   i. CT noise
   j. NCRP
2. What is the dose limit for diagnostic imaging personnel?
3. During what two examination procedures is occupational radiation exposure usually the highest?
4. Why is diagnostic medical radiation exposure to patients commanding increased attention?
5. List the three ways patient dose is reported.
6. What is the estimated GSD caused by diagnostic x-ray examination?
7. Why are measurements of gonadal dose important?
8. Why is ESE not used in values stated for patient dose in mammography?
9. What is the difference between ESE in CT versus ESE in routine radiography?
10. What is the required length of the exposure cord on the mobile radiographic unit?

11. When must personnel radiation monitoring be provided?
12. Describe the design of film badges. How are they to be worn and where are they placed on the body?
13. List the exposure data that must be included in the personnel monitoring report.
14. What is an appropriate thicknesses of protective apparel?
15. What is the procedure for holding patients during an x-ray examination?
16. What four types of screening x-rays are no longer recommended?
17. Discuss the factors that should be considered when planning a routine x-ray examination room.

18. An obstetric and gynecologic hospital contains 250 beds and runs at a 75% occupancy rate. Forty percent of the inpatients are referred for x-ray examination. The normal period of hospitalization for these patients is 5 days. How many x-ray rooms would be needed for inpatient care?
19. A new clinic anticipates 10,000 patients each year with 90% requiring an x-ray examination. Of these patients, 20% require reexamination. How many x-ray rooms would be needed to handle the patient load in this clinic?
20. Describe the features of optically stimulated dosimetry that make it particularly effective for occupational radiation monitoring.

Glossary

Abrasion layer The protective covering of gelatin enclosing an emulsion.

Absolute age-response relationship The increased incidence of a disease is a constant number of cases after a minimal latent period.

Absolute risk The incidence of malignant disease in a population within 1 year for a given dose; it is expressed as number of cases/10^6 persons/rem.

Absorbed dose **a.** The energy transferred from ionizing radiation per unit mass of irradiated material; expressed in rad (100 erg/g) or gray (1 J/kg). **b.** The thermalization of tissue by the absorption of ultrasound energy; expressed as a rise in temperature (°C).

Absorption **a.** The transfer of energy from an electromagnetic field to matter. Removal of x-rays from a beam via the photoelectric effect. **b.** Process by which ultrasound transfers energy to tissue by the conversion of acoustic energy to heat.

Absorption blur The characteristic of the subject affecting subject contrast.

Acceleration (a) The rate of change of velocity with time.

Acceleration of gravity The constant rate at which objects falling to the Earth accelerate.

Acetic acid The chemical used in the stop bath.

Activator Chemical, usually acetic acid in the fixer and sodium carbonate in the developer, used to neutralize the developer and swell the gelatin.

Active memory Data can be stored or accessed at random from anywhere in main memory in approximately equal amounts of time, regardless of where the data are located.

Actual focal-spot size The area on the anode target that is exposed to electrons from the tube current.

Acute radiation syndrome Radiation sickness that occurs in humans after whole-body doses of 1 Gy (100 rad) or more of ionizing radiation delivered over a short time.

Adenine A nitrogenous organic base that attaches to a deoxyribose molecule.

Adhesive layer A protective covering of gelatin that encloses the emulsion.

Units are shown in parenthesis: for example, (Joules), (mHz), (m/s).

Aerial oxidation Oxidation that occurs when air is introduced into the developer when it is mixed, handled, and stored.

Afterglow Phosphorescence in an intensifying screen.

Age-response function The pattern of change in radiosensitivity as a function of phase in the cell cycle.

Air-gap technique The practice of moving the image receptor 10 to 15 cm from the patient so that fewer scattered x-rays interact with the image receptor, enhancing contrast.

ALARA The principle that radiation exposure should be kept as low as reasonably achievable, economic and social factors being taken into account.

Algorithm A computer-adapted mathematical calculation applied to raw data during image reconstruction.

Alnico An alloy of aluminum, nickel, and cobalt; one of the more useful magnets produced from ferromagnetic material.

Alpha particle (α particle) The particulate form of ionizing radiation consisting of two protons and two neutrons. The nucleus of helium. Emitted from the nucleus of a radioactive atom.

Alternating current (AC) The oscillation of electricity in both directions in a conductor.

Amber filter A filter that transmits light with wavelengths longer than 550 nm, which is above the spectral response of blue-sensitive film.

American Association of Physicists in Medicine (AAPM) The scientific society of medical physicists.

American College of Medical Physicists (ACMP) The professional society of medical physicists.

American College of Radiology (ACR) The professional society of radiologists and medical physicists.

American Society of Radiologic Technologists (ASRT) The scientific and professional society of radiographers.

Ammeter A device that measures current.

Ampere (A) The SI unit of electric charge. 1A = 1C/s.

Amplitude The width of a waveform.

Anabolism The process of synthesizing smaller molecules into a larger macromolecule.

Anaphase The second phase of mitosis, during which chromatids repel one another and migrate along the mitotic spindle to opposite sides of the cell.

Anatomically programmed radiography (APR) Rather than have the technologist select a desired kVp and mAs, graphics on the console guide the technologist.

Angiography Fluoroscopy in which the x-ray examination is applied toward the visualization of vessels.

Angstrom (Ån) The unit of measure of wavelength. 1 Ån = 10^{-10} m.

Anode Positively charged side of an x-ray tube, which contains the target.

Anthropomorphic Human characteristics.

Antibodies Proteins produced by the body in response to the presence of foreign antigens, such as bacteria or viruses.

Antigen The molecular configuration of an antibody that attacks a particular type of invasive or infectious agent.

Aperture a. A circular opening for the patient in the gantry of a computed tomographic or magnetic resonance imaging system. **b.** The fixed collimation of a diagnostic x-ray tube, as in an aperture diaphragm. **c.** The variable opening before the lens of a cine or photospot camera.

Aperture diaphragm A simple beam-restricting device that attaches a lead-lined metal diaphragm to the head of the x-ray tube.

Archival quality Referring to the fact that the image does not deteriorate with age but remains in its original state.

Area beam The x-ray beam pattern that is usually shaped like a square or rectangle and that is used in conventional radiography and fluoroscopy.

Array processor The part of a computer that handles raw data and performs the mathematical calculations necessary to reconstruct a digital image.

Artifact An unintended optical density on a radiograph or another film-type image receptor.

Asthenic Referring to a body habitus of a patient who is small and frail.

Atom The smallest particle of an element that cannot be divided or broken by chemical means.

Atomic mass The relative mass of a specific isotope of an element.

Atomic mass number (A) The number of protons plus the number of neutrons in the nucleus.

Atomic mass unit (amu) The mass of a neutral atom of an element, expressed as one twelfth the mass of carbon, which has an arbitrarily assigned value of 12.

Atomic number (Z) The number of protons in the nucleus.

Atrophy The shrinking in size of a tissue or organ.

Attenuation The reduction in radiation intensity as a result of absorption and scattering.

Automatic brightness control (ABC) A feature on a fluoroscope that allows the radiologist to select an image-brightness level that is subsequently maintained automatically by varying the kVp, the mAs, or both.

Automatic exposure control (AEC) A feature that determines radiation exposure during radiography in most x-ray imaging systems.

Autotransformer A transformer located in the operating console that controls the kVp; it has one winding of wire and varies voltage and current by self-induction.

Autotransformer law The principle stating that the voltage received and the voltage provided are in direct relation to the number of turns of the transformer enclosed by the respective connections.

Average gradient   Measure of radiographic contrast.

Axial   Perpendicular to the long axis of the body.

Axial tomography   Conventional tomography in which the plane of the image is parallel with the long axis of the body and results in sagittal and coronal images.

Backscatter radiation   X-rays that have interacted with an object and are deflected in backward.

Bandpass   The number of times per second that the electron beam can be modulated.

Basal cells   The stem cells that mature as they migrate to the surface of the epidermis.

Base   Area that serves as a mechanical support for the active phosphor layer in a radiographic intensifying screen.

Base density   The optical density inherent in the base of the film.

Baseline mammography   A woman's first radiographic examination of her breasts, used for comparison with all future mammograms.

Base plus fog (B+F)   The average density from an unexposed area of the strips.

Battery cell   Each zinc-copper plate formation in a voltaic pile.

Beam axis   The central line representing maximal ultrasound or x-ray intensity.

Beam-limiting device   A device that provides a means of restricting the size of an x-ray field.

Beam penetrability   The ability of an x-ray beam to penetrate tissue.

Beam restrictor   A device that restricts the size of the x-ray field to only the anatomic structure of interest.

Becquerel (Bq)   Special name for the SI units of radioactivity. One becquerel is equal to disintegration per second.

Beta particle (β particle)   Ionizing radiation with characteristics of an electron; emitted from the nucleus of a radioactive atom.

Binary number system   A number system with only two digits, 0 and 1.

Biochemistry   Chemical reactions at the molecular level.

Biplane imaging   A configuration of pairs of serial changers used with two orthogonal x-ray sources.

Bipolar   A magnet that has two poles.

Bit   The smallest unit of measure in computer storage capacity.

Bit depth   The number of bits used to reproduce image gray levels (e.g., 8 bits = 2^8 = 256 gray levels).

Body habitus   The general size and shape of a patient.

Brachytherapy   Radiation oncology in which the source of radiation is on or in the body.

Bremsstrahlung x-ray   An x-ray resulting from interaction of the projectile electron with a target nucleus; braking radiation.

Brightness gain   The ability of the image intensifier to increase the illumination level of the image.

Bucky factor (B)   The ratio of incident radiation to transmitted radiation through a grid; the ratio of patient dose with and that without a grid.

Bucky slot cover   A protective cover that automatically shields the Bucky slot opening during fluoroscopic examinations when the Bucky tray is at the foot of the table.

Buffer   Acetate added to the fixer to maintain a constant pH.

Buffering agent   An alkali compound in the developer that enhances the action of the developing agent by controlling the concentration of hydrogen ions.

Byte   A group of eight bits; represents one character or digit.

Calipers   An instrument with two bent or curved legs used for measuring the thickness of a solid.

Calorie (c)   The energy necessary to raise the temperature of 1 g of water 1° C.

C-arm fluoroscope   A portable device for fluoroscopy. The opposite ends of the C-shaped support arm hold the image intensifier and the x-ray tube.

Cassette   The rigid holder that contains the film and screens.

Cassette-loaded spot film   The conventional method of capturing images used with image-intensified fluoroscopes.

Catabolism   The process that creates energy for a cell by breaking down molecular nutrients that are brought to and diffused through the cell membrane.

Cathode   The negative side of the x-ray tube; contains the filament and focusing cup.

Cathode rays   A stream of electrons.

Cathode ray tube (CRT)   An electron beam tube designed for a two-dimensional display of signals.

Cell   The basic unit of all living matter.

Cell cloning   The process of normal cells producing a visible colony in a short time.

Cell cycle time   The average time from one mitosis to another.

Cell theory   The principle that all plants and animals contain cells as their basic functional units.

Center for Diseases and Radiological Health (CDRH)   Agency responsible for a national electronic radiation-control program. Known as the **Bureau of Radiological Health (BRH)** before 1982.

Central axis x-ray beam   An x-ray beam composed of x-rays traveling along the center of the useful x-ray beam.

Central nervous system (CNS) syndrome   A form of acute radiation syndrome caused by radiation doses of 50 Gy (5000 rad) or more of ionizing radiation that results in failure of the central nervous system, followed by death within a few hours to several days.

Central processing unit (CPU)   The processing hardware in large computers.

Central ray   The center of the x-ray beam that interacts with the image receptor.

Centrifugal force   The force that causes an electron to travel straight and leave the atom.

Centripetal force   The force that keeps an electron in orbit.

Characteristic curve   A graph of optical density vs. log relative response; H&D curve.

Characteristic x-ray   The x-ray released as a result of the photoelectric effect and whose discrete energies are determined by the respective electron binding energy.

Charge coupled device (CCD)   A solid-state device that converts visible light photons to electrons.

Chelate   A sequestering agent.

Chemical energy   The energy released by a chemical reaction.

Chemical fog   An artifact produced by chemical contamination of the developer.

Chemical symbol   The alphabetical abbreviation of an element.

Chip   A tiny piece of semiconductor material.

Chromatid deletion   The breakage of a chromatid.

Cine film   The film used in cinefluorography.

Cinefluorography   The recording of fluoroscopic images on movie film.

Classical scattering   The scattering of x-rays with no loss of energy. Also called **coherent, Rayleigh, or Thompson scattering**

Clearing agent   A chemical, usually ammonium thiosulfate, added to the fixer to remove undeveloped silver bromine from the emulsion.

Clinical tolerance   Moist desquamation in radiation therapy.

Closed-core transformer   A square core of ferromagnetic material built up of laminated layers of iron, which helps reduce energy losses caused by eddy currents.

Coast time   The time it takes the rotor to rest after use.

Codon   A series of three base pairs in the DNA.

Collimation   Restriction of the useful x-ray beam to reduce patient dose and improve image contrast.

Collimator   A device used to restrict x-ray beam size and shape.

Commutator   A device that acts like a switch, converting an alternating-current generator to a direct-current generator.

Compensating filter   Material inserted between an x-ray source and a patient to shape the intensity of the x-ray beam. An x-ray beam filter is designed to make the remnant beam more uniform in intensity.

Compression   The act of flattening soft tissue to improve optical density.

Compression device   A device that maintains close screen-film contact when the cassette is closed and latched.

Compton effect   The scattering of x-rays, resulting in ionization and loss of energy.

Compton scattering   The interaction between an x-ray and a loosely bound outer-shell electron, resulting in ionization and x-ray scattering.

Computed radiography (CR)   Radiographic technique that uses a photostimulable phosphor as the image receptor and an area beam.

Computed tomography (CT)   Creation of a cross-section tomographic section of the body using a rotating fan beam, detector array, and computed reconstruction.

Computed tomography dose index (CTDI)   The radiation dose in a single lice over a 10 cm length so that dose delivered beyond the selected slice thickness is included.

Conduction   The transfer of heat by molecular agitation.

Conductor   A material that allows heat or electric current to flow.

Cone   A circular metal tube that attaches to x-ray tube housing to limit the beam size and shape.

Cone cutting   Misalignment of cones that causes one side of the radiograph to not be exposed because the edge of the cone may interfere with the x-ray beam.

Cones and cylinders   Modifications of the aperture diaphragm.

Connective tissue   Tissue that binds tissue and organs together.

Contact shields   Shields that are flat and are placed directly on the patient's gonads.

Continuous quality improvement (CQI)   A program that includes administrative protocols for the continual improvement of mammographic quality.

Contrast   The degree of difference between the light and dark areas of a radiograph.

Contrast agent   A compound used as an aid for imaging internal organs with x-rays.

Contrast improvement factor   The ratio of radiographic contrast with a grid to that without a grid.

Contrast index   The difference between the step with an average optical density closest to 2.2 and the step with an average optical density closest to, but not less than, 0.5.

Contrast medium   An agent that enhances differences in anatomic structures.

Contrast resolution   The ability to distinguish between and to image similar tissues.

Controlled area   An area where personnel occupancy and activity are subject to control and supervision for the purpose of radiation protection.

Convection   The transfer of heat by the movement of hot matter to a colder place.

Conversion efficiency (CE)   The rate at which x-ray energy is transformed into light in an intensifying screen.

Conversion factor The ratio of the illumination intensity at the output phosphor to the radiation intensity incident on the input phosphor.

Coolidge tube A type of vacuum tube in use today that allows x-ray intensity and energy to be separately and accurately selected.

Cosmic rays Particulate and electromagnetic radiation emitted by the sun and the stars.

Coulomb (C) The SI unit of electric charge.

Coulomb per kilogram (C/kg) The SI unit of radiation exposure. 2.58×10^{-4} C/kg = 1 R.

Coupling The joining of magnetic fields produced by the primary and secondary coils.

Covalent bond The chemical union between atoms formed by sharing one or more pairs of electrons.

Covering power The more efficient use of silver in an emulsion to produce the same optical density per unit exposure.

Crookes tube The forerunner of modern fluorescent, neon, and x-ray tubes.

Crossed grid A grids that has lead strips running parallel to both the long and short axes.

Cross-linking The process of side spurs created by irradiation and attaching to a neighboring macromolecule or to another segment of the same molecule.

Crossover The process occurring during meiosis when chromatids exchange chromosomal material.

Crossover rack A device in an automatic processor that transports film from one tank to the next.

Cryogen An extremely cold liquid.

Crystal lattice A three-dimensional, cross-linked structure of silver, bromine, and iodine atoms.

Curie (Ci) The former unit of radioactivity. Expressed as 1 Ci = 3.7×10^{10} disintegrations per second = 3.7×10^{10} Bq.

Cutie pie The nickname for an ionization chamber–type survey meter.

Cytoplasm The protoplasm existing outside the cell's nucleus.

Cytosine A nitrogenous organic base that attaches to a deoxyribose molecule.

Data acquisition system (DAS) A computer-controlled electronic amplifier and switching device to which the signal from each radiation detector of a multislice spiral computed tomographic scanning system is connected.

Decimal system A system of numbers based on multiples of 10.

Densitometer Instrument that measures the optical density of exposed film.

Density difference (DD) The difference between the step with an average optical density closest to 2.2 and the step with an average optical density closest to, but not less than, 0.5.

Deoxyribonucleic acid (DNA) Molecule that carries the genetic information necessary for cell replication. The target molecule of radiobiology.

Derived quantities Any secondary quantity derived from a combination of one or more of the three base quantities, such as mass, length, and time.

Desquamation Ulceration and denudation of the skin.

Detail The degree of sharpness of structural lines on a radiograph.

Detective quantum efficiency (DQE) The percentage of x-rays absorbed by the screen.

Detector array Group of detectors and interspace material used to separate them. The image receptor in computed tomography.

Deterministic effect A biologic response whose severity varies with radiation dose. A dose threshold usually exists.

Developing The stage of processing during which the latent image is converted to a manifest image.

Developing agent A chemical, usually phenidone, hydroquinone, or Metol, that reduces exposed silver ions to atomic silver.

Development fog An artifact that results from crystals that had not been exposed reducing to metallic silver as a result of the lack of a restrainer.

Diagnostic mammography Examination performed on patients with symptoms or elevated risk factors for breast cancer.

Diagnostic-type protective tube housing Lead-lined housing enclosing an x-ray tube that shields leakage radiation to less than 100 mR/hr at 1 m.

Diaphragm A device that restricts an x-ray beam to a fixed size.

Dichroic stain A two-colored stain that appears as a curtain effect on the radiograph.

DICOM Digital Imaging and Communications in Medicine Standard to enable imaging systems from different manufacturers to communicate.

Differential absorption Different degrees of absorption in different tissues that results in image contrast and formation of the x-ray image.

Digital fluoroscopy (DF) A digital x-ray imaging system that produces a series of dynamic images obtained with an area x-ray beam and an image intensifier.

Digital radiography (DR) Static images produced with either a fan x-ray beam intercepted by a linear array of radiation detectors or an area x-ray beam intercepted by a photostimulable phosphor plate or a direct-capture solid-state device.

Dimagnetic Nonmagnetic materials that are unaffected when brought into a magnetic field.

Dimensional stability The property that allows the base of radiographic film to maintain its size and shape during use and processing so that it does not contribute to image distortion.

Diode Vacuum tube with two electrodes, a cathode, and an anode.

Dipolar Referring to a molecule with areas of opposing electric charges.

Direct current (DC)   The flow of electricity in only one direction in a conductor.

Direct-current motor   An electric motor in which many turns of wire are used for the current loop and many bar magnets are used to create the external magnetic field.

Direct effect   Effect of radiation that occurs when the ionizing radiation interacts directly with a particularly radiosensitive molecule.

Direct-exposure film   Film used without intensifying screens.

Disaccharide   A sugar.

Dissociation   The process of separating a whole into parts.

Distortion   Unequal magnification of different portions of the same object.

Dose   The amount of radiant energy absorbed by an irradiated object.

Dose equivalent (H)   The radiation quantity that is used for radiation protection and that expresses dose on a common scale for all radiations. Expressed in rem or sievert (Sv).

Dose length product (DLP)   The product of the CTDI and the slice thickness. Depends only on the selected Ct parameters and does not reflect patient dose.

Dose limit (DL)   The maximum permissible dose.

Dosimeter   An instrument that detects and measures exposure to ionizing radiation.

Dosimetry   The practice of measuring the intensity of radiation.

Double-contrast examination   An examination of the colon that uses air and barium for contrast.

Double-emulsion film   Radiographic film that has an emulsion coating on both sides of the base and a layer of supercoat over each emulsion.

Double-helix   The configuration of DNA that is shaped like a ladder twisted about an imaginary axis like a spring.

Doubling dose   That dose of radiation expected to double the number of genetic mutations in a generation.

Duplicating film   A single-emulsion film that is exposed to ultraviolet light or blue light through the existing radiograph to produce a copy.

Dynamic range   The range of values that can be displayed by an imaging system; shades of gray.

Early effect   A radiation response that occurs within minutes or days after radiation exposure.

Eddy current   A current opposing the magnetic field that induced it, creating a loss of transformer efficiency.

Edge enhancement   The accentuation of the interface between different tissues.

Edge-response function (ERF)   The mathematical expression of the ability of the computed tomographic scanner to reproduce a high-contrast edge with accuracy.

Effective atomic number   The weighted average atomic number for the different elements of a material.

Effective dose (E)   The sum over specified tissues of the products of the equivalent dose in a tissue (H_T) and the weighting factor for the tissue (W_T). Effective dose is a method of converting a nonuniform radiation dose, as when a protective apron is worn, to a dose, with respect to risk, as if the whole body were exposed.

Effective dose equivalent (H_E)   The sum of the products of the dose equivalent to a tissue (H_T) and the weighting factors (W_T) applicable to each of the tissues irradiated. The values (W_T) are different for effective dose and effective dose equivalent.

Effective focal-spot size   The area projected onto the patient and the image receptor.

Elective booking   A safeguard against the irradiation of an unsuspected pregnancy.

Electrical energy   The work that can be done when an electron or an electronic charge moves through an electric potential.

Electric circuit   The path of the electron flow from the generating source through the various components and back again.

Electric current   The flow of electrons.

Electric field   The lines of force exerted on charged ions in the tissues by the electrodes that cause charged particles to move from one pole to another.

Electricity   A form of energy created by the activity of electrons and other subatomic particles in motion.

Electrification   The process of adding or removing electrons from a substance.

Electrified object   An object that has too few or too many electrons.

Electrode   An electrical terminal or connector.

Electromagnet   A coil or wire wrapped around an iron core, which intensifies the magnetic field.

Electromagnetic energy   The type of energy in x-rays, radio waves, microwaves, and visible light.

Electromagnetic radiation   Oscillating electric and magnetic fields that travel in a vacuum with the velocity of light. Includes x-rays, gamma rays, and some nonionizing radiation (such as ultraviolet, visible, infrared, and radio waves).

Electromagnetic spectrum   The continuum of electromagnetic energy.

Electromotive force   Electric potential; measured in volts (V).

Electron   Elementary particle with one negative charge. Electrons surround the positively charged nucleus and determine the chemical properties of the atom.

Electron binding energy   The strength of attachment of an electron to the nucleus.

Electron optics   The engineering aspects of maintaining proper electron travel.

Electron spin   The momentum of a particle of an atom in a fixed pattern.

Electron volt (eV)   The unit of energy equal to that which an electron acquires from a potential difference of 1 V.

Electrostatics   Study of fixed or stationary electric charge.

Element   An atom having the same atomic number and same chemical properties. A substance that cannot be broken down further without changing its chemical properties.

Elemental mass   The characteristic mass of an element, determined by the relative abundance of isotopes and their respective atomic masses.

Elongation   An image made to appear longer than it really is because the inclined object is not located on the central x-ray beam.

Embryologic effect   Damage occurring as a result of an organism being exposed to ionizing radiation during its embryonic stage of development.

Emulsion   The material with which x-rays or light photons from screens interact and transfer information.

Endoplasmic reticulum   A channel or series of channels that allows the nucleus to communicate with the cytoplasm.

Energy   The ability to do work; measured in joules (J).

Energy levels   The orbits around the nucleus that contain a designated number of electrons.

Energy subtraction   A technique that uses the two x-ray beams alternately to provide a subtraction image resulting from differences in photoelectric interaction.

Entrance roller   A roller that grips the film to begin its trip through the processor.

Entrance skin exposure (ESE)   X-ray exposure to the skin; expressed in milliroentgen (mR).

Enzyme   A molecule that is necessary in small quantities to allow a biochemical reaction to continue even though it does not directly enter into the reaction.

Epidemiology   The study of the occurrence, distribution, and causes of disease in humans.

Epilation   The loss of hair.

Epithelium   The covering tissue that lines all exposed surfaces of the body, both exterior and interior.

Erg (Joule)   The unit of energy and work.

Erythema   A sunburnlike reddening of the skin.

Erythrocyte   A red blood cell.

EUR/OPE   *E*lectrons *u*sed in *r*eduction/*o*xidation *p*rocedure *e*lectrons.

Excess risk   The difference between the observed and the expected number of cases.

Excitation   The addition of energy to a system by raising the energy of electrons with the use of x-rays.

Exit radiation   The x-rays that remain after the beam exits through the patient.

Exponent   Superscript or power to which 10 is raised in scientific notation.

Exponential form   Power-of-10 notation.

Exposed matter   The matter that intercepts radiation and absorbs part or all of it; irradiated matter.

Exposure   The measure of the ionization produced in air by x-rays or gamma rays. The quantity of radiation intensity expressed in roentgen (R), Coulombs per kilogram (C/kg), or air kerma (Gy).

Exposure factors   The factors that influence and determine the quantity and quality of x-radiation to which the patient is exposed.

Exposure linearity   The ability of a radiographic unit to produce a constant radiation output for various combinations of mA and exposure time.

Extinction time   The time required to end an exposure.

Extrafocal radiation, off-focus radiation   Electrons that bounce off the focal spot and land on other areas of the target.

Extrapolation   The estimation of a value beyond the range of known values.

Falling-load generator   A design in which exposure factors are automatically adjusted to the highest mA at the shortest exposure time allowed by the high-voltage generator.

Fan beam   An x-ray beam pattern used in computed tomography and digital radiograph; projected as a slit.

Feed tray   The start of the transport system where the film to be processed is inserted into the automatic processor in the darkroom.

Ferromagnetic material   Material that is strongly attracted by a magnet and that can usually be permanently magnetized by exposure to a magnetic field.

Field   The interactions among different energies, forces, or masses that cannot be seen but can be described mathematically.

Field of view (FOV)   The image matrix size provided by digital x-ray imaging systems.

Fifteen-percent rule   A principle stating that if the optical density on a radiograph is to be increased using kVp, an increase in kVp by 15% is equivalent to doubling the mAs.

Filament   The part of the cathode that emits electrons, resulting in a tube current.

File   A collection of data or information that is treated as a unit by the computer.

Film badge   A pack of photographic film used for approximate measurement of radiation exposure to radiation workers. It is the most widely used and most economical type of personnel radiation monitor.

Film graininess   The distribution of silver halide grains in an emulsion.

Filtered back projection   The process by which an image acquired during computed tomography and stored in computer memory is reconstructed.

Filtration   The removal of low-energy x-rays from the useful beam with aluminum or another metal. It results in increased beam quality and reduced patient dose.

First-generation computed tomographic scanner A finely collimated x-ray beam, single-detector assembly that translates across the patient and rotates between successive translations.

Five-percent rule A principle stating that an increase of 5% in the kVp may be accompanied by a 30% reduction in the mAs to produce the same optical density at a slightly reduced contrast scale.

Fixing The stage of processing during which the silver halide not exposed to radiation is dissolved and removed from the emulsion.

Fluorescence The emission of visible light only during stimulation.

Fluorescent screen The cycle in a television-picture tube when the electron beam creates the television optical signal and then immediately fades.

Fluoroscope A device used to image moving anatomic structures with x-rays.

Fluoroscopy An imaging modality that provides a continuous image of the motion of internal structures while the x-ray tube is energized. Real-time imaging.

Flux gain The ratio of the number of light photons at the output phosphor to the number of x-rays at the input phosphor.

Focal spot The region of anode target where electrons interact to produce x-rays.

Focal-spot blur A blurred region on the radiograph over which the technologist has little control.

Focused grid A radiographic grid constructed so that the grid strips converge on an imaginary line.

Focusing cup A metal shroud surrounding the filament.

Fog An unintended optical density on a radiograph that reduces contrast because of light or chemical contamination.

Fog density The development of silver grain that contains no useful information.

Force That which changes the motion of an object; a push or a pull. Expressed in newtons (N).

Foreshortening The reduction in image size; related to the angle of inclination of the object.

4% voltage ripple Three-phase, 12-pulse power whose voltage supplied to the x-ray tube never falls below 96% of the peak value.

14% ripple Three-phase, six pulse power whose voltage supplied to the x-ray tube never falls below 86% of the peak value.

Fourth-generation computed tomographic scanner A unit in which the x-ray source rotates but the detector assembly does not.

Fraction A numerical value expressed by dividing one number by another.

Fractionated A radiation dose delivered at the same dose in equal portions at regular intervals.

Free radical An uncharged molecule containing a single unpaired electron in the valence shell.

Frequency The number of cycles or wavelengths of a simple harmonic motion per unit time. Expressed in Hertz (Hz). 1 Hz = 1 cycle/s.

Fulcrum The imaginary pivot point about which the x-ray tube and the image receptor move.

Full-wave rectification A circuit in which the negative half-cycle corresponding to the inverse voltage is reversed so that a positive voltage is always directed across the x-ray tube.

Full width at half maximum (FWHM) The width of the profile at half its maximum value.

Fundamental laws of motion The three principles of inertia, force, and action/reaction established by Isaac Newton.

Fundamental particles The three primary constituents of an atom: electrons, photons, and neutrons.

Gantry The portion of the computed tomographic or magnetic resonance imaging system that accommodates the patient and source or the detector assemblies.

Gastrointestinal (GI) syndrome A form of acute radiation syndrome that appears in humans at a threshold dose of about 10 Gy (1000 rad). It is characterized by nausea, diarrhea, and damage to the cells lining the intestines.

Geiger-Muller (G-M) counter Radiation-detection and radiation-measuring instrument that detects individual ionizations. It is the primary radiation survey instrument for nuclear medicine facilities.

Gelatin The part of the emulsion that provides mechanical support for the silver halide crystals by holding them uniformly dispersed in place.

Generation time See cell cycle time.

Genetically significant dose (GSD) The average gonadal dose to members of the population who are of childbearing age.

Genetic cell The oogonium or the spermatogonium.

Genetic effect Effects of radiation that affects and individual and subsequent unexposed generations.

Germ cell A reproductive cell.

Glandular dose The average radiation dose to glandular tissue.

Glow curve A graph that shows the relationship of light output to temperature change.

Glycogen A human polysaccharide.

Gonadal dose The exposure to the reproductive organs.

Gradient The slope of the tangent at any point on the characteristic curve.

Granulocyte A scavenger cell used to fight bacteria.

Gray (Gy) Special name for the SI unit of absorbed dose and air kerma. 1 Gy = 1 J/kg = 100 rad.

Gray scale An image display in which intensity is recorded as variations in brightness.

Grid   A device used to reduce the intensity of scatter radiation in the remnant x-ray beam.

Grid clean-up   The ability of a grid to absorb scatter radiation.

Grid-controlled tube   An x-ray tubes designed to be turned on and off very rapidly for situations requiring multiple exposures at precise exposure times.

Grid cutoff   The absence of optical density on a radiograph because of unintended x-ray absorption in a grid.

Grid frequency   The number of grid lines per inch or centimeter.

Grid lines   A series of sections of radiopaque material.

Grid ratio   The ratio of grid height to grid strip separation.

Guanine   A nitrogenous organic base that attaches to a deoxyribose molecule.

Guide shoe   A device in an automatic processor that is used for steering film around bends.

Guidewire   A device that allows the safe introduction of the catheter into the vessel.

Halation   The reflection of screen light transmitted through the emulsion and base.

Half-life   The time required for a quantity of radioactivity to be reduced to half its original value.

Half-valve layer (HVL)   The thickness of absorber necessary to reduce an x-ray beam to half its original intensity.

Half-wave rectification   A condition in which the voltage is not allowed to swing negatively during the negative half of its cycle.

Hard copy   A permanent image on film or paper, as opposed to an image on a cathode ray tube, disk, or magnetic tape.

Hardener   A chemical, usually potassium glutaraldehyde alum in the fixer, that is used to stiffen and shrink the emulsion.

Hard x-ray   An x-ray that has high penetrability and therefore is of high quality.

Hardware   The visible parts of the computer.

Health physics   The science concerned with the recognition, evaluation, and control of radiation hazards.

Heel effect   The absorption of x-rays in the heel of the target, resulting in reduced x-ray intensity to the anode side of the central axis.

Hematologic syndrome   A form of acute radiation syndrome after whole-body exposure to doses ranging from approximately 1 to 10 Gy (100 to 1000 rad). It is characterized by the reduction in white cells, red cells, and platelets in the circulating blood.

Hertz (Hz)   The unit of frequency; the number of cycles or oscillations each second of a simple harmonic motion.

Hexadecimal number system   Number system used by low-level applications to represent a set of four bits.

High-contrast resolution   The ability to image small objects having high subject contrast; spatial resolution.

High-voltage generator   One of three principal parts of an x-ray imaging system; it is always close to the x-ray tube.

Hit   A radiation interaction with the target.

Homeostasis   a. A state of equilibrium among tissue and organs. b. The ability of the body to return to normal function despite infection and environmental changes.

Hormone   A protein manufactured by various endocrine glands and carried by the blood to regulate body functions such as growth and development.

Horsepower (hp)   The British unit of power.

Houndsfield unit (HU)   The scale of computed tomographic numbers used to judge the nature of tissue.

Hybrid subtraction   A technique that combines temporal and energy subtraction.

Hydroquinone   The principal compound used in the chemical composition of film developers.

Hypersthenic   Referring to a body habitus of a patient who is big in frame and overweight.

Hypo   Sodium thiosulfate, a fixing agent that removes unexposed and undeveloped silver halide crystals from the emulsion.

Hypo retention   The undesirable retention of the fixer in the emulsion.

Hyposthenic   Referring to a body habitus of a patient who is thin but healthy looking.

Hysteresis   The additional resistance created by the alternate reversal of the magnetic field caused by the alternating current.

Image detail   The sharpness of small structures on the radiograph.

Image-forming x-ray   An x-ray that exits from the patient and enters the image receptor.

Image intensifier   An electronic vacuum tube that amplifies a fluoroscopic image to reduce patient dose.

Image matrix   A layout of cells in rows and columns.

Image noise   The deterioration of the radiographic image.

Image receptor (IR)   The medium that transforms the x-ray beam into a visible image; radiographic film or a phosphorescent screen.

Image receptor contrast   Contrast that is inherent in the film and is influenced by processing of the film. See also **subject contrast**.

Improper fraction   A fraction in which the quotient is greater than 1.

Indirect effect   The effect of radiation that results from the production of free radicals produced by the interaction of radiation with water.

Induction   The process of making ferromagnetic material magnetic.

Induction motor   An electric motor in which the rotor is a series of wire loops but the external magnetic field is supplied by several fixed electromagnets called stators.

Inertia   The property of matter that resists change in motion or at rest.

Infrared light A light consisting of photons with wavelengths longer than those of visible light but shorter than those of microwaves.

Infrared radiation Electromagnetic radiation just lower in energy than visible light, with a wavelength in the range of 0.7 to 1000 μm.

Inherent filtration The filtration of useful x-ray beams provided by the permanently installed components of an x-ray tube housing assembly and the glass window of an x-ray tube.

Initiation time The time required to start an exposure.

Input The process of transferring information into primary memory.

Insulator A material that inhibits the flow of electrons in a conductor or in heat transfer.

Integrate mode A function of an instrument designed to measure the total accumulated intensity of radiation over a period of time.

Intensification factor (IF) The ratio of exposure without screens to that with screens to produce the same optical density.

Intensifying screen A sensitive phosphor that converts x-rays to light to shorten exposure time and reduce patient dose.

Intensity profile The projection formed by the intensity of radiation detected according to the attenuation pattern.

Internally deposited radionuclide A naturally occurring radionuclide in the human body.

International System of Units (SI) Standard system of units based on the meter, kilogram, and second; it has been adopted by all countries and is used in all branches of science.

Interface Hardware and software that enable imaging systems to interconnect and to connect with printers.

Interphase The period of growth of the cell between divisions.

Interpolation The estimation of a value between two known values.

Interrogation time Time during which the signal from an image detector is sampled.

Interspace material The sections of radiolucent material in a grid.

Interstitial Referring to the area between cells.

Inverse square law Law stating that the intensity of the radiation at a location is inversely proportional to the square of its distance from the source of radiation.

Inverse voltage Current flowing from the anode to the cathode.

Inverter High-speed switches that convert direct current into a series of square pulses.

In vivo In the living cell.

Ion An atom with too many or too few electrons; an electrically charged particle.

Ion chamber An instrument that detects and measures the radiation intensity in areas outside of protective barriers.

Ionic bonds A bonding that occurs because of an electrostatic force between ions.

Ionization The removal of an orbital electron from an atom.

Ionization potential The amount of energy (34 eV) necessary to ionize tissue atoms.

Ionized Referring to an atom that has an extra electron or has had an electron removed.

Ionizing radiation Radiation capable of ionization.

Ion pair Two oppositely charged particles.

Irradiated Referring to matter that intercepts radiation and absorbs part or all of it; exposed.

Isobars Atoms having the same number of nucleons but different numbers of protons and neutrons.

Isochromatid A fragment in a chromosome aberration.

Isomers Atoms having the same number of protons and neutrons but a different nuclear energy state.

Isotones Atoms having the same number of neutrons.

Isotopes Atoms that have the same number of protons but a different number of neutrons.

Isotropic Equal intensity in all directions; having the same properties in all directions.

Joule (J) The unit of energy; the work done when a force of 1 N acts on an object along a distance of 1 m.

Karotype A chromosome map.

Kerma (k) The energy absorbed per unit mass from the initial kinetic energy released in matter of all the electrons liberated by x-rays or gamma rays. Expressed in gray (Gy). 1 Gy = 1 J/kg.

Kilo- Prefix meaning "one thousand."

Kiloelectron volt (keV) The kinetic energy of an electron equivalent to 1000 eV. 1 keV = 1000 eV.

Kilogram (kg) The scientific unit of mass that is unrelated to gravitational effects; 1000 g.

Kilovolt (kV) Electric potential equal to 1000 V.

Kinetic energy The energy of motion.

Kilovolt peak (kVp) A measure of the maximum electrical potential across an x-ray tube; expressed in kilovolts.

Lag Phosphorescence.

Laser disk A removable disk that uses laser technology to write and read data.

Late effect A radiation response that is not observed for 6 months or more after the exposure.

Latent image An unobservable image stored in the silver halide emulsion; it is made manifest by processing.

Latent image center A sensitivity center that has many silver ions attracted to it.

Latent period The period after the prodromal stage of the acute radiation syndrome during which there is no visible sign of radiation sickness.

Lateral decentering The improper positioning of the grid that results in cutoff.

Latitude The range of x-ray exposure over which a radiograph is acceptable.

Law of Bergonié and Tribondeau   The principle stating that the radiosensitivity of cells is directly proportional to their reproductive activity and inversely proportional to their degree of differentiation.

Law of conservation of energy   The principle stating that energy may be transformed from one form to another but cannot be created or destroyed; the total amount of energy is constant.

Law of conservation of matter   The principle stating that matter can be neither created nor destroyed.

Law of inertia   The principle stating that a body will remain at rest or continue to move with a constant velocity in a straight line unless acted on by an external force.

LD$_{50/60}$ Dose of radiation expected to cause death within 60 days to 50% of those exposed.

Leakage radiation   Secondary radiation emitted through the tube housing.

Limiting resolution   The spatial frequency at a modulation transfer function equal to 0.1.

Linear energy transfer (LET)   A measure of the rate at which energy is transferred from ionizing radiation to soft tissue. Expressed in kiloelectron volts per micrometer of soft tissue.

Linear, nonthreshold   Referring to the dose-response relationship that intersects the dose axis at or below zero.

Linear, threshold   Referring to the dose-response relationship that intercepts the dose axis at a value greater than zero.

Linear tomography   The imaging modality in which the x-ray tube is mechanically attached to the image receptor and moves in one direction as the image receptor moves in the opposite direction.

Line focus   The projection of an inclined line into a surface, resulting in a smaller size.

Line focus principle   A design incorporated into x-ray tube targets to allow a large area for heating while maintaining a small focal spot.

Line pair   One bar and its interspace of equal width.

Lodestone   A leading stone.

Logic function   A computer-recognized command that evaluates an intermediate result and performs subsequent computations depending on that result.

Log relative exposure (LRE)   The change in optical density over each exposure interval.

Long gray scale   A low-contrast radiograph that has many shades of gray.

Look-up-table (LUT)   A matrix of data that manipulates the values of gray levels, converting an image input value to a different output value.

Low-contrast resolution   The ability to image objects with similar subject contrast.

Luminescence   The emission of visible light.

Lymphocyte   The white blood cell that plays an active role in providing immunity for the body by producing antibodies; it is the most radiosensitive blood cell.

Lysosome   Cell that contains enzymes capable of digesting cellular fragments.

Magnetic dipole   Current flowing in an infinitesimally small loop.

Magnetic dipole moment   Vector with a magnitude equal to the product of the current flowing in a loop and the area of the current loop.

Magnetic domain   An accumulation of many atomic magnets with their dipoles aligned.

Magnetic permeability   The property of a material causing it to attract the imaginary lines of the magnetic field.

Magnetic susceptibility   The ease with which a substance can be magnetized.

Magnetite   The magnetic oxide of iron.

Magnetism   The polarization of a material.

Magnetization   The relative magnetic flux density in a material compared with that in a vacuum.

Magnification   The condition in which the images on the radiograph are larger than the object they represent.

Magnitude   A number representing a quantity.

Main-chain scission   The breakage of the long-chain macromolecule that divides the long, single molecule into smaller ones.

Mainframe computer   A fast, medium to large, large-capacity system that has multiple microprocessors.

Mammographer   A radiologic technologist specializing in breast x-ray studies.

Mammography   Radiographic examination of the breast using low kilovoltage.

Manifest illness   The stage of the acute radiation syndrome during which signs and symptoms are apparent.

Manifest image   The observable image formed when the latent image undergoes the proper chemical processing.

Man-made radiation   X-rays and artificially produced radionuclides used for nuclear medicine.

Mask image   The image obtained from mask mode.

Masking   The act of ensuring that no extraneous light from the viewbox enters the viewer's eyes.

Mask mode   The method of temporal subtraction that results in successive subtraction images of contrast-filled vessels.

Mass   A quantity of matter; expressed in kilograms.

Mass density   The quantity of matter per unit volume.

Mass-energy equivalence   Energy equals mass multiplied by the square of the speed of light.

Matrix   The rows and columns of pixels displayed on a digital image.

Matter   Anything that occupies space and has form or shape.

Maximum-intensity projection (MIP)   Reconstruction of an image by selecting the highest-value pixels along any arbitrary line through the data set and exhibiting only those pixels.

Maximum permissible dose (MPD)   The dose of radiation that would be expected to produce no significant radiation effects.

Mean lethal dose   A constant related to the radiosensitivity of a cell.

Mean marrow dose (MMD)   The average radiation dose to the entire active bone marrow.

Mean survival time   The average time between exposure and death.

Mechanical energy   The ability of an object to do work. See also **kinetic energy** and **potential energy**.

Medical physicist   A physicist who examines and monitors the performance of imaging equipment.

Meiosis   The process of germ cell division that reduces the chromosomes in each daughter cell to half the number of chromosomes in the parent cell.

Metabolism   Anabolism and catabolism.

Metaphase   The phase of cell division during which the chromosomes are divisible.

Metol   A secondary constituent used in the chemical composition of developing agents.

Microcalcifications   Calcific deposits that appear as small grains of varying sizes on the x-ray film.

Microcomputer   A personal computer or electronic organizer.

Microcontroller   A tiny computer installed in an appliance.

Microfocus tube   A tubes that has a very small focal spot and that is specifically designed for imaging very small microcalcifications at relatively short source-to-image distances.

Microwave   A short-wavelength radiofrequency.

Mid-density (MD) step   The step that has an average optical density closest to, but not less than, 1.2.

Milliampere (mA)   The measure of x-ray tube current.

Milliampere-second (mAs)   The product of exposure time and x-ray tube current; a measure of the total number of electrons.

Minification gain   The ratio of the square of the diameter of the input phosphor to the square of the diameter of the output phosphor.

Misregistration   Misalignment of two or more images because of patient motion between image acquisition.

Mitochondrion   A structure that digests macromolecules to produce energy for the cell.

Mitosis (M)   The process of somatic cell division wherein a parent cells divides to form two daughter cells identical to the parent cell.

Modem   A device that converts digital information into analog information.

Modulation   A changing of the magnitude of a video signal; the magnitude is directly proportional to the light intensity received by the television-camera tube.

Modulation transfer function (MTF)   A mathematical procedure for measuring resolution.

Molecule   A group of atoms of various elements held together by chemical forces; the smallest unit of a compound that can exist by itself and retain all its chemical properties.

Molybdenum   A target material for x-ray tubes that is used in mammography.

Momentum   The product of the mass of an object and its velocity.

Monoenergetic   A beam containing x-rays or gamma rays that all have the same energy.

Monosaccharide   A sugar.

Motherboard   The main circuit board in a system unit.

Motion blur   The blurring of the image that results from movement of either the patient or the x-ray tube during exposure.

Moving grid   A grid that moves while the x-ray exposure is being made.

Multiplanar reformation (MPR)   Process in which transverse images are stacked to form a three-dimensional data set.

Multislice computed tomography   An imaging modality that uses two detector arrays to produce two spiral slices at the same time.

Multitarget or single-hit model   A model of radiation dose-response relationship for more complicated biologic systems, such as human cells.

Muscle   A tissue capable of contracting.

Mutual induction   The process of producing electricity in a secondary coil by passing an alternating current through a nearby primary coil.

National Council on Radiation Protection and Measurement (NCRP)   The organization that continuously reviews the recommended dose limits.

Natural   A zero dose of radiation exposure.

Natural environmental radiation   Naturally occurring ionizing radiation, including cosmic rays, terrestrial radiation, and internally deposited radionuclides.

Natural magnet   A magnet that gets its magnetism from the Earth.

Nervous tissue   Tissue that consists of neurons and is the avenue through which electrical impulses are transmitted throughout the body for control and response.

Neuron   A cell of the nervous system that has long, thin extensions from the cell to distant parts of the body.

Neutron   Uncharged elementary particle, with a mass slightly greater than that of the proton, found in the nucleus of every atom heavier than hydrogen and in the nucleus of an atom.

Newton (N)   The unit of force in the SI system; 1 N < 1/4 lb.

Node   One of many stations or terminals of a computer network.

Noise   a. The grainy or uneven appearance of an image caused by an insufficient number of primary x-rays. b. A uniform signal produced by scattered x-rays.

Nonionizing radiation   Radiation for which the mechanism of action in tissue does not directly ionize atomic or molecular systems through a single interaction.

Nonlinear, nonthreshold   Referring to varied responses that are produced from varied doses, with any dose expected to produce a response.

Nonlinear, threshold   Referring to varied responses that are produced from varied doses, with a particular level below which there is no response.

Nonscheduled maintenance   Maintenance that becomes necessary because of a failure in the system that necessitates processor repair.

Nonstochastic effects   Biologic effects of ionizing radiation that demonstrate the existence of a threshold. The severity of the biologic damage increases with increased dose.

North pole   A magnetic pole that has a positive electrostatic charge.

Nuclear energy   The energy contained in the nucleus of an atom.

Nucleolus   A rounded structure that is often attached to the nuclear membrane and controls the passage of molecules, especially RNA, from the nucleus to the cytoplasm.

Nucleon   A proton or a neutron.

Nucleotide   The unit formed from a nitrogenous base, a five-carbon sugar molecule, and a phosphate molecule.

Nucleus   a. The center of a living cell; a spherical mass of protoplasm containing the genetic material (DNA), which is stored in its molecular structure. b. The center of an atom containing neutrons and protons.

Nuclide   General term referring to all know isotopes, both stable and unstable, of chemical elements.

Object plane   The plane in which the anatomic structures that are to be imaged lie.

Occupational dose   The dose received by an individual in a restricted area during the course of employment in which the individual's assigned duties involve exposure to radiation.

Occupational exposure   Radiation exposure received by radiation workers.

Off-focus radiation   X-rays produced in the anode but not at the focal spot.

Off-level grid   An artifact produced by having an improperly positioned radiographic tube, not by having an improperly positioned grid.

Object-to-image receptor distance (OID)   The distance from the image receptor to the object that is to be imaged.

1% voltage ripple   High-frequency generators that have higher x-ray quantity and quality.

100% voltage ripple   Single-phase power in which the voltage varies from zero to its maximum value.

Oocytes   Primordial follicles that grow to encapsulate oogonia.

Opaque   A surface that does not allow the passage of light.

Open filament   A condition that results when the filament becomes thinner and breaks.

Operating console   Console that allows the radiologic technologist to control the x-ray tube current and voltage so that the useful x-ray beam is of proper quantity and quality.

Operating system   The series of instructions that organizes the course of data through the computer to solve a particular problem.

Optical density   The degree of blackening of a radiograph.

Optical disk   A removable disk that uses laser technology to write and read data.

Ordered pairs   Notation for coordinates in which the first number of the pair represents a distance along the x-axis and the second number indicates a distance up the y-axis.

Origin   The point where two axes meet on a graph.

Organs   A collection of tissues of similar structure and function.

Organ system   A combination of tissues and organs that forms an overall integrated organization.

Organic molecule   A molecule that is life supporting and contains carbon.

Orthochromatic   Referring to blue- or green-sensitive film; usually exposed with rare earth screen.

Outcome analysis   Image interpretation that involves reconciling the patient's ultimate disease condition with the radiologist's diagnosis.

Output   The process of transferring the results of a computation from primary memory to storage or the user.

Overcoat   A protective covering of gelatin that encloses the emulsion.

Overexposed   Referring to a radiograph that is too dark because too much x-radiation reached the image receptor.

Ovum   The mature germ cell found in a female.

Oxidation   A reaction that produces an electron.

Oxygen enhancement ratio (OER)   The ratio of the dose necessary to produce a given effect under anoxic conditions to the dose necessary to produce the same effect under aerobic conditions.

Pair production   The interaction between the x-ray and the nuclear electric field that causes the x-ray to disappear and causes two electrons, one positive and one negative, to take its place.

Panchromatic   Referring to film that is sensitive to the entire visible light spectrum.

Parallel circuit   A circuit that contains elements that bridge conductors rather than lie in a line along a conductor.

Parallel grid   A simple grid in which all lead grid strips are parallel.

Paramagnetic Referring to materials slightly attracted to a magnet and loosely influenced by an external magnetic field.

Parenchymal Referring to part of the organ that contains tissues representative of that particular organ.

Partial volume effect Distortion of the signal intensity from a tissue because it extends partially into an adjacent slice thickness.

Particle accelerator An atom "smasher."

Particulate radiation Radiation distinct from x-rays and gamma rays; examples are alpha particles, electrons, neutrons, and protons.

Penetrability The ability of an x-ray to penetrate tissue; the range in tissue; x-ray quality.

Penetrometer An aluminum step wedge.

Penumbra Image blur result from the size of the focal spot; geometric unsharpness.

Permanent magnet A magnet whose magnetism is artificially induced.

Phantom A device that simulates some parameters of the human body for evaluating imaging system performance.

Phenidone A secondary constituent used in the chemical composition of developing agents.

Phosphor The active layer of the radiographic intensifying screen closest to the radiographic film.

Phosphorescence The emission of visible light during and after stimulation.

Photoconductor A material that conducts electrons when illuminated.

Photodiode A solid-state device that converts light into an electric current.

Photodisintegration The process by which very-high-energy x-rays can escape interaction with electrons and the nuclear electric field and can be absorbed directly by the nucleus.

Photoelectron An electron that has been removed during the process of photoelectric absorption.

Photoelectric effect The absorption of an x-ray by ionization.

Photoemission Electron emission after light stimulation.

Photographic effect The formation of the latent image.

Photometer An instrument that measures light intensity.

Photomultiplier tube An electron tube that converts visible light into an electrical signal.

Photon Electromagnetic radiation that has neither mass nor electric charge but interacts with matter as though it is a particle; x-rays and gamma rays.

Photospot camera A camera that exposes only one frame when active, receiving its image from the output phosphor of the image-intensifier tube.

Photostimulation The emission of visible light after excitation by laser light.

Photothermographic A printing process in which film is exposed to light, forming a latent image, which is made visible by heat.

Phototimer A device that allows automatic exposure control.

Pitch See **spiral pitch ratio.**

Pixel A picture element; the cell of a digital image matrix.

Planck's constant (h) A fundamental physical constant that relates the energy of radiation to its frequency.

Planetary rollers Rollers positioned outside the master roller and guideshoes.

Pluripotential stem cell A stem cell that has the ability to develop into several different types of mature cells.

Pocket ionization chamber (pocket dosimeter) A personnel radiation-monitoring device.

Point lesion Any change that results in the impairment or loss of function at the point of a single chemical bond.

Point mutation A molecular lesion caused by the change or loss of a base that destroys the triplet code and may not be reversible.

Polarity The existence of opposing negative and positive charges.

Pole The magnetically charged end of a material.

Polyenergetic Referring to radiation, such as x-rays, having a spectrum of energies.

Polysaccharide A large carbohydrate that includes starches and glycogen.

Positive beam limiting (PBL) A feature of radiographic collimators that automatically adjusts the radiation field to the size of the image receptor.

Potassium bromide A compound used as a restrainer in the developer.

Potassium iodide A compound used as a restrainer in the developer.

Potential energy The ability to do work by virtue of position.

Power Time rate at which work (W) is done. 1 W = 1 J/s.

Power-of-10 notation Exponential form.

Precursor cell An immature cell.

Predetector collimator A collimator that restricts the x-ray beam viewed by the detector array.

Prepatient collimator A collimator that consists of several sections so that a nearly parallel x-ray beam results.

Prereading voltmeter A kVp meter that registers even though an exposure is not being made and no current is flowing in the circuit; this allows the voltage to be monitored before an exposure.

Preservative A chemical additive, usually sodium sulfide, that maintains the chemical balance of the developer and fixer.

Preventative maintenance   A planned program of parts replacement at regular intervals.

Primary coil   The first coil through which the varying current in an electromagnet is passed.

Primary protective barrier   Any wall to which the useful beam can be directed.

Processing   Chemical treatment of the emulsion of a radiographic film to change a latent image to a manifest image.

Processor   The electronic circuitry that does the actual computations and the memory that supports it.

Prodromal period   The first stage of the acute radiation syndrome, which occurs within hours after radiation exposure.

Proper fraction   A fraction in which the quotient is less than 1.

Prophase   The phase of cell division during which the nucleus and the chromosomes enlarge and the DNA begins to take structural form.

Proportion   The relation of one part to another.

Proportional counter   A sensitive instruments used primarily as stationary laboratory instruments for the assay of small quantities of radioactivity.

Protective coating   The layer of the radiographic intensifying screen closest to the radiographic film.

Protective housing   A lead-lined metal container into which the x-ray tube is fitted.

Protein synthesis   The metabolic production of proteins.

Proton   An elementary particle with a positive electric charge equal to that of an electron and a mass approximately equal to that of a neutron. It is located in the nucleus of an atom.

Protracted dose   A dose of radiation delivered continuously but at a lower dose rate.

Pulse mode/rate mode   Instruments designed to detect the presence of radiation.

Quality assurance (QA)   All planned and systematic actions necessary to provide adequate confidence that a facility, system, or administrative component will perform safely and satisfactorily in service to a patient. It includes scheduling, preparation and promptness in the examination or treatment, reporting of results, and quality control.

Quality control (QC)   All actions necessary to control and verify the performance of equipment. It is included in quality assurance.

Quantum   An x-ray photon.

Quantum mottle   Radiographic noise produced by the random interaction of x-rays with an intensifying screen. This effect is more noticeable when very high rare-earth systems are used at a high kVp.

Quantum theory   The theory in the physics of matter smaller than an atom and of electromagnetic radiation.

Rad (radiation absorbed dose)   Special unit for absorbed dose and air kerma. 1 rad = 100 erg/g = 0.01 Gy.

Radiation   The energy emitted and transferred through matter.

Radiation biology   The branch of biology concerned with the effects of ionizing radiation on living systems.

Radiation exposure   X-ray quantity or intensity, measured in roentgens.

Radiation fog   Artifact caused by unintentional exposure to radiation.

Radiation hormesis   The theory that suggests that very low radiation doses may be beneficial.

Radiation quality   The relative penetrability of an x-ray beam determined by its average energy; usually measured by half-value layer or kilovolt peak.

Radiation quantity   The intensity of radiation; usually measured in milliroentgen (mR).

Radiation standards   The recommendations, rules, and regulations regarding permissible concentrations, safe handling, techniques, transportation, industrial control of radioactive material.

Radiation (thermal)   The transfer of heat by the emission of infrared electromagnetic radiation.

Radiation weighting factor (W_R)   The factor used for radiation-protection that accounts for differences in biologic effectiveness between different radiations. Formerly called **quality factor.**

Radioactive decay   A naturally occurring process whereby an unstable atomic nucleus relieves its instability through the emission of one or more energetic particles.

Radioactive disintegration   The process by which the nucleus spontaneously emits particles and energy and transforms itself into another atom to reach stability.

Radioactive half-life   The time required for a radioisotope to decay to half its original activity.

Radioactivity   The rate of decay or disintegration of radioactive material. Expressed in curie (Ci) or becquerel (Bq). 1 Ci = 3.7×10^{10} Bq.

Radiofrequency (RF)   Electromagnetic radiation having frequencies from 0.3 kHz to 300 GHz; magnetic resonance imaging uses RF in the range of approximately 1 to 100 mHz.

Radiographer   A radiologic technologist who deals specifically with x-ray imaging.

Radiographic contrast   The combined result of image receptor contrast and subject contrast.

Radiographic intensifying screen   A device that converts the energy of the x-ray beam into visible light to increase the brightness of an x-ray image.

Radiographic noise   The undesirable fluctuation in the optical density of the image.

Radiographic technique   The combination of settings selected on the control panel of the x-ray imaging system to produce a quality image on the radiograph.

Radiographic technique chart   A guide that describes standard methods for consistently producing high-quality images.

Radiography An imaging modality that uses x-ray film and usually an x-ray tube mounted from the ceiling on a track that allows the tube to be moved in any direction and provides fixed images.

Radioisotopes Radioactive atoms having the same number of protons. They are changed into a different atomic species by disintegration of the nucleus accompanied by the emission of ionizing radiation.

Radiological Society of North America (RSNA) The scientific society of radiologists and medical physicists.

Radiologist A physician specializing in medical imaging using x-rays, ultrasound, and magnetic resonance imaging.

Radiolucent Referring to a tissue or material that transmits x-rays and appears dark on a radiograph.

Radiolysis of water The dissociation of water into other molecular products as a result of irradiation.

Radionuclides Any nucleus that emits radiation.

Radiopaque Referring to a tissue or material that absorbs x-rays and appears bright on a radiograph.

Radiosensitivity The relative susceptibility of cells, tissues, and organs to the harmful action of ionizing radiation.

Radon A colorless, odorless, naturally occurring radioactive gas (^{222}Ra) that decays via alpha emission and has a half-life of 3.8 days.

RAID (redundant array of inexpensive disks) system A system consisting of at least disk drives within a single cabinet that collectively act as a single storage system.

Random access memory (RAM) Data that can be stored or accessed at random from anywhere in main memory in approximately equal amounts of time, regardless of where they are located.

Rare earth element An element that is a transitional metal found in low abundance in nature.

Rare earth screen A radiographic intensifying screen made from rare earth elements, making it more useful for radiographic imaging.

Raster pattern The pattern produced on the screen of a television picture tube by the movement of an electron beam or on film by a laser scan.

Ratio The mathematical relationship between similar quantities.

Read-only memory (ROM) A data-storage device that contains information supplied by the manufacturer and cannot be written on or erased.

Real time A display for which the image is continuously renewed, often to view anatomic motion, in fluoroscopy and ultrasound.

Reciprocity law The principle stating that optical density on a radiograph is proportional only to the total energy imparted to the radiographic film.

Reconstruction The creation of an image from data.

Reconstruction time The time needed for the computer to present a digital image after an examination is completed.

Recorded detail The degree of sharpness of structural lines on a radiograph.

Recovery Repair and repopulation.

Rectification The process of converting alternating current to direct current.

Rectifier The electronic device that allows current flow in only one direction.

Red filter A filter that transmits light only above 600 nm; it is used with both green- and blue-sensitive film.

Redox Simultaneous reduction and oxidation reactions.

Reducing agent The chemical responsible for reduction.

Reduction The process by which an electron is given up by a chemical to neutralize a positive ion.

Reflection The return or reentry of an x-ray.

Reflective layer The layer of the intensifying screen that intercepts light headed in other directions and redirects it to the film.

Refraction The deviation of course when photons of visible light traveling in straight lines pass from one transparent medium to another.

Region of interest (ROI) The area of an anatomic structure on a reconstructed digital image as defined by the operator using a cursor.

Relative age-response relationship The increased incidence of a disease proportional to its natural incidence.

Relative biologic effectiveness (RBE) The ratio of the dose of standard radiation necessary to produce a given effect to the dose of test radiation needed for the same effect.

Relative risk The estimation of late radiation effects in large populations without having any precise knowledge of their radiation dose.

Relay An electrical device based on electromagnetic induction that serves as a switch.

Rem (radiation equivalent man) The special unit for dose equivalent and effective dose. It has been replaced by the sievert (Sv) in the SI system. 1 rem = 0.01 Sv.

Remnant radiation The x-rays that pass through the patient and interact with the image receptor.

Replenishment The replacement of developer and of fixer in the automatic processing of film.

Repopulation Replication by surviving cells.

Resistance An opposition to a force.

Resolution A measure of the ability of a system to image two separate objects and visually distinguish one from the other.

Restrainer A compound that restricts the action of the developing agent to only irradiated silver halide crystals.

Ribonucleic acid (RNA) Molecules that are involved in the growth and development of a cell through a number of small, spherical cytoplasmic organelles that attach to the endoplasmic reticulum.

Ribosomes The site of protein synthesis.

Right-hand rule   The rule by which the direction of the magnetic field lines can be determined.

Roller subassembly   One of three principal film-transport subsystems in an imaging system.

Rotating anode   Anode used in general-purpose x-ray tubes because the tubes must be capable of producing high-intensity x-ray beams in a short time.

Rotor   The rotating part of an electromagnetic induction motor; it is located inside the glass envelope.

Saccharide   A carbohydrate.

Safe industry   An industry that has an associated annual fatality accident rate of no more than 1 per 10,000 workers.

Safelight   An incandescent lamp with a color filter that provides sufficient illumination in the darkroom while ensuring that the film remains unexposed.

Sagittal plane   Any anterior-posterior plane parallel to the long axis of the body.

Saturation current   A filament current that has risen to its maximum value because all of the available electrons have been used.

Scalar   Referring to a quantity or a measurement that has only magnitude.

Scanned projection radiography (SPR)   Generalized method of making a digital radiograph; used in computed tomography for precision localization.

Scatter radiation   X-rays scattered back in the direction of the incident x-ray beam.

Scheduled maintenance   Procedures performed on a routine basis.

Scientific notation   Exponential form.

Scintillation detector   An instrument used in the detector arrays of many computed tomographic scanners.

Screen-film   The most commonly used film; used with intensifying screens.

Screening mammography   An imaging examination performed on the breasts of asymptomatic women using a two-view protocol to detect unsuspected cancer.

Screen lag   The phosphorescence in an intensifying screen.

Screen speed   A relative number used to identify the efficiency of conversion of x-rays into usable light.

Second (s)   The standard unit of time.

Secondary coil   The coil in which the induced current in an electromagnet flows.

Secondary electron   The ejected electron from the outer shell of an atom.

Secondary memory   Data stored on tape drives, diskettes, and hard disk drives.

Secondary protective barrier   Barriers designed to shield areas from secondary radiation.

Secondary radiation   Leakage and scatter reaction.

Second-generation computed tomographic scanner   A unit that incorporates the natural extension of the single-detector to a multiple-detector assembly inter-

cepting a fan-shaped rather than a pencil-shaped x-ray beam.

Section thickness   The thickness of tissue that will not be blurred by tomography.

Selectivity   The ratio of primary radiation to scattered radiation transmitted through grid.

Self-induction   The magnetic field produced in a coil of wire that opposes the alternating current being conducted.

Self-rectified system   An imaging system in which the x-ray tube serves as the vacuum-tube rectifier.

Semiconductor   Material that can serve both as a conductor and as an insulator of electricity.

Sensitivity   The ability of an image receptor to respond to x-rays.

Sensitivity center   The physical imperfections in the lattice of the emulsion layer that occur during the film manufacturing process.

Sensitivity profile   The slice thickness.

Sensitizing agent   An agent that enhances the effect of radiation.

Sensitometer   An optical step wedge that is used to construct a characteristic curve.

Sensitometry   The study of the response of an image receptor to x-rays.

Sequestering agent   An agents introduced in the developer to form stable complexes with metallic ions and salts.

Shaded surface display (SSD)   A computer-aided technique that identifies a narrow range of values as belonging to the object to be imaged and displays that range.

Shadow dose equivalent (HS)   The dose of radiation to which the external skin or an extremity is exposed.

Shadow shield   A shields that is suspended over the region of interest and that casts a shadow over the patient's reproductive organs.

Shape distortion   A kind of distortion caused by elongation or foreshortening.

Shells   The orbital energy levels surrounding the nucleus of an atom.

Shell-type transformer   A transformer that confines more of the magnet field lines of the primary winding because there are essentially two closed cores.

Short gray scale   A high-contrast radiograph that exhibits black to white in just a few apparent steps.

Sievert (Sv)   Special name for the SI unit of dose equivalent and effective dose. $1 \text{ Sv} = 1 \text{ Jkg}^{-1} = 100 \text{ rem}$.

Sigmoid-type (S-type) dose-response relationship   A nonlinear, threshold radiation dose-response relationship.

Silver bromide   The material that makes up 98% of the silver halide crystals in a typical emulsion.

Silver halide crystals   The active ingredient of the radiographic emulsion. It is instrumental in creating a latent image on the radiograph.

Silver iodide   The material that makes up 2% of the silver halide crystals in a typical emulsion.

Sine wave   The variation of movement of photons in electrical and magnetic fields

Single-target hit model   A model of radiation dose-response relationships for enzymes, viruses, and bacteria.

Sinusoidal   Simple motion; a sine wave.

Skin erythema dose (SED)   A dose of radiation, usually about 200 rad or 2 Gy, that causes a redness of the skin.

Slice thickness   The thickness of the tissue being imaged.

Slice-acquisition rate (SAR)   A measure of the efficiency of a multislice spiral computed tomographic scanner.

Slip ring technology   Technology that allows the gantry to rotate continuously without interruption, making spiral computed tomography possible.

Sludge   Deposits on the film resulting from dirty or warped rollers, causing emulsion pick-off and gelatin buildup.

Sodium carbonate   An alkali compound contained in the developer.

Sodium hydroxide   An alkali compound contained in the developer.

Sodium sulfite   The preservative added to the developer that keeps it clear.

Soft copy   The output on a display screen.

Soft tissue radiography   Radiography in which only muscle and fat structures are imaged.

Software   The computer programs that tell the hardware what to do and how to store data.

Soft x-ray   An x-ray that has low penetrability and therefore is of low quality.

Solenoid   Helical winding of current-carrying wire that produces a magnetic field along the axis of the helix.

Solid-state diode   A diode that passes electric current in only one direction.

Solution   A suspension of particles or molecules in a fluid.

Solvent   A liquid into which various solids and powders can be dissolved.

Somatic cells   All the cells of the body except the oogonium and spermatogonium.

Somatic effects   Effects of radiation, such as cancer and leukemia, limited to an exposed individual. See also **genetic effect.**

Source-to-image receptor distance (SID)   The distance from the x-ray tube to the image receptor.

Source-to-skin distance (SSD)   The distance from the patient's skin to the fluoroscopic tube.

Space charge   The electron cloud near the filament.

Space-charge effect   The phenomenon of the space charge that makes it difficult for subsequent electrons to be emitted by the filament because of the electrostatic repulsion.

Spatial distortion   The misrepresentation in the image of the actual spatial relationships among objects.

Spatial frequency   The measure of resolution; usually expressed in line pairs per millimeter (lp/mm).

Spatial resolution   The ability to image small objects that have high subject contrast.

Spatial uniformity   The constancy of pixel values in all regions of the reconstructed image.

Special quantities   Additional quantities designed to support measurement in specialized areas of science and technology.

Spectrum   Graphic representation of the range over which a quantity extends.

Spectrum matching   Use of rare earth screens only in conjunction with film emulsions that have light absorption characteristics matched to the light emission of the screen.

Speed   Term used to loosely describe the sensitivity of film to x-rays.

Speed index   The step that has an average optical density closest to, but not less than, 1.2.

Sperm   See **spermatozoa.**

Spermatocyte   A mature spermatogonia.

Spermatogonium   The male germ cell.

Spermatozoa   A functionally mature male germ cell.

Spindle fibers   The fibers that connect a centromere and two chromatids to the poles of the nucleus during mitosis.

Spindles   The poles of the nucleus.

Spinning top   A device used to check exposure timers.

Spiral/helical   The term given to computed tomography because it is the apparent motion of the x-ray tube during the scan.

Spiral pitch radio   The relationship between the patient couch movement and x-ray beam collimation.

Spot film   Static image in small-format image receptor taken during fluoroscopy.

Square law   The principle stating that one can compensate for a change in the source-to-object distance by changing the mAs by the factor SID squared.

Starch   A plant polysaccharide.

Stationary anode   An anode used in imaging systems in which high tube current and power are not required.

Stator   Stationary coil windings located in the protective housing but outside the x-ray tube glass envelope. It is part of the electromagnetic induction motor.

Stem cell   An immature or a precursor cell.

Step-down transformer   A transformer in which the voltage is decreased from the primary side to the secondary side.

Stepping   A computer-controlled capability on a patient table that allows imaging from the abdomen to the feet after a single injection of contrast media.

Step-up transformer   A transformer in which the voltage is increased from the primary side to the secondary side.

Step wedge   A filter used when radiographing a body part, such as the foot, that varies in thickness from one end to the other.

Stereoradiography   The practice of making two radiographs of the same object and viewing through a device which allows each eye to view a different radiograph.

Sthenic   Referring to a body habitus of a patient who is strong and active; the average body habitus.

Stochastic effects   The probability or frequency of the biologic response to radiation as a function of radiation dose. Disease incidence increases proportionally with dose, and there is no dose threshold.

Storage memory   The main computer memory where the program and data files are stored.

Straight-line portion   The portion of a sensitometric curve where the diagnostic or most useful range of density is produced.

Stromal   Referring to part of an organ that is composed of connective tissue and vasculature that provides structure to the organ.

Structure mottle   Distribution of phosphor crystals in an intensifying screen.

Subatomic particle   A particle smaller than the atom.

Subject contrast   The part of radiographic contrast determined by the size, shape, and x-ray attenuating characteristics of the subject being examined and the energy of the x-ray beam. See also **image receptor contrast.**

Substance   Any drug, chemical, or biologic entity.

Subtraction technique   A method of removing all unnecessary anatomic structures from an image and enhancing only those of interest.

Supercomputer   One of the fastest and highest-capacity computers, containing hundreds to thousands of microprocessors.

Superconductivity   The property of some materials to exhibit no resistance below a critical temperature.

Supporting tissue   Tissue that binds tissues and organs together.

Target   a. The region of an x-ray tube anode struck by electrons emitted by the filament. b. The molecule (DNA) that is most sensitive to radiation.

Target molecule   Molecule (DNA) that is few in number yet essential for cell survival and is particularly sensitive to the effects of ionizing radiation.

Target theory   The theory that a cell will die if of target molecules are inactivated as a result of radiation exposure.

Technique factors   The kVp and mA as selected for a given radiographic examination.

Teleradiology   The transfer of images and patient reports to remote sites.

Telophase   The final subphase of mitosis that is characterized by the disappearance of the structural chromosomes into a mass of DNA and the closing off of the nuclear membrane into two nuclei.

Temperature   A measure of heat and cold.

Temporal subtraction   Computer-assisted technique whereby an image obtained at one time is subtracted from an image obtained at a later time.

Temporary magnet   A magnet that retains the properties of a magnet only while its magnetism is being induced.

Tenth-value layer (TVL)   The thickness of absorber necessary to reduce an x-ray beam to one tenth its original intensity. 1 TVL = 3.3 half-value layers.

Terminal   An input and output device that uses a keyboard for input and a display screen for output.

Terrestrial radiation   The radiation emitted from deposits of uranium, thorium, and other radionuclides in the Earth.

Tesla (T)   The SI unit of magnetic field intensity. An older unit is the gauss (G). 1 T = 10,000 G.

Test object   a. A passive device that provides echoes and permits evaluation of one or more parameters of an ultrasound system but does not necessarily duplicate the acoustic properties of the human body. b. A passive device of geometric shapes designed to evaluate the performance of x-ray and magnetic resonance imaging systems. See also **phantom.**

Thermal energy   The energy of molecular motion; heat; infrared radiation.

Thermal radiation   The transfer of heat by infrared emission.

Thermaluminescence dosimetry   The emission of light by a thermally stimulated crystal after irradiation.

Thermionic emission   The emission of electrons from a heated surface.

Thermographic   A process that uses only heat to produce a visible image on film.

Thermometer   A device that measures temperature.

Thiosulfate   The fixing agent that removes unexposed and undeveloped silver halide crystals from the emulsion.

Three-phase electric power   The generation of three simultaneous voltage waveforms out of step with one another, thus never dropping the voltage to zero during exposure.

Threshold dose   The dose below which a person has a negligible chance of sustaining specific biologic damage or the dose at which a response to an increasing x-ray intensity first occurs.

Thrombocyte   A circular or oval disk called a **platelet** found in the blood that initiates blood clotting and prevents hemorrhage.

Throughput   Number of patients imaged per day. Number of films imaged per hour.

Thymine   A nitrogenous organic base that attaches to a deoxyribose molecule.

Time-interval-difference (TID) mode   Technique that produces subtracted images from progressive masks and the frames that follow.

Time-of-occupancy factor (T) The amount of time the area being protected is used.

Tissue A collection of cells of similar structure and function.

Tissue weighting factor (W_T) The proportion of the risk of stochastic effects resulting from irradiation of the whole body when only an organ or tissue is irradiated. It accounts for the relative radiosensitivity of various tissues and organs.

Tomogram An x-ray image of a coronal, sagittal, transverse, or oblique section through the body.

Tomography Imaging modality that brings into focus only the anatomic structure lying in a plane of interest while blurring structures on either side of that plane.

Total effective dose (TED) The recommendation by the National Council on Radiation Protection and Measurement that a radiation worker's lifetime effective dose be limited to the worker's age in years multiplied by 10 mSv.

Total filtration Inherent filtration plus added filtration.

Transaxial Across the body; transverse.

Transcription The process of constructing mRNA.

Transfer An addition of an amino acid during translation.

Transformer An electrical device operating on the principle of mutual induction to change the magnitude of current and voltage.

Translation The process of forming a protein molecule from messenger RNA.

Translucent A surface that allows light to be transmitted but greatly alters and reduces its intensity.

Transmission The passing of an x-ray beam through the anatomic part without any interaction with the atomic structures.

Transparent A surface that allows light to be transmitted almost unaltered.

Transport roller An agents that moves the film through the chemical tanks and dryer assembly.

Transverse Across the body; axial.

Transverse image An image perpendicular to the long axis of the body.

Tungsten A metal element that is the principal component of the cathode and the anode.

Turnaround assembly A device in the automatic processor for reversing the direction of the film.

Turns ratio The quotient of the number of turns in the secondary coil to the number of turns in the primary coil.

Ultraviolet light Light that is located at the short end of the electromagnetic spectrum between visible light and ionizing x-rays; it is beyond the range of human vision.

Uncontrolled area Area occupied by anyone; the maximum exposure rate allowed in this area is based on the recommended dose limit for the public.

Underexposed Referring to a radiograph that is too light because too little x-radiation reached the image receptor.

Undifferentiated cell An immature or a nonspecialized cell.

Unified field theory The theoretical combination of magnetic, electric, gravitational, and strong nuclear forces along with weak interaction to explain the physical laws of magnetism.

Unit A standard of measurement.

Use factor (U) The proportional amount of time during which the x-ray beam is energized or directed toward a particular barrier.

Useful beam The primary radiation used to form the image.

Valence electron An electron in the outermost shell.

Variable aperture collimator A box-shaped device containing a radiographic beam-defining system. It is the device most often used to decline the size and shape of a radiographic beam.

VDT Abbreviation for **video display terminal.**

Vector A quantity or measurement that has magnitude, unit, and direction.

Velocity (v) The rate of change of an object's position with time; speed.

Video display terminal A monitor similar to a television screen.

Vidicon The television-camera tube most often used in television fluoroscopy.

Vignetting A reduction in brightness at the periphery of the image.

Visible light The radiant energy in the electromagnetic spectrum that is visible to the human eye.

Volt (V) The SI unit of electric potential and potential difference.

Voltage ripple A way to characterize voltage waveforms.

Voltaic pile A stack of copper and zinc plates that produces an electric current; a precursor of the modern battery.

Voxel A three-dimensional pixel; volume element.

Washing The stage of processing during which any remaining chemicals are removed from the film.

Watt (W) One ampere of current flowing through an electric potential of one volt.

Wave equation The formula stating that velocity equals frequency multiplied by wavelength.

Waveform The graphic representation of a wave.

Wavelength The distance between similar points on a sine wave; the length of one cycle.

Wave-particle duality The principle stating that both wave and particle concepts must be retained, since wavelike properties are exhibited in some experiments and particle-like are exhibited properties in others.

Wave theory   The theory that electromagnetic energy travels through space in the form of waves.

Weight   The force on a mass caused by the acceleration of gravity. Properly expressed in newtons (N), but commonly expressed in pounds (lb).

Wetting   A process that makes the emulsion film swell so that subsequent chemical baths can reach all parts of the emulsion uniformly.

Wetting agent   The agent, usually water, that treats the radiograph so that the chemicals can penetrate the emulsion.

Whole body   For purposes of external exposure, the head, trunk (including gonads), arms above the elbow, and leg above the knee.

Whole-body exposure   A radiographic exposure in which the whole body, rather than an isolated part, is irradiated.

Window   A thin section of glass envelope through which the useful beam emerges.

Windowing   The technique that allows one to see only a "window" of the entire dynamic range.

Window level   The location on a digital image number scale where the levels of grays are assigned. It regulates the optical density of the displayed image and identifies the type of tissue to be imaged.

Window width   A specific number of gray levels or digital image numbers assigned to an image. It determines the gray-scale rendition of the imaged tissue and therefore the image contrast.

Word   Two bytes of information.

Work (W)   The product of the force on an object and the distance over which the force acts. Expressed in Joules (J). $W = F \times d$.

Workload (W)   The product of the maximum milliamperage (mA) and the number of x-ray examinations performed per week. Expressed in milliamperes per minute per week (mA/min/wk).

Workstation   A powerful desktop system, often connected to larger computer systems so that users can transfer and share information.

X-axis   The horizontal line of a graph.

X-ray   Penetrating, ionizing electromagnetic radiation having a wavelength much shorter than that of visible light.

X-ray imaging system   An x-ray system designed for radiography, tomography, or fluoroscopy.

X-ray quality   The penetrability of an x-ray beam.

X-ray quantity   The output intensity of an x-ray imaging system, measured in roentgens (R).

X-ray tube rating charts   Charts that guide the technologist in the use of x-ray tubes.

Y-axis The vertical line of a graph.

Zonography Thick-slice tomography with a tomographic angle of less than 10 degrees.

PHOTO CREDITS

Figure 1-8   From Eisenberg RL: *Radiology: an illustrated history,* St Louis, 1992, Mosby.

Figure 16-15   From *Mosby's radiographic instructional series: radiographic imaging,* St Louis, 1998, Mosby.

Figure 20-7   From Fauber T: *Radiographic imaging and exposure,* St Louis, 2000, Mosby.

Figure 27-8   Seeram E: *Computed tomography: physical principals, clinical applications, and quality control,* ed 2, Philadelphia, 2000, WB Saunders.

Figure 32-4   From Papp J: *Quality management in the imaging sciences,* St Louis, 1998, Mosby.

Figure 32-5   From Papp J: *Quality management in the imaging sciences,* St Louis, 1998, Mosby.

Figure 40-11   From *Mosby's radiographic instructional series: radiographic imaging,* St Louis, 1998, Mosby.

Figure 40-12, A   Sherer MA: *Radiation protection in medical radiology,* ed 3, St Louis, 1998, Mosby.

Index

Page numbers followed by f indicate figures; t, tables; b, boxes.

Conversion Tables

Length

Unit	Equivalent in Meters
1 centimeter (cm)	10^{-2}
1 micron (μm)	10^{-6}
1 nanometer (nm)	10^{-9}
1 angstrom (Å)	10^{-10}
1 mile (mi)	1609

Mass-energy*

Electron Volts	Joules	Kilograms	Atomic Mass Units
1.0	1.60×10^{-19}	1.78×10^{36}	1.07×10^{-9}
6.24×10^{18}	1.0	1.11×10^{17}	6.69×10^{9}
5.61×10^{32}	8.99×10^{13}	1.0	6.02×10^{23}
9.32×10^{8}	1.49×10^{-10}	1.66×10^{27}	1.0

*(1J = 10^7 ergs; 4.19 J = 1 calorie; 1 BTU = 1.06×10^{10} ergs.)

Time

Years	Days	Hours	Minutes	Seconds
1	365	8.75×10^3	5.26×10^5	3.15×10^7
	1	24	1.44×10^3	8.64×10^4
		1	60	3.6×10^3
			1	60